Multimedia CD-ROM
Single-User License Agreement

1. NOTICE. READ THE TERMS AND CONDITIONS OF THIS LICENSE AGREEMENT CAREFULLY BEFORE OPENING THE SEALED PACKAGE CONTAINING THE MULTIMEDIA CD-ROM AND THE COMPUTER SOFTWARE THEREIN (ENTITLED STUDENT SOFTWARE CHALLENGE TO ACCOMPANY MEDICAL INSURANCE BILLING AND CODING: AN ESSENTIALS WORKTEXT), AND THE ACCOMPANYING USER DOCUMENTATION (THE SOFTWARE IS REFERRED TO AS THE "SOFTWARE," THE USER DOCUMENTATION IS REFERRED TO AS THE "USER DOCUMENTATION," AND THESE ARE ALL COLLECTIVELY REFERRED TO AS THE "MULTI-MEDIA PRODUCT"). THE MULTIMEDIA PRODUCT IS COPYRIGHTED AND LICENSED (NOT SOLD). WE ARE WILLING TO LICENSE THE MULTIMEDIA PRODUCT TO YOU ONLY ON THE CONDITION THAT YOU ACCEPT ALL OF THE TERMS CONTAINED IN THIS LICENSE AGREEMENT. BY OPENING THIS PACKAGE YOU ARE AGREEING TO BE BOUND BY ALL OF THE TERMS OF THIS AGREEMENT. IF YOU DO NOT AGREE TO THESE TERMS WE ARE UNWILLING TO LICENSE THE MULTIMEDIA PRODUCT TO YOU, AND YOU SHOULD NOT OPEN THE SEALED PACKAGE. IN SUCH CASE, PROMPTLY RETURN THE UNOPENED PACKAGE WITH ALL ACCOMPANYING MATERIAL, ALONG WITH PROOF OF PAYMENT, TO THE AUTHORIZED DEALER FROM WHOM YOU OBTAINED IT FOR A FULL REFUND OF THE PRICE YOU PAID.

   THIS LICENSE AGREEMENT SUPERSEDES ALL PRIOR AGREEMENTS, REPRESENTATIONS, OR UNDERSTANDINGS BETWEEN THE PARTIES CONCERNING THE MULTIMEDIA PRODUCT.

   "WE," "US," "OUR," AND SIMILAR PRONOUNS REFER TO THE W.B. SAUNDERS COMPANY.

2. **Ownership and License.** Upon all of the terms and conditions herein, we hereby grant to you, and you accept, a non-exclusive limited license to use the Multimedia Product. The Software contained therein is licensed to you in machine-readable, object code form only. This is a license agreement and NOT an agreement for sale. Except as is otherwise specifically provided herein, this license permits you to install and/or use one copy of the Software on a single personal computer that is owned, leased, or otherwise controlled by you. You may change such computers from time to time, so long as the Software is not installed or used on more than a single computer at a time. The Multimedia Product is owned by us or our licensors, and is protected by U.S. and international copyright laws. Your rights to use the Multimedia Product are specified in this Agreement, and we retain all rights not expressly granted to you in this Agreement.

3. **Transfer and Other Restrictions.** You may not rent, lend, or lease the Multimedia Product. You may not and you may not cause or allow others to (a) disassemble, decompile, or otherwise derive source code from the Software), (b) reverse engineer the Software, (c) modify or prepare derivative works of the Multimedia Product or any portion thereof, (d) use the Software in an on-line or Internet system, or (e) use the Multimedia Product in any manner that infringes on the intellectual property rights or other rights of another party.

   Notwithstanding the foregoing, you may transfer this license to use the Multimedia Product to another party on a permanent basis by transferring this copy of the license agreement, the Multimedia Product, and all documentation, provided that you provide us with written notification of the transfer and the transferee agrees to be bound by the terms of this license agreement. Such transfer of possession terminates your license with us. Such other party shall be licensed under the terms of this Agreement upon its acceptance of this agreement by its clear written assent (acceptable to us) and initial use of the Multimedia Product. If you transfer the Multimedia Product, you must remove any and all installation files from your computers, hard disks, etc., and you may not retain any copies of those files for your own use.

4. **Limited Warranty and Limitation of Liability.** For a period of sixty (60) days from the date you acquired the Multimedia Product from us or our authorized dealer, we warrant to you, for your benefit alone, that the media containing the Software will be free from defects that prevent you from installing and/or using the Software on your computer. If the Multimedia CD you may, as your sole and exclusive remedy, obtain a replacement free of charge if you return the defective disk to us with a dated proof of purchase. Otherwise, the Multimedia Product is licensed to you on an "AS IS" basis without any warranty of any nature.

   WE DO NOT WARRANT THAT THE MULTIMEDIA PRODUCT WILL MEET YOUR REQUIREMENTS OR THAT ITS OPERATION WILL BE UNINTERRUPTED OR ERROR-FREE. WE EXCLUDE AND EXPRESSLY DISCLAIM ALL EXPRESS AND IMPLIED WARRANTIES NOT STATED HEREIN, INCLUDING THE IMPLIED WARRANTIES OF MERCHANTABILITY AND FITNESS FOR A PARTICULAR PURPOSE.

   WE SHALL NOT BE LIABLE FOR ANY DAMAGE OR LOSS OF ANY KIND ARISING OUT OF OR RESULTING FROM YOUR POSSESSION OR USE OF THE MULTIMEDIA PRODUCT (INCLUDING DATA LOSS OR CORRUPTION), REGARDLESS OF WHETHER SUCH LIABILITY IS BASED IN TORT, CONTRACT OR OTHERWISE AND INCLUDING, BUT NOT LIMITED TO, ACTUAL, SPECIAL, INDIRECT, INCIDENTAL, EXEMPLARY, AND/OR CONSEQUENTIAL DAMAGES OR ANY LOST PROFITS OR LOST DATA. IF THE FOREGOING LIMITATION IS HELD TO BE UNENFORCEABLE, OUR MAXIMUM LIABILITY TO YOU SHALL NOT EXCEED THE AMOUNT OF THE LICENSE FEE PAID BY YOU FOR THE MULTIMEDIA PRODUCT. THE REMEDIES AVAILABLE TO YOU AGAINST US AND THE LICENSORS OF MATERIALS INCLUDED IN THE MULTIMEDIA PRODUCT ARE EXCLUSIVE.

   Some states do not allow the limitation or exclusion of implied warranties or liability for incidental or consequential damages, so the above limitations or exclusions may not apply to you.

   The terms of this Section 4 shall survive termination of this license agreement for any reason.

5. **United States Government Restricted Rights.** The Multimedia Product and documentation are provided with Restricted Rights. Use, duplication, or disclosure by the U.S. Government or any agency or instrumentality thereof is subject to the restrictions in F.A.R. 52.227-14 (June 1987) Alternate III (June 1987), F.A.R. 52.227-19 (June 1987), or D.F.A.R.S. 252.227-7013 (b)(3) (November 1995), or applicable successor clauses, and/or similar provisions of the Federal Acquisition Regulations, as applicable. Manufacturer is the W.B. Saunders Company, the Curtis Center, Suite 300, Independence Square West, Philadelphia, PA 19106.

6. **Term and Termination.** This license is effective upon your opening of the sealed package and continues until terminated. This license and your right to use this Multimedia Product automatically terminate if you fail to comply with any provisions of this Agreement, destroy the copy of the Multimedia Product in your possession, or voluntarily return the Multimedia Product to us. Upon termination you will destroy any and all authorized copies of the Multimedia Product and all related documentation and any and all authorized copies thereof.

7. **Miscellaneous Provisions.** This Agreement will be governed by and construed in accordance with the substantive laws of the State of Missouri, and the parties will submit to and will not oppose venue in Missouri state or federal court. This is the entire agreement between us relating to the Multimedia Product, and supersedes any purchase order, communications, advertising or representations concerning the contents of this package. No change or modification of this Agreement will be valid unless it is in writing and is signed by us.

   The license fee paid by you is paid in consideration of the license granted under this license agreement.

   Should any term of this license agreement be declared void or unenforceable by any court or tribunal of competent jurisdiction, such declaration shall have no effect on the remaining terms hereof. The failure of either party to enforce any rights granted hereunder or to take action against the other party in the event of any breach hereunder shall not be deemed a waiver by that party as to the subsequent enforcement of rights or subsequent actions in the event of future breaches.

Medical Insurance Billing and Coding

AN ESSENTIALS WORKTEXT

Marilyn Takahashi Fordney, CMA-AC, CMT
Formerly Instructor of Medical Insurance, Medical Terminology,
Medical Machine Transcription, and Medical Office Procedures
Ventura College
Ventura, California

Linda L. French, CMA-C, NCICS
Business Consultant and Instructor of Medical Insurance Procedures,
Administrative Medical Assisting, and Medical Terminology
Simi Valley Adult School and Career Institute
Simi Valley, California;
Ventura College
Ventura, California;
Oxnard College
Oxnard, California

Medical Insurance Billing and Coding

AN ESSENTIALS WORKTEXT

SAUNDERS
An Imprint of Elsevier Science
Philadelphia London New York St. Louis Sydney Toronto

SAUNDERS
An Imprint of Elsevier Science

The Curtis Center
Independence Square West
Philadelphia, Pennsylvania 19106

Library of Congress Cataloging-in-Publication Data

Fordney, Marilyn Takahashi.
Medical insurance billing and coding: an essentials worktext / Marilyn Takahashi Fordney, Linda L. French.

p. cm.

ISBN 0–7216–9516–7

1. Medical offices—Management. 2. Insurance, Health—Finance. 3. Health insurance claims. I. French, Linda L. II Title.

R728.5 .F67 2003
651′.961—dc21 2002070600

All the material included in figures, tables, examples, and assignments have been altered to prevent identification of the cases or parties involved. The names and addresses are fictitious, and no reference to a person living or dead is intended. No evaluation of medical practice, or medical advice is to be inferred from the patient/medical records, nor is any recommendation made toward alternative treatment methods or prescribed medications.

Legal information appears in chapters where it applies to insurance billing and coding. The information presented is not a substitute for legal advice, and the physician and his or her insurance billing specialist should always seek the counsel of an attorney about specific questions of law as they relate to the medical practice.

Rules, regulations, and guidelines for private insurance and government programs, diagnostic and procedure coding, completing the Health Insurance Claim Form, along with other information described in this publication and found on the publisher's web site are based on research of current literature, medical seminars, and consultation with knowledgeable persons in the field. Care has been taken to verify the accuracy of all information presented; however, this information cannot and should not be relied on as necessarily applicable to a given individual's case or to a specific region in the United States. The authors, editors, and publisher cannot accept responsibility for errors or omissions or for consequences from application of the information in this worktext and make no warranty, expressed or implied, with respect to its content. The authors, editors, and publisher cannot accept any responsibility for changes in published addresses or telephone numbers, or subject matter or content received while accessing the web sites listed in this publication (e-mail, newsgroup, or chatroom). The reader is expressly warned to consider and adopt all safety precautions that might be indicated by the application of information herein and to avoid all potential hazards. By following the instructions contained herein, the reader willingly assumes all risks in connection with such instructions.

MEDICAL INSURANCE BILLING AND CODING: An Essentials Worktext ISBN 0–7216–9516–7

Executive Editor: Adrianne Cochran
Senior Developmental Editor: Rae L. Robertson
Project Manager: Tina K. Rebane

Printed in the United States of America.

Last digit is the print number: 9 8 7 6 5 4 3 2 1

I gratefully recognize the special friendship and strong connection I share with my coauthor, Linda French, which goes far beyond this worktext. Because of my experience in education after working as a medical assistant for many years, I wish to dedicate this work to you, the student, for you are the reason for its existence.

MARILYN T. FORDNEY, CMA-AC, CMT

To my mother, Eleanor Campbell Barnes,
and to my husband of 37 years, Dick,
who always supported me,
never doubted my success,
and patiently awaited the completion of this worktext.
To my students,
who inspired me to be a better teacher,
challenged me to reach for higher goals,
and ignited my creativity to produce original material,
to present straightforward concepts,
and to offer simple solutions to their many questions.
To my mentor and coauthor, Winkie,
who always encouraged me,
respected my viewpoint,
gave me the opportunity,
and served as my anchor in difficult times.
I am ever grateful!!!

LINDA L. FRENCH, CMA-C, NCICS

Preface

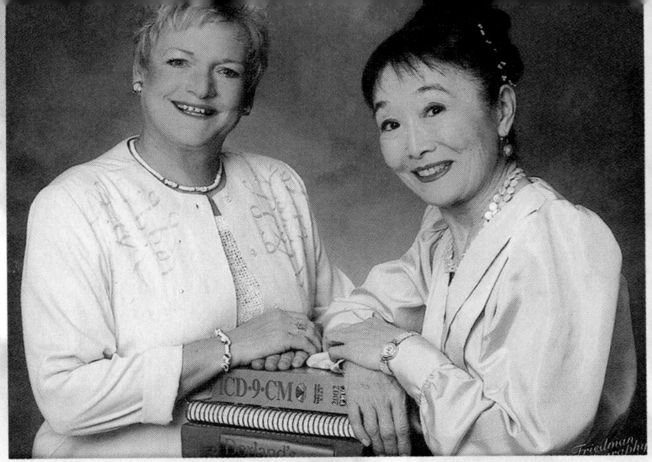

Medical Insurance Billing Specialist the Life Support of the Medical Office

TO THE STUDENT

Just as vessels in the human body carry life-sustaining blood to every organ, vessels in a physician's office carry *currency* needed to sustain life in a medical practice. Consistent cash flow is critical in a healthy outpatient medical practice, and the HCFA-1500 insurance claim form represents from 85% to 95% of the reimbursement that travels through these vessels. The form is driven by the medical insurance billing specialist and can travel on the freeway (electronic billing) and get to the insurance company and back in 2 to 7 days. Or, it can take the highway (computer-generated or typewritten optical character recognition [OCR] billing) and get there on a slower route and return in 2 to 4 weeks. Sometimes it takes the side roads (non-OCR billing), gets caught in traffic, gets lost, gets into an accident, and never arrives in one piece, or at all.

This worktext is designed to help you learn all of the clerical functions that a medical biller performs in order to process the HCFA-1500 insurance claim form and have it arrive in a safe and expedient way. You will learn how to avoid traffic snags and travel the complicated freeway system to deliver a clean claim. The reward for this is increased reimbursement and consistent cash flow for the physician.

To monitor the billing system, you may be the one who needs to take the pulse of the practice on a regular basis and make sure that all vital signs are fine. If something goes wrong, you may need to diagnose and prescribe treatment. The medical insurance biller is a key player in the financial operations of the medical office, and it may be necessary to write a prescription that goes into office policy to institute standards for the medical practice.

The physician is familiar with noncompliant patients. Such patients do not follow a recommended treatment plan and put themselves at risk for further illness. You need to know insurance rules and regulations for various plans and may need to speak to office staff and the physician regarding his or her compliance with billing regulations. Teamwork is necessary. The practice is at risk if the staff or physician is noncompliant with billing rules.

As you work your way through the worktext, you will see many of the faces behind medical insurance billing that provide this life support function in a variety of medical settings. By meeting these professionals and having them share their thoughts with you, it is our hope that you will be able to get a glimpse from behind the scenes and gain a real-world perspective so that you will be encouraged and motivated in your new career. Their professional profiles are included to illustrate different ways of getting started, variances in job duties, and highlights of the profession.

To do assignments in this worktext and gain expertise in coding and insurance claim completion, an individual must have access to reference material. Refer to the Resources section at the end of the following chapters to locate suggested reference information needed for this course: medical dictionary, pharmaceutical and word codebooks (Chapter 1); diagnostic codebook (Chapter 4); procedural codebooks (Chapters 5 and 6); books or booklets on the topics of Medicaid, Medicare, TRICARE, CHAMPVA, workers' compensation, and state disability plans (see corresponding program chapters).

In addition to resource material you will need a set of highlight pens, some 3″ by 5″ reference cards, pen, pencil, and an attitude of adventure. You are setting forth in the great adventure of learning how to find your way around the maze of insurance rules and regulations. Have fun!

Student Portfolio

Completed exercises and assignments may be kept in a separate folder to be used as a job portfolio or reference manual for the physician's office. You may wish to re-do exercises in perfect form for this purpose. The portfolio can be used to show future employers job functions for which you have been trained, and also as a reference guide when completing job tasks in a work setting and completing claim forms for various insurance programs. Class handouts, such as insurance program newsletters and compliance issue alerts, may be added.

TO THE INSTRUCTOR

The first edition of *Medical Insurance Billing and Coding: An Essentials Worktext* is addressed to the student who is preparing for a career as a medical insurance billing specialist in an outpatient setting (physician's office or clinic), or who wishes to work in or establish an independent billing service and needs a basic understanding of the reimbursement process. This worktext includes the BEST from the well-established, comprehensive companion text, *Insurance Handbook for the Medical Office*, 7th edition, which has been used by thousands of students over the past 25 years. This worktext strives to duplicate the high standards set by the *Insurance Handbook*. It has more than 150 new figures, tables, and examples developed in full color to enhance visual learning and added to approximately 200 that have been expanded from the *Insurance Handbook*.

This worktext was born out of a need to create a combined insurance text/workbook that presents basic concepts, yet includes comprehensive information for students who are studying in a short or one-semester program. The worktext may be used as a learning tool for courses offered at private post-secondary, vocational, or commercial learning institutions, community colleges, and regional occupational and welfare-to-work programs. Seminar-style classes and independent home study are possible using this worktext.

Competency objectives from the American Association of Medical Assistants curriculum guidelines that address the medical insurance billing specialist have been used where applicable.

LAYOUT OF THE WORKTEXT

Concepts and exercises are arranged from simple to complex throughout the worktext to allow students to master basic skills before attempting complicated tasks. The first two chapters cover information needed to build a strong insurance foundation. Medical/insurance terminology, medicolegal issues, health insurance contracts, and an overview of different types of health insurance programs are the cornerstones for this foundation.

As job skills are learned they become the building blocks that are put upon the foundation of insurance knowledge. Instructions and exercises for the first skills are found in Chapter 2 (e.g., composing a letter, envelope preparation, completing an insurance precertification form) and additional skills are presented in all subsequent chapters. All skills needed to process claims in the billing cycle are taught using a step-by-step approach and are continually reinforced with exercise sessions as described in key features.

Handling source documents and the billing cycle are presented in Chapter 3. All documents are illustrated as they might appear in the physician's office; however, some may be abbreviated due to page size constraints.

Diagnostic coding and procedural coding are the focus of the next three chapters, featuring many examples and opportunities to practice. Diagnostic and procedure codebooks published for the year 2002 have been used for all exercises. Abstracting from the medical record is presented in Chapter 7, with a chance to code from chart notes. In Chapter 8, the HCFA-1500 insurance claim form is presented, and all of the previously learned skills are put to practice while completing the claim form and learning submission rules.

Various insurance plans and programs are presented in Chapters 9 through 13 with eligibility and enrollment requirements, plan benefits, program options and guidelines, and HCFA-1500 claim form requirements. The "roof" is constructed in the last two chapters (14 and 15), which include handling reimbursement, the credit/collection process, and tracking unpaid insurance claims. It is this knowledge that protects all of the previous work that a medical insurance biller does when submitting clean claims and ensures maximum reimbursement.

KEY FEATURES

- **Objectives**—are divided into "learning objectives," clearly stated for each chapter to help set goals, and "performance objectives," incorporated into exercises that develop job skills.
- **Key Terms**—are listed in bold colored type with full definitions in the glossary located in Appendix E. To help students master the vocabulary of insurance claims processing and study for quizzes and tests, it is suggested that while reading chapter material each term be recorded on a 3″ by 5″ flash card with its definition. Special notes regarding the term may be recorded during lectures.
- **Chapter Outlines**—are detailed and found at the beginning of the worktext. They can be used to help locate information quickly and organize note taking during class lectures.
- **Professional Profiles**—are written by working medical insurance billing specialists and offer an inside look into the exciting profession that the student is about to embark upon.
- **Time Lines**—offer a quick glance at historical insurance events, with dates.
- **Expressions from Experience**—are interspersed throughout the chapters and offer insight and suggestions from a working professional regarding the topic that is presented.

- **Full color**—is used to teach visually and add interest to figures, tables, examples, flow sheets, and decision trees.
- **Figures, Tables, and Examples**—are presented throughout the worktext. Each is titled for clear identification and location; many depict coding examples and realistic scenarios.
- **Summation and Previews**—are presented at the end of each chapter, summarizing key points from the chapter and giving a preview of what's ahead.
- **Golden Rules**—were created to reinforce important concepts presented in each chapter and may be memorized for future use.
- **Resources**—are listed at the end of each chapter and include reference books, code books, Internet addresses, and other information pertinent to each chapter topic.
- **Claim Form Instructions**—are comprehensive and color coded with payer icons located in Appendix D for quick reference; each basic program includes an insurance template.

LEARNING AND PRACTICING JOB SKILLS

You will have an opportunity to pause and practice **CPR,** the life support of medical insurance billing, which is integrated throughout the worktext and taught through:

- **Challenge Sessions,** which demand critical thinking skills. These sessions involve problem solving using more than one learned concept;
- **Practice Sessions,** which allow you to practice task-oriented job skills and offer an opportunity for repetitive skill building; and
- **Review Sessions,** which will help you reinforce technical material and review new concepts.

By offering a variety of self-study sessions, students will maximize learning opportunities.

Check Your Heartbeat—instructions will guide students to turn to the end of each chapter for answers to CPR sessions.

Get an Examination—after checking your heartbeat to review areas of deficiency, clarify new concepts, and rehearse new skills.

Study Sessions—offered at the end of each chapter, after you have read chapter segments and paused to practice CPR, include review questions to reinforce key concepts for each topic, assist in studying insurance billing and coding theory, and present a comprehensive review of chapter material using a variety of question formats.

Billing Breaks—occur whenever an insurance case is assigned so students gain experience completing the HCFA-1500 claim form. Realistic patient registration forms, encounter forms, and medical record documents are used for students to abstract data, code diagnoses and procedures, and complete claim forms for private, managed care, and a variety of government programs.

Exercise Exchange—sessions offer competency-based simulated assignments to practice job skills needed when working as an insurance billing specialist, including diagnostic and procedure coding. A complete list of job skills follows. Diagnostic coding exercises and codes used in case scenarios have been chosen from a common list of diagnostic codes. Procedure coding exercises and codes used in case scenarios have been selected from a list of the top 50 codes billed to Medicare in 1999. Worksheets used when learning to code diagnoses and abstract information from the medical record to code services and procedures have been designed to help students organize and record complex information.

JOB SKILLS

Chapter 1

None

Chapter 2

Exercise Exchange

2–1 Compose a Letter of Discharge
Prepare a Business Envelope for Mailing
Complete U.S. Postal Service Forms
2–2 Complete an Insurance Predetermination Form

Chapter 3

Exercise Exchange

3–1 Complete a Patient Registration Form
3–2 Abstract Information from an Insurance Identification Card
3–3 Post Transactions on a Ledger Card

Chapter 4

Exercise Exchange

4–1 through 4–25
Code Diagnoses

Chapter 5

Exercise Exchange

5–1 through 5–24
Code Evaluation and Management Services

Chapter 6

Exercise Exchange

6–1 through 6–20
Code Procedures and Services from the:
Surgery Section
Radiology Section
Pathology/Laboratory Section
Medicine Section

Apply modifiers to appropriate procedure codes

Chapter 7

Exercise Exchange

7–1 Abstract Information from a Chart Note
7–2 Abstract Information from a Progress Report
7–3 Abstract Information from a Medical Record

Chapter 8

Exercise Exchange

8–1 Abstract Information and Complete Top Portion of HCFA-1500 Claim Form
8–2 Abstract Information and Complete Bottom Portion of HCFA-1500 Claim Form

Chapter 9

Billing Break

9–1 Complete the HCFA-1500 claim form for a private insurance case abstracting information from a Patient Registration form and an Encounter form.
9–2 Complete the HCFA-1500 claim form for a private insurance case abstracting information from a Patient Registration form and an Encounter form.
9–3 Complete the HCFA-1500 claim form for a managed care case abstracting information from a Patient Registration form and an Encounter form.
9–4 Complete the HCFA-1500 claim form for a managed care case abstracting information from a Patient Registration form and Medical Record; coding diagnoses and procedures/services.

Exercise Exchange

9–1 Complete Managed Care Plan Authorization Request.

Chapter 10

Billing Break

10–1 Complete the HCFA-1500 claim form for a Medicaid case abstracting information from a Patient Registration form and Medical Record; coding diagnoses and procedures/services.
10–2 Complete two HCFA-1500 claim forms for a Medicare case abstracting information from a Patient Registration form and Medical Record; coding diagnoses and procedures/services.

Chapter 11

Billing Break

11–1 Complete the HCFA-1500 claim form for a Medicare case abstracting information from a Patient Registration form and Medical Record; coding diagnoses and procedures/services.
11–2 Complete the HCFA-1500 claim form for a Medicare/Medigap case abstracting information from a Patient Registration form and Medical Record; coding diagnoses and procedures/services.
11–3 Complete the HCFA-1500 claim form for a Medicare/Medicaid case abstracting information from a Patient Registration form and Medical Record; coding diagnoses and procedures/services.
11–4 Complete the HCFA-1500 claim form for a Medicare Secondary Payer (MSP) case abstracting information from a Patient Registration form and Medical Record; coding diagnoses and procedures/services.

Exercise Exchange

11–1 Calculate Medicare Fees
11–2 Complete an Advance Beneficiary Notice
11–3 Code Using HCPCS Level II

Chapter 12

Billing Break

12–1 Complete the HCFA-1500 claim form for a TRICARE case abstracting information from a Patient Registration form and Medical Record; coding diagnoses and procedures/services.
12–2 Complete the HCFA-1500 claim form for a CHAMPVA case abstracting information from a Patient Registration form and Medical Record; coding diagnoses and procedures/services.

Exercise Exchange

12–1 Complete a TRICARE Preauthorization/Referral Request Form.
12–2 Edit a HCFA-1500 Claim Form Prior to Electronic Submission for a TRICARE Case.

Chapter 13

Billing Break

13–1 Complete the HCFA-1500 claim form for a workers' compensation case abstracting information from a Patient Registration form and Medical Record; coding diagnoses and procedures/services.
13–2 Complete the HCFA-1500 claim form for a workers' compensation case abstracting information from a Patient Registration form and Medical Record; coding diagnoses and procedures/services.

Exercise Exchange

13–1 Complete a Doctor's First Report of Occupational Injury and Illness Form.

Chapter 14

Exercise Exchange

14–1 Calculate the Accounts Receivable Ratio for College Clinic.
14–2 Determine How Much of College Clinic's A/R is Over 90 Days
14–3 Calculate the Collection Rate for College Clinic for the Month of March 2002
14–4 Prepare a Credit Card Voucher
14–5 Complete a Financial Agreement

Chapter 15

Exercise Exchange

15–1 Trace a Delinquent Claim
15–2 Compose a Letter of Appeal
15–3 Interpret an Explanation of Benefits, Abstract Data, Calculate and Post Payments and Adjustments to Three Patients' Ledger Cards

Computer Sessions—are offered in appropriate chapters to direct students to practice completing insurance cases using Student Software Challenge on CD-ROM. The goal of using this software is to give the user a hands-on, realistic approach as though working in a medical setting by selecting appropriate patient files to obtain needed information to complete the HCFA-1500 insurance claim form. Key terms and abbreviations are incorporated into patient records for the last 5 cases, and definitions may be accessed through a linked glossary. The skill of extracting data from these source documents, coding diagnoses, services and procedures, as well as claim form completion for various programs is developed. Immediate feedback is received while completing the claim form, and block instructions are linked for easy reference. The claim form can be printed and all Billing Break assignments may also be completed using the "Other Patients" file in the software. Forms can be easily corrected for resubmission. This simulated learning methodology makes possible an easier transition from classroom to workplace. Full instructions for installing and operating the software are found in Appendix G.

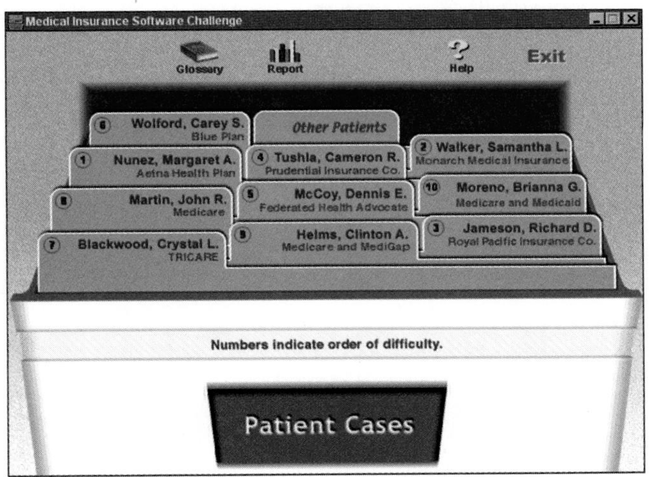

Weigh Your Progress—by keeping a written record of all homework assignments, test scores, and class projects using the Assignment Score Sheet found in Appendix F.

APPENDICES

Tabs—mark appendices for easy reference.

Appendix A—contains the College Clinic simulation; the clinic includes ten staff physicians and employs all students.

Appendix B—contains the mock fee schedule for private carriers, Medicare participating fees, nonparticipating fees, and limited charges, as well as global follow-up days for surgical procedures to be used with Billing Break exercises.

Appendix C—contains a complete list of CPT modifiers and a sample list of Medicare's HCPCS Level II modifiers and codes.

Appendix D—contains comprehensive block by block instructions for completing the HCFA-1500 insurance claim form. Each block is set apart with colored numbers and each insurance plan or program has its own colored icon to help locate information quickly.

Appendix E—contains a comprehensive glossary of all key terms.

Appendix F—contains blank forms and sample documents that are easily removable for students to use with exercises to enhance typing skills and form completion.

Appendix G—presents the installation and operating instructions for the Student Software Challenge found on the CD-ROM that accompanies the worktext.

SUPPLEMENTARY MATERIALS

Instructor's Curriculum Resource to Accompany Medical Insurance Billing and Coding: An Essentials Worktext in Print and on CD-ROM

The following features are included in the *Instructor's Curriculum Resource:*

- Assistance in developing a course on medical insurance billing for varied-length programs (i.e., curriculum for a 12-week, 16-week, 18-week, and 20-week course).
- Lesson plans and suggestions on lecture material to facilitate lesson preparation and ensure complex concepts are covered and discussed.
- Suggestions for additional classroom activities, including games and drills.
- Teaching tips and ideas for instructors on how to make medical insurance billing FUN!
- Exercise Exchange answer keys with rationales.
- Billing Break exercise answer keys with optional codes for difficult cases and rationales.
- Quick Quiz designed for all chapters includes between 10 and 15 questions on key points.
- Test Case for HCFA-1500 insurance claim form may be used to test claim completion for private insurance carriers and/or Medicare (may be used for final examination).
- Test Bank includes 200 questions in variable formats to assist the instructor in test construction.
- Lecture slides for use in overhead projection or in Power Point presentation for all chapters.

MERLIN Web Site—sign on at http://www.wbsaunders.com/MERLIN/Fordney/insurancebook/ for free website companion. Established for instructors and students for *Medical Insurance Billing and Coding: An Essentials Worktext* to post technical updates when available, errors and corrections in the worktext, additional exercises for students, links to related websites, author information, and more. Use your unique passcode to access active websites keyed specifically to the contents of this worktext. The weblinks are updated continually, with new ones added as they develop.

Insurance videos—available. Tape One discusses legal, ethical, and professional concepts (ISBN 0–7216–8833–0). Tape Six discusses claim completion and common claim errors (ISBN 0–7216–8838–1). Call Customer Service to order at 1-800-545-2522. ***Insurance Handbook for the Medical Office, Student Workbook*, 7th edition,** may be used with this worktext if more exercises are desired. A special "test section" at the end of the workbook can be used for quizzing students. The College Clinic simulation uses the same physicians and fee schedule; no exercises have been repeated in the worktext.

Acknowledgments

This worktext has been a vision for many years, and without the help and support of numerous people it could not have become a reality. Professional colleagues, educators, and friends generously offered their ideas, suggestions, and encouragement, which helped form this worktext. Students from Simi Valley Adult School thoughtfully gave their suggestions and criticisms, volunteered to work on developing exercises, lent technical subject matter, and asked many questions that spurred the quest to find answers. We are grateful for their willing participation.

We would like to thank the many professionals who contributed their expertise on various topics for the *Insurance Handbook for the Medical Office*, 7th edition, which were incorporated into the technical content of this worktext. Experts reviewed chapters of the *Insurance Handbook*, and all improvements for clarity of topics and deletions were considered when writing this worktext. A special note of appreciation to our assistant, Ginger Daugherty, who helped with computer technology and did various tasks that supported the ongoing writing and editing process.

We gratefully acknowledge the staff of Saunders who helped create, produce, and market this worktext. Special thanks go to Bill Donnelly and Ellen Zanolle, the artists involved with the design of the cover, and Marie Gardocky-Clifton, the artist who helped develop the full-color format from the Saunders Design Department.

The photograph for the preface was taken by Friedman Photography, Ventura, California. Many other photographers were involved in supplying professional photography for the Professional Profiles and Expressions from Experience, and we value their artistic contributions.

Particular appreciation is given to Andrew Allen, Publishing Director; Adrianne Cochran, Executive Editor; and Rae Robertson, Senior Developmental Editor, for their help in making this become a reality. Others who participated in making this worktext are: Tina Rebane, Project Manager, and Elizabeth Melchor, Editorial Assistant. Our gratitude is extended to Norman Stellander, Senior Project Manager.

Special appreciation is expressed to Jenny Alicandri and Sarahlynn Lester of the Marketing Department, and the Elsevier Science marketing staff across the United States who put the worktext into the hands of those who are in need of this educational tool.

Names of supply companies and organizations who provided material may be found throughout the worktext. Special thanks to Bibbero Systems, Inc., Petaluma, California, for supplying up-to-date business forms and medical documents, and to Rhino Graphics, Port Hueneme, California, for their expert graphic suggestions.

Acknowledgments for Professional Profiles and Expressions from Experience

We would like to thank the medical insurance billing specialists and coders who offered their insight to be used as Professional Profiles and Expressions from Experience. Without their contributions, it would not have been possible to give an "inside look" into the profession of medical insurance billing. We are grateful for their participation and reflections.

Kara Chang
Workers' Compensation Billing Specialist
Ventura, California

Laura M. Garcia
President
LMG Medical Management
Duarte, California

Katrina Ginn
Emergency Room Ward Clerk/Transcriptionist
Woodland Hills, California

Tamra Hollins
Collection Specialist
Ventura, California

Maureen Jackson
Medical Insurance Billing Student
Camarillo, California

Sharon LaScala, NCICS
Insurance Billing Specialist/Office Manager
Simi Valley and Thousand Oaks, California

Sue Manion
Medical Transcriptionist/Medical Insurance Biller
Valencia, California

Elizabeth Palace
Diagnostic Coder
Conejo Valley, California

Cathy Petersen
Pediatric Billing Specialist
Lincoln, Nebraska

Deborah Pitts
Medical Insurance Billing Specialist
Medical Billing Company
Canoga Park, California

Charline Rambaud, CPC
AccuQuik Billing Service–Owner
Oak Park, California

Holley Romero
Operations Manager
Irvine, California

Jane Seelig, CMA-A
Medical Insurance Billing Specialist
Columbus, Indiana

Jimetria Smith
Student/Medical Insurance Billing Specialist
Moorpark, California

Lateisha Ware
Medical Insurance Billing Specialist—Radiology
Simi Valley, California

Consultants

Without the knowledge of expert consultants who provided technical assistance and vital information about private, state, and federal insurance programs, the massive task of compiling an insurance worktext with up-to-date information might never have been accomplished. Although the names of all those who graciously assisted are too numerous to mention, we would like to list the principal consultants for this first edition:

American Academy of Professional Coders
Conejo Chapter
Thousand Oaks, California

Verna Bueschen, CPC-H
Simi Valley, California

Lily Chen
Simi Valley, CA

Rose Crawford
Medical Insurance Billing Specialist
Simi Valley, California

Diana Davis
Manager, Contracting and Data Support
TRICARE Programs
Ventura, California

Ann Hill
Pharmacy Technician Program
Simi Valley Adult School and Career Institute
Simi Valley, California

Gloria Huang
Ventura, California

Pat McElhaney
Provider Network Coordinator
TRICARE Programs
Ventura, California

Alfredo Ocampo
Oxnard, California

Daniela Steines
Aefligen, Switzerland

Griff Stelzner
Assistant Claims Manager
State Compensation Insurance Fund
Oxnard, California

Pauline Triebenbacher
Health Net Federal Services
Marketing and Military Treatment Facilities
Provider Health Relations
Port Hueneme Naval Base, California

Contents

SECTION III

Coding Insurance Claims

SECTION IV

Claim Submission

SECTION VI

Receiving Payment and Problem Solving

Appendices

Medical Insurance Billing and Coding

AN ESSENTIALS WORKTEXT

Objectives

After reading this chapter and completing the exercise sessions, you should be able to:

- ✔ Analyze how previous education, experience, and skills will enhance learning and future employment opportunities.
- ✔ Describe the variety of career possibilities and areas of specialization open to those trained as insurance billing specialists.
- ✔ Name job responsibilities assigned to insurance billing and coding specialists.
- ✔ List personal and professional qualifications required by an insurance billing specialist.
- ✔ Describe what aspects of medical insurance billing are affected by medicolegal issues.
- ✔ Define medical insurance terms and abbreviations presented in this chapter.
- ✔ Differentiate between medical ethics and medical etiquette.
- ✔ Define confidential information.
- ✔ List various types of insurance fraud and abuse as they relate to insurance claims.
- ✔ Specify types of certification and registration available to insurance billers, coders, and administrative medical assistants.
- ✔ Explain how medical and insurance knowledge can be kept current.
- ✔ Summarize how insurance billing and the insurance billing specialist are the "life support" of the medical office.

Key Terms

abuse
American Association of Medical Assistants (AAMA)
blanket bond
bonding
cash flow
certification
churning
coding specialist
confidential communication
continuity of care
embezzlement
ethics
etiquette
fraud
medical insurance billing specialist
mentor
multiskilled health practitioner (MSHP)
networking
nonprivileged information
password
personal bond
phantom billing
ping-ponging
position-schedule bond
privileged information
registration
respondeat superior
yo-yoing

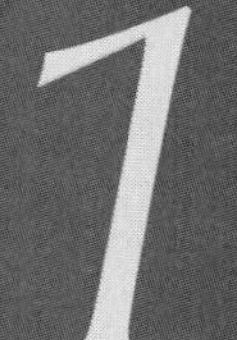

Chapter 1

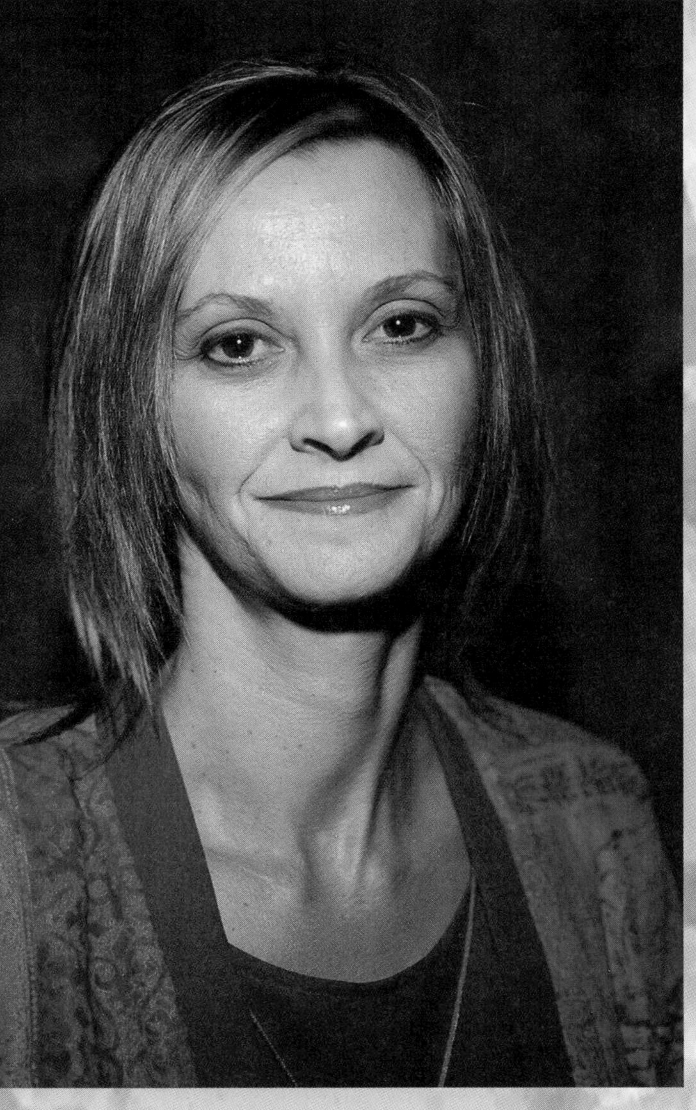

I am a Nationally Certified Insurance Coding Specialist and graduate of a medical insurance billing vocational program. Before completion of the course, I was hired by a two-doctor internal medicine practice that specializes in pulmonology.

Six years ago I suffered a traumatic below-the-knee amputation in a motorcycle accident and during my rehabilitation I had difficulty getting the insurance to cover my prosthetic leg. People I was dealing with had limited knowledge in this area and seemed unconcerned with how important it was that I get a leg so that I could return to work. Care, concern, compassion, and competence (the 4 Cs) were all but absent and replaced by an indifference and "burned out" attitude.

It has been very satisfying and rewarding working in this field, applying the 4 Cs and having a positive impact in people's lives.

Sharon LaScala, NCICS
Billing Specialist, Office Manager
Internal Medicine—Pulmonology

A Career as an Insurance Billing Specialist

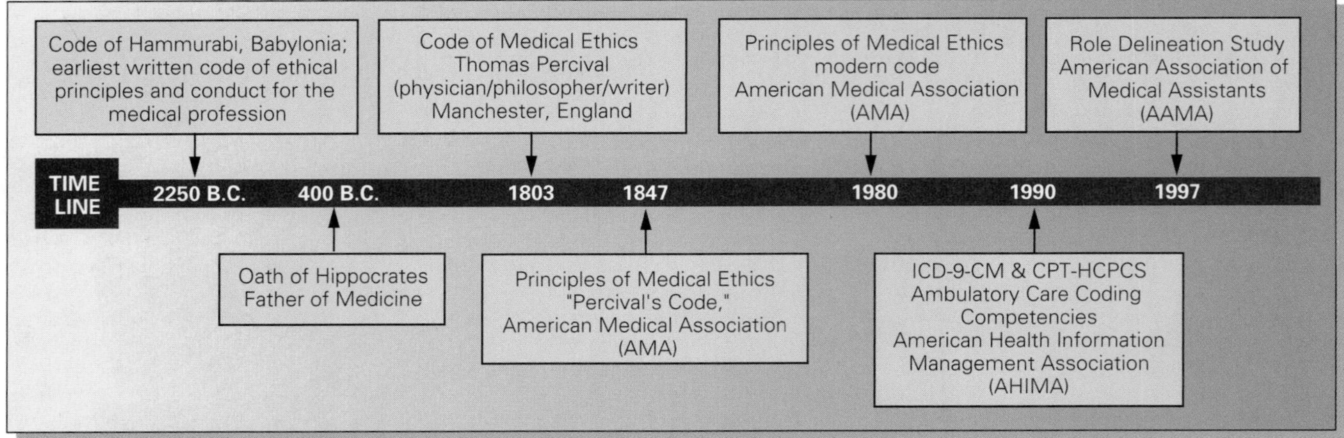

ROLE AND RESPONSIBILITIES OF THE INSURANCE BILLING SPECIALIST

Congratulations! You have selected a career path in one of the fastest-growing areas of the 21st century—healthcare. The profession you have chosen, medical insurance billing, is a vital part of all healthcare facilities because it brings in the currency that is needed to operate the practice. That is why it is referred to as the "life support of the medical office." Regardless of whether it is a solo physician's practice, multispecialty medical group, large clinic, or hospital facility, they all require medical insurance billers to process claims. Services in all medical facilities are provided to patients in exchange for reimbursement. With the increasing cost of healthcare, many patients have medical health insurance to cover these costs. The expedient processing of the health insurance claim form to receive maximum reimbursement is the goal of the **medical insurance billing specialist** and the focus of this worktext.

There is basic insurance information, billing rules, and practical skills that must be learned before a claim form can be processed. This worktext will give you background information and teach you individual skills in a simplified step-by-step fashion, as if they were building blocks necessary to build a structure. The first essential when constructing a building is a stable foundation. Medical terminology and medicolegal terms are two cornerstones that you will need to construct this foundation. Basic terms in this and subsequent chapters appear in boldface or italicized type. Refer to the glossary in Appendix E at the end of the worktext for a comprehensive list of key terms with detailed definitions to help broaden your knowledge. Each learned task is reinforced with practice sessions throughout this worktext. Simple solutions are offered for reimbursement problems, as well as for other challenging tasks.

This chapter will introduce you to the role and responsibilities of the insurance billing specialist. Later chapters will build on this foundation and will guide you through the entire process of insurance billing—from handling source documents, to abstracting information from the medical record, to coding procedures and diagnoses, to completing the ledger, and finally to filling out the claim form. Once these building blocks are in place, you will have all the necessary skills to process insurance claims. The final chapter deals with following up after claim submission. This is the covering (or roof) that is placed on the foundation of insurance knowledge that protects and ensures that all of the hard work you have done filing claims will bring maximum reimbursement. All of the above will help you obtain a position as a medical insurance billing specialist.

Job Titles

In the past, the medical assistant working in a physician's office performed both administrative (front office) and clinical (back office) duties. Then, as decades passed, he or she performed either one or the other. Next, due to ever-changing government regulations and variations in insurance industry standards, medical assisting job tasks became specialized. During this phase it was commonplace to find administrative duties divided and shared by a number of employees, for example, receptionist, bookkeeper, file clerk, insurance billing specialist, transcriptionist, and so on.

Soon, downsizing occurred in industry and corporations across America. In the healthcare setting, **multiskilled health practitioners (MSHPs)** became cross-trained to once again perform a variety of job tasks, thereby offering more flexibility to the employer. By doing so, the x-ray technician in an orthopedic office could perform phlebotomy when needed, the transcriptionist could process laboratory tests, and the insurance billing specialist could take over for the receptionist at the front desk during the lunch hour. The diversity of job duties makes the MSHP more employable. Knowledge of insurance claims completion and assignment of accurate codes enhances skills so that the MSHP can offer more flexibility in a medical setting.

Just as the administrative medical assistant's job duties became more specialized, so did the various roles of the medical insurance biller. Job titles changed to reflect this specialization and are listed and described in Table 1–1. The larger the practice, the more likely you are to find these specialized positions. The smaller the practice, the more likely that one person will perform diversified job duties and may need to be cross-trained in other areas.

Table 1–1 Roles of the Medical Insurance Billing Specialist

Specialized Job Title	Job Duties
Claims assistant professional (CAP) or claims manager	Assists consumer to obtain maximum benefits. Helps patients understand, organize, file, and negotiate health insurance claims.
Coding specialist	Codes diagnoses and procedures with expertise, using diagnostic and procedural codebooks.
Collection manager	Answers inquiries regarding account balances and insurance submission dates. Has knowledge of collection laws and collection techniques used to collect on accounts and minimize accounts receivable.
Electronic claims processor	Processes claims via the computer using telecommunication lines.
Insurance billing specialist	Handles source documents, codes procedures and diagnoses, processes insurance claims, and follows up on delayed reimbursement in a healthcare facility.
Insurance coordinator	Answers insurance questions and obtains preauthorization for patients.
Insurance counselor	Speaks confidentially with patients to discuss treatment plans, insurance coverage, and payment options. Verifies eligibility, precertification, preauthorization, or second opinion requirements.
Medical biller	Processes insurance claims for a variety of insurance plans and government programs.
Medical and financial records manager	Interprets explanation of benefits and remittance advice documents; posts payments to accounts receivable.
Medicaid billing specialist	Submits claims for state Medicaid programs.
Medicare billing specialist	Submits claims for the federal Medicare program.
Reimbursement manager or specialist	Focuses on coding issues and billing practices to receive maximum reimbursement from insurance plans and programs.
Self-employed insurance billing specialist	Processes insurance claims from outside the physician's office using computer software to upload or download medical files. May handle the accounts receivable.

Job Responsibilities

One of the reasons that the job of medical insurance billing specialist is so attractive is that it is diversified and offers a broad spectrum of tasks to be performed. If you like variety, you will be constantly challenged because there are many facets to insurance claim completion. On the other hand, if you would like to handle just one aspect of medical billing, larger offices hire specialized billers.

Some of the job responsibilities include patient contact. There is a need for a new breed of people to interact with patients. Patients need to be treated as valued clients, not just as sick people. Insurance coverage and payment problems may often be overwhelming for patients who are already dealing with poor health. Personal service and the ability to demonstrate compassion and be a patient advocate are skills used to deal with such situations. You need to have the ability to measure what matters to the patient and to serve the patient's needs. In a traditional business setting, these might be called customer service skills. If you enjoy interacting with people, you may seek a position that offers patient contact. Following are some job responsibilities and their importance to the insurance billing process.

Data collection from patients, hospitals, laboratories, and other physicians needs to be exact and complete. Documentation is critical to good patient care and must be done comprehensively for proper reimbursement. Diagnostic and procedure coding must be precise and reviewed for correctness prior to sending out claims. Insurance claims must be generated promptly and submitted accurately to ensure timely payment and continuous cash flow. **Cash flow** is the amount of money received that is actually available to the medical practice for business operations. Without money coming in, overhead expenses cannot be met and the practice would fold. Keeping up-to-date on specific insurance plans, rules, and regulations allows the insurance specialist to process claims according to the latest guidelines. Bookkeeping transactions, such as posting charges for services and procedures, posting payments from patients and insurance companies, calculating deductions and adjustments, and balancing patient accounts and daily ledger sheets, provide the practice with an accurate description of its financial status. Following up on claims is critical to obtaining maximum reimbursement. The well-rounded and versatile medical insurance billing specialist will be able to perform all of these tasks.

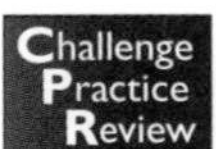

Pause and Practice CPR

REVIEW SESSIONS 1–1 THROUGH 1–3

Directions: *Complete the following questions as a review of information you have just read.*

1–1 State the goal of the medical insurance billing specialist. ________________________________

____

1–2 Name two key elements necessary to construct a stable foundation for a medical insurance billing specialist.

(1) ______________________________

(2) ______________________________

1–3 State the full title and define the abbreviation (acronym) MSHP. ______________________________

____

CHECK YOUR HEARTBEAT! Turn to the end of the chapter for answers to these review sessions.

Educational and Training Requirements

Generally, a high-school diploma or general equivalency diploma (GED) is required for entry into an insurance billing and/or **coding specialist** accredited program. An accredited program usually offers additional education, as well as more complex training in medical terminology, anatomy and physiology, ethics and medicolegal issues, procedural and diagnostic coding, insurance claims completion, general office skills, and computer proficiency.

For one who seeks a job as an insurance billing specialist, experience in coding and insurance claims completion and/or completion of a 1-year insurance specialist certificate program is usually required. However, prior work experience also facilitates an accelerated level of learning. You may have worked in another healthcare career field and want to transfer that knowledge to the insurance arena. Or, you may have extensive computer knowledge, experience with bookkeeping, or familiarity with the human body or medical language. All of these, and perhaps other skills you obtain, will help accelerate your level of learning and, along with the training you receive, will prepare you for a wide range of employment opportunities. Many accredited programs include an externship experience (on-the-job training) that you can add to your resume. Whether you begin this course without skills and know nothing about the healthcare profession or you have previous skills and/or have worked in some other area of healthcare, this worktext is designed to help develop the necessary skills that will be needed as an entry-level medical insurance billing specialist.

For one who seeks a job as a coder, completion of an accredited program for coding certification or an accredited health information medical record technology program is recommended. Ambulatory (outpatient) coding competencies for ICD-9-CM (diagnostic coding) and CPT-HCPCS (procedural coding) may be found at the American Health Information Management Association web site www.ahima.org. Click on "Certification," then "Employer Resources" for an inclusive list of training requirements.

Certification and Registration

To reach a professional level, certification and registration are available from many national associations. Becoming certified or registered is certainly an essential goal if one seeks career advancement. **Certification** is a statement issued by a board or association verifying that a person meets professional standards. **Registration** may be accomplished by two methods: (1) as a person whose name has been entered in an official registry that lists names of persons in an occupation who have satisfied specific requirements, or (2) by attaining a certain level of education and paying a registration fee.

A number of certifications are available on a national level, depending on how you wish to specialize. Refer to Table 1–2 for a list of certified/registered titles with abbreviations, a brief description of how to obtain the certification/registration, and the mailing address, web site, and e-mail address to obtain more information.

Keeping Current

The Industrial Age has given way to the Information Age, which has resulted in more information being produced in the past 30 years than in the previous 5,000. In the fast-paced world of insurance billing, it is imperative to keep abreast of changes. Following are suggestions to help you keep current.

1. Join a professional organization (see Table 1–2) to network with others in the same career field such as classmates, instructors, relatives, friends, and professional contacts. **Networking** is the exchange of information or services among individuals, groups, and institutions.
2. Read newsletters and journals published by the aforementioned organizations.
3. Attend meetings and workshops in this career field to learn about and exchange the latest information.
4. Attend state (Medicaid) and federal (Medicare, TRICARE, and CHAMPVA) insurance program seminars.
5. Keep in contact with your local medical society.
6. Select a mentor in the insurance field whose background, values, and style are similar to yours. A **mentor** is a guide or teacher who offers advice, criticism, wisdom, guidance, and perspective to an inexperienced but promising protégé to help reach a life goal.

Career Opportunities and Advantages

Jobs in medical insurance billing are on the rise and are available in every state, both in large cities and small. Salaries range greatly, depending on knowledge, experience, duties, responsibilities, locale, and size of the employing institution. Check in your area to discover the exact range.

Job sites requiring a knowledgeable medical insurance biller are expanding and are available in offices of doctors, chiropractors, physical therapists, and anesthesiologists, as well as outpatient clinics, laboratories,

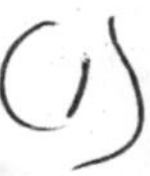

Table 1–2 Certification and Registration

Title	Abbreviation	Description to Obtain Certification or Registration	Professional Association Mailing Address	Telephone Number	E-Mail Address Web Site
Certified Claims Assistance Professional	CCAP	Self-study program and pass certification examination	Alliance of Claims Assistance Professionals (ACAP) 873 Brentwood Drive West Chicago, IL 60185	(877) 275-8765	askus@claims.org Web site: www.claims.org
Certified Coding Specialist *or*	CCS	Self-study program and pass certification examination	American Health Information Management Association (AHIMA)*	(800) 335-5535	info@ahima.mhs.compuserve.com Web site: www.ahima.org
Certified Coding Specialist—Physician-based	CCS-P	Self-study program and pass certification examination	PO Box 97349 Chicago, IL 60690-7349		
Certified Electronic Claims Professional	CECP	Self-study program and pass certification examination	Alliance of Claims Assistance Professionals (ACAP) 873 Brentwood Drive West Chicago, IL 60185	(877) 275-8765	askus@claims.org Web site: www.claims.org
Certified Medical Assistant	CMA	Graduate from accredited medical assisting program; apply to take national certifying examination	American Association of Medical Assistants (AAMA) 20 North Wacker Drive Chicago, IL 60606	(800) 228-2262	Web site: www.aama.ntl.org
Certified Medical Biller	CMB	Pass 2-hour examination written for physician's office billers and other outpatient facilities	American Association of Medical Billers (AAMB) PO Box 44614 Los Angeles, CA 90044-0614	(323) 778-4352 Fax: (323) 778-2814	AAMB@aol.com Web site: billers.com/aamb/page2.html
Certified Medical Billing Association	CMBA	Complete comprehensive program and pass ` proficiency test	International Billing Association, Inc. (IBA) 7315 Wisconsin Ave, Suite 424 E Bethesda, MD 20814	(301) 961-8680	micheles@biller.com Web site: www.biller.com
Certified Medical Billing Specialist	CMBS	Pass 3-hour examination written for physician's office billers and other outpatient facilities	American Association of Medical Billers (AAMB) PO Box 44614 Los Angeles, CA 90044-0614	(323) 778-4352 Fax: (323) 778-2814	AAMB@aol.com Web site: billers.com/aamb/page2.html
Certified Medical Office Manager	CMOM	Examination for supervisors or managers of small-group and solo practices	Professional Association of Health Care Office Managers (PAHCOM) 461 East Ten Mile Rd. Pensacola, FL 32534-9712	(800) 451-9311	pahcom@pahcom.com Web site: www.pahcom.com
Certified Medical Practice Executive Nominee 1st level Certification 2nd level Fellow 3rd level	CMPE	Eligible group managers join; membership/nominee—1st level Complete 6- to 7-hour examination—2nd level Mentoring project or thesis—3rd level	Medical Group Management Association (MGMA), American College of Medical Practice Executives (affiliate) 104 Inverness Terrace East Englewood, CO 80112	(303) 397-7869	acmpe@mgma.com Web site: www.mgma.com/acmpe
Certified Professional Coder *or*	CPC	Independent study program and examination (approximately 5 hours [CPC] and 8 hours [CPC-H] in length)	American Academy of Professional Coders (AAPC) 309 West 700 South Salt Lake City, UT 84101	(800) 626-CODE	aapc@worldnet.att.net Web site: www.aapcnatl.org
Certified Professional Coder—Hospital	CPC-H				

Table continued on following page

*Beginning in 2002, an entry-level coding credential (CCA) is offered.

Beginning in 2002, an entry-level coding credential (CCA) is offered.

Table 1–2 **Certification and Registration *Continued***

Title	Abbreviation	Description to Obtain Certification or Registration	Professional Association Mailing Address	Telephone Number	E-Mail Address Web Site
Certified Patient Account Technician *or*	CPAT	Complete self-study course and pass standard examination; administered twice yearly	American Guild of Patient Account Management (AGPAM) National Certification Examination Program 1101 Connecticut Ave. NW, Suite 700 Washington, DC 20036	(202) 857-1179	Scott-Hall@dc.sba.com Web site: www.agpam.org
Certified Clinic Account Technician *or*	CCAT				
Certified Clinic Account Manager	CCAM				
Healthcare Reimbursement Specialist	HRS	Successfully complete open-book examination	National Electronic Biller's Alliance (NEBA) 2226-A Westborough Blvd. #504 South San Francisco, CA 94080	(415) 577-1190 Fax: (415) 577-1290	mmedical@aol.com Web site: www.nebazone.com
National Certified Insurance and Coding Specialist	NCICS	Graduate from an insurance program and sit for certification examination given by independent testing agency at many school sites across the nation	National Center for Competency Testing 7007 College Blvd. Suite 250 Overland Park, KS 66211	(800) 875-4404 Fax: (913) 498-1243	Web site: www.ncctinc.com
Registered Medical Assistant	RMA	Take certification offered by the American Medical Technologists (AMT)	Registered Medical Assistant/ AMT 710 Higgins Rd. Park Ridge, IL 60068	(847) 823-5169	amtmail@aol.com Web site: www.amtl.com
Registered Medical Coder	RMC	Yearly correspondence program governed by the National Coding Standards Committee and pass an examination	Medical Management Institute 1125 Cambridge Square Alpharetta, GA 30004-5724	(800) 334-5724	bobby.carvell @ipractice.md Web site: www.theinstitute.com

radiology centers, long-term care facilities, and acute care hospitals. In this exciting and ever-changing career field, job opportunities also exist in insurance companies and managed care organizations as well as billing services, consulting firms, and schools or organizations who are looking for instructors or lecturers. You can also set a future goal, after you have obtained experience, to be your own boss by either setting up an in-home billing service or establishing an office for billing services.

A great advantage in this career field is the opportunity to have flexible hours. Many healthcare institutions are open 24 hours a day and 7 days a week; however, physicians' offices usually maintain a more traditional schedule. Most employees in the physician's office must adhere to the physician's schedule; however, the medical insurance billing specialist may be able to come in early to transmit electronic claims during nonpeak hours or stay late to make collection calls. It may be advantageous to both the physician and the insurance specialist to vary his or her schedule according to the needs of the practice.

Opportunities for someone visually or hearing impaired may be available in this career field with the use of special equipment. The American Collectors Association (ACA) in Minneapolis, Minnesota, has developed a training program for the visually impaired, and many schools now have special equipment to accommodate the visually and hearing impaired. Figure 1–1 illustrates a number of employment opportunities for someone trained in insurance billing. Jobs are listed according to job title with necessary requirements.

Personal and Professional Qualifications

Attributes

There are many characteristics or qualities that an individual should have to function well as an insurance billing specialist. It is important to be a logical and practical thinker as well as creative in problem solving. To have a curious nature and an inquisitive mind helps the medical biller investigate issues and be dissatisfied until all questions have been answered. Efficiency hinges on organization, and a person with good organizational skills can track the multitudes of paperwork that accompany this job and follow up on insurance claims in a methodical fashion. Being meticulous and neat is critical in completing various forms sent to the physician's office and posted entries to the ledger or day sheet. Strong critical thinking and reasoning skills will help evaluate and prioritize the day-to-day workload and solve problems as they occur. One who is honest, conscientious, loyal, and trustworthy is always an asset to the employer. Some qualities, like enthusiasm and self-motivation, cannot be measured, but they can be observed by others. Someone who notices that something needs to be done and takes the initiative to do it will be a valued employee.

Perhaps the most important attribute is being reliable. No one is born with this characteristic but you can develop and practice this as part of your training. There are three aspects to being a reliable person. First, be punctual; show up for class and/or work on time. Second, come prepared and ready to work. A medical biller usually works independently and a plan must be made in advance regarding work that is to be done on a daily basis. And third, follow through on what you say you will do. These qualities are evident in a person and will be welcomed by a future employer and coworkers.

Skills

Completing insurance claims encompasses many skills. To be proficient, you will need the following skills, which are listed with situations demonstrating how they apply:

- A solid foundation and working knowledge of medical terminology, including abbreviations, laboratory tests, clinical procedures, pathologic conditions, anatomy, and physiology.

  Application: Interpretation of patients' chart notes, operative reports, and coding manuals; communicating with insurance companies and other allied health professionals.

- Good listening skills and an ability to learn quickly.

  Application: Listening carefully is the first step in communicating effectively. An eagerness and willingness to learn new tasks will help make your job easier and more interesting.

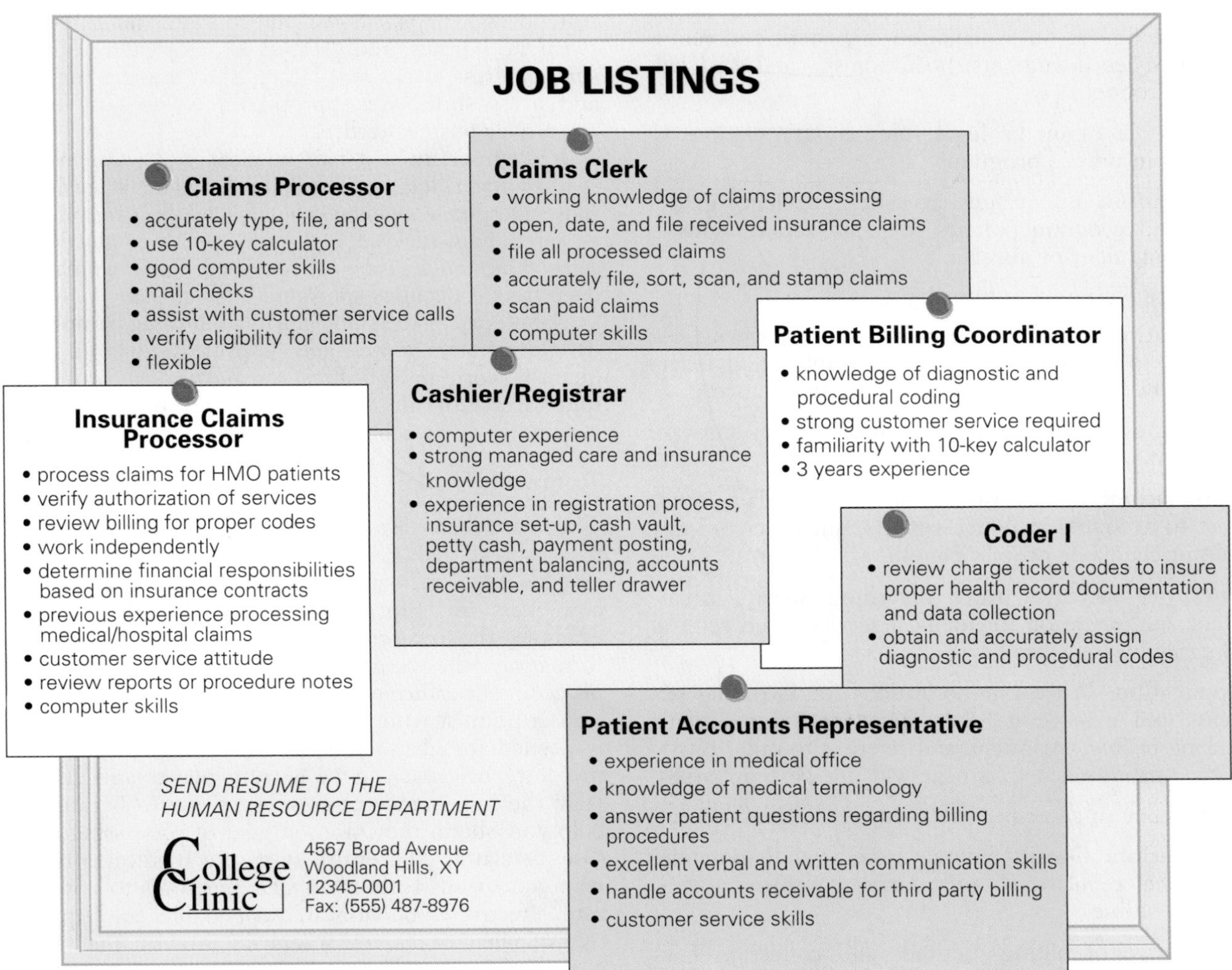

Figure 1–1. Job listings, showing job titles and qualifications as they would be posted for a large medical clinic.

- Knowledge of current billing regulations for each insurance program and managed care plan in which the practice participates.

  Application: File insurance claims with each insurance company or managed care plan according to specific rules and regulations. Without adhering to these rules, claims will not be processed and paid correctly.

- Proficient use of procedural and diagnostic codebooks and other related resources.

  Application: Accurately code procedures, services, and diagnoses for each case billed to obtain maximum reimbursement.

- Precise reading skills with good comprehension.

  Application: Interpret chart notes, operative reports, coding manuals, insurance program manuals, bulletins, and newsletters.

- Basic mathematics, bookkeeping skills, and accurate computation.

  Application: Total fees on insurance claim forms; evaluate figures on explanation of benefit and remittance advice documents; post, adjust, total, and balance accounts.

- Knowledge of medicolegal rules and regulations of various insurance programs.

  Application: File claims according to legal guidelines and program policies to avoid actions considered fraudulent or abusive.

- Accurate typing or keying skills.

  Application: Type at least 35 to 45 words per minute to accurately input demographic and insurance data and/or complete insurance claim forms.

- Basic knowledge of computer and medical software program.

  Application: Locate various screens for data input, post to accounts, produce reports, and electronically submit claims or process computerized claims.

- Interpret insurance rules regarding specific treatment, authorization for medical services, and referral of patients.

  Application: Process authorizations for incoming patients and manage necessary paperwork for patients seeking testing, treatment, and referrals to other physicians; unauthorized treatment will not be reimbursed.

- Proficiency in accessing information via the Internet.

  Application: Obtain federal, state, and commercial insurance regulations and current information as needed online.

- Knowledge of billing methods and collection laws and techniques.

  Application: Apply latest billing and collection ideas to keep cash flow constant and to avoid delinquent accounts; avoid lawsuits by applying state and federal collection laws.

- Generate insurance claims with accuracy and speed.

  Application: Submit correct claims and produce them quickly for fast payment; rate of production and accuracy are both measures of proficiency.

It is important to remember that both personal attributes and job skills are necessary to attain a job as a medical insurance biller. Once job skills are learned and presented on a resume to a future employer, your attitude and determination may be what gets you hired.

Personal and Professional Image

A professional image can be conveyed to a patient within a split second. Body language reflects attitude without any words being spoken. Being confident of your abilities adds to your image of professionalism, as does the way you appear. Be attentive to apparel and grooming. In a work setting, a uniform may be required or business attire that is conservative and stylish but not trendy. For women, this may include a business suit, dress, or skirts of appropriate length; slacks; sweaters; blouses; and dress shoes. For men, a business suit, or dress slacks and jacket; shirt and tie (optional); and dress shoes are appropriate. A lab coat may be worn over business attire.

It is important that hair be clean and worn in a style that flatters. Because fragrances can be offensive and cause allergies, they should be avoided. Fingernails should be carefully manicured, and bright polish or glued-on designs/rhinestones should not be used. For a woman, subdued facial makeup is appropriate for day use.

For either gender, jewelry should be simple, and dangling earrings avoided. A professional pin is frequently worn in an office setting and at professional functions. Consult the employer for office policy regarding body piercing and tattoos.

Teamwork

There are many aspects to what makes an individual a true professional. Getting along with people rates high on the list. An insurance specialist depends on many coworkers for information needed to bill claims; for example, the receptionist who collects the patient information, the clinical medical assistant who circles procedures performed on the encounter form, and the transcriptionist who transcribes the medical record that is needed for abstracting information for billing. It is therefore necessary to be a team player and acknowledge the importance of coworkers' duties because they help you obtain the common goal of processing the insurance claim. The entire staff in a medical office is a team and needs to hold regular meetings to communicate effectively. Be honest, dependable, and appreciative of what other coworkers do for you that enables you to do your job better. Never take part in office gossip or politics. Be willing to do all jobs that you are asked to do and be efficient in how you carry them out.

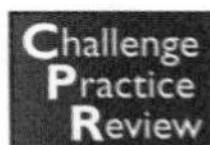

Pause and Practice CPR

REVIEW SESSIONS 1–4 THROUGH 1–6

Directions: *Complete the following questions as a review of information you have just read.*

1–4 Specify the educational requirements for entry into an accredited program for an insurance billing and/or coding specialist. ____________________

____

1–5 List four advantages the career of medical insurance billing specialist offers.

(1) ____________________

(2) ____________________

(3) ____________________

(4) ____________________

1–6 State why you think teamwork is important for a medical insurance billing specialist.

____

____

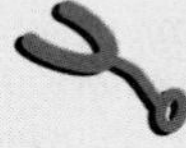

CHECK YOUR HEARTBEAT! Turn to the end of the chapter for answers to these review sessions.

Medical Etiquette

Before beginning work as an insurance billing specialist, it is wise to have a basic knowledge of medical etiquette as it pertains to the medical profession, the insurance industry, and the medical coder. Medical **etiquette** has to do with how the medical professional conducts him- or herself. Customs, courtesy, and manners of the medical profession can be expressed in three simple words—consideration for others. Several points about medical etiquette bear mentioning:

1. Keep a professional demeanor and maintain a certain amount of formality when interacting with others.
2. Acknowledge people who enter your office with eye contact and if busy, say "I'll be with you in a moment."
3. Identify yourself, by name and title, to callers and to those you call.
4. Treat outside physicians with respect. Never keep them waiting in the office or on the telephone (unless a patient's chart needs to be pulled). Connect them promptly to the physician or usher them into the doctor's office and notify the physician that they are waiting.
5. Address physicians, using the title doctor (e.g., Dr. Practon), and do not be too casual by using first names with patients, coworkers, and supervisors unless you have been asked to address them by their first name.
6. Always be friendly and courteous, thanking others for their help when they assist you with your job.
7. Have a positive attitude. Negative remarks and behavior can be infectious and contaminate the entire office environment. Look for the good instead of the bad when you regard people and situations.

Medical Ethics

Medical **ethics** are not laws but are standards of conduct generally accepted as a moral guide for behavior by which an insurance billing or coding specialist may determine the appropriateness of his or her conduct in a relationship with patients, the physician, coworkers, the government, and insurance companies. Acting with ethical behavior means to carry out responsibilities with integrity, decency,

Expressions from Experience

Working in this field reminds me a lot of being on an athletic team. You must be competitive, have a desire to overcome challenges, and do your best, thus bringing unity, prosperity, and success to your team. Performing well in my dual position as insurance specialist and office manager benefits all team members of the practice.

Sharon LaScala, NCICS
Billing Specialist, Office Manager
Internal Medicine—Pulmonology

AMERICAN ASSOCIATION OF MEDICAL ASSISTANTS CODE OF ETHICS

The Code of Ethics of AAMA shall set forth principles of ethical and moral conduct as they relate to the medical profession and the particular practice of medical assisting.

A. Render service with full respect for the dignity of humanity;

B. Respect confidential information obtained through employment unless legally authorized or required by responsible performance of duty to divulge such information;

C. Uphold the honor and high principles of the profession and accept its disciplines;

D. Seek to continually improve the knowledge and skills of medical assistants for the benefit of patients and professional colleagues;

E. Participate in additional service activities aimed toward improving the health and well-being of the community.

Figure 1–2. Code of ethics for medical assistants as established and printed in the bylaws of the American Association of Medical Assistants (AAMA), revised October 2000, Chicago, IL. (Reprinted with permission.)

honesty, competence, respect, fairness, trust, and courage. Moral standards are often referred to as the values one has and frequently involve religious views or spiritual beliefs. Moral standards impact all aspects of daily living, for example, violating the confidence of a coworker or patient, breaking marital vows, or cheating on a tax return. You cannot disconnect your personal morality from your business morality. Your personal and business decisions generally are consistent with your moral standards. A question to ask yourself is, Why should I comply with often meaningless government rules and regulations? Your answer will depend on your moral standards and if you can violate the confidence of coworkers, why would you comply with such seemingly silly regulations?

The timeline at the beginning of this chapter lists the origins and history of medical ethics for the health professional. The preamble of the American Medical Association (AMA) Principles of Medical Ethics was developed primarily for the benefit of the patient. It states "the physician must recognize responsibility not only to patients, but also to society, to other health professionals, and to self."

Expressions from Experience

Our practice reflects quality patient care, but patient care does not stop in the treatment room. When patients' insurance and financial issues are dealt with in a professional and compassionate manner, they feel that the medical office is a team, on their side, supporting all aspects of their care.

Sharon LaScala, NCICS
Billing Specialist, Office Manager
Internal Medicine—Pulmonology

It is the insurance biller's responsibility to inform the supervisor in charge if unethical or possible illegal practices are taking place. Illegal activities are subject to penalties, fines, and/or imprisonment. They may also result in loss of morale, reputation, and the goodwill of the community.

Some principles of ethics for the medial assistant and insurance billing specialist are as follows:

- Never make critical remarks about a physician.
- Never belittle patients.
- Maintain a dignified, courteous relationship with all persons with whom you speak.
- Do not make critical statements about the treatment given a patient by another physician.
- Notify your physician if you discover that a patient may have questionable issues regarding care, conduct, or treatment with your office or another physician's practice.

Reporting incorrect information may be considered fraud or abuse which can possibly damage the individual's future benefits, impair the integrity of the insurance company's database, allow incorrect reimbursement for services, or deny payment. In some cases there may be distinctions between illegal and unethical behavior, depending on where it occurs. For instance, it is *illegal* to report incorrect information to government-funded programs, such as Medicare, Medicaid, and TRICARE. However, it is *unethical* to report incorrect information to private insurance carriers.

The **American Association of Medical Assistants (AAMA)** has established a code of ethics. Because the job of an insurance billing specialist is part of the administrative medical assistant's role, this code is appropriate, whether one is a member or nonmember, and regardless of whether administrative or clinical duties are being performed (Figure 1–2).

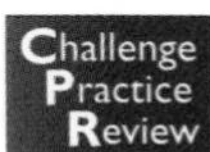

Pause and Practice CPR

REVIEW SESSION 1–7

Directions: *Differentiate between ethics and etiquette by listing the letter "A" or "B" by the words used to describe these terms.*

1–7 A. Ethics ______ values ______ manners

B. Etiquette ______ courtesy ______ consideration

______ morals ______ standards of conduct

PRACTICE SESSION 1–8

Directions: *Remember—you cannot disconnect your personal morality from your business morality. The following questions are designed to help you analyze your* personal moral standard, *which has at one extreme "absolute good/ethical" and at the other "absolute bad/immoral." Determining where you fall on the morality scale will help you understand how you react to certain issues and situations in the medical office. Moral standards impact all aspects of your daily life and whatever standards you have cannot be disconnected from the business decisions you will make in the physician's office. Please be honest with your answers.*

1–8 (1) You discover after returning home from a shopping trip that you received two items but only paid for one. Would you keep the extra item? ______________

(2) You gave the sales clerk $10 and were given change for $20. Would you keep the extra change? ______________

(3) A coworker disclosed personal information to you in confidence. Would you tell your best friend? ______________

(4) A coworker has an unexcused absence. Would you lie to your supervisor to protect the coworker? ______________

(5) You are in a nonsmoking building. If you are a smoker, would you smoke in the bathroom? ______________

(6) A family member has committed a crime. Would you lie to protect him or her? ______________

(7) The cable company made a mistake and you received premium channels with no charge. Would you view these extra channels until the cable company corrected its mistake? ______________

(8) Salary information is confidential at your company. Would you look at a coworker's employment file to determine the fairness of your compensation? ______________

(9) If you had an affair, would you lie to your spouse? ______________

(10) You are attending a medical conference and the airline made a mistake and placed you in first class although you paid for a coach ticket. Would you order a drink and fly first class? ______________

CHECK YOUR HEARTBEAT! Turn to the end of the chapter for answers to these review and practice sessions.

CONFIDENTIAL COMMUNICATION

When working with patients and their medical records, the insurance billing specialist must be responsible for maintaining confidential communication. **Confidential communication** is privileged communication that may be disclosed only with the patient's permission. Everything you see, hear, or read about patients remains confidential and does not leave the office. Never talk about patients or data contained in medical records where others may overhear. Some employers require employees to sign a confidentiality agreement (Fig. 1–3). Such agreements should be updated periodically to address issues raised by the use of new technologies.

Nonprivileged Information

Nonprivileged information consists of ordinary facts unrelated to the treatment of the patient. This might include the patient's name, city of residence, and dates of admission or discharge. The patient's authorization is not needed unless the record is in a specialty hospital (e.g., alcohol treatment center), or in a special service unit of a general hospital (e.g., psychiatric unit).

Privileged Information

All information (whether oral or recorded in any form or medium) that is related to the treatment and progress of the patient is **privileged information,** also referred to as *protected health information* (PHI). The patient record, including photocopies and all confidential documents, requires a signature to release information.

The federal Health Insurance Portability and Accountability Act (HIPAA) privacy rule, which applies to health plans, healthcare clearinghouses, and providers who transmit any health information in electronic form, went into effect in April 2001. The HIPAA definition of PHI expands the application of this law beyond electronic health information to include health information that is:

- Transmitted by electronic media.
- Maintained in any medium described in HIPAA's definition of electronic media.
- Transmitted or maintained in any other form or medium.

Electronic media includes dial-up lines, leased lines, private networks, the Internet, Extranet, and those transmissions that are physically moved from one location to another using magnetic tape, disk, or compact disk media. Two different types of forms to protect disclosure of information are:

1. *Consent form*—signed prior to treatment for use or disclosure of information pertaining to treatment, payment, and healthcare operations (e.g., disclosure to other providers to allow **continuity of care** for a patient, or disclosure to payers to allow reimbursement provisions—see Fig. 1–4).
2. *Authorization form*—that will direct the release of specific information to an identified recipient on a one-time basis for purposes other than treatment, payment, or operations (e.g., release of information to a physician in another city—see Fig. 1–5).

A member of the office staff needs to act as the *policy official* who is responsible for the development and implementation of privacy policies and procedures, staff training regarding the policies, and a complaint process for patients. Signed documents need to be retained for 6 years, or until the date when it was last in effect, whichever is later.

For most providers, this rule is scheduled to be enforced in April 2003. Medical offices, at this point, are making necessary changes so that they will be in compliance. Alterations and modifications may be made to

EMPLOYEE CONFIDENTIALITY STATEMENT

As an employee of College Clinic (employer), and having been trained as an insurance billing specialist with employee responsibilities and authorization to access personal medical and health information, I recognize that violation of confidentiality statutes and rules may lead to immediate dismissal from employment and, depending on state laws, criminal prosecution. I understand that such violation may cause irreparable damage to my employer, and the employer and any other injured party may seek legal action against me. I acknowledge that this signed document will be placed in my personnel file at this facility.

Mary Doe
Signature

Brenda Sheila
Witness signature

Mary Doe
Print name

September 14, 20XX
Date

Figure 1–3. An example of an employee confidentiality agreement that may be used by an employer when hiring an insurance billing specialist.

the rule prior to the enforcement date, so watch for updates regarding this issue.

A written *notice of privacy practices for protected health information* should be given to patients and displayed in the waiting room. The notice must contain:

- Uses and disclosures of health information the practice permits, including examples.
- Notice of information that will be used by the practice to contact individuals to provide appointment reminders and other uses (e.g., fund raising, approved marketing information, or release to the individual's health plan).
- The individual's rights to request restrictions, receive confidential information, and receive a copy of the notice.
- Information on how to file a complaint associated with the notice.

When releasing medical information, never let an original patient record leave the office; release copies only. If the consent or authorization is a photocopy, it

College Clinic
4567 Broad Avenue
Woodland Hills, XY
12345-0001

Phone: 555/486-9002 **Fax: 555/487-8976**

CONSENT TO THE USE AND DISCLOSURE OF HEALTH INFORMATION

I understand that this organization originates and maintains health records which describe my health history, symptoms, examination, test results, diagnoses, treatment, and any plans for future care or treatment. I understand that this information is used to:

- plan my care and treatment
- communicate among health professionals who contribute to my care
- apply my diagnosis and services, procedures, and surgical information to my bill
- verify services billed by third-party payers
- assess quality of care and review the competence of healthcare professionals in routine healthcare operations

I further understand that:

- a complete description of information uses and disclosures is included in a *Notice of Information Practices* which has been provided to me
- I have a right to review the notice prior to signing this consent
- the organization reserves the right to change their notice and practices
- any revised notice will be mailed to the address I have provided prior to implementation
- I have the right to object to the use of my health information for directory purposes
- I have the right to request restrictions as to how my health information may be used or disclosed to carry out treatment, payment, or health care operations
- the organization is not required to agree to the restrictions requested
- I may revoke this consent in writing, except to the extent that the organization has already taken action in reliance thereon.

☐ I request the following restrictions to the use or disclosure of my health information.

____

Date ____________ Notice Effective Date ____________

Signature of Patient or Legal Representative ____________ Witness ____________

Signature ____________ Title ____________

Date ____________ __ Accepted __ Rejected

Figure 1–4. An example of a consent form used to disclose and use health information for treatment, payment, or healthcare operations.

AUTHORIZATION FOR RELEASE OF INFORMATION

Section A: Must be completed for all authorizations.

I hereby authorize the use or disclosure of my individually identifiable health information as described below.
I understand that this authorization is voluntary. I understand that if the organization authorized to receive the information is not a health plan or health care provider, the released information may no longer be protected by federal privacy regulations.

Patient name: Chloe E. Levy **ID Number:** 3075

Persons/organizations providing information:
College Clinic, Gerald Practon, MD
4567 Broad Avenue
Woodland Hills, XY 12345-0001

Persons/organizations receiving information:
Margaret L. Lee, MD
328 Seward Street
Anytown, XY 45601-0731

Specific description of information [including date(s)]: Initial history and physical and complete medical records for last 3 years

Section B: Must be completed only if a health plan or a health care provider has requested the authorization.

1. The health plan or health care provider must complete the following:
   a. What is the purpose of the use or disclosure? Patient relocating to another city
   b. Will the health plan or health care provider requesting the authorization receive financial or in-kind compensation in exchange for using or disclosing the health information described above? Yes ___ No X
2. The patient or the patient's representative must read and initial the following statements:
   a. I understand that my health care and the payment for my health care will not be affected if I do not sign this form. Initials: CEL
   b. I understand that I may see and copy the information described on this form if I ask for it, and that I get a copy of this form after I sign it. Initials: CEL

Section C: Must be completed for all authorizations.

The patient or the patient's representative must read and initial the following statements:

1. I understand that this form will expire on 09/01/20XX (DD/MM/YR) Initials CEL
2. I understand that I may revoke this authorization at any time by notifying the providing organization in writing, but if I do not it will not have any effect on any actions they took before they received the revocation. Initials: CEL

Chloe E Levy June 1, 20XX

Signature of patient or patient's representative **Date**
(Form MUST be completed before signing)

Printed name of patient's representative: ______

Relationship to the patient: ______

YOU MAY REFUSE TO SIGN THIS AUTHORIZATION
You may not use this form to release information for treatment or payment except when the information to be released is psychotherapy notes or certain research information.

Figure 1–5. Completed Authorization for Release of Information form for patient relocating to another city. Note: This form is used on a one-time basis for reasons other than treatment, payment, or healthcare operations. When the patient arrives at the new physician's office, a consent for treatment, payment, and healthcare operations form will need to be signed. (From Federal Register, Vol. 64, No. 212, Appendix to Subpart E of Part 164—Model Authorization Form, November 3, 1999.)

is necessary to state that the photocopy is approved by the patient, or contact the patient and arrange to obtain an original signed document. Unauthorized release of information is called *breach of confidential communication.* Some forms of medical records, such as mental health records, have an even greater degree of privacy. Several states have passed laws allowing certain test results and other sensitive information (e.g., human immunodeficiency virus [HIV] test, alcoholism, or substance abuse) to be placed separate from the patient's medical record. A special form to release this information is used. If you are ever in doubt about when to obtain a consent or authorization, always take the safe route and secure the patient's signature.

A patient has a right to see his or her record. However, to avoid misunderstanding of technical terms, it is preferable not to allow laypersons to examine records without the presence of the physician. If the patient requests to review his or her medical record, inform the physician so that he or she can help interpret the language and abbreviations used in the documentation.

Right to Privacy

All patients have a right to privacy. Following are guidelines to help you honor the patient's right to privacy and guard privileged information.

1. Discuss patient information only with the patient's physician or office personnel that need to have the information to do their job.
2. Obtain a consent to release medical information before discussing patient information with an insurance company or other individual.
3. Respond to telephone inquiries by asking that the request be in writing and include the patient's signed authorization.
4. Refer people who are uncooperative about signing a consent or authorization form to the physician.
5. Leave only your name, office name, and return telephone number when speaking on voice mail because the call may inadvertently be received at a wrong number or by someone other than the patient.
6. Never attempt to interpret a report or provide information regarding test results.
7. Turn over or cover patients' records when left on your desk so that they are not exposed to passersby.
8. Use a privacy screen, clear patient information from the screen, turn the computer screen off, or log off the computer terminal before leaving a workstation.
9. Use a password for each individual computer user and change passwords at regular intervals. A **password** is a combination of letters, numbers, or both assigned to access computer data.
10. Shred notes, papers, messages, memos, and other private information that are not being kept in the patient's permanent record.
11. Remove original records from the copy machine when finished photocopying.

Since the advent of Internet access, federal laws address confidentiality issues, not only in the doctor's office but outside the walls of hospital departments and physician offices. They cover contractors and other entities who have access to health information. Some states are developing their own bills aimed at stricter laws to protect health information, not only for the benefit of healthcare providers but also for marketing and contract negotiation purposes. Example 1–1 illustrates four scenarios where a breach of verbal confidential information has occurred.

Example 1–1

Verbal Communication Confidentiality Examples

Scenario #1—A coding clerk overhears two employees discussing a patient by name. Because the clerk had been working on the medical record of that patient and is now familiar with the patient's history, he or she realizes that the information being discussed is not accurate. The coding clerk then interrupts, making a comment about the patient's diagnosis.

COMMENT—Information should not be discussed with coworkers or other employees and must never be relayed to anyone other than a person who has a valid need to provide care for the patient.

Scenario #2—In reviewing an insurance claim, the insurance billing specialist realizes that he or she knows the individual who has a diagnosis that indicates a mental condition. The specialist discusses this with a friend at lunch.

COMMENT—This is a violation. An employee must never give anyone information on a patient's diagnosis.

Scenario #3—A Marilyn Monroe impersonator is scheduled to receive surgery. Over dinner at home, an insurance billing specialist relates the diagnosis and name of the surgery to his or her spouse.

COMMENT—Never discuss confidential information about patients to family, even a spouse.

Scenario #4—A physician in private practice calls the billing clerk via cellular telephone to answer a question about a patient's diagnosis that is to be listed on an insurance claim.

COMMENT—Cellular transmission may be intercepted by anyone with inexpensive eavesdropping equipment. In this scenario, a traditional telephone line must be used when relating confidential information about a patient's diagnosis.

Exceptions to the Right to Privacy

The following are exceptions, with rationales, to the patient's right to privacy when the confidentiality between the physician and the patient is automatically waived.

1. Workers' compensation medical and financial records.

   Rationale: Because the physician is examining the patient at the request of a third party.
2. Communicable disease reports.

   Rationale: For the protection of the public.
3. Child abuse information and records.

   Rationale: For the protection of the child.
4. Gunshot wound information and records.

   Rationale: For the good of society.
5. Stabbings resulting from criminal actions.

   Rationale: For the good of society.
6. Diseases and ailments of newborns and infants.

   Rationale: For the gathering of information to improve and protect future infants.
7. Subpoenaed records.

   Rationale: Because the court has already obtained permission.
8. Search warrants to obtain medical records.

   Rationale: Because law enforcement has already obtained permission.
9. Medical records of managed care organizations (MCOs) which have a contract with the physician that states "for quality care purposes, the MCO has the right to audit those patients' records."

   Rationale: The MCO has the right to audit those patients' records.

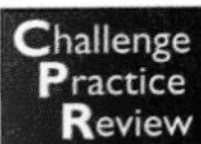

Pause and Practice CPR

REVIEW SESSION 1–9

Directions: *Fill in the blanks for the following statements as a review regarding confidential information.*

1–9 (1) Information such as the patient's name, address, and dates of discharge from the hospital is called ______________________

(2) Information related to the treatment of patients is called ______________________

____

(3) Unauthorized release of information is called ______________________

____

(4) The patient record, including photocopies, and all confidential documents require a/an ______________________ to allow a third party access to the information.

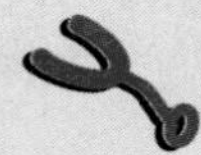

CHECK YOUR HEARTBEAT! Turn to the end of the chapter for answers to this review session.

PROFESSIONAL LIABILITY

Employer Liability

Physicians are legally responsible for their own conduct and for any actions of their employees performed within the context of their employment. This is referred to as vicarious liability, also known as **respondeat superior,** which literally means "let the master answer." However, this does not mean that an employee cannot be sued or brought to trial. Actions by the insurance biller may have a legal ramification for the employer. For example, if an employee knowingly submits a fraudulent Medicaid or Medicare claim at the direction of the employer, and subsequently the practice is audited, the employer and the employee can be brought into litigation by the state or federal government.

For protection, the physician-employer maintains medical professional liability insurance, otherwise known as malpractice insurance. It is also the physician's responsibility to make certain all staff members are protected under this policy. It is prudent for the medical biller to check with his or her physician-employer to be sure that he or she is covered under this type of insurance policy; otherwise he or she could be sued as an individual.

Employee Liability

Individual protection against loss of monies that occurs through error or unintentional omission on the part of the individual or service submitting the insurance claims may be obtained through a policy known as an *errors and omissions insurance policy*. If the physician asks you as an insurance biller to do something that is in the least bit questionable, such as write off patient balances for certain patients automatically, then make sure you have a legal document or signed waiver of liability relieving you of the responsibility for such actions.

Scope of Practice

The term *scope of practice* is commonly used in the insurance industry to define the parameters of a professional's regular duties and activities. In March 2000, the AAMA Board of Trustees approved a Scope of Practice for Medical Assistants. A Role Delineation Chart analyzing the many job functions of the medical assistant is presented in Table 1–3.

A medical insurance billing specialist's duties fall under the job description of an administrative medical assistant. It is the medical assistant's responsibility to know what he or she can and cannot do based on their education and training, their job description, the policies and procedures of their employer, and the laws, rules, and regulations in their state. If the procedure or job task in question does not fall within the scope of practice for medical assistants, it will not be covered by the professional liability policy. Having your own policy assures that the policy's maximum limit will be used to defend you and you alone.

When employed as a medical assistant who is submitting insurance claims, information on professional liability insurance may be obtained from the AAMA. To contact this association, see Table 1–2 for the address and web site.

Fraud

Fraud is *knowing* and *intentional* deception (lying) or misrepresentation that could result in some unauthorized benefit to the deceiver or some other person. It is a felony, and if detected, financial penalties or a prison term can be imposed, depending on the laws of the state. Claims are audited by state and federal agencies as well as private insurance companies. If a Medicare or TRICARE case is involved, then fraud becomes a federal offense and federal laws apply.

Usually fraud involves careful planning. Some examples are shown in Table 1–4. The concept of *intent* is key to the definition of Medicare and Medicaid fraud. Two types of intent must be proven: intent to agree to practice a fraudulent act, and intent to knowingly and willfully commit a major offense. When an insurance billing specialist completes the insurance claim form with billing information that does not reflect the true situation, then he or she may be found guilty of conspiring to commit fraud. It is not necessary to receive monetary profit from a fraudulent act to be judged guilty of participating in a criminal conspiracy.

Unintentional fraud may occur when completing the insurance claim form. For example, in a Medicare case, if payment of benefits are assigned to the physician and the statement "signature on file" (SOF) is inserted on the claim form (Block 12) instead of a written signature, and the office records do not contain the patient's signature authorization assigning benefits to the physician, this is a federal violation. To safeguard against this, the insurance billing specialist must verify that a Medicare signature authorization assigning benefits to the physician is on file before submitting a claim with the SOF statement.

A coder or biller who has knowledge of fraud or abuse should take the following measures:

1. Document the false statement or representation of the facts.
2. Notify the provider both personally and with a dated, written memorandum.
3. Follow up with a memorandum to the office manager or employer stating your concern if no change is made.
4. Keep a written audit trail with dated memorandums.
5. Do not discuss the problem with anyone who is not immediately involved.

If the person in charge does not seem concerned about suspected fraud and abuse, it may be time to look for a new job. A physician or office manager who is unethical and knowingly allows fraud and abuse to occur would not hesitate to disclaim all knowledge of what was taking place and point the finger elsewhere. For up-to-date information on fraud alerts, see Resources at the end of this chapter.

Abuse

The concept of abuse is harder to define, because those committing abuse also knowingly submit claims they know (or should know) are unacceptable. **Abuse** entails incidents or practices by physicians that are inconsistent with accepted sound medical business or fiscal practices that are not usually considered fraudulent. Though an abuse charge is less serious than one of fraud, a fine of as much as $10,000 per claim, plus an assessment of up to three times the amount improperly claimed, can be imposed. Some examples are shown in Table 1–5.

In subsequent chapters about various insurance programs, additional information about fraud and abuse pertinent to each program is given.

Compliance Program

A compliance program is a written plan that outlines good billing practices. Its purpose is to cut down on fraud and abuse by having written rules and regulations in the physician's office for employees to refer to and be guided by. Refer to Chapter 7 for a complete discussion regarding compliance.

Embezzlement

Embezzlement is stealing money that has been entrusted to one's care. In many cases of insurance claims embez-

Table 1–3 Medical Assistant Role Delineation Chart

Administrative

Administrative Procedures

- Perform basic clerical functions
- Schedule, coordinate, and monitor appointments
- Schedule inpatient/outpatient admissions and procedures
- Understand and apply third party guidelines
- Obtain reimbursement through accurate claims submission
- Monitor third party reimbursement
- Perform medical transcription
- Understand and adhere to managed care policies and procedures
- Negotiate managed care contracts (adv*)

Practice Finances

- Perform procedural and diagnostic coding
- Apply bookkeeping principles
- Document and maintain accounting and banking records
- Manage accounts receivable
- Manage accounts payable
- Process payroll
- Develop and maintain fee schedules (adv*)
- Manage renewals of business and professional insurance policies (adv*)
- Manage personal benefits and maintain records (adv*)

Clinical

Fundamental Principles

- Apply principles of aseptic technique and infection control
- Comply with quality assurance practices
- Screen and follow up patient test results

Diagnostic Orders

- Collect and process specimens
- Perform diagnostic tests

Patient Care

- Adhere to established triage procedures
- Obtain patient history and vital signs
- Prepare and maintain examination and treatment areas
- Prepare patient for examinations, procedures, and treatments
- Assist with examinations, procedures, and treatments
- Prepare and administer medications and immunizations
- Maintain medication and immunization records
- Recognize and respond to emergencies
- Coordinate patient care information with other healthcare providers

General (Transdisciplinary)

Professionalism

- Project a professional manner and image
- Adhere to ethical principles
- Demonstrate initiative and responsibility
- Work as a team member
- Manage time efficiently
- Prioritize and perform multiple tasks
- Adapt to change
- Promote the CMA credential
- Enhance skills through continuing education

Communications Skills

- Treat all patients with compassion and empathy
- Recognize and respect cultural diversity
- Adapt communications to individual's ability to understand
- Use professional telephone technique
- Use effective and correct verbal and written communications
- Recognize and respond to verbal and nonverbal communications
- Use medical terminology appropriately
- Receive, organize, prioritize, and transmit information
- Serve as liaison
- Promote the practice through positive public relations

Legal Concepts

- Maintain confidentiality
- Practice within the scope of education, training, and personal capabilities
- Prepare and maintain medical records
- Document accurately
- Use appropriate guidelines when releasing information
- Follow employer's established policies dealing with the healthcare contract
- Follow federal, state, and local legal guidelines
- Maintain awareness of federal and state healthcare legislation and regulations
- Maintain and dispose of regulated substances in compliance with government guidelines
- Comply with established risk management and safety procedures
- Recognize professional credentialing criteria
- Participate in the development and maintenance of personnel, policy, and procedure manuals
- Develop and maintain personnel, policy, and procedure manuals (adv*)

Instruction

- Instruct individuals according to their needs
- Explain office policies and procedures
- Teach methods of health promotion and disease prevention
- Locate community resources and disseminate information
- Orient and train personnel (adv*)
- Develop educational materials
- Conduct continuing education activities (adv*)

Operational Functions

- Maintain supply inventory
- Evaluate and recommend equipment and supplies
- Apply computer techniques to support office operations
- Supervise personnel (adv*)
- Interview and recommend job applicants (adv*)
- Negotiate leases and prices for equipment and supply contracts (adv*)

Green-colored blocks represent skills taught in this worktext.
White-colored blocks represent additional skills an insurance billing specialist may need.
* Denotes advanced skills.
Reprinted by permission of the American Association of Medical Assistants from the AAMA Role Delineation Study. Occupational Analysis of the Medical Assisting Profession.

zlement, the physician is held as the guilty party and ends up paying huge sums of money to the insurance carrier when false claims are submitted by an employee. If an undiscovered embezzler leaves the employer and you are hired to replace that person, you could be accused, some months down the line, of doing something that you did not do. Take the following precautions to protect yourself as an employee and to protect the medical practice:

Table 1–4 Examples of Fraud

- Bill for services or supplies not provided (**phantom billing** or invoice ghosting), or for an office visit if a patient fails to keep an appointment and is not notified ahead of time that this is office policy
- Alter fees on a claim form to obtain higher payment
- Forgive the deductible or copayment routinely
- Alter medical records to generate fraudulent payments
- Leave relevant information off a claim (e.g., failing to reveal whether a spouse has health insurance coverage through an employer)
- Upcode (e.g., submitting a code for a complex fracture when the patient had a simple fracture)
- Shorten (e.g., dispensing less medication than billed for)
- Split billing schemes (e.g., billing procedures over a period of days when all treatment occurred during one visit)
- Use another person's insurance card in obtaining medical care
- Change a date of service
- Post enhanced amounts to generate fraudulent payments
- Offer free items or services in exchange for a Medicare or Medicaid number
- Provide cheap equipment and bill for expensive equipment
- Complete Certificate of Medical Necessity by someone other than the physician
- Post adjustments instead of payments to pocket money (cash)
- Solicit, offer, or receive a kickback, bribe, or rebate in return for referring a patient to a physician, physical therapist, or pharmacy or for referring a patient to obtain any item or service that may be paid for in full or in part by Medicare or Medicaid
- Restate the diagnosis to obtain insurance benefits or better payment
- Apply deliberately for duplicate payment (e.g., billing Medicare twice, billing Medicare and the beneficiary for the same service, or billing Medicare and another insurer in an attempt to get paid twice)
- Unbundle or explode charge (e.g., billing a multichannel laboratory test as if individual tests were performed)
- Collusion between a physician and a carrier employee when the claim is assigned (if the physician deliberately overbilled for services, overpayments could be generated with little awareness on the part of the Medicare beneficiary)
- Bills based on gang visits (e.g., a physician visits a nursing home and bills for 20 visits without furnishing any specific service to, or on behalf of, individual patients)

- Ask the physician or supervisor to initial all posting entries for adjustments, discounts, and write-offs on either the ledger card or day sheet.
- Ask the physician to periodically check an entire day's records (patient sign-in log, appointment schedule, encounter forms, ledger cards, day sheet, deposit slip, and cash receipts).
- Run a daily trial balance of accounts receivable; verify encounter forms against charges posted and monies received against money on hand.
- Run a monthly balance of accounts receivable, balancing all ledger cards with the month's end total on the day sheet.
- Review the monthly bank statement to verify that all deposits tally with receipts for each business day.
- Bring poor bookkeeping and record-keeping methods to your employer's attention.
- Stamp all insurance checks immediately with a *restrictive* endorsement, "For Deposit Only," on the back.
- Use prenumbered encounter forms, transaction slips, and cash receipts to track all transactions; when errors occur, void and keep in the financial file.
- Use prenumbered insurance claim forms if a signature stamp is allowed, to ensure no false claims are being filed.
- Type your initials at the bottom left corner of the insurance claim form to identify who completed and submitted the claim.
- Retain Explanation of Benefits or Remittance Advice documents that accompany checks from insurance companies.

Only a few of the many precautions for protection are mentioned here. Embezzlement can occur in accounts receivable, accounts payable, petty cash, use of computers, and in various other aspects of a medical practice.

Bonding

Insurance billers, or anyone who handles checks or cash should be bonded or insured. **Bonding** is an in-

Table 1–5 Examples of Medical Billing Abuse

- Refer excessively to other providers for unnecessary services; also called **ping-ponging**
- Charge excessively for services or supplies
- Perform a battery of diagnostic tests when only a few are required for services; also called **churning**
- Violate Medicare's physician participating agreement
- Call patients back for repeated and unnecessary follow-up visits; also called **yo-yoing**
- Bill Medicare beneficiaries at a higher rate than other patients
- Submit bills to Medicare instead of to third party payers (e.g., claims for injury from an automobile accident, or taking place in a store, or the workplace)
- Breach assignment of benefits agreement
- Fail to make required refunds when services are not reasonable and necessary
- Require patients to contract to pay their physician's full charges, in excess of the Medicare charge limits
- Require a patient to waive rights to have the physician submit claims to Medicare and obligate a patient to pay privately for Medicare-covered services
- Require patients to pay for services not previously billed, including telephone calls with the physician, prescription refills, and medical conferences with other professionals
- Require patients to sign a global waiver agreeing to pay privately for all services that Medicare will not cover, and using these waivers to obligate patients to pay separately for a service that Medicare covers as part of a package or related procedures

surance contract by which a bonding agency guarantees payment of a certain sum to a physician in case of a financial loss caused by an employee or some contingency over which the payee has no control. Bonding methods for a practice with three or more office employees are:

- **Blanket bond**—provides coverage for all employees regardless of job title.
- **Position-schedule bond**—covers a designated job title, such as a bookkeeper or insurance biller, rather than a named individual. If one employee in a job category leaves, the replacement is automatically covered.
- **Personal bond**—provides coverage for individuals who handle large sums of money. A thorough background investigation is required.

Such bonding contracts may be obtained from a casualty insurance agent or broker. Bond coverage should be reviewed periodically with the insurance agent to ensure that coverage is keeping pace with the expansion of the medical practice.

SUMMATION AND PREVIEW

You have now begun your study to become an insurance billing specialist. Remember that the job that you are training for will have a direct influence on the profitability of the medical practice. In subsequent chapters you will learn important information and the skills to help you achieve this goal. Throughout this course you will have the opportunity to form a positive professional and personal image.

The medical terminology that is presented throughout this worktext and the medicolegal issues that you have learned in this chapter are two cornerstones in the foundation on which you will be placing the building blocks which represent each skill and task that you will learn. In the next chapter, you will be learning about health insurance contracts and different types of health insurance programs and coverage, which are the two final cornerstones of this vital foundation. In the next chapter you will also start building skills as you learn how to compose a letter, prepare a business envelope, complete U.S. Postal Service forms, and how to complete an insurance precertification form.

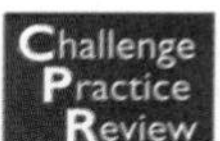

Pause and Practice CPR

REVIEW SESSIONS 1–10 THROUGH 1–14

Directions: *Complete the following questions as a review of information you have just read.*

1–10 Define *respondeat superior.* ______________________________

____

1–11 State the biggest difference between the definitions of fraud and abuse in the medical office.

____

____

1–12 What is the maximum fine for insurance abuse? ______________________________

____

1–13 A written plan that outlines good billing practices is called a/an ______________________________

____

1–14 How should an insurance claim be marked to identify who is responsible for filling it out and submitting it? ______________________________

____

CHECK YOUR HEARTBEAT! Turn to the end of the chapter for answers to these review sessions.

GOLDEN RULE

Be professional, personable, punctual, and employ ethical behavior.

Chapter 1 Review and Practice

Study Session

Directions: *Review the objectives, key terms, and chapter information before completing the following questions.*

1–1 List six job sites where career opportunities exist for a medical insurance billing specialist and indicate where you would like to seek employment and why.

(1) ______________________________

(2) ______________________________

(3) ______________________________

(4) ______________________________

(5) ______________________________

(6) ______________________________

I would like to seek employment at the site I have listed in # ____ because ____________

____

____

1–2 Name three skills needed to interact with patients.

(1) ______________________________

(2) ______________________________

(3) ______________________________

1–3 Name job responsibilities assigned to a medical insurance biller and coder.

(1) ______________________________

(2) ______________________________

(3) ______________________________

(4) ______________________________

(5) ______________________________

(6) ______________________________

(7) ______________________________

1–4 Name three ways to keep current in the profession of medical insurance billing.

(1) ______________________________

(2) ______________________________

(3) ______________________________

1–5 According to the preamble of the AMA Principles of Medical Ethics, who should the physician recognize responsibility to? ______________________________

____

1–6 List six possible outcomes of illegal activity in the physician's office.

(1) ______________________________

(2) ______________________________

(3) ______________________________

(4) ______________________________

(5) ______________________________

(6) ______________________________

1–7 Why is it preferable not to allow laypersons to examine their medical records without the presence of the physician? ______________________________

____

1–8 What should you do if a person is uncooperative regarding the need for a signed consent or authorization to release medical information? ______________________________

____

1–9 List five exceptions to the right to privacy.

(1) ______________________________

(2) ______________________________

(3) ______________________________

(4) ______________________________

(5) ______________________________

1–10 List two types of professional liability insurance that protect the medical insurance billing specialist. (1) ______________________________

(2) ______________________________

1–11 Read the following statements and determine which kind of bond is appropriate.

(1) Jane works in an office that carries a bond that covers her because she has the title "medical insurance billing specialist."

____

(2) John is bonded because all employees at the clinic where he works are bonded.

____

(3) Jill went through an extensive background investigation before obtaining a bond to cover the large deposits she makes for the doctor.

____

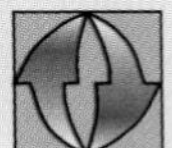

Exercise Exchange

Directions: Answer the following questions to perform a self-evaluation which will help you determine what education, experience, and skills you already possess that can be used in your new career field. Set goals by exploring the possibilities of future certification/registration.

1–1 Search Various Certified/Registered Job Titles, and (1) Choose One that Describes the Position You Would Like to Obtain in the Future, and (2) State Why You Have Chosen It.

(1) ______________________________

(2) ______________________________

____

1–2 List Previous Education and Experience and Analyze How Each Will Enhance Learning and Future Employment Opportunities.

____

____

____

1–3 In the First Column List the Three Most Important Attributes that You Possess, and in the Second Column Briefly State How These Characteristics Will Help You Function as a Medical Insurance Billing Specialist.

(1) ______________ ______________________________

(2) ______________ ______________________________

(3) ______________ ______________________________

1–4 List Three Skills that You Already Possess From the Ones Listed in Chapter 1.

(1) ______________________________

(2) ______________________________

(3) ______________________________

NOTES

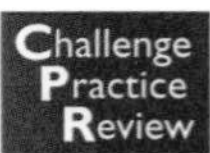

CPR Session: Answers

REVIEW SESSIONS 1–1 THROUGH 1–3

1–1 The expedient processing of the health insurance claim form to receive maximum reimbursement.

1–2 (1) Medical terminology.
(2) Medicolegal terms.

1–3 Multiskilled health practitioner—a cross-trained medical assistant who performs a variety of job tasks offering flexibility to the employer.

REVIEW SESSIONS 1–4 THROUGH 1–6

1–4 High-school diploma or general equivalency diploma (GED)

1–5 Possible answers:
(1) Jobs are on the rise and available in all states.
(2) Jobs sites are expanding.
(3) Flexible hours.
(4) Opportunities for visually or hearing impaired.
(5) Self-employment.

1–6 Possible answers:
(1) An insurance specialist depends on many coworkers for information needed to bill claims.
(2) Coworkers help you obtain the common goal of processing the insurance claim to attain maximum reimbursement for the patient and physician.
(3) Coworkers enable you to do your job better.

REVIEW SESSION 1–7

1–7 A. Ethics—values, morals, standards of conduct.
B. Etiquette—manners, courtesy, consideration.

PRACTICE SESSION 1–8

1–8 If you answered *yes* to:
8 to 10 questions—You may be entering into a career field that you are not suited for.
5 to 7 questions—You are ethically challenged and should think about how the situations you answered yes to would impact the world if everyone answered yes.
2 to 4 questions—You fall into the normal range, even though you may not be proud of the situations where you answered yes.
0–1 question—You are a rare moral person. Keep your standards high and do not be afraid to set an example for others with your decision making and actions.

REVIEW SESSION 1–9

1–9 (1) Nonprivileged information.
(2) Confidential communication, privileged information, or protected health information.
(3) Breach of confidential communication.
(4) Signed consent or authorization to release information.

REVIEW SESSIONS 1–10 THROUGH 1–14

1–10 Vicarious liability ("let the master answer"); physicians are legally responsible for their own conduct and for any actions of their employees performed within the context of their employment.

1–11 Fraud is an intentional deception (felony).

1–12 $10,000 per claim plus an assessment of up to three times the amount improperly claimed.

1–13 Compliance program.

1–14 Type the initials of the person who filled out the claim form and processed it on the bottom left corner of the claim

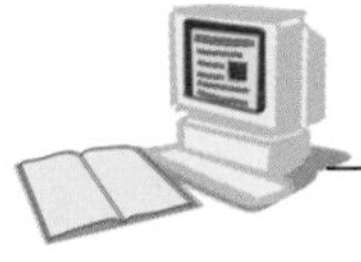

Resources

Good resource material is critical to a medical insurance billing specialist. You are not expected to remember all the rules and regulations or to know all of the answers; however, you are expected to know where to look to locate answers and determine solutions to insurance questions and problems.

The AAMA has chapters in many states that feature educational workshops and lectures. Become a member of this organization or one of the other organizations listed in Table 1–2. The AAMA has a JobSource that allows you to browse and reply to active job postings, check for new jobs, deliver your resume, and research participating employers. You can also receive e-mail notices as new jobs that meet your criteria are added.

Since this chapter emphasizes the job of a medical insurance billing specialist, information about job openings are included here. You may look at this information now to investigate possibilities, and mark it to refer to again after you have completed this course.

There are many ways to obtain information on job openings. The Internet is one source and if you subscribe to a monthly online service, you can network by posting a notice on a bulletin board with your resume or a note stating that you are looking for a particular type of position in a given locale.

You may also register with a computerized job search company. Often, registration can be done without charge. An extensive profile questionnaire is completed online and the firm acts as a liaison between employer and applicant. First, connect online and then go to a web index to locate a search engine that lists different options to explore, such as Yahoo (www.yahoo.com/), Infoseek (infoseek.go.com), or Alta Vista (www.altavista.com). Next go to one of the sites below listing job openings and/or salary information. In addition to job search information, following are resource materials to help you build a strong foundation and obtain information on fraud alerts.

Internet Job Sites

America's Job Bank—job postings
Web site: http://www.ajb.dni.us

Career Magazine—hundreds of national job openings are listed in a variety of fields
Web site: http://www.career-mag.com/careermag/

E-Span Employment Database Search—job posting
Web site: http://www.espan.com/

MedSearch America—employment service posts jobs for hospitals, managed care organizations, and pharmaceutical companies
Web site: http://www.medsearch.com or gopher://gopher.medsearch.com

PracticeNet—provides descriptions of medical practice opportunities
Web site: http://www.practice-net.com

Salary Wizard—salary ranges for thousands of job titles in a comprehensive set of career fields, sorted by occupation, and region.
Web site: http://www.salary.com

Fraud Alerts

Office of the Inspector General (OIG) and Federal Bureau of Investigation OIG national hotline—(800) HHS-TIPS

Healthcare Fraud and Abuse, A Physician's Guide to Compliance, 2000. American Medical Association, (800) 621-8335

Reference Books

Hook Up, Get Hired! The Internet Job Search Revolution. Kennedy, Joyce Lain. New York, John Wiley & Sons.

Medical Dictionaries, Pharmacy, and Wordbooks

Dorland's Illustrated Medical Dictionary. Updated periodically (available on CD-ROM). Philadelphia, W.B. Saunders, (800) 545-2522

Medical Language Instant Pocket Translator. Chabner, Davi-Ellen. Philadelphia, W.B. Saunders, 2001, (800) 545-2522

Miller-Keane Encyclopedia and Dictionary of Medicine, Nursing, and Allied Health. Updated periodically. Philadelphia, W.B. Saunders, (800) 545-2522

Mosby's GenRx, A Comprehensive Reference for Generic and Brand Prescription Drugs, Published annually. St. Louis, Mosby–Year Book, (800) 545-2522

Mosby's Medical, Nursing, and Allied Health Dictionary. Updated periodically. Anderson, Ken; Anderson, Lois; Glanze, Walter. St. Louis, Mosby–Year Book, (800) 545-2522

Sloane's Medical Word Book. Updated periodically. Sloane, Sheila. Philadelphia, W.B. Saunders, (800) 545-2522

Stedman's Medical Dictionary. Updated periodically. Philadelphia, Lippincott Williams & Wilkins

NOTES

Objectives

After reading this chapter and completing the exercise sessions, you should be able to:

Learning Objectives

- ✔ Differentiate between a group, individual, and prepaid health insurance contract.
- ✔ State how an individual applies for a health insurance policy.
- ✔ Define the standard terms of an insurance policy.
- ✔ Explain coordination of benefits and the birthday law.
- ✔ Discuss the elements of precertification and preauthorization requirements.
- ✔ Name five types of policy renewal provisions and cite their conditions and stipulations.
- ✔ List different types of health insurance coverage and their benefit provisions.
- ✔ Explain the physician/patient contract for various types of patients.
- ✔ Discuss four major categories all health insurance programs fall under.
- ✔ Describe in general terms the important features of federal, state, and private health insurance plans and workers' compensation.

Performance Objectives

- ✔ Complete an Insurance Predetermination Form.
- ✔ Compose a letter of withdrawal by a physician from the treatment of a patient.
- ✔ Prepare a business envelope for mailing.
- ✔ Complete U.S. Postal Service forms used for mailing.

Key Terms

birthday law
claim
coinsurance
contract
coordination of benefits
copayment (copay)
deductible
dependents
eligibility
emancipated minor
exclusions
expressed contract
guarantor
health insurance
implied contract
indemnity
insurance policy
insured
major medical
preauthorization
precertification
predetermination
premium
prepaid health plan
subscriber
time limit
waiting period

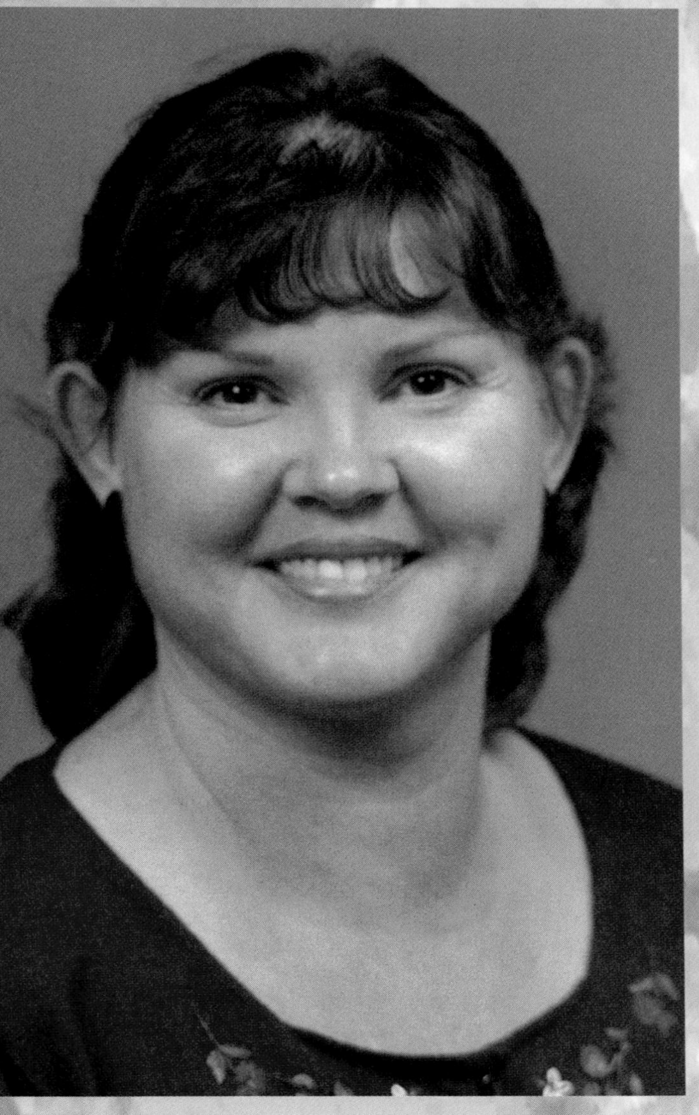

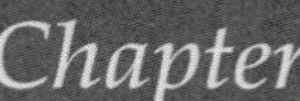

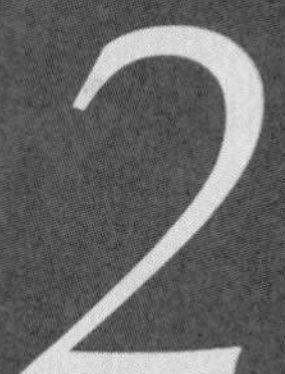

Chapter 2

I previously worked as an LVN and gave up nursing to stay home and raise my children. I am now ready to re-enter the workforce and chose medical insurance billing to add to my nursing background. As a nurse, I used to audit charts and enjoyed the detail work. I find that medical insurance billing is much the same; filling out forms with accuracy is the main objective. Some of the role playing we did in class to practice collection calls helped me build confidence.

I feel ready to embark upon the work world because I have a broader understanding of the medical field. I understand what happens to patients from the time they come into the office until they leave, and not just what happens in the treatment room. I am busy working on my resume and am excited about the career that is ahead of me.

Maureen Jackson
Medical Insurance Billing Student
Adult School Vocational Program

Fundamentals of Health Insurance Coverage

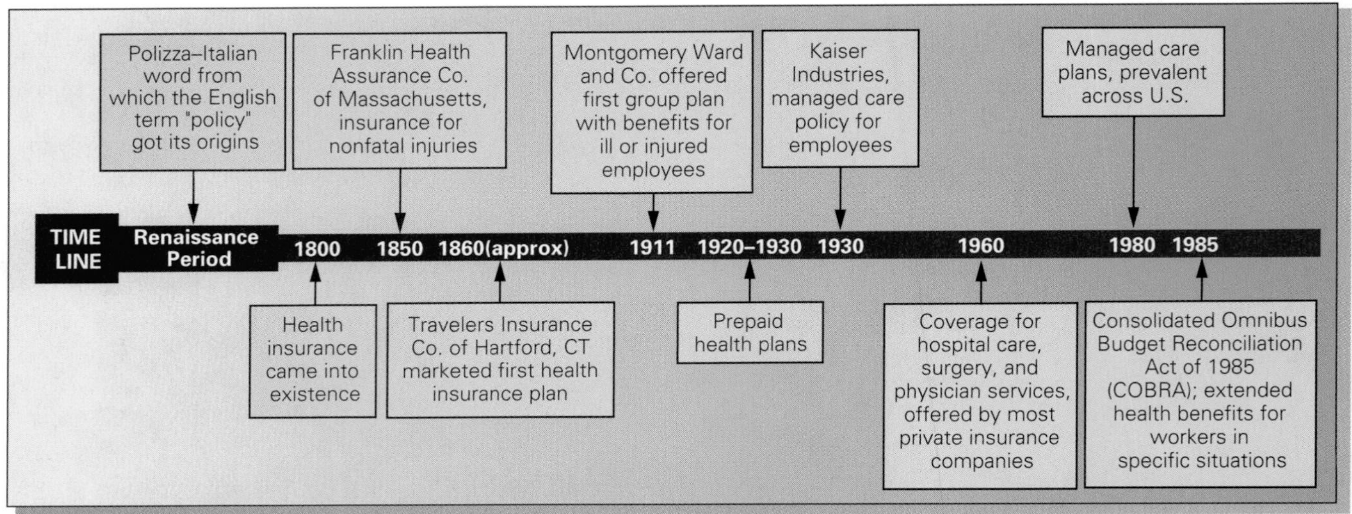

HEALTH INSURANCE CONTRACTS

Understanding health insurance contracts, policy terms and provisions; the physician/patient contract, along with different types of health insurance programs and coverage, will be the focus of this chapter. This information lays the two final cornerstones to secure a strong foundation of insurance knowledge.

Although this worktext is designed to present the basics of medical insurance billing, it is packed full of technical data and provides a comprehensive background of insurance knowledge while teaching practical job skills. As you progress through this worktext, remember—you are not expected to know all of the answers; however, you are expected to know where to look to locate answers and determine solutions to insurance questions and problems.

Health insurance is a contract between a policyholder and an insurance carrier or government program to reimburse the policyholder for all or a portion of the cost of medical care rendered by healthcare professionals. This care includes that which is medically necessary and preventive treatment. The purpose of health insurance is to help offset some of the high costs accrued from an injury or illness. In the last decade, medical care costs have escalated, forcing insurance companies to reduce types of coverage and the federal government to adopt cost-containment policies for government-sponsored programs. Patients may be covered under different types of private, state, or federal programs and because individual needs vary, each patient may have a different type of health insurance policy with various benefits.

There are three ways in which a person can acquire health insurance: (1) obtain insurance through a group plan, (2) pay the premium on an individual basis, or (3) enroll in a prepaid health plan.

Group Contract

A group contract is any insurance plan by which a group of employees (and their eligible dependents) or other group with members having like interests (e.g., American Association of Medical Assistants, United States Tennis Association, and so forth) is insured under a single policy issued to their employer or leader. Individual certificates are given to each insured individual or family unit and the coverage is the same for each person in the group. A group policy is usually less expensive and provides better benefits. If a new employee declines enrollment, he or she must sign a waiver stating this fact.

Many physicians can obtain comprehensive group coverage through plans sponsored by the professional organization to which they belong. This is sometimes called a *blanket contract.*

Conversion Privilege

If a person is covered under a group contract and leaves the employer or organization, or the group contract is terminated, the insured may continue the same or lesser coverage under an individual policy if the group contract has a *conversion privilege.* Usually, conversion from a group policy to an individual policy increases the premium and reduces the benefits. However, a physical examination is not required and this may be beneficial to someone having a preexisting condition and considered *high-risk.*

Consolidated Omnibus Budget Reconciliation Act

Under the Consolidated Omnibus Budget Reconciliation Act of 1985 (COBRA), when an employee is laid off or has work hours reduced from a company with 20 or more workers, federal law requires that the group health insurance coverage be extended to the employee and his or her dependents at group rates for up to 18 months. However, the COBRA premium rates are usually higher than the rates the employee was previously paying for the same insurance. In some circumstances, the continuation of benefits can extend up to 36 months.

Medical Savings Account

The federal government established the *Medical Savings Account (MSA)* as a pilot project. It is a type of tax-free savings account that may be offered to employees by a limited type of employer (e.g., small employers) to help pay healthcare costs. Individuals set aside money to pay for healthcare expenses before taxes are added on to their income. Employers may also make tax-free contributions. MSA balances accumulate from year to year tax-free. MSAs developed for the Medicare program are discussed in Chapter 11.

Another type of medical savings account offered by large group employers is referred to as a *flex account;* however, unused funds may *not* be carried over from year to year. In this plan, the employee projects the amount of healthcare dollars that he or she will spend in a calendar year to be set aside, over and above insurance-covered amounts. When healthcare services are provided, the patient files a claim to receive reimbursement from these funds and uses the explanation of benefits (EOB) from the insurance company as documentation. If the funds are not used in the calendar year, the monies will not be returned.

Processing of insurance claims with large deductibles (i.e., over $1,000), even though you know the insurance company will not be paying for the services, is necessary so that the patient/employee may submit documentation and recoup funds from the MSA. It may also be necessary to provide EOB documents from the insurance company to patients who do not receive them for this same purpose.

Individual Contract

Any health insurance plan issued to an individual (and dependents) is called an *individual contract.* Usually, the cost for this type of policy is more, and often benefits are less than those obtainable under a group plan. Sometimes an individual contract is called *personal insurance.*

Prepaid Health Plan

A healthcare program in which a specified set of health benefits is provided in exchange for a yearly fee or fixed periodic payments is called a **prepaid health plan.** Prepaid health plans were the forerunner of today's managed care plans and will be defined later in this chapter and discussed in Chapter 9.

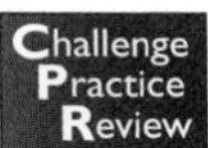

Pause and Practice CPR

PRACTICE SESSIONS 2–1 THROUGH 2–3

Directions: *Complete the following questions by applying the information you have just read.*

2–1 Emile Madison works for the National Telephone Corporation and has elected to obtain their health insurance plan. What *type* of insurance coverage does she have?

____

2–2 Emile has money taken out of her paycheck every month and put into an account to pay for uncovered insurance expenses. What *type* of account does she have?

____

2–3 Emile's boyfriend does not have insurance from his employer so he has elected to purchase a policy for health insurance coverage. What *type* of insurance coverage does he have?

____

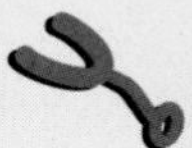

CHECK YOUR HEARTBEAT! Turn to the end of the chapter for answers to these practice sessions.

LEGAL PRINCIPLES OF INSURANCE

The role of the medical insurance billing specialist is to complete the insurance claim accurately and to facilitate **claim** submission so that prompt and maximum reimbursement is received. The claim is essentially a bill sent to the insurance company requesting payment for services rendered. It cannot be overemphasized that keeping up-to-date on policies and procedures of individual healthcare plans is essential to accomplish this. An insurance biller cannot escape liability by pleading ignorance. Most legal issues of health insurance claims fall under civil law because health insurance is regulated by state laws. It is not considered a federally regulated industry.

Before developing the skill of coding and completion of the insurance claim form, it is necessary to know the legalities of the job, frequently encountered legal situations, and simple solutions for handling them. Legal situations, as well as fraud and abuse issues, occur daily in the performance of job duties and involve confidentiality of medical records, accurate insurance claim completion, credit and collection laws, and so on. Legal requirements for the process of insurance billing will be interlaced throughout this worktext. Following, legal contracts will be discussed.

The Insurance Policy

The first legal item in the business of handling medical insurance is the **insurance policy.** An insurance policy is a legally enforceable agreement, or **contract.** Regardless of whether the contract is a group, individual, or prepaid contract, there is no standard health insurance contract; however, state laws regulate the way policies are written and minimum requirements of coverage.

To obtain a health insurance policy, the applicant answers questions and provides information on the *policy application* which usually has two sections, the first containing basic information about the applicant, and the second concerning the health history of the individual. The insurance company then decides whether it will accept the risk and enter into a contract with the applicant.

Individuals who take out a policy receive an original document composed by the insuring company. When a fraudulent statement has been made by the policyholder on the application, a policy can be challenged and coverage may not be in effect. After a policy has been in force for 2 or 3 years, a policy becomes *incontestable* and may not be challenged.

The Insured

The **insured** is the individual (enrollee) or organization protected in case of loss under the terms of an insurance policy. The insured is known as a **subscriber** or, in some insurance programs, a *member, policyholder,* or *recipient,* and may not necessarily be the patient seen for the medical service. In group insurance, the employer is considered the insured, and the employees are the risks. However, when calling to verify insurance coverage or when completing the insurance claim form, the covered employee is referred to as the insured.

A policy might also include **dependents** of the insured. Generally, this term refers to the spouse and children of the insured, but under some contracts, parents, other family members, and domestic partners may be covered as dependents.

Expressions from Experience

As a student who completed a Medical Insurance Billing program, I can't emphasize enough the need for understanding medical terminology. Even though I received this as part of my LVN training, I felt that I needed a good review. This became evident when we got into coding. It is important to have a full understanding of the body parts in order to understand procedures and diagnoses.

Maureen Jackson
Medical Insurance Billing Student
Adult School Vocational Program

Policy Renewal Provisions

Health insurance policies may have renewal provisions written into the contract stating the circumstances wherein the insurance company may refuse to renew, may cancel coverage, or may increase the premium. Following are five classifications with descriptions:

1. *Cancelable policy*—grants the insurer the right to cancel the policy at any time and for any reason. In some states, this type of policy is illegal.
2. *Optionally renewable policy*—affords the insurer the right to refuse to renew the policy on a date specified in the contract, such as a premium due date or anniversary date. At that time, new coverage limitations may be added or premium rates increased.
3. *Conditionally renewable policy*—grants the insurer a limited right to refuse to renew a health insurance policy at the end of a premium payment period for reasons of age and/or employment status, but not because of the insured's health status.
4. *Guaranteed renewable policy*—requires the insurer to renew coverage as long as premium payments are made. These policies may be renewable for life, or may have age limits of 60, 65, or 70 years.
5. *Noncancelable policy*—ensures that the insurer cannot increase premium rates and must renew the policy until the insured reaches the age specified in the contract. Some disability income policies have noncancelable terms.

General Policy Limitations

Health insurance policies contain **exclusions**—some more than others. Following are some possible exclusions or *limitations:*

- Acquired immunodeficiency syndrome (AIDS)
- Attempted suicide
- Cancer
- Losses due to injury on the job
- Losses resulting from military service
- Pregnancy
- Self-inflicted injuries

Be aware that some insurance policies may state that a procedure or service is not covered (excluded) when a state law says that the procedure is a "mandated benefit." Some examples are reconstructive breast surgery after mastectomy, surgical procedures affecting the upper and lower jawbones, and infertility coverage under group policies. Thus, beyond reading the policy, further investigation of state laws may be necessary.

Many policies do not provide benefits for *preexisting conditions* which are conditions that existed and were treated before the policy was issued. In some instances, such conditions might be covered after a specified period of time following the issuance of the policy provided no further treatment of the condition was rendered.

Some policies have a *waiver,* or *rider,* which is an attachment to a policy that modifies clauses and provisions of the policy by either adding coverage or excluding certain illnesses or disabilities that would otherwise be covered. Generally, waivers are used to eliminate benefits for specific preexisting conditions.

Waiting Period

A **waiting period,** or *elimination period,* is (1) the period of time that an individual must wait to become eligible for insurance coverage (e.g., the employee must be with a firm for 30 days before coverage commences, or (2) the amount of time that an individual must wait to become eligible for a specific benefit (e.g., an employee must wait 9 months prior to seeking maternity benefits).

Time Limit

The **time limit** is the amount of time from the date of service (DOS—date when the illness or injury was treated) to the date (deadline) the claim can be filed with the insurance company. Each insurance plan or program has specific time limits that must be adhered to, or payment, also called reimbursement or **indemnity,** from the insurance carrier will not be generated. The insurance billing specialist must know various time limits of state and federal programs as well as those of private insurance carriers. For managed care plans, the contract that has been signed between the physician and the managed care organization contains this information.

Case Management Requirements

Eligibility

Since the majority of patients will be using some type of health insurance to help pay for medical expenses, it is prudent to find out about the patient's coverage before expenses are incurred. The first step is to find out if the patient is eligible for the coverage he or she claims to have. Insurance **eligibility** is obtained by contacting the insurance company and verifying that the patient is indeed covered. This may be done over the telephone, via a voice automated system, using computer software, over the Internet, or with a managed care plan by checking an eligibility list. Depending on the type of practice you are working in, eligibility may be verified for all patients prior to their first visit, or only for high dollar services and procedures such as surgery and expensive testing.

Precertification

Once eligibility is verified, the next step is to substantiate whether a specific diagnostic test, surgery, or hospitalization is covered under a patient's contract. This is referred to as **precertification** and is usually done prior to scheduling a service/procedure. You may telephone the insurance company for this information, or send a precertification form via mail or fax machine. Sometimes a number is given to verify that precertification has been obtained.

Predetermination

Once you know that the patient is eligible for insurance coverage, and the specific service/procedure the doctor has recommended is covered, it is advisable to find out the maximum dollar amount that the carrier will pay. This information is obtained through **predetermination** and may be done when a service/procedure is tentatively scheduled. After the dollar amount is received from the insurance carrier, give the patient an estimate of fees for the proposed service/procedure. A form may be used so that the patient has a copy of the quoted amounts (Fig. 2–1). This written estimate expedites collection because the patient sees his or her actual financial responsibility. At this point a payment plan may be arranged if necessary.

Preauthorization

Many private insurance carriers and prepaid health plans have certain requirements that must be met before they will approve diagnostic testing, hospital admissions, inpatient or outpatient surgeries, and specific procedures. **Preauthorization** is the process used to determine medical necessity and obtain permission from the insurance carrier to admit a patient or perform a service/procedure and ensure reimbursement. The insurance specialist needs to be aware of all services/procedures requiring preauthorization. A list containing that information is usually included in the insurance or managed care contract. Various types of prior approval are discussed in Chapter 9 along with an illustration of a preauthorization form (see Fig. 9–6).

Policy Terms and Financial Obligation

Premium

The policy becomes effective only after the company offers the policy and the person accepts it and pays the initial premium. The **premium** is the cost of the coverage that the insurance policy contains and may vary

College Clinic
4567 Broad Avenue
Woodland Hills, XY
12345-0001

Phone: 555/486-9002 Fax: 555/487-8976

INSURANCE PREDETERMINATION FORM

Perry Cardi MD
physician

Patient: Leslee Austin Telephone # (555) 486-8452
Address: 209 Refugio Road Date of Birth 04-07-44
City Woodland Hills State XY ZIP 12345-0001
Social Security # 629-XX-9260 Accident Yes ___ No X
Insurance Company American Insurance Member # Am 45692
Insurance Co. Address 4040 Broadway Ave Group # 123P
Valley Vista, XY 12345 Telephone # (555) 238-5000
Policy holder Leslee Austin
Relationship to insured: Self X Spouse ___ Child ___ Other ___
Type of coverage: HMO X PPO ___ 80/20 ___ 70/30 ___ Other: ___
Procedure/Service Cardioversion (CPT 92960)
Diagnosis Atrial fibrillation (ICD-9-CM 427.31)

BENEFITS:
Coverage effective date: From 02/01/XX To 01/31/XX
Pre-existing exclusions: Lupus erythematosus
Major medical Yes X No ___
Deductable Yes ___ No X Amount $ ___
Per family: Yes ___ No X Amount $ ___
Deductable paid to date: Amount $ ___
Out of pocket expense limit: Amount $ ___
Per: ___

Maximum benefit or benefit limitation: $1,000,000 lifetime
Second opinion requirements: Yes ___ No X
Precertification/Preauthorization Yes X No ___
Reference # 432786
Authorized by: Lucille Vasquez

COVERAGE:

Procedures/Services	YES	NO	COVERAGE DETAILS AND LIMITS
Office visits	X		Physical exam; one per year
Consultations	X		
ER visits	X		
X-ray	X		
Laboratory	X		Need authorization
Office surgery	X		Need authorization
Hospital surgery	X		
Anesthesia	X		Need authorization
DME			

Physician payment schedule: RVS ___ RBRVS ___ UCR ___ Other X

Payment sent to: Provider X Patient ___ Time limit after submssion? 30 days
Verification by: Karen Reynolds Date: 07-14-XX

Figure 2–1. Insurance Predetermination Form. This form can be used when telephoning an insurance company or sent to an insurance company to find out the maximum dollar amount that will be paid for consulting services, surgery, x-ray and laboratory tests, and so on.

greatly depending on the age and health of the individual and the type of insurance protection. If the premium is paid at the time the application is submitted, then the insurance coverage can be put into force before the policy is delivered. Premiums are then paid monthly, quarterly, biannually, or annually to keep the policy in force. If the premium is not paid, a *grace period* of from 10 to 30 days is usually given before insurance coverage ceases.

Deductible

If a policy has a **deductible,** a specific amount of money must be paid each year before the policy benefits begin (e.g., $100, $250, $500). The higher the deductible, the lower the cost of the policy, and the lower the deductible, the higher the cost of the policy. Some policies have family deductibles so that in the case of a family of more than two people, each one will not have to reach his or her deductible to receive benefits. For example, a mother and father have four children and have a health insurance policy with a $250 individual deductible and a $500 family deductible. If the mother is ill and reaches her individual deductible of $250, and one of the children has an accident and reaches his or her individual deductible of $250, then the family deductible ($500) has been met and if the father or one of the other three children becomes ill, the deductibles need not be met before benefits begin.

Coinsurance and Copayment

Most policies have a **coinsurance,** or *cost-sharing* requirement, which is the responsibility of the insured. Following are two types of coinsurance requirements:

1. Percentage of the fee that is approved by the insurance company (e.g., 20%). This amount is paid after the deductible has been met.
2. Specific dollar amount to be collected when covered services are received (e.g., $5, $10, or $25 for physician services, $50 for emergency room, $25 for pharmacy). Managed care plans as well as state and federal programs refer to this as a **copayment (copay).**

It is not advisable to routinely waive coinsurance and copayment amounts. Most insurance companies do not tolerate this practice because it is a breach of contract. They may view it as giving the patient a discount and making the insurance company pay 100% of the fee. If audited, the federal government can assess penalties for not collecting coinsurance payments for patients seen under the Medicare program. However, if coinsurance payments are waived for legitimate reasons on a case-by-case basis, and documentation stating the reason appears in the patient's record, there should not be any problems. Generally, coinsurance payments are collected after the insurance company has paid. Deductibles and copayments should be collected at the time of service, and copayments collected prior to the patient's being seen.

Guarantor

A **guarantor** is the individual who is responsible for payment of the medical bill. Usually a form, indicating an agreement to pay, is signed by the guarantor, or the patient accepts treatment, which constitutes an expressed promise. Most of the time the patient is the guarantor and must be of legal age, 18 or 21 years, depending on state law.

Individual state laws vary governing financial responsibility; however, many declare that a husband is responsible for his wife's debts; a wife is not always responsible for her husband's debts. A father is ordinarily responsible for his children's debts if they are minors and are not emancipated, unless husband and wife are divorced and a court of law declares a responsible party. Children may or may not be responsible for the debts of their parents, depending on the circumstances.

Emancipated Minor

An **emancipated minor** is a child who falls out of the jurisdiction and custody of his or her parents or guardians. They may personally consent to medical, surgical, or hospital treatment and parents are not liable for their medical expenses. Minors are considered emancipated when they:

1. Live apart from their parents or guardians and manage their financial affairs.
2. Marry or are divorced at any age.
3. Serve on active duty in the military service.
4. Live away from home as a college student, even if they are financially dependent on their parents.
5. Become a parent (married or unmarried).

The patient record should contain the minor's signed statement that the minor is responsible for oneself.

Coordination of Benefits

When the patient has more than one insurance policy, a **coordination of benefits** (COB) statement helps in the determination of primary (first) and secondary coverage. This clause requires insurance companies to coordinate the reimbursement of benefits, thus preventing the duplication or overlapping of payments for the same medical expense.

In general, if both a husband and wife work and both have their spouses included in their insurance coverage, the *patient's* insurance plan would be considered primary and the spouse's plan would be secondary. This is the rule regardless of the amount of deductibles, copayments, or benefits.

Expressions from Experience

To put my best foot forward, I needed to study the subject matter each week. By doing so, I felt better prepared to ask questions in class about material that wasn't clear to me. When everyone shared, regardless of whether they had the right or wrong answer, it seemed to give a clearer picture and better understanding to all of the students.

Maureen Jackson
Medical Insurance Billing Student
Adult School Vocational Program

Birthday Law

When a child is covered under an insurance plan from both parents, in the majority of states the **birthday law** determines which plan is primary. The health plan of the person whose birthday (month and day, *not year*) falls earlier in the calendar year will pay first, and the plan of the other person covering the dependent will be the secondary payer. If both mother and father have the same birthday, the plan of the person who has had coverage longer is the primary payer. Most states have adopted this birthday rule; however, if one of the two plans has not adopted this rule (i.e., if one plan is in another state), the rules of the plan not abiding by the birthday law determine which plan is primary and which is secondary.

In the case of divorce, the plan of the parent with custody of the children is the primary payer unless the court determines differently and it is so stated in the divorce settlement.

Unions and companies that self-insure their employees do not fall under this birthday law. The states that do not have birthday laws are Georgia, Hawaii, Idaho, Massachusetts, Mississippi, Vermont, and Virginia, and Washington, D.C.

INSURANCE COVERAGE AND BENEFITS

Since insurance policies are complex and contain a great deal of technical jargon, a basic understanding of coverage is needed. Although benefits vary from policy to policy, *basic health insurance coverage* includes benefits for hospitalization, surgical care, physician services, and other medical expenses. **Major medical** or *extended benefits* contracts are designed to offset large medical expenses caused by prolonged illness or serious injury. Supplemental insurance and other coverage and benefits (e.g., dental, vision, disability, and so forth) are also available, as presented in Table 2–1.

Table 2–1 Types of Insurance Coverage and Benefits

Insurance Type	Benefit
BASIC MEDICAL COVERAGE	
Hospitalization	Room and board; specialized hospital services.
Surgical care	Surgeon and assistant surgeon's fee (e.g., aspiration, excision, incision, reduction of fractures, removal of foreign bodies).
Physician services	Physician's fee for nonsurgical services; office, home, and hospital visits.
Other medical expenses	Diagnostic laboratory and radiology tests; pathology; physical therapy; chiropractic treatment.
MAJOR MEDICAL COVERAGE	
Catastrophic coverage	After a certain dollar amount (e.g., $2,000) is reached, either paid by patient (out-of-pocket) or by another insurance plan, major medical becomes effective and picks up a percentage of or all of the remaining amount.
Prolonged illness coverage	After a certain number of days in hospital (e.g., 10 days), major medical becomes effective and picks up a percentage of or all of the remaining amount.
SUPPLEMENTAL COVERAGE	
Secondary insurance	Policy written to provide benefits in addition to primary policy. Medigap is a type of supplemental insurance for the Medicare program.
LIABILITY COVERAGE	
Automobile, business, homeowner policies	Insurance coverage specific to where an accident occurred (e.g., car accident, at place of business, or on the premises of a home).
DISABILITY PROTECTION	
Loss of income insurance	Weekly or monthly cash benefits provided to policyholders who are employed and become unable to work due to an accident or illness (does not pay for medical bills).
LONG-TERM COVERAGE	
Long-term healthcare facility insurance	Room and board coverage; skilled nursing (e.g., IV fluids), or routine nonmedical care such as bathing, feeding, catheter change, and so forth.
HOME HEALTHCARE COVERAGE	
Home healthcare insurance	Nursing care in the home for the chronically ill, disabled, and developmentally disabled.
DENTAL COVERAGE	
Dental plan	Usually includes preventive teeth cleaning and x-ray examinations. Copayments of fixed amounts (e.g., $10–$25), or percentage amounts (e.g., 70%, 80%, or 90%) are charged for services on coverage list.
VISION COVERAGE	
Vision care	Reimbursement for all or a percentage of cost (within a limit) for refraction, lenses, and frames.
SPECIAL RISK COVERAGE	
Special risk insurance	Protection against a specific risk from a type of accident (e.g., auto accident, airplane crash, cruise ship accident) or illness (e.g., cancer).
SPECIAL CLASS COVERAGE	
Special class insurance	Limited coverage for individuals who cannot qualify for a standard policy due to poor health.

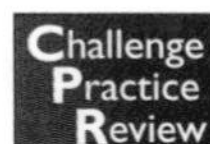

Pause and Practice CPR

REVIEW SESSIONS 2–4 THROUGH 2–5

Directions: *Complete the following questions as a review of the information you have just read.*

2–4 Circle the correct answer: Most legal issues of health insurance claims [fall under federal law] [fall under civil law] [are not governed by federal and state laws].

2–5 Refer to Table 2–1 and state what type of insurance coverage applies to the following statements:

(a) An employed individual becomes ill and receives weekly benefits from a private insurance company. ______________________________

(b) An individual becomes sick and has an insurance plan that pays for the doctor's visit.

____

(c) An individual is going to have surgery. Basic medical coverage will cover most of the expenses; however, the patient has another health insurance plan that will pick up the remaining costs. ______________________________

(d) An individual has a lengthy illness and has received treatment for 6 months. Out-of-pocket expenses have reached $2,500 at this time and the remaining costs will be paid through this type of insurance coverage. ______________________________

CHALLENGE SESSION 2–6

Directions: *Refer to the "birthday law" and the definition of "guarantor" in the previous section and determine which parent's policy is primary for the following scenario.*

2–6 Amy Atwater is 12 years old and has an appointment to see Dr. Practon. Her parents (Gail and Gene) both have her included on their insurance policies. Gail's birthday is 12/3/66 and Gene's is 5/12/67. Which parent's policy is considered primary when billing Amy's insurance claim and why? ______________________________

____

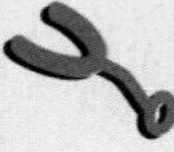

CHECK YOUR HEARTBEAT! Turn to the end of the chapter for answers to these review and challenge sessions.

PHYSICIAN/PATIENT CONTRACT

The majority of contracts in the business world are written; however, the physician/patient contract is usually expressed, or implied. The contract begins when the physician accepts the patient and agrees to treat the patient. This **implied contract** is defined as not manifested by direct words but implied or deduced from the circumstance, the general language, or the conduct of the patient. For example, if Mary Johnson goes to Dr. Doe's office and Dr. Doe gives Ms. Johnson professional services that she accepts, this is an implied contact. When the office agrees to make an appointment for a new patient, and the patient arrives to be seen, enters the treatment room, allows himself or herself to be examined, and accepts the physician's recommendations, the actions of the patient and physician indicate that both accept the other's role in this contract. An **expressed contract** is usually verbal but may be written. However, the majority of physician/patient contracts are implied.

Private Patients

The contract for treatment of a private patient is between the physician and the patient. This is true even if the patient is covered by medical insurance;

thus the patient is liable for the entire bill. Insurance coverage is meant to help offset the expense. It is the patient's responsibility to pay the physician and bill the insurance company to receive reimbursement, or to assist and intervene with the insurance company if the physician's office is billing and payment is not received.

Managed Care Patients

A physician under contract with a managed care plan receives an updated list of current enrollees every month. The physician is obligated to see those individuals who are enrolled, should one of them call for an appointment or arrive in the hospital's emergency room; however, the contract for treatment occurs when the patient is first seen.

A managed care organization (MCO) contract contains the terms by which it will pay the physician. The physician, in turn, is responsible for following the managed care plan's requirements to receive reimbursement. Managed care patients are usually responsible for fixed copayment amounts and services excluded from the contract (e.g., cosmetic surgery, eyeglasses, and so forth). Details on different types of managed care contracts which use fixed prepayment systems will be discussed in Chapter 9.

Assignment of Medical Benefits

If payment is to go directly from the insurance company to the physician, then the patient must sign a document granting permission when first seen at the

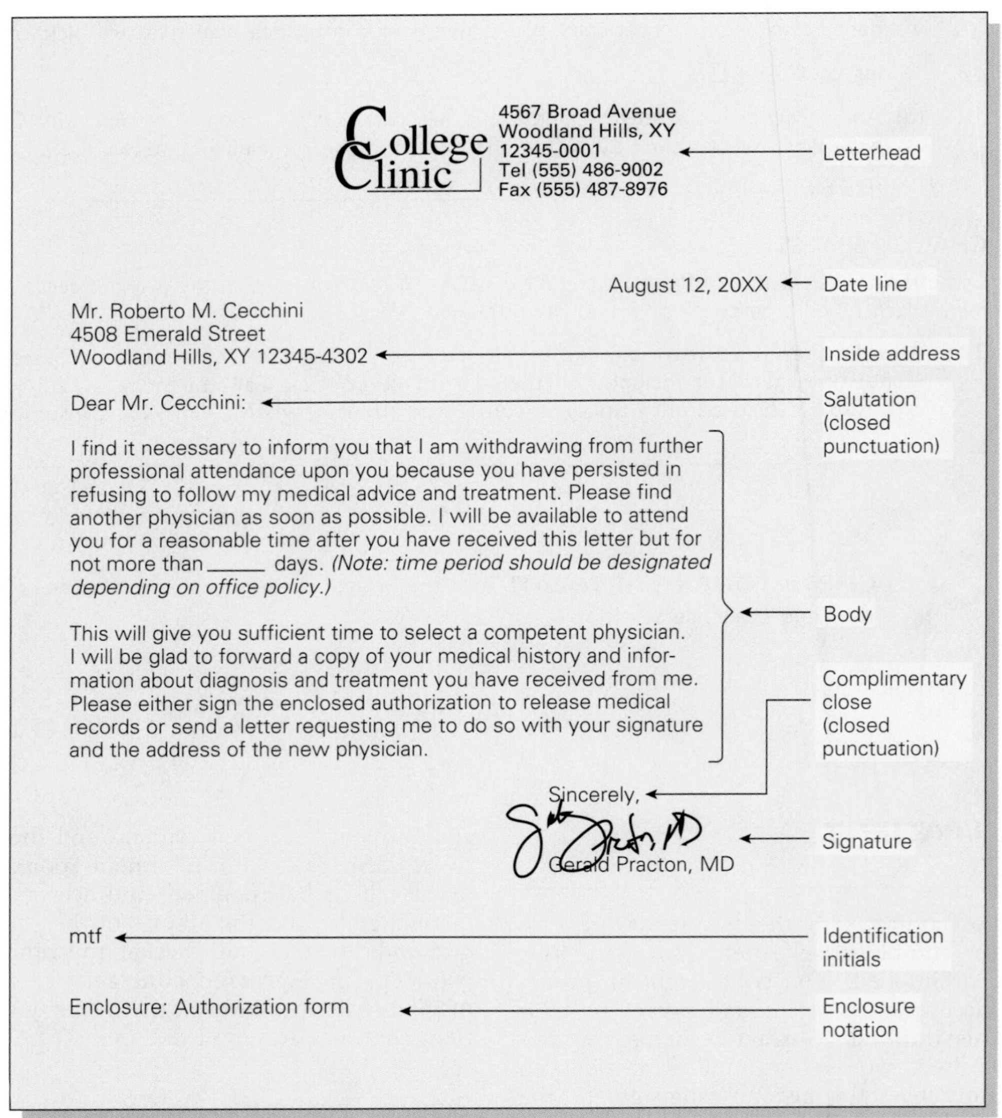

College Clinic
4567 Broad Avenue
Woodland Hills, XY
12345-0001
Tel (555) 486-9002
Fax (555) 487-8976

August 12, 20XX

Mr. Roberto M. Cecchini
4508 Emerald Street
Woodland Hills, XY 12345-4302

Dear Mr. Cecchini:

I find it necessary to inform you that I am withdrawing from further professional attendance upon you because you have persisted in refusing to follow my medical advice and treatment. Please find another physician as soon as possible. I will be available to attend you for a reasonable time after you have received this letter but for not more than _____ days. *(Note: time period should be designated depending on office policy.)*

This will give you sufficient time to select a competent physician. I will be glad to forward a copy of your medical history and information about diagnosis and treatment you have received from me. Please either sign the enclosed authorization to release medical records or send a letter requesting me to do so with your signature and the address of the new physician.

Sincerely,

Gerald Practon, MD

mtf

Enclosure: Authorization form

Figure 2–2. Example letter informing a patient the physician is withdrawing from his case. Letter typed in modified block style (dateline, complimentary close, and signature indented) with closed punctuation and enclosure notation.

doctor's office. This is referred to as an *assignment of medical benefits* and will be discussed in detail in Chapter 3.

Patients Examined for Employment or Disability

Courts in most jurisdictions have ruled that there is no physician/patient relationship in an employment or disability examination and the doctor does not owe a duty of care to the person being examined, chiefly because the insurance company is requesting the examination and the patient is not seeking the medical services of the physician. For this reason, an assignment of benefits is not necessary and the physician receives payment directly from the insurance company.

Workers' Compensation Patients

When a person is injured on the job or becomes sick because of a job-related illness, this is referred to as a workers' compensation case. It may also be called an industrial accident or illness. In this type of case, the contract exists between the physician and the insurance company. This is because the patient's employer is providing medical services through a workers' compensation health insurance policy, and the patient is not financially responsible. The physician receives payment directly from the workers' compensation insurance carrier.

Termination of Physician/Patient Contract

A physician may wish to withdraw formally from further care of a patient because the patient did not follow instructions, failed to return for an appointment, walked out of a hospital without being discharged, or discontinued payments on an overdue account. The patient may also decide to discharge the physician and seek care elsewhere. A physician may terminate a patient contract by:

- Sending a formal letter of withdrawal to the patient, allowing enough time for the patient to find a new physician (Fig. 2–2).
- Sending a letter of confirmation of discharge when the patient states that he or she no longer desires care (Fig. 2–3).
- Sending a letter confirming that the patient left the hospital against medical advice (AMA). If there is a signed statement in the patient's hospital records to this effect, it is not necessary to send a letter.

College Clinic
4567 Broad Avenue
Woodland Hills, XY
12345-0001
Tel (555) 486-9002
Fax (555) 487-8976

September 3, 20XX

Mrs. Gregory Putnam
4309 North E Street
Woodland Hills, XY 12345-4398

Dear Mrs. Putnam

This will confirm our telephone conversation today during which you discharged me from attending you as your physician in your present illness. In my opinion, your medical condition requires continued treatment by a physician. If you have not already obtained the services of another physician, I suggest you do so without further delay.

You may be assured that, upon your written authorization, I will furnish your new physician with information regarding the diagnosis and treatment you have received from me.

Very truly yours

Gerald Procton, MD

mtf

Figure 2–3. Example letter sent to patient to confirm discharge by patient. Letter typed in modified block style (dateline, complimentary close, and signature indented) with open punctuation (no commas after salutation or complimentary close).

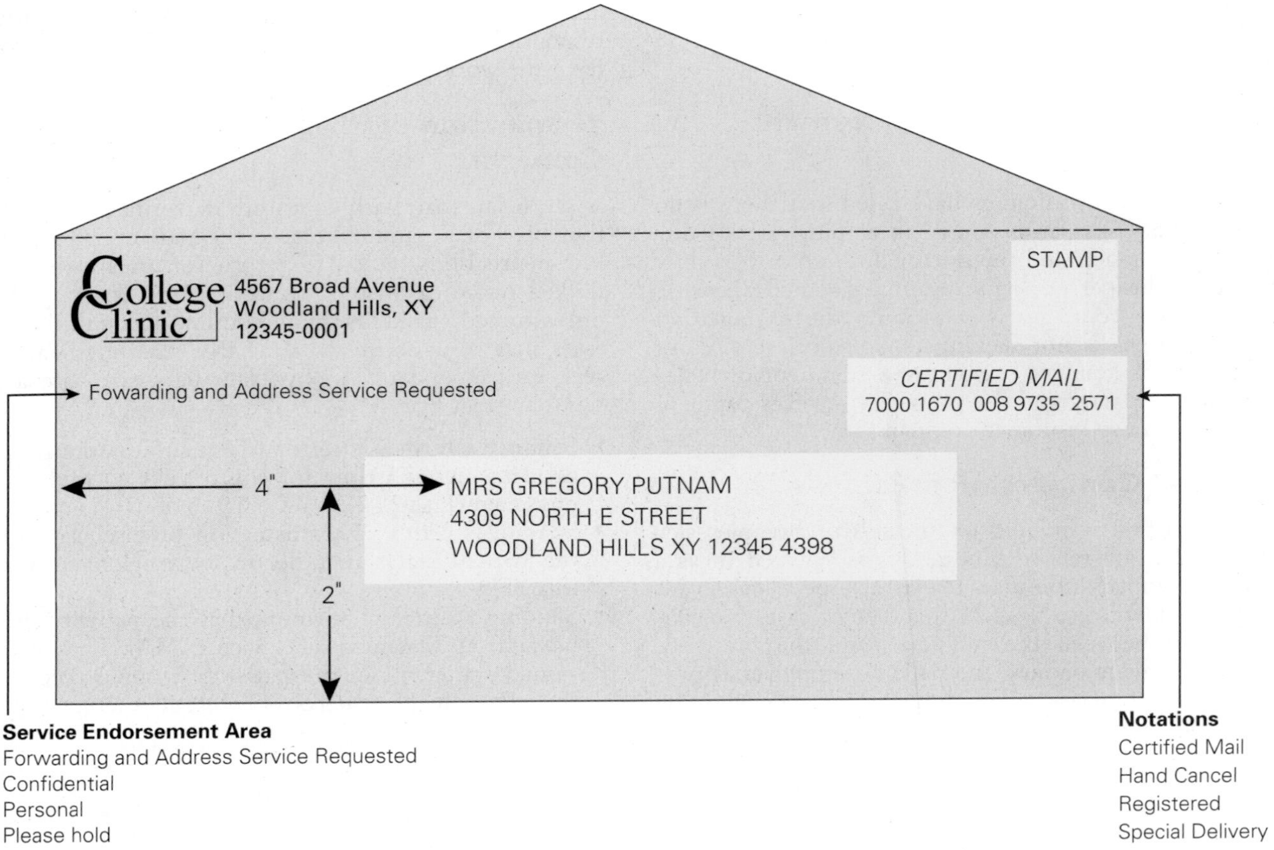

College Clinic 4567 Broad Avenue
Woodland Hills, XY
12345-0001

STAMP

Fowarding and Address Service Requested

CERTIFIED MAIL
7000 1670 008 9735 2571

4"

MRS GREGORY PUTNAM
4309 NORTH E STREET
WOODLAND HILLS XY 12345 4398

2"

Service Endorsement Area
Forwarding and Address Service Requested
Confidential
Personal
Please hold

Notations
Certified Mail
Hand Cancel
Registered
Special Delivery

Figure 2–4. Example of a #10 ($9^1/_2 \times 4^1/_8''$) business envelope used for professional correspondence illustrating placement of address, return address, service endorsement area, and area for notations. United States Postal Service Optical Character Recognition (OCR) equipment reads both upper and lower case; however, they recommend using all capital letters.

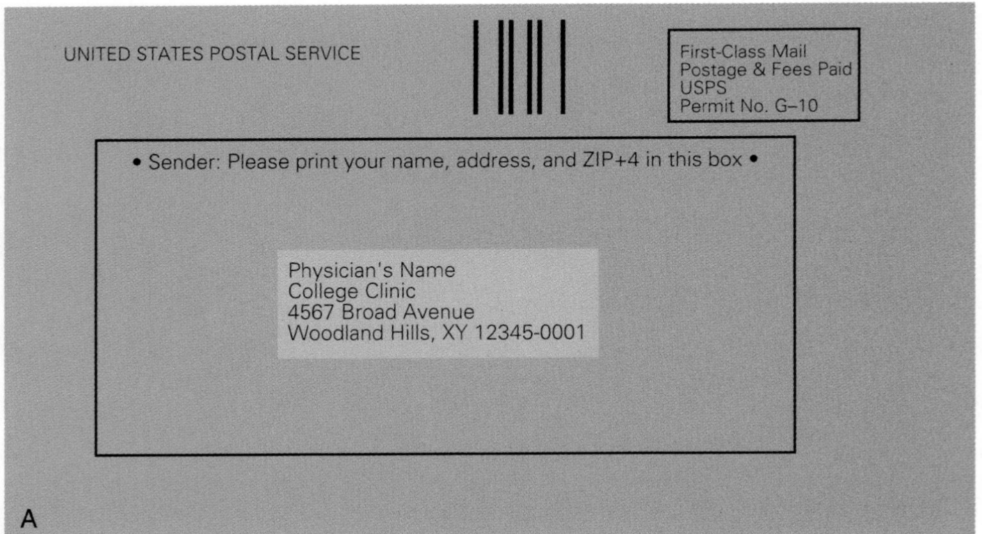
UNITED STATES POSTAL SERVICE

First-Class Mail
Postage & Fees Paid
USPS
Permit No. G-10

• Sender: Please print your name, address, and ZIP+4 in this box •

Physician's Name
College Clinic
4567 Broad Avenue
Woodland Hills, XY 12345-0001

A

Figure 2–5 A–C. Example of the front (A) and back (B) of a completed return receipt for domestic mail (Postal Service Form 3811) and completed receipt for certified mail (C) (Postal Service Form 3800). (Provided by the U.S. Government Printing Office.)

SENDER: *COMPLETE THIS SECTION*

- ☐ Complete items 1,2, and 3. Also complete item 4 if Restricted Delivery is desired.
- ☐ Print your name and address on the reverse so that we can return the card to you.
- ☐ Attach this card to the back of the mailpiece, or on the front if space permits.

1. Article Addressed to:

Mr. John Doe
2761 Fort Street
Woodland Hills, XY 12345

COMPLETE THIS SECTION ON DELIVERY

A. Received by (*Please Print Clearly*) B. Date of Delivery

C. Signature
X ☐ Agent ☐ Addressee

D. Is delivery address different from item1? ☐ Yes
If YES, enter delivery address below: ☐ No

3. Service Type
☒ Certified Mail ☐ Express Mail
☐ Registered ☐ Return Receipt for Merchandise
☐ Insured Mail ☐ C.O.D.

4. Restricted Delivery? (*Extra Fee*) ☐ Yes

2. Article number (*Copy from service label*)
7000 0520 0020 3886 3129

PS Form 3811, July 1999 Domestic Return Receipt 102595-00-M-0952

Figure 2–5 A–C. B *Continued*

C
 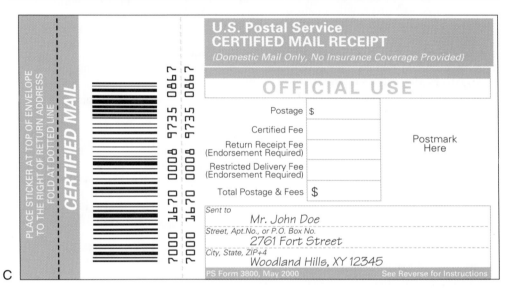
PLACE STICKER AT TOP OF ENVELOPE TO THE RIGHT OF RETURN ADDRESS
FOLD AT DOTTED LINE
CERTIFIED MAIL

7000 1670 0008 9735 0867
7000 1670 0008 9735 0867

U.S. Postal Service
CERTIFIED MAIL RECEIPT
(Domestic Mail Only, No Insurance Coverage Provided)

OFFICIAL USE

Postage	$
Certified Fee	
Return Receipt Fee (Endorsement Required)	
Restricted Delivery Fee (Endorsement Required)	
Total Postage & Fees	$

Postmark Here

Sent to Mr. John Doe
Street, Apt.No., or P.O. Box No. 2761 Fort Street
City, State, ZIP+4 Woodland Hills, XY 12345

PS Form 3800, May 2000 See Reverse for Instructions

Managed care patients may be discharged in the same manner as patients with private insurance or government plans. An example of a #10 envelope used to send professional correspondence is seen in Figure 2–4. All correspondence should be dated and sent by registered or certified mail with return receipt requested (Fig. 2–5). This document is kept in the patient's medical record as proof that the patient was notified.

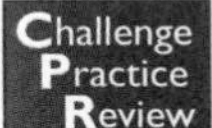

Pause and Practice CPR

REVIEW SESSIONS 2–7 THROUGH 2–9

Directions: *Circle or write in the correct answer for the following questions as a review of the information you have just read.*

2–7 Physician/patient contracts are usually [written] [expressed] [implied].

2–8 The contract for private patients is between the [patient and insurance company] [patient and physician] [insurance company and physician].

2–9 What are the proper procedures to follow when the physician decides to formally withdraw from treating a patient? ______________________________

____

____

CHECK YOUR HEARTBEAT! Turn to the end of the chapter for answers to these review sessions.

TYPES OF HEALTH INSURANCE PROGRAMS

Many forms of health insurance coverage are in effect in the United States. Categories of health insurance include private insurance, government plans, managed care contracts, and workers' compensation—all referred to as third party payers. Although income continuation benefit plans do not provide medical coverage, they are also considered a form of health insurance.

The U.S. Census Bureau collected data indicating that in the calendar year 2000, 86% of Americans had some type of health insurance; therefore, payments from third party payers account for a large percent of physician payments. Only 14% of Americans do not have some kind of health insurance. Table 2–2 illustrates the mix of payer sources and percentages from the 2000 census. An overview and brief explanation of various programs to be discussed in this worktext are given here. For an in-depth explanation, refer to the appropriate chapters that follow.

Government Plans

CHAMPVA

CHAMPVA (Civilian Health and Medical Program of the Department of Veterans Affairs) is a federal program that covers medical expenses of spouses and children of veterans with total, permanent, service-connected disabilities, or of the surviving spouses and children of veterans who died as a result of service-connected disabilities. Medical and dental services may be rendered to veterans at a *Veterans Affairs (VA) Outpatient Clinic* (see Chapter 12).

Medicaid

Medicaid is a program sponsored jointly by federal, state, and local governments to provide healthcare benefits to indigent persons on welfare (public assistance), aged individuals who meet certain financial requirements, and the disabled. Some states have expanded coverage for other medically needy individuals who meet special state-determined criteria. Coverage and benefits vary widely from state to state (see Chapter 10). In California, this program is known as *Medi-Cal.*

Table 2–2 Sources of Third Party Payers

Health Insurance Type	U.S. Population with Coverage (%)
Private insurance plans	72.4%
Medicare program	13.4%
Medicaid program	10.4%
Military healthcare coverage (active duty, TRICARE, CHAMPVA)	3.0%

Medicare

Medicare coverage is for individuals over 65 years of age. It is sponsored by the federal government and has three parts: Part A—hospital insurance, Part B—supplementary medical insurance, and Part C—Medicare Plus (+) Choice Program. Benefits are also extended to certain disabled people (e.g., the blind or totally disabled), those requiring kidney dialysis, and kidney transplant patients (see Chapter 11).

TRICARE

TRICARE is a government-sponsored program that provides hospital and medical services for dependents of active service personnel and retired service personnel, as well as dependents of members who died on active duty. There are three (TRI) different healthcare plans available (see Chapter 12).

Managed Care Contracts

Managed Care Organizations

Managed care organizations have evolved in definition and increased in number since the original Health Maintenance Organization was formed. Generally, MCOs are prepaid health plans that deliver a full range of services to voluntarily enrolled members, with an emphasis on preventive medicine. Physicians are usually reimbursed by a fixed periodic payment, called *capitation*, regardless of the amount of actual services used. Network providers and facilities are utilized and care is managed by primary care physicians (PCPs). In various plans, patients may be given a choice as to how to receive services, and physicians may receive separate reimbursement through fee-for-service structures. Types of MCOs include Competitive Medical Plans (CMPs), Exclusive Provider Organizations (EPOs), Foundations for Medical Care, Health Maintenance Organizations (HMOs), Independent Practice Associations (IPAs), Physician Provider Groups, Point of Service (POS) plans, Preferred Provider Organizations (PPOs), and Triple Option Health Plans. Details and descriptions of each type of MCO are found in Chapter 9.

Commerical Carriers

Private Insurance

There are numerous insurance companies that offer group and individual insurance to persons, either through employment or independently. Collectively, these are referred to as *commercial* or *private insurance carriers*. The fee structure for these types of plans is covered in Chapter 9.

Industrial Insurance

Workers' Compensation

Workers' compensation insurance is a contract purchased by the employer that insures the employee against on-the-job injury or illness (see Chapter 13).

Income Continuation Benefits

Disability Income Insurance

Disability Income Insurance provides periodic payments to replace income when the insured is unable to work as a result of illness, injury, or disease (see Chapter 13). This type of insurance should not be confused with workers' compensation, which provides work-related coverage.

Unemployment Compensation Disability

Unemployment Compensation Disability (UCD) covers off-the-job injury or sickness that is paid by deductions from a person's paycheck. This program is administered by a state agency (see Chapter 13).

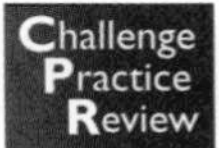

Pause and Practice CPR

REVIEW SESSIONS 2–10 THROUGH 2–12

Directions: *Write in the correct answer for the following questions as a review of the information you have just read.*

2–10 What type of insurance is available for individuals over the age of 65?

____

2–11 What types of insurance are referred to as "prepaid health plans"?

____

2–12 What type of insurance is available for an individual who suffers an injury on the job?

____

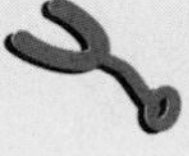

CHECK YOUR HEARTBEAT! Turn to the end of the chapter for answers to these review sessions.

SUMMATION AND PREVIEW

Now that you understand the various terms and provisions of a health insurance contract and different types of health insurance programs and coverage, you have laid the last two cornerstones of the foundation of insurance knowledge. You are now ready to begin experiencing the development of the first practical skills: letter composition, envelope preparation using Optical Character Recognition (OCR) guidelines, completion of U.S. Postal Service forms for mailing, and completion of an insurance predetermination form. You will encounter additional skills as you progress through this worktext and master the practical side of medical insurance billing. As each task is completed and each skill is learned, they become building blocks which you will set upon the foundation of insurance knowledge you have built. They will not only broaden your foundation, but will also help you execute the job of medical insurance billing.

As you progress in this course you may feel like there is too much information to remember. Golden Rules were chosen to help you throughout this course and in your future position. Learning each task is your short-term goal. As you learn one task at a time, you will soon put them all together and reach your long-term goal of becoming a medical insurance billing specialist.

GOLDEN RULE

You are not expected to know all of the answers; you are expected to know where to find solutions.

Chapter 2 Review and Practice

Study Session

Directions: *Review the objectives, key terms, and chapter information before completing the following questions.*

2–1 When several employees have a contract under a single insurance policy issued by their employer, this health coverage is called a ________________ contract.

2–2 The individual enrolled in the health insurance plan is known as the ________________ and may also be called the ________________, ________________, ________________.

2–3 Conditions that existed prior to a health insurance contract may not be covered and would be referred to as ________________.

2–4 The amount of time from the date of service to the date an insurance claim may be submitted according to an insurance contract is called a/an ________________.

2–5 When the insurance company pays the physician, this may also be referred to as ________________.

2–6 Fill in the correct case management requirement that fits the following definitions:

(a) Determining the maximum dollar amount the insurance plan will pay for a specific procedure or service. ________________

(b) Determining if the patient has insurance coverage. ________________

(c) Determining if the service or procedure requested is medically necessary. ________________

(d) Determining if a specific procedure or service is covered under the insurance contract. ________________

2–7 The amount paid for the coverage under an insurance policy is called the ________________.

2–8 A specific amount of money that must be paid each year before policy benefits begin is called the ________________.

2–9 The individual responsible for payment of the medical bill is called the ________________.

2–10 When a patient has more than one insurance policy, the primary and secondary payers are determined by a provision called the ________________.

2–11 The type of insurance that provides coverage for room and board in a skilled nursing facility is called ________________.

2–12 A patient buys an insurance policy to cover a cruise accident before sailing for Tahiti. This policy is called ______________________.

2–13 Insurance that covers a patient who slips and falls while opening the door to the physician's office is called ______________________.

2–14 Insurance coverage that provides care for a home-bound patient is called ______________________.

2–15 In a workers' compensation case, the contract exists between ______________________.

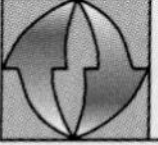

Exercise Exchange

2–1 Write a Letter of Withdrawal, Address a Business Envelope, and Complete a U.S. Postal Service Form.

Scenario: Evan Campbell is negligent about following Dr. Perry Cardi's advice after he had a myocardial infarction. He continues to smoke, will not take his medication regularly, and refuses to lose weight or exercise. He is belligerent when speaking to Dr. Cardi and the office staff. He caused quite a commotion yelling at the nurses when he was in the hospital and left the hospital against medical advice.

Directions

1. Use the patient demographic information provided below and write a letter of withdrawal directed to Mr. Campbell. Dr. Cardi would like to give Mr. Campbell 30 days notice to find a new physician.

2. Use the College Clinic letterhead (Form 01 in Appendix F) or design a similar letterhead on your computer. Dr. Cardi will sign the letter. Use modified block style, referring to Figure 2–2 for an example.

3. Type Evan Campbell's address on a #10 envelope (Form 02 in Appendix F), referring to Figure 2–4 for placement of correct information.

4. Send the letter by certified mail, return receipt requested (Form 03 in Appendix F). Refer to Figure 2–5 for placement of correct information.

Patient Demographic Information

Date: Use current date

Patient: Evan B. Campbell

Address: 429 Atwater Street, Woodland Hills, XY 12345-0001

2–2 Complete an Insurance Predetermination Form.

Scenario: Dr. Raymond Skeleton recommends an aspiration and injection for treatment of a solitary bone cyst for patient Mason Roberts. The insurance specialist calls ABC Insurance Company to predetermine surgical expenses and records the information on an Insurance Predetermination Form (see Fig. 2–1).

Directions

1. Abstract data from the conversation given below and complete Form 04 (Appendix F) as if you were the insurance specialist working for College Clinic.
2. Sign your name as the person verifying coverage and use today's date.

Telephone Conversation

Medical Insurance Billing Specialist: *Hello, I would like to predetermine benefits for patient Mason Roberts; date of birth 11-15-60; member number 215497T; group number 1201.*

Insurance Company Representative: *Is the patient the insured?*

Medical Insurance Billing Specialist: *Yes, can you tell me what type of coverage he has?*

Insurance Company Representative: *He has a traditional 80/20 plan.*

Medical Insurance Billing Specialist: *What is the effective date of his coverage?*

Insurance Company Representative: *March, 21, 20XX though March 20, 20XX.*

Medical Insurance Billing Specialist: *The procedure in question is an aspiration and injection for a solitary bone cyst, CPT number 20615, ICD-9-CM number 733.21. Can you give me a predetermination for this procedure?*

Insurance Company Representative: *He has a major medical plan, with a deductible of $200 which has already been met. Is this procedure going to be done in the office?*

Medical Insurance Billing Specialist: *Yes.*

Insurance Company Representative: *Office surgery is covered and the benefit for this procedure is 80% of $496 which is the usual and customary charge.*

Medical Insurance Billing Specialist: *Are there any requirements, such as a second opinion, precertification, or preauthorization?*

Insurance Company Representative: *A second opinion is not needed and I can give you a precertification number. Just one moment please. Hello, it is 135792A.*

Medical Insurance Billing Specialist: *What is your name please?*

Insurance Company Representative: *Holly Hampton.*

Medical Insurance Billing Specialist: *Will the payment be sent directly to the provider, and how long after submission of the claim can we expect payment?*

Insurance Company Representative: *The provider will be sent payment approximately 30 days after submission of the insurance claim.*

Medical Insurance Billing Specialist: *I forgot to ask, does he have any preexisting exclusions in his policy?*

Insurance Company Representative: *No.*

Medical Insurance Billing Specialist: *Thank you, Holly, for the information.*

Insurance Company Representative: *You are welcome. Goodbye.*

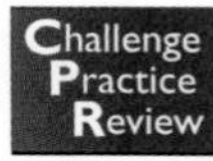

CPR Session: Answers

PRACTICE SESSIONS 2–1 THROUGH 2–3

2–1 Group contract/coverage.
2–2 Medical Savings Account.
2–3 Individual contract/personal insurance.

REVIEW SESSIONS 2–4 THROUGH 2–5

2–4 Fall under civil law. **Rationale:** *Because health insurance is regulated by state laws, it is not considered a federally regulated industry.*
2–5 (a) disability protection/loss of income insurance.
(b) basic medical coverage/physician services.
(c) supplemental coverage/secondary insurance.
(d) major medical coverage/catastrophic coverage.

CHALLENGE SESSION 2–6

2–6 Amy's father Gene's insurance plan is primary because by month and day (5/12), his birthday falls in the calendar year before that of Amy's mother (Gail's birthday—12/3).

REVIEW SESSIONS 2–7 THROUGH 2–9

2–7 implied.
2–8 patient and physician.
2–9 Send a formal letter of withdrawal by certified mail (return receipt requested), allowing enough time for the patient to find a new physician.

REVIEW SESSIONS 2–10 THROUGH 2–12

2–10 Medicare.
2–11 managed care organizations.
2–12 workers' compensation insurance.

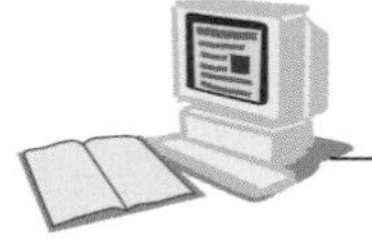

Resources

Internet Sites

Web sites for government health insurance programs such as Medicare, TRICARE, and CHAMPVA; state and federal Medicaid and disability benefit programs; and workers' compensation insurance are listed at the end of chapters discussing those topics in this worktext.

Specific health insurance plans may be located by searching for their names. A health insurance web site that may give you information and links to other health insurance web sites is:

Health Insurance Association of America
Web site: http://www.hiaa.org/about/about.htm

To obtain up-to-date information on domestic/foreign mailing/shipping regulations, ZIP codes, and other information go to the following web sites:

U.S. Postal Service
Web site: http://www.usps.com

Objectives

After reading this chapter and completing the exercise sessions, you should be able to:

Learning Objectives

- ✔ Name source documents used in the physician's office.
- ✔ State information included on a patient registration form.
- ✔ List three patient signature requirements.
- ✔ Identify the purpose of an encounter form and enumerate alternative names for this form.
- ✔ Define a patient account/ledger and day sheet.
- ✔ Describe an insurance pending file.
- ✔ Explain what happens to a claim at the insurance carrier.
- ✔ Memorize steps in processing an insurance claim.

Performance Objectives

- ✔ Complete a patient registration form.
- ✔ Abstract information from an insurance identification card.
- ✔ Post transactions on a ledger card.

Key Terms

accounts receivable
assignment
balance
credit
creditor
day sheet
debtor
encounter form
explanation of benefits (EOB)
ledger card
patient registration form
physician extenders
post
provider
reimbursement
remittance advice (RA)
running balance

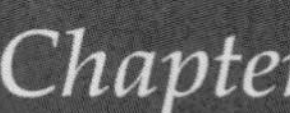

Chapter

3

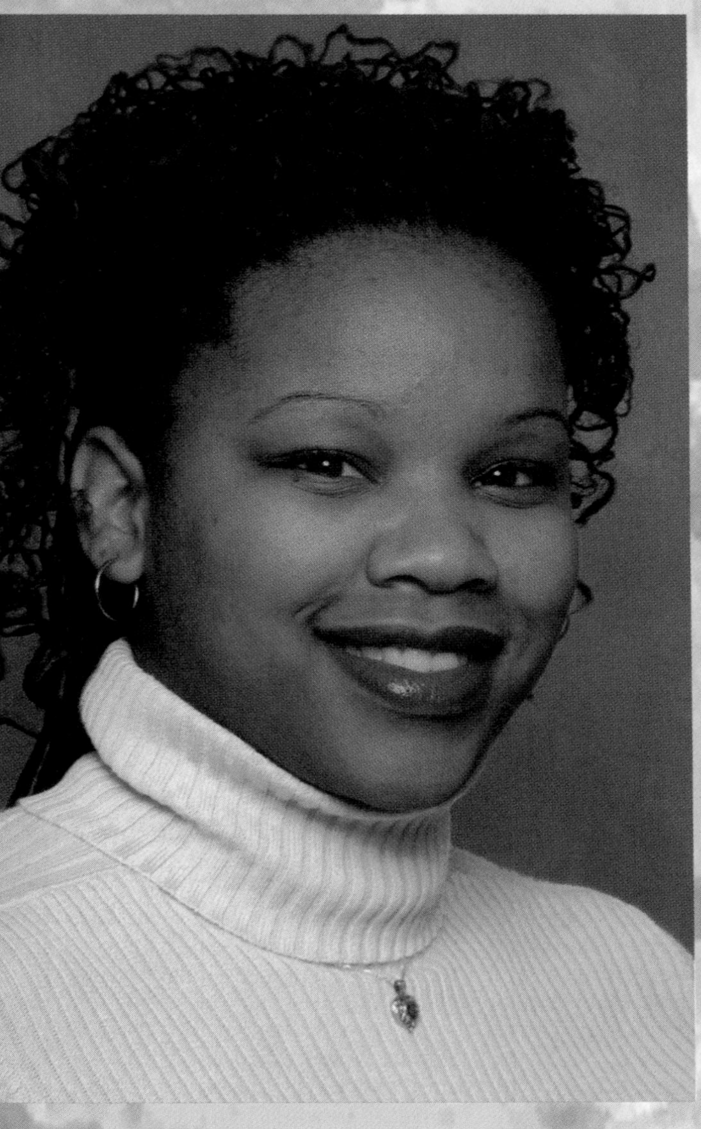

I am a medical insurance billing specialist and work in a medical billing office filing claims for several radiologists. My duties include performing data entry, processing HCFA-1500 claim forms, posting insurance payments, and writing letters of appeal. I also code medical reports, post monthly write-offs, follow-up on patient accounts, and train coworkers. I love the look of understanding on a coworker's face after I have trained them on a task.

The office manager asked that I develop a letter for the company requesting patient insurance information. This was an interesting challenge and I collected everyone's opinion and brain-stormed for an entire day. I came up with a finished product that the owner loved and that is used by our company as an official request for patient insurance information.

Lateisha Ware
Medical Insurance Billing/Coding Specialist
Billing Center—Radiology

Source Documents and the Insurance Claim Cycle

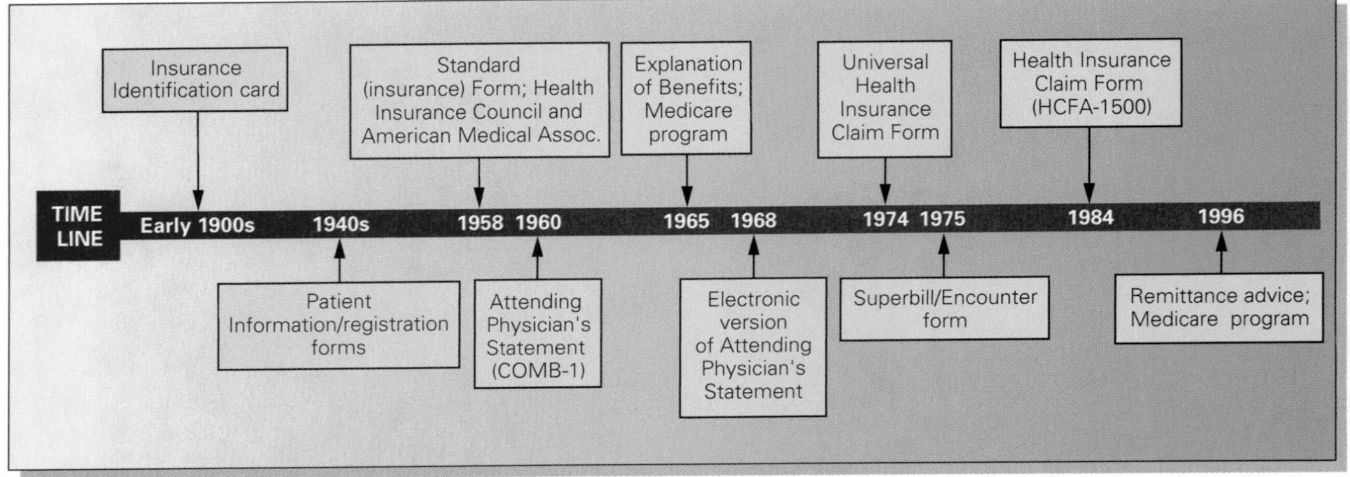

THE REIMBURSEMENT CYCLE

There are many staff members involved and numerous source documents used in the reimbursement cycle. This cycle refers to the process, from start to finish, used to collect money in the physician's office. It may also be referred to as the *cash flow cycle* or the *revenue cycle*. **Reimbursement** means repayment. In times past, the patient paid for medical services and the insurance company reimbursed the patient. Now, often, the physician files the insurance claim and waits to receive payment directly from the insurance company; however, the term is still used when insurance payment is pending.

To make claims submission and reimbursement a success, it is necessary to identify all of the office staff and understand the functions that each individual performs in the reimbursement process. Figure 3–1 illustrates the reimbursement cycle as it follows each staff member, and the task he or she performs, through the medical office. Steps to process an insurance claim are listed indicating what *action* is taken by each staff member and what source document is used. Each member is a vital part of the healthcare team and plays a role in sustaining the life of the medical practice. The orchestration of this cycle in a smooth and efficient manner is key to a healthy medical practice. If staff members do not obtain accurate documentation, coders do not capture services and verify codes, or billers do not generate clean claims quickly, teamwork breaks down and the cash flow is affected, putting the medical practice at risk. Examine Figure 3–1 now and again after all of the various functions have been explained.

Patient Education

The patient is the first and last person involved in the reimbursement cycle. During the initial contact with the patient, information should be provided about office fees and payment policies. This will decrease the number of billing statements sent and increase collections. Regardless of insurance coverage, always make the patient realize that he or she is responsible for the bill. A new patient information pamphlet or brochure and confirmation letter (Fig. 3–2) may be sent to welcome the new patient to the medical practice. This letter will inform the patient about the practice, clearly outline payment expectations, provide collection policies and procedures in printed form, establish a contact person, invite questions, and confirm all specific details discussed.

SOURCE DOCUMENTS

The insurance claim form is a compilation of information that has been collected from the patient prior to submission. This information needs to be accurate and complete; otherwise the claim will not be processed correctly. The forms containing these pieces of information will be referred to in this chapter as source documents. Data that appear on the insurance claim form are only as reliable as the source document from which the data came. Part of learning how to be a good insurance biller is knowing where to look for information. In this chapter you will be learning which source documents contain necessary information that will eventually end up on the health insurance claim form.

Patient Registration Form

The **patient registration form,** also called the patient information form (Fig. 3–3), is used to collect personal data (patient's name, address, telephone number) and essential facts about his or her medical health insurance coverage. There is no substitute for good information-gathering techniques at the time of initial patient registration. Some medical practices preregister new patients during the initial telephone call or have a designated staff member contact the patient prior to the first appointment. Learn as much as possible about the patient and his or her ability to pay before any services are provided. This is when the patient is likely to be the most cooperative. As questions are asked over the telephone, office personnel input information into the computer system and the patient is registered prior to coming to the office.

If preregistration is not done in this manner, the patient either needs to be sent a registration form to fill out, or needs to be advised to arrive at the office early

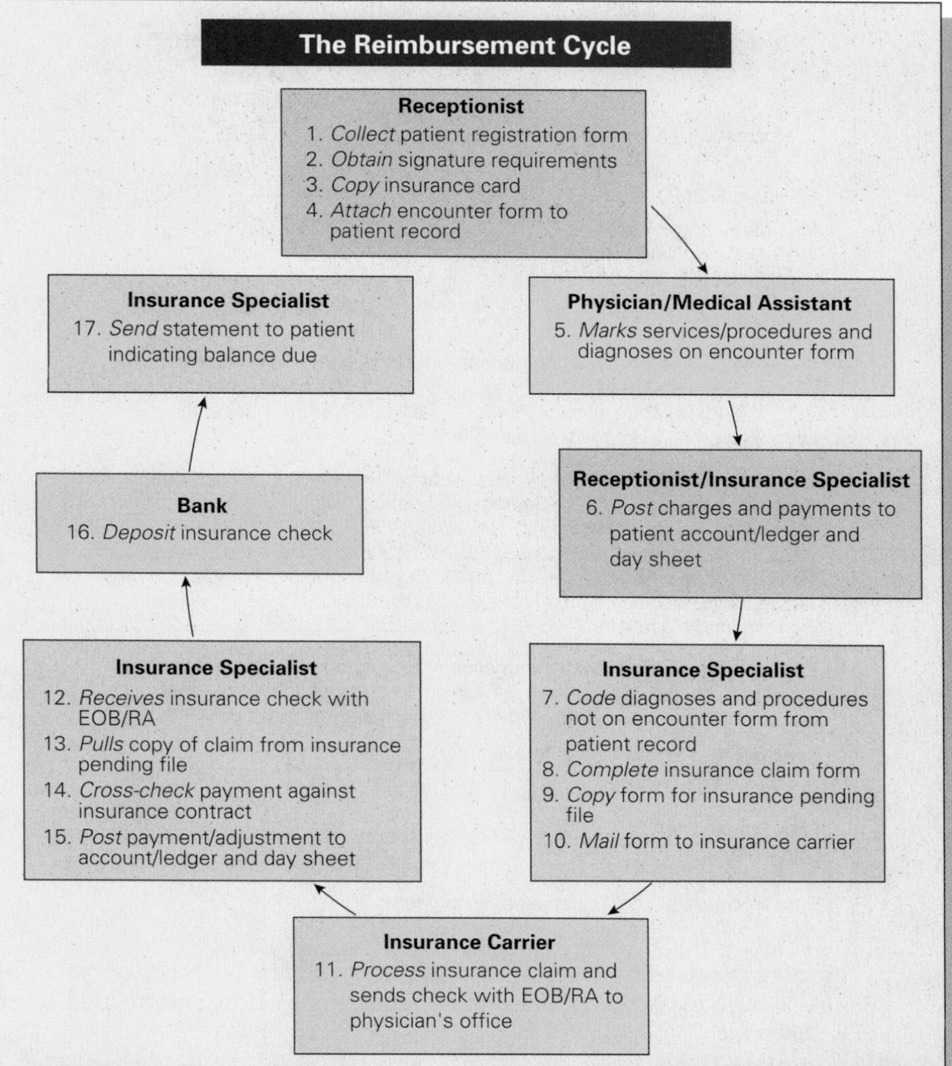

Figure 3–1. Diagram of the reimbursement cycle as it takes place in the physician's office. Each step along the reimbursement path is numbered, listing the staff member, the task he or she performs, and the source document used, from the time the patient arrives at the reception desk to the time a statement is sent to collect the balance due after the insurance company has paid.

to complete the patient registration form. A practice information brochure, history information sheet, and a letter confirming the appointment can be sent together with the patient registration form. This packet of information advises the patient about office policies and allows the patient time in his or her home to look up specific dates related to their health history prior to arriving at the office. One of these methods and time need to be allowed to collect this vital information and to discuss the patient's responsibility with respect to payment policies prior to becoming a new patient.

The patient registration form can be one that is developed by the physician and personalized to his or her practice, or a generic form purchased from a medical stationery company. If the patient is aged or has a language problem or disability, it may be necessary for the medical assistant to interview the patient to obtain current, complete, and correct information. These data will be used to set up a medical and financial record for the patient, complete the health insurance claim form, communicate with the patient at future dates, and collect on the account.

Instruct the patient to answer all questions and indicate any spaces on the form that do not apply by marking "N/A" (not applicable). Review of the completed patient information sheet will ensure that all blanks have been addressed and accurate data have been collected. It will also alert office staff to an account that may be a future problem. If the form is returned with blank spaces, assist the patient in completing them. Items often overlooked are the street address, when a post office box is given; an apartment or mobile home number; and a business telephone number with department and extension. These will help to trace a patient who moves. If the patient refuses to divulge any information, invoking the privacy laws, it should be policy to require payment for services at the time care is rendered.

Verify insurance and all other data that may have changed at each visit, as patients may transfer from one

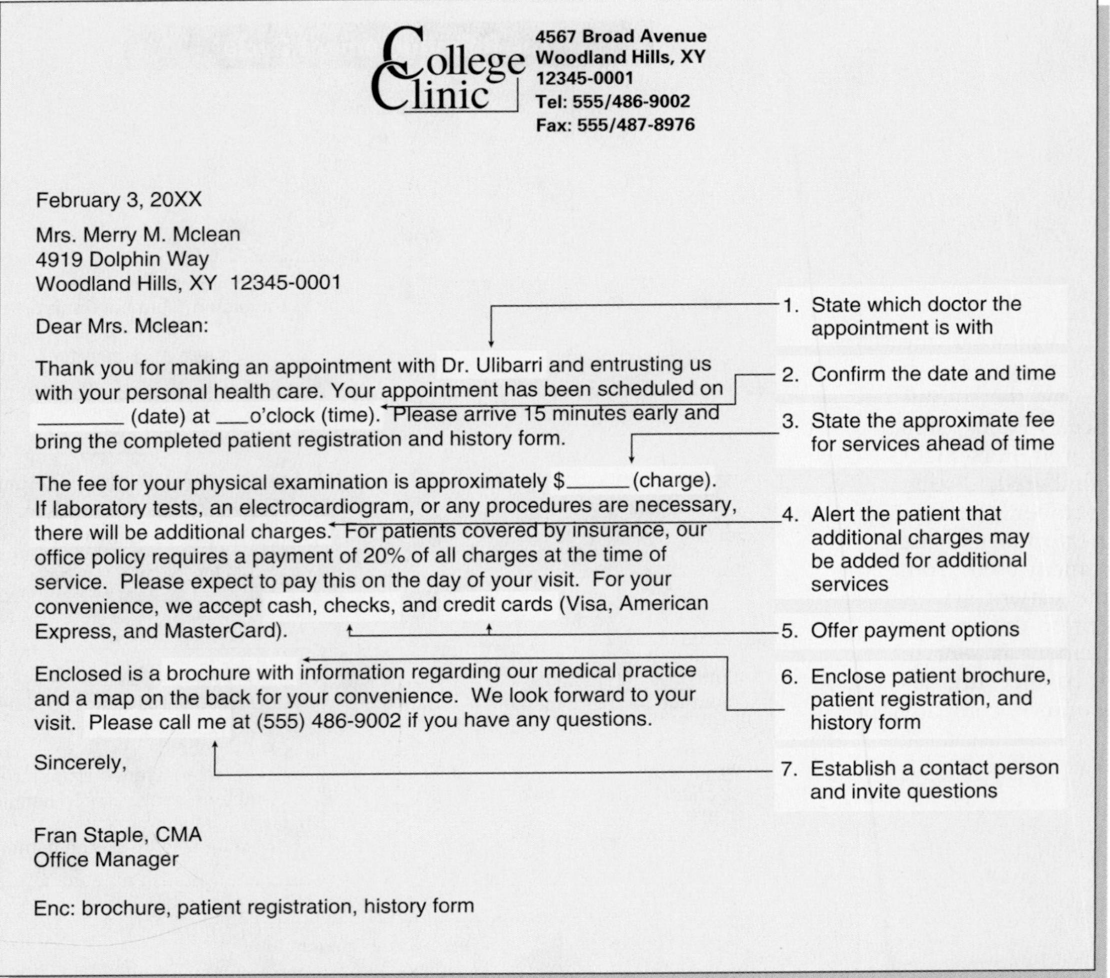

College Clinic
4567 Broad Avenue
Woodland Hills, XY
12345-0001
Tel: 555/486-9002
Fax: 555/487-8976

February 3, 20XX

Mrs. Merry M. Mclean
4919 Dolphin Way
Woodland Hills, XY 12345-0001

Dear Mrs. Mclean:

Thank you for making an appointment with Dr. Ulibarri and entrusting us with your personal health care. Your appointment has been scheduled on ______ (date) at ___o'clock (time). Please arrive 15 minutes early and bring the completed patient registration and history form.

The fee for your physical examination is approximately $______ (charge). If laboratory tests, an electrocardiogram, or any procedures are necessary, there will be additional charges. For patients covered by insurance, our office policy requires a payment of 20% of all charges at the time of service. Please expect to pay this on the day of your visit. For your convenience, we accept cash, checks, and credit cards (Visa, American Express, and MasterCard).

Enclosed is a brochure with information regarding our medical practice and a map on the back for your convenience. We look forward to your visit. Please call me at (555) 486-9002 if you have any questions.

Sincerely,

Fran Staple, CMA
Office Manager

Enc: brochure, patient registration, history form

Figure 3–2. New patient confirmation letter emphasizing information to incorporate when writing to a new patient.

insurance plan to another, move, marry, divorce, or change jobs. This may be done by giving the patient either an update form or a copy of the previously completed patient registration form and providing him or her with a red pen to add new information, correct any incorrect data, initial all changes, and date the form.

The following facts should be recorded:

- *Name*—First, middle initial, and last name. Verify that they are identical to how they appear on the insurance identification card. Keep a cross-reference file to find names of people recently married, children with different last names than parents, and so forth.
- *Address and telephone number*—Street address, including apartment number and ZIP code; telephone number with area code.
- *Business information*—Name of business and department, if applicable; street address; telephone number with area code and extension; and occupation.
- *Date of birth (DOB)*
- *Guarantor*—Person responsible for payment of account.
- *Social Security Number (S.S.#)*—All children age 2 years old and above should have a S.S.#.
- *Spouse's name and occupation*—Include spouse's job title and business telephone number with extension.
- *Referring physician*—Name and title or other referral source.
- *Driver's license number*—Ask how long the person has been living at his or her address if the driver's license is from out of state.
- *Emergency contact*—Close relative or friend with name, address, and daytime telephone number.
- *Insurance information*—Name, address, and telephone number of insurance company; policy and group number; name of insured party for *all* insurance carriers covering the patient. Ask older patients on Medicare if they have traditional Medicare or a Medicare managed care program.

Insurance cards copied ☒
Date: Jan. 20, 20XX

Patient Registration

Account #: 84516
Insurance #: H-550-XX-5172-02
Co-Payment : $OV $10 ER $50

Please PRINT AND complete ALL sections below!

Is your condition the result of a work injury? YES (NO) An auto accident? YES (NO)
Date of injury: ______

PATIENT'S PERSONAL INFORMATION Marital status ☐ Single X Married ☐ Divorced ☐ Widowed
Sex: ☐ Male X Female
Name: FUHR (last name) LINDA (first name) L. (initial)
Street Address: 3070 Tipper Street (Apt # 4) City: Oxnard State: CA Zip: 93030
Home phone: (555) 276-0101 Work phone: (555) 372-1151 Social Security # 550-XX-5172
Date of Birth: 11/05/65 Driver's License: (State & Number) G00750XX
Employer/Name of School Electronic Data Systems ☒ Full Time ☐ Part Time
Spouse's Name: FUHR (last name) GERALD (first name) T. (initial) Spouse's Work phone: (555) 921-0075
How do you wish to be addressed? LINDA Social Security # 545-XX-2771

PATIENT'S/RESPONSIBLE PARTY INFORMATION
Responsible party: GERALD T. FUHR Date of Birth: 06-15-64
Relationship to patient: ☐ Self ☒ Spouse ☐ Other Social Security # 545-XX-2771
Responsible party's home phone: ((555) 276-0101 Work phone: (555) 921-0075
Address: 3070 Tipper Street (Apt # 4) City: Oxnard State: CA Zip: 93030
Employer's Name: General Electric Phone number: ((555) 485-0121
Address: 317 East Main City: Oxnard State: CA Zip: 93030
Your occupation: Technician
Spouse's Employer's Name: Electronic Data Systems Spouse's Work phone: ((555) 372-1151
Address: 2700 West 5th Street City: Oxnard State: CA Zip: 93030

PATIENT'S INSURANCE INFORMATION *Please present insurance cards to receptionist.*
PRIMARY insurance company's name: ABC Insurance Company
Insurance address: P.O. Box 12340 City: Fresno State: CA Zip: 93765
Name of insured: Linda L. Fuhr Date of Birth: 11/05/65 Relationship to insured: ☒ Self ☐ Spouse ☐ Other ☐ Child
Insurance ID number: H-550-XX-5172-02 Group number: 17098-020-00004
SECONDARY insurance company's name: None
Insurance address: ______ City: ______ State: ______ Zip: ______
Name of insured: ______ Date of Birth: ______ Relationship to insured: ☐ Self ☐ Spouse ☐ Other ☐ Child
Insurance ID number: ______ Group number: ______
Check if appropriate: ☐ Medigap policy ☐ Retiree coverage

PATIENT'S REFERRAL INFORMATION *(Please circle one)*
Referred by: Margaret Taylor (Mrs. W. T.) If referred by a friend, may we thank her or him? (Yes) No
Name(s) of other physician(s) who care for you: Jason Smythe, MD

EMERGENCY CONTACT
Name of person not living with you: Hannah Gildea Relationship: Aunt
Address: 4621 Lucretia Avenue City: Oxnard State: CA Zip: 93030
Phone number (home): (555) 274-0132 Phone number (work): ( ) ______

Assignment of Benefits • Financial Agreement

I hereby give lifetime authorization for payment of insurance benefits be made directly to Gerald Practon, MD, and any assisting physicians, for services rendered. I understand that I am financially responsible for all charges whether or not they are covered by insurance. In the event of default, I agree to pay all costs of collection, and reasonable attorney's fees. I hereby authorize this healthcare provider to release all information necessary to secure the payment of benefits.
I further agree that a photocopy of this agreement shall be as valid as the original.
Date: Jan 20, 20XX Your signature: Linda L Fuhr
Method of payment: ☐ Cash ☒ Check ☐ Credit Card

Figure 3–3. Patient registration form showing a comprehensive listing of personal and financial information obtained from the patient prior to or on his or her first visit to the office. (Form courtesy of Bibbero Systems, Inc., Petaluma, CA. Phone: [800] 242-2376; FAX: [800] 242-9330; www.bibbero.com.)

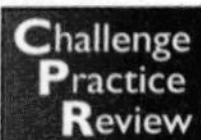

Pause and Practice CPR

REVIEW SESSIONS 3–1 THROUGH 3–3

Directions: *Complete the following questions as a review of information you have just read.*

3–1 At an office meeting, the office manager states that the patient information being collected is not complete and patients are taking too much time in the waiting room filling out the necessary forms. Give suggestions on several ways that patient data can be collected to help obtain more accurate information and keep the physician's schedule on course.

(1) ______________________________

(2) ______________________________

(3) ______________________________

(4) ______________________________

3–2 Name three pieces of personal information.

(1) ______________________________

(2) ______________________________

(3) ______________________________

3–3 List four ways in which the information from the patient registration form is used.

(1) ______________________________

(2) ______________________________

(3) ______________________________

(4) ______________________________

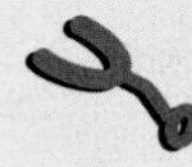

CHECK YOUR HEARTBEAT! Turn to the end of the chapter for answers to these review sessions.

Insurance Identification Card

Photocopy the front and back of the insurance identification cards for all insurance plans that the patient belongs to (Fig. 3–4). Date the photocopy and place it in the patient's file. A copy produces error-free insurance data and can be used in lieu of completing the insurance section on the patient registration form. Information such as deductible or copayment amounts, preapproval provisions, and insurance company name, address, and telephone number may be listed on the front or back of the card.

On a return visit, ask to see the card and check it against data on file. If it differs, photocopy both sides of the card and write the date on the copy, using this as the base for revising data on file.

Patient Signature Requirements

After the patient information has been gathered and the insurance card photocopied, several signature requirements must be obtained to allow processing of all information necessary to complete the insurance claim form and receive reimbursement. Following are the requirements and definitions for the release of medical information, assignment of benefits, and financial agreement. Most patient registration forms include a statement for these signature requirements (see bottom of Fig. 3–3). The standard insurance claim form (HCFA-1500) also contains a space for the first two requirements as shown in Figure 3–5, Blocks 12 and 13.

Release of Medical Information

If the physician is submitting an insurance claim for the patient, the patient must sign a release of information (also known as a consent) before information can be given to an insurance company. An authorization release needs to be obtained before information is given to *any* third party, including an attorney or family member.

Release of medical information was discussed in Chapter 1 under Privileged Information and the consent and authorization forms were illustrated in Figures 1–4 and 1–5. Date all forms and keep them in the patient's file for future reference. On the HCFA-1500 insurance claim form, the signature to release medical information is found in Block 12 (see Fig. 3–5).

Assignment of Benefits

If the physician wishes to receive the insurance check instead of having it sent directly to the patient, he or she needs to have the patient assign benefits to the physician. The general definition of **assignment** is the transfer, after an event insured against, of an individual's legal right to collect an amount payable under an insurance contract. This signature requirement is called an *assignment of benefits* and, when obtained, may be referred to as the physician *accepting assignment.*

INSURANCE IDENTIFICATION NUMBER

CALMED CO.

	HOSPITAL	EMERGENCY ROOM
GROUP NUMBER	CO-PAY	CO-PAY
17098-020-00004	$ .00	$ 50.00

MEMBER
LINDA L. FUHR

MEMBER NUMBER
H-550-XX-5172-02

MC

PRIMARY CARE PHYSICIAN
GEOFF LOMAN

OFFICE VISIT
CO-PAY
$10.00

ABC INSURANCE COMPANY
P.O. BOX 12340
FRESNO CA 93765

IMPORTANT INFORMATION ON REVERSE

FOR BENEFITS, ELIGIBILITY AND CLAIMS CALL MEMBER SERVICES: 1-800-988-0652
FOR PRECERTIFICATION AND REFERRALS CALL: 1-800-736-7799

PAYOR NUMBER 60054 0106

GROUP NUMBER; MEMBER NAME; MANAGED CARE PLAN; PRIMARY CARE PHYSICIAN; INSURANCE COMPANY NAME AND BILLING ADDRESS; COPAYMENT/ OFFICE VISIT; TOLL-FREE TELEPHONE NUMBERS

PRESCRIPTION INFORMATION → RX COPAY $10.00 RX GROUP NUMBER 0067-0000 PHARMACY PLAN

For mental health services, call 1-800-424-4047

INSTRUCTIONS TO PATIENT → **Member**: Co-pays and higher benefits apply to services rendered by your primary care physician (PCP) or through your PSP's referral. Call your PCP in advance for an appointment. If a life threatening emergency exists, seek immediate attention. If admitted, call Member Services within 48 hours. When not referred by your PCP, you are responsible for any precertification required by your plan. For you or your physician to obtain precertification, call Member Services. Failure to obtain precertification may result in reduced benefits.

INSTRUCTIONS TO PHYSICIANS → **Providers**: Call Member Services to verify eligibility; this card does not guarantee coverage. In case of an emergency, notify Member Services the next business day.
This plan is administered by ABC Insurance Company.

ABC Health Plans

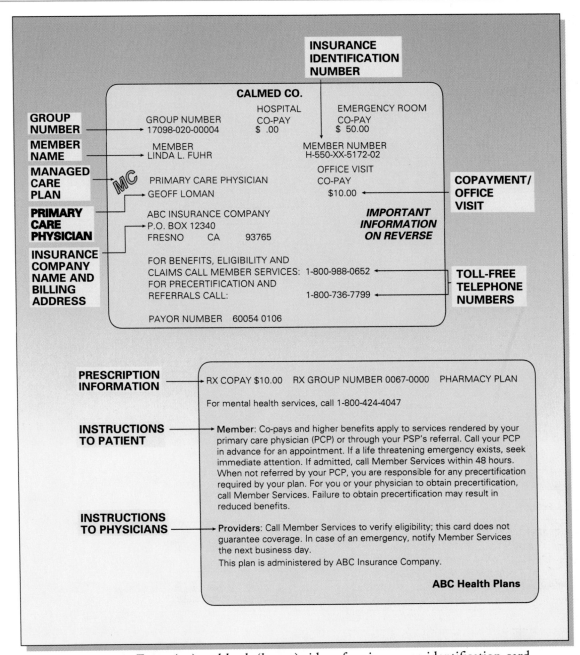

Figure 3–4. Front (*top*) and back (*bottom*) sides of an insurance identification card.

An assignment of benefits becomes a legally enforceable document; however, each course of treatment (specific hospitalization, testing service, or office visits pertaining to one diagnosis) may need to have an assignment document executed by the patient unless an annual or lifetime signature authorization is accepted by the insurance carrier. When the signature is obtained separate from the insurance form and kept in the patient's medical file, it may be referred to on the insurance claim form by typing "signature on file," or the abbreviation "SOF," in

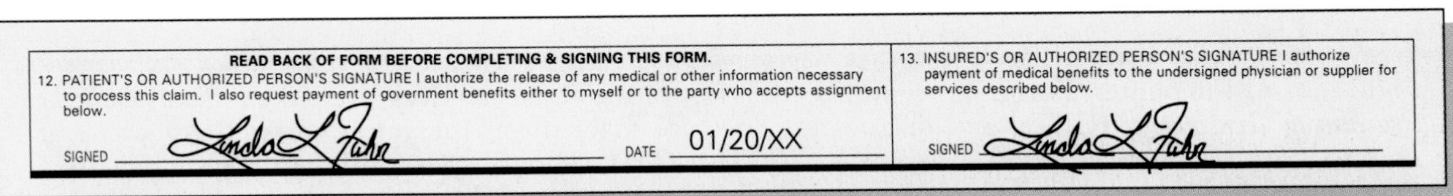

READ BACK OF FORM BEFORE COMPLETING & SIGNING THIS FORM.

12. PATIENT'S OR AUTHORIZED PERSON'S SIGNATURE I authorize the release of any medical or other information necessary to process this claim. I also request payment of government benefits either to myself or to the party who accepts assignment below.

SIGNED Linda L. Fuhr DATE 01/20/XX

13. INSURED'S OR AUTHORIZED PERSON'S SIGNATURE I authorize payment of medical benefits to the undersigned physician or supplier for services described below.

SIGNED Linda L. Fuhr

Figure 3–5. Sections 12 and 13 from the Health Insurance Claim Form (HCFA-1500), illustrating consent for release of information and assignment of benefits.

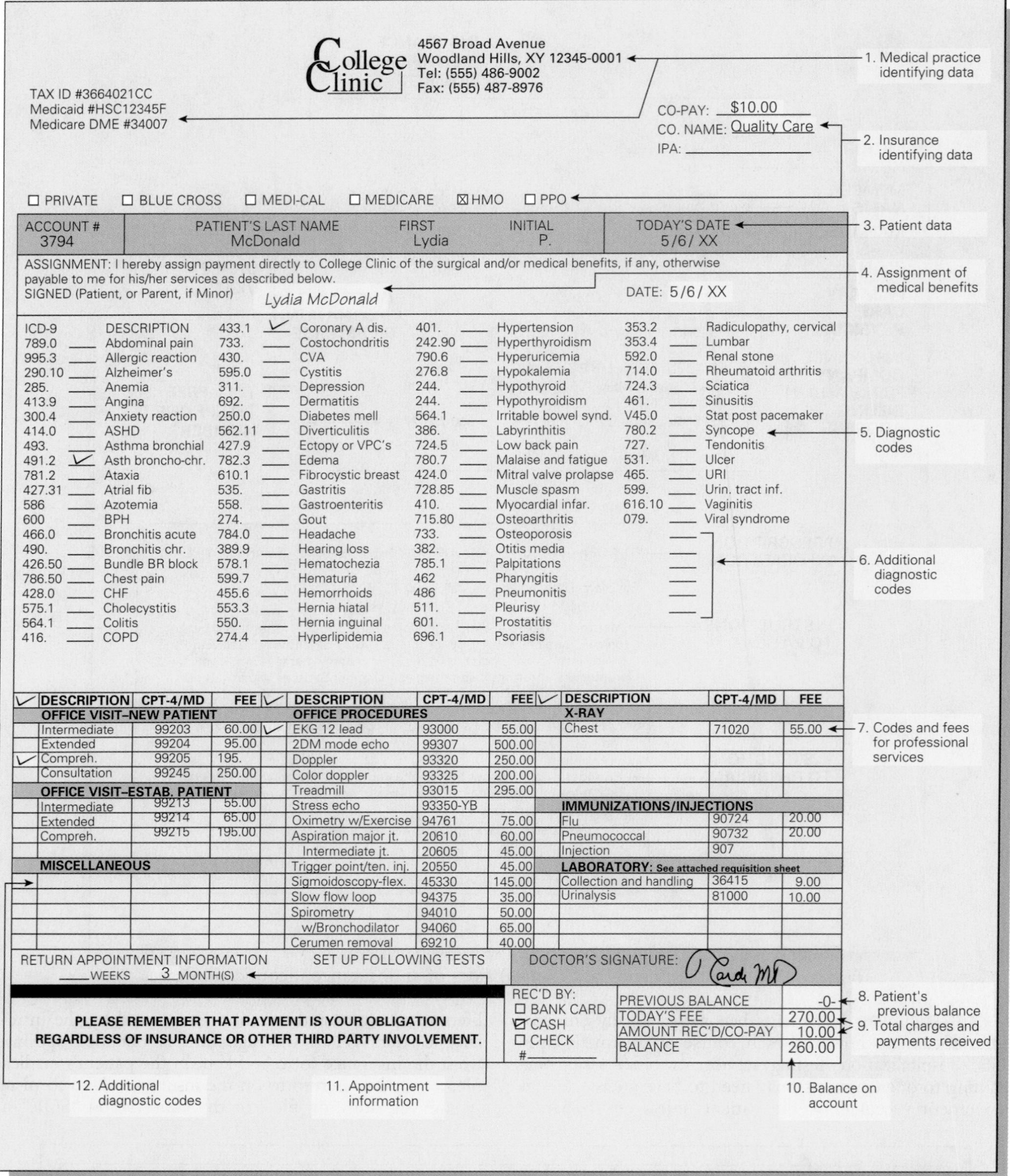

College Clinic
4567 Broad Avenue
Woodland Hills, XY 12345-0001
Tel: (555) 486-9002
Fax: (555) 487-8976

TAX ID #3664021CC
Medicaid #HSC12345F
Medicare DME #34007

CO-PAY: $10.00
CO. NAME: Quality Care
IPA:

☐ PRIVATE ☐ BLUE CROSS ☐ MEDI-CAL ☐ MEDICARE ☒ HMO ☐ PPO

ACCOUNT #	PATIENT'S LAST NAME	FIRST	INITIAL	TODAY'S DATE
3794	McDonald	Lydia	P.	5/6/ XX

ASSIGNMENT: I hereby assign payment directly to College Clinic of the surgical and/or medical benefits, if any, otherwise payable to me for his/her services as described below.
SIGNED (Patient, or Parent, if Minor) *Lydia McDonald* DATE: 5/6/ XX

ICD-9	✓	DESCRIPTION	Code	✓	Description	Code	✓	Description	Code	✓	Description
789.0		Abdominal pain	433.1	✓	Coronary A dis.	401.		Hypertension	353.2		Radiculopathy, cervical
995.3		Allergic reaction	733.		Costochondritis	242.90		Hyperthyroidism	353.4		Lumbar
290.10		Alzheimer's	430.		CVA	790.6		Hyperuricemia	592.0		Renal stone
285.		Anemia	595.0		Cystitis	276.8		Hypokalemia	714.0		Rheumatoid arthritis
413.9		Angina	311.		Depression	244.		Hypothyroid	724.3		Sciatica
300.4		Anxiety reaction	692.		Dermatitis	244.		Hypothyroidism	461.		Sinusitis
414.0		ASHD	250.0		Diabetes mell	564.1		Irritable bowel synd.	V45.0		Stat post pacemaker
493.		Asthma bronchial	562.11		Diverticulitis	386.		Labyrinthitis	780.2		Syncope
491.2	✓	Asth broncho-chr.	427.9		Ectopy or VPC's	724.5		Low back pain	727.		Tendonitis
781.2		Ataxia	782.3		Edema	780.7		Malaise and fatigue	531.		Ulcer
427.31		Atrial fib	610.1		Fibrocystic breast	424.0		Mitral valve prolapse	465.		URI
586		Azotemia	535.		Gastritis	728.85		Muscle spasm	599.		Urin. tract inf.
600		BPH	558.		Gastroenteritis	410.		Myocardial infar.	616.10		Vaginitis
466.0		Bronchitis acute	274.		Gout	715.80		Osteoarthritis	079.		Viral syndrome
490.		Bronchitis chr.	784.0		Headache	733.		Osteoporosis			
426.50		Bundle BR block	389.9		Hearing loss	382.		Otitis media			
786.50		Chest pain	578.1		Hematochezia	785.1		Palpitations			
428.0		CHF	599.7		Hematuria	462		Pharyngitis			
575.1		Cholecystitis	455.6		Hemorrhoids	486		Pneumonitis			
564.1		Colitis	553.3		Hernia hiatal	511.		Pleurisy			
416.		COPD	550.		Hernia inguinal	601.		Prostatitis			
			274.4		Hyperlipidemia	696.1		Psoriasis			

✓	DESCRIPTION	CPT-4/MD	FEE	✓	DESCRIPTION	CPT-4/MD	FEE	✓	DESCRIPTION	CPT-4/MD	FEE
	OFFICE VISIT–NEW PATIENT				**OFFICE PROCEDURES**				**X-RAY**		
	Intermediate	99203	60.00	✓	EKG 12 lead	93000	55.00		Chest	71020	55.00
	Extended	99204	95.00		2DM mode echo	99307	500.00				
✓	Compreh.	99205	195.		Doppler	93320	250.00				
	Consultation	99245	250.00		Color doppler	93325	200.00				
	OFFICE VISIT–ESTAB. PATIENT				Treadmill	93015	295.00				
	Intermediate	99213	55.00		Stress echo	93350-YB			**IMMUNIZATIONS/INJECTIONS**		
	Extended	99214	65.00		Oximetry w/Exercise	94761	75.00		Flu	90724	20.00
	Compreh.	99215	195.00		Aspiration major jt.	20610	60.00		Pneumococcal	90732	20.00
					Intermediate jt.	20605	45.00		Injection	907	
	MISCELLANEOUS				Trigger point/ten. inj.	20550	45.00		**LABORATORY:** See attached requisition sheet		
					Sigmoidoscopy-flex.	45330	145.00		Collection and handling	36415	9.00
					Slow flow loop	94375	35.00		Urinalysis	81000	10.00
					Spirometry	94010	50.00				
					w/Bronchodilator	94060	65.00				
					Cerumen removal	69210	40.00				

RETURN APPOINTMENT INFORMATION ___ WEEKS 3 MONTH(S)
SET UP FOLLOWING TESTS
DOCTOR'S SIGNATURE:

PLEASE REMEMBER THAT PAYMENT IS YOUR OBLIGATION REGARDLESS OF INSURANCE OR OTHER THIRD PARTY INVOLVEMENT.

REC'D BY:
☐ BANK CARD
☑ CASH
☐ CHECK
#

PREVIOUS BALANCE	-0-
TODAY'S FEE	270.00
AMOUNT REC'D/CO-PAY	10.00
BALANCE	260.00

Figure 3–6. Encounter Form; procedure codes for professional services are taken from *Current Procedural Terminology* (CPT), and diagnostic codes are taken from the *International Classification of Diseases, 9th Revision, Clinical Modification* (ICD-9-CM). (Courtesy of Bibbero Systems, Inc., Petaluma, CA. Phone: [800] 242-2376; FAX: [800] 242-9330; www.bibbero.com.)

the signature block. In Figure 3–5, Block 12 contains the assignment of benefits for government programs (Medicare, TRICARE, CHAMPVA), and Block 13 contains the assignment for private insurance plans. When using an insurance claim form with no printed assignment, attach a separate signed form authorizing the patient to assign benefits to the physician and keep a copy for your records. Assignment of benefit requirements for individual insurance plans will be discussed within each chapter that relates to specific insurance programs.

Financial Agreement

As mentioned in Chapter 2, the guarantor needs to sign a statement indicating full responsibility for payment of the account. This is necessary, even if there is insurance coverage from one or more carriers. This signature requirement may be obtained on a separate form; however, it is usually included on the patient registration form (see bottom of Fig. 3–3). When the patient has completed the patient registration form, be sure this is signed and filed in the patient's medical record.

Encounter Form

An **encounter form,** also called a charge slip, communicator, fee ticket, multipurpose billing form, patient service slip, routing form, superbill, and transaction slip, contains areas to check off or write in diagnoses and procedures, along with basic information about the patient and patient's account (e.g., name, date, previous balance, return appointment, and so forth). This form (Fig. 3–6) is attached to the patient's medical record when the chart is prepared for the patient's visit.

Encounter forms vary greatly, depending on the type of practice, but may serve as a combination bill, insurance form, and routing document used in both computer and pegboard (manual) bookkeeping systems. This multipurpose billing form may be generated from computer software, printed by a medical stationery supply company as a two- or three-part form, and/or contain bar codes that may be scanned to input charges and diagnoses into the patient's computerized account. Unique sequential numbers should be assigned to each encounter form so that all forms are accounted for at the end of the day.

Many medical practices use this form as a routing sheet and it often becomes a source document for insurance claim data. The encounter form's procedure and diagnostic code sections should be reviewed and updated annually to include new codes and delete old or unused codes.

After examination and treatment, the physician completes the encounter form by checking off procedure codes for services and treatment, writing in diagnoses or checking off diagnostic codes, and indicating when the patient will return. A clinical medical assistant may be involved with checking off services he or she has performed on the patient at the direction of the physician such as an injection, laboratory work, electrocardiogram (ECG), or other diagnostic testing.

The encounter form is then carried by the physician, medical assistant, or patient to the reception desk, where fees are determined for services performed. The patient is advised that the insurance company will be billed and the patient is given the opportunity to pay and make a future appointment.

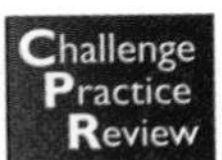

Pause and Practice CPR

REVIEW SESSIONS 3–4 THROUGH 3–6

Directions: *Complete the following questions as a review of information you have just read.*

3–4 Why is the insurance card copied and used in lieu of the patient filling out the insurance section on the patient registration form?

____

3–5 Match the definition with the correct signature requirement for (a) release of medical information, (b) assignment of benefits, (c) financial agreement:

________ The transfer, after an event insured against, of an individual's legal right to collect an amount payable under an insurance contract.

________ Statement indicating full responsibility for payment of the account.

________ A consent to send information to a third party.

3–6 What are three main functions of an encounter form?

(1) ____________________________________

(2) ____________________________________

(3) ____________________________________

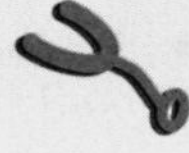

CHECK YOUR HEARTBEAT! Turn to the end of the chapter for answers to these review sessions.

Patient Account/Ledger

The bookkeeping system in a physician's office may be computerized or done manually using a *pegboard bookkeeping* method. In either case, a financial accounting record is maintained for each patient who receives professional services. The medical assistant or insurance billing specialist may use a copy of the encounter form to **post** (record) transactions. Posting entries include:

- Professional fees—credits (e.g., charges)
- Payments—debits (e.g., cash, check, or credit card)
- Adjustments—debits (e.g., insurance contract write-offs or courtesy adjustments)
- Balance due—to each patient's account

The **balance** of the account is the amount owed on a credit transaction. If the service or procedure is not paid for at the time of service, **credit** is extended and the patient has an *unpaid* balance or *outstanding* balance. The physician is referred to as the **creditor** and the patient as the **debtor.**

A **ledger card** (Fig. 3–7) is the name for the individual account used in the pegboard bookkeeping system. It may double as a *statement* (bill) and be copied and sent to the patient requesting payment. In this worktext, a ledger card will be used to post transactions so that you will have an understanding of all computations. Each service must be posted on a single line with a **running balance** calculated in the right column. When the front side of

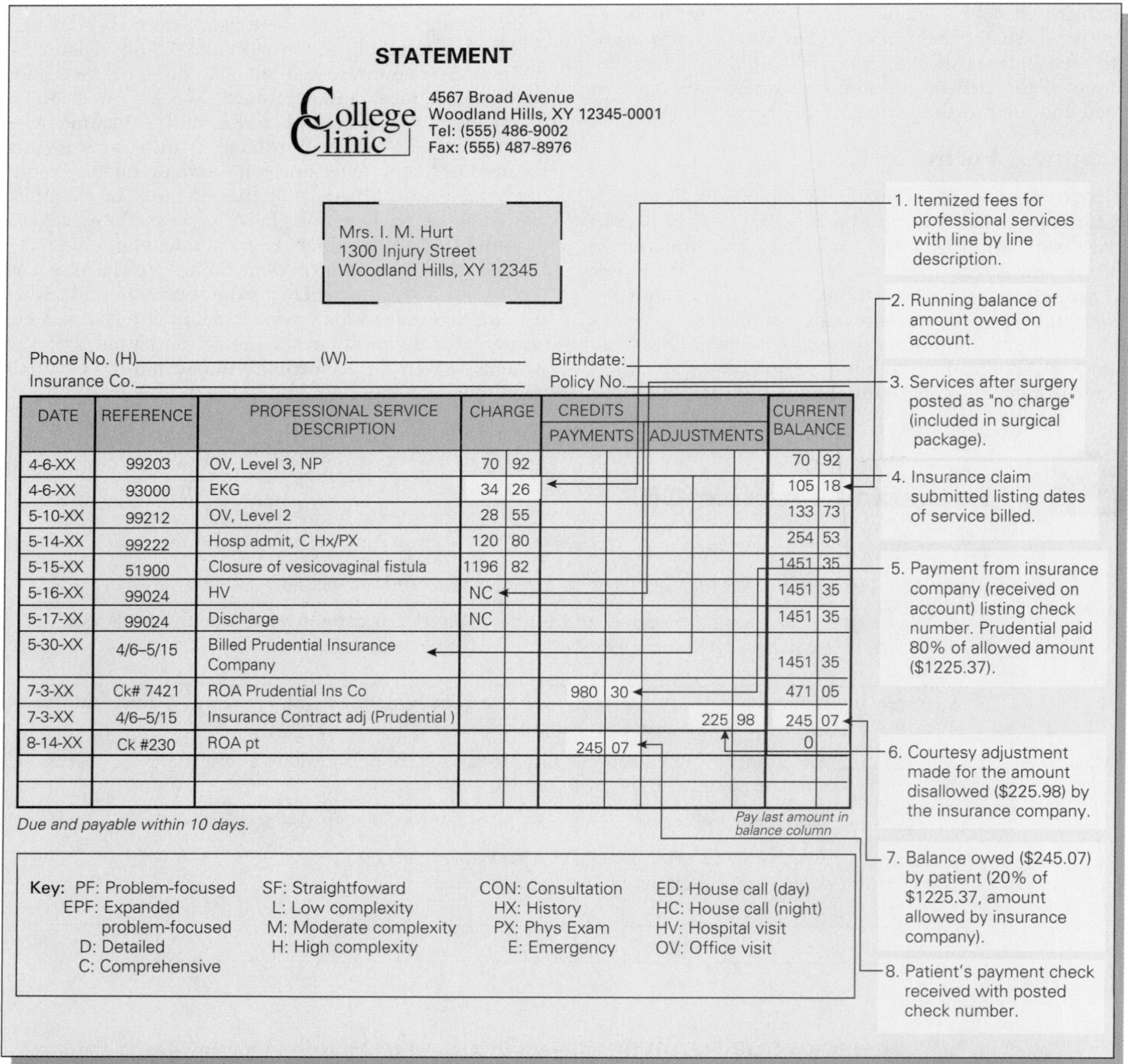

STATEMENT

College Clinic
4567 Broad Avenue
Woodland Hills, XY 12345-0001
Tel: (555) 486-9002
Fax: (555) 487-8976

Mrs. I. M. Hurt
1300 Injury Street
Woodland Hills, XY 12345

Phone No. (H)______ (W)______ Birthdate:______
Insurance Co.______ Policy No.______

DATE	REFERENCE	PROFESSIONAL SERVICE DESCRIPTION	CHARGE	CREDITS: PAYMENTS	CREDITS: ADJUSTMENTS	CURRENT BALANCE
4-6-XX	99203	OV, Level 3, NP	70 92			70 92
4-6-XX	93000	EKG	34 26			105 18
5-10-XX	99212	OV, Level 2	28 55			133 73
5-14-XX	99222	Hosp admit, C Hx/PX	120 80			254 53
5-15-XX	51900	Closure of vesicovaginal fistula	1196 82			1451 35
5-16-XX	99024	HV	NC			1451 35
5-17-XX	99024	Discharge	NC			1451 35
5-30-XX	4/6–5/15	Billed Prudential Insurance Company				1451 35
7-3-XX	Ck# 7421	ROA Prudential Ins Co		980 30		471 05
7-3-XX	4/6–5/15	Insurance Contract adj (Prudential)			225 98	245 07
8-14-XX	Ck #230	ROA pt		245 07		0

Due and payable within 10 days.

Pay last amount in balance column

Key: PF: Problem-focused; EPF: Expanded problem-focused; D: Detailed; C: Comprehensive; SF: Straightfoward; L: Low complexity; M: Moderate complexity; H: High complexity; CON: Consultation; HX: History; PX: Phys Exam; E: Emergency; ED: House call (day); HC: House call (night); HV: Hospital visit; OV: Office visit

Figure 3–7. Ledger card illustrating posting of professional services with references and descriptions, fees, payments, adjustments, and balance due.

the ledger is completely filled up, the account balance is brought forward (extended) to the back side or to a new card. The date an insurance claim is sent, including the name of the insurance carrier and date(s) of service(s) billed, should be recorded on the ledger card.

If a medical practice is computerized, all financial transactions are executed using billing software. Patients who are private 1 month and on the Medicaid program the next month, or who are injured on the job and covered under workers' compensation, will require more than one account to keep private and state records separate. Table 3–1 describes how to make various entries to each column on the ledger card.

Post all charges on the same day or the day following services. Timely posting of charges is increasingly essential as insurance carriers may refuse to pay on claims not submitted within 90 days from the date of service. Post each professional service, referencing the procedure code, as a separate line item (on a separate line).

Day Sheet/Daily Log

Transactions (charges, payments, adjustments) for all patients seen in one day are recorded on a **day sheet** or *daily log* (Fig. 3–8). This register shows how much money the practice generated in charges and payments as well as how much money is adjusted for patients' accounts on any given day. Each day's totals are carried forward and another day sheet is set up to receive posting for the following day. At the end of the month, the monthly total is brought forward to the next month. The total amount of money *owed* for professional services rendered, that is, the combined charges minus all payments, is called the **accounts receivable.** This is not money that is available to the practice, but is the amount of money to be collected from insurance companies and patients.

In a pegboard bookkeeping system and in a computer system, entries on the patient's ledger and day sheet are made at the same time. A pegboard bookkeeping system is also called a "write-it-once" bookkeeping system because it allows the overlay of several documents (e.g., encounter form, ledger card, deposit slip, cash receipt) on the day sheet. By using no-carbon-required (NCR) paper for these documents, you can write on the top document and record on all the documents under it. This decreases errors and saves time in posting. In a computer system, transactions are posted to the patient's account on a charge screen and are automatically added or subtracted in the daily log. Balances are also automatically brought forward from day to day, month to month, and year to year.

Expressions from Experience

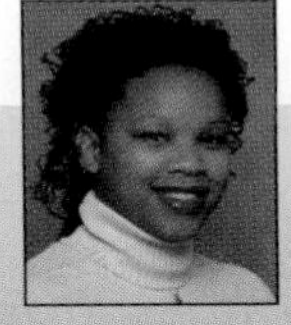

I love learning anything new and there is always something new to learn in this field.

Lateisha Ware
Medical Insurance Billing/Coding Specialist
Billing Center—Radiology

Table 3–1 Posting to a Patient's Ledger

Column	Entry
Address box	Insert patient's name and address, including ZIP code.
Personal data	Enter home and work telephone numbers, birth date, insurance company's name, and policy number.
Date	Post the *date of service* (DOS), payment, adjustment, or date insurance or patient was billed. The posting date is the *actual date* the transaction is recorded. If the DOS differs from the posting date, reference the DOS in the reference or description column.
Reference	Indicate: (1) Procedure code number when posting charges. (2) Check number, "cash," or credit card number when posting payments. (3) Date(s) of service when posting an adjustment. (4) Date(s) of service when indicating the insurance was billed.
Professional service description	Enter: (1) Description of service using key at bottom of ledger when posting charges. (2) Received on account (ROA) and who made payment (e.g., patient [pt], name of insurance co., or name of credit card) when posting payments. (3) Type of adjustment (e.g., ins. contract adj., courtesy adj.). (4) Name of insurance carrier billed.
Charge	Enter each fee (charge) on a separate line from the mock fee schedule
Payments	Enter amount paid
Adjustment	Enter amount Optional: posted on the same line as the payment
Current balance	Line by line add (credit) charges to the running balance and subtract (debit) payments and adjustments from the running balance to determine the current balance. When an entry is made without a charge, payment, or adjustment (e.g., date insurance company or patient was billed), carry down the running balance from the previous line.

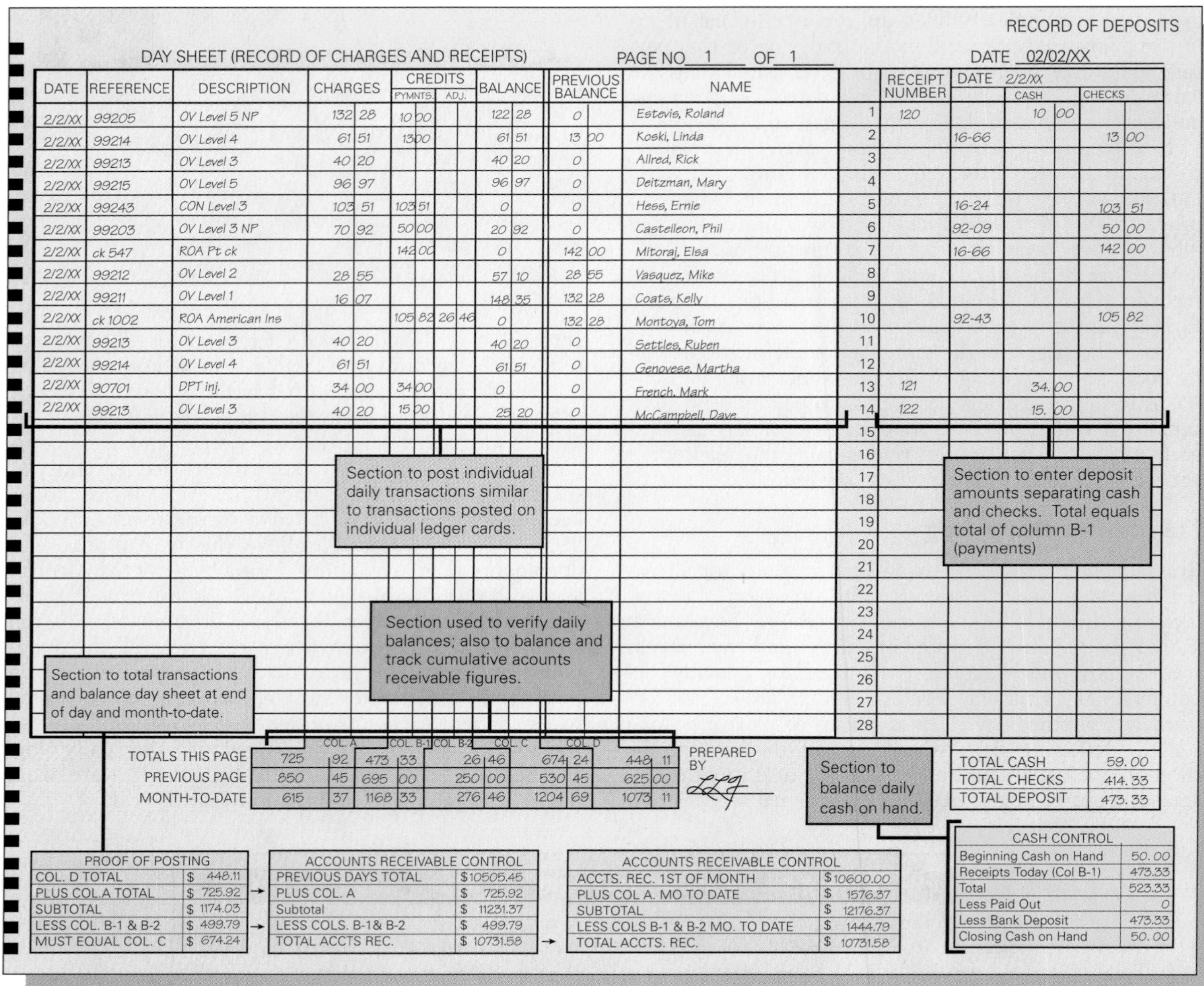

RECORD OF DEPOSITS

DAY SHEET (RECORD OF CHARGES AND RECEIPTS) PAGE NO 1 OF 1 DATE 02/02/XX

DATE	REFERENCE	DESCRIPTION	CHARGES	CREDITS PYMNTS.	CREDITS ADJ.	BALANCE	PREVIOUS BALANCE	NAME		RECEIPT NUMBER	DATE 2/2/XX	CASH	CHECKS
2/2/XX	99205	OV Level 5 NP	132 28	10 00		122 28	0	Estevis, Roland	1	120		10 00	
2/2/XX	99214	OV Level 4	61 51	13 00		61 51	13 00	Koski, Linda	2		16-66		13 00
2/2/XX	99213	OV Level 3	40 20			40 20	0	Allred, Rick	3				
2/2/XX	99215	OV Level 5	96 97			96 97	0	Deitzman, Mary	4				
2/2/XX	99243	CON Level 3	103 51	103 51		0	0	Hess, Ernie	5		16-24		103 51
2/2/XX	99203	OV Level 3 NP	70 92	50 00		20 92	0	Castelleon, Phil	6		92-09		50 00
2/2/XX	ck 547	ROA Pt ck		142 00		0	142 00	Mitoraj, Elsa	7		16-66		142 00
2/2/XX	99212	OV Level 2	28 55			57 10	28 55	Vasquez, Mike	8				
2/2/XX	99211	OV Level 1	16 07			148 35	132 28	Coats, Kelly	9				
2/2/XX	ck 1002	ROA American Ins		105 82	26 46	0	132 28	Montoya, Tom	10		92-43		105 82
2/2/XX	99213	OV Level 3	40 20			40 20	0	Settles, Ruben	11				
2/2/XX	99214	OV Level 4	61 51			61 51	0	Genovese, Martha	12				
2/2/XX	90701	DPT inj.	34 00	34 00		0	0	French, Mark	13	121		34. 00	
2/2/XX	99213	OV Level 3	40 20	15 00		25 20	0	McCampbell, Dave	14	122		15. 00	
									15				
									16				
									17				
									18				
									19				
									20				
									21				
									22				
									23				
									24				
									25				
									26				
									27				
									28				

	COL. A	COL. B-1	COL. B-2	COL. C	COL. D
TOTALS THIS PAGE	725 92	473 33	26 46	674 24	448 11
PREVIOUS PAGE	850 45	695 00	250 00	530 45	625 00
MONTH-TO-DATE	615 37	1168 33	276 46	1204 69	1073 11

PREPARED BY LLG

TOTAL CASH	59. 00
TOTAL CHECKS	414. 33
TOTAL DEPOSIT	473. 33

PROOF OF POSTING	
COL. D TOTAL	$ 448.11
PLUS COL.A TOTAL	$ 725.92
SUBTOTAL	$ 1174.03
LESS COL. B-1 & B-2	$ 499.79
MUST EQUAL COL. C	$ 674.24

ACCOUNTS RECEIVABLE CONTROL	
PREVIOUS DAYS TOTAL	$10505.45
PLUS COL. A	$ 725.92
Subtotal	$ 11231.37
LESS COLS. B-1& B-2	$ 499.79
TOTAL ACCTS REC.	$ 10731.58

ACCOUNTS RECEIVABLE CONTROL	
ACCTS. REC. 1ST OF MONTH	$10600.00
PLUS COL A. MO TO DATE	$ 1576.37
SUBTOTAL	$ 12176.37
LESS COLS B-1 & B-2 MO. TO DATE	$ 1444.79
TOTAL ACCTS. REC.	$ 10731.58

CASH CONTROL	
Beginning Cash on Hand	50. 00
Receipts Today (Col B-1)	473.33
Total	523.33
Less Paid Out	0
Less Bank Deposit	473.33
Closing Cash on Hand	50. 00

Figure 3–8. Example of a day sheet (daily log) illustrating various sections used to post and monitor transactions in a physician's office.

The Insurance Claim Form

The insurance billing specialist completes the universal insurance claim form obtaining necessary information from the patient registration form, insurance card, encounter form, and/or patient record. Accurate procedural and diagnostic codes are included, necessary signatures are obtained, and the form is mailed to the correct insurance carrier. The claim should be processed in a timely manner to stay within insurance program/plan time limits and ensure prompt payment. The minimum information required by third party payers is:

1. What was done? — Services and procedures—coded using CPT-HCPCS procedural codes, which are presented in Chapters 5 and 6.
2. Why was it done? — Diagnoses—coded using ICD-9-CM diagnostic codes, which are presented in Chapter 4.
3. When was it performed? — Date(s) of service (DOS)—codes, which are defined in Chapter 8 and listed in Appendix D.
4. Where was it performed? — Place(s) of service (POS)—codes, which are defined in Chapter 8 and listed in Appendix D.
5. Who did it? — Provider name(s) and identifying number(s)—these are obtained from the encounter form or medical record and listed in Appendix A.

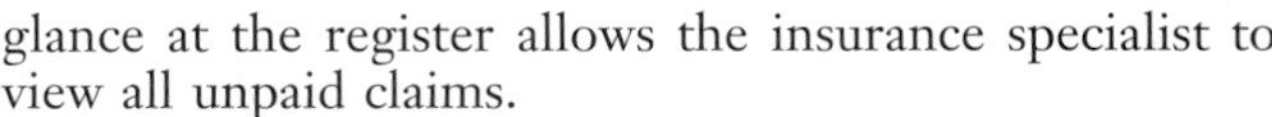

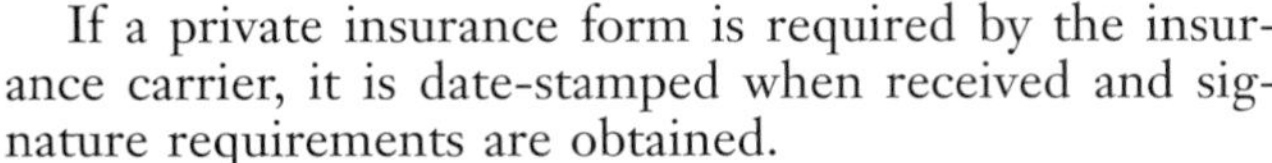

Expressions from Experience

There is a sense of stability in this field because it will always exist.

Lateisha Ware
Medical Insurance Billing/Coding Specialist
Billing Center—Radiology

If a private insurance form is required by the insurance carrier, it is date-stamped when received and signature requirements are obtained.

Patients who submit their own insurance claims are given two copies of the encounter form. The patient attaches one copy to the insurance claim form after completing the top portion (patient's information) and forwards it to the insurance carrier, retaining one copy for personal records.

Provider's Signature

The completed insurance claim form is reviewed for accuracy and signed by the provider of services or the provider's representative. A **provider** is any individual or organization that provides healthcare services. Providers may be physicians, chiropractors, physical therapists, medical equipment suppliers, or facilities such as urgent care centers, surgery centers, hospitals, and pharmacies. **Physician extenders** are also considered providers and include nurse practitioners, nurse midwives, physician assistants, and nurse anesthetists. Details regarding physician signature requirements are covered in Chapter 8.

Insurance Pending File and Claims Register

A duplicate of the claim is saved in the computer system, or retained in an insurance pending file in the event payment is not received and the claim must be followed up. This file may also be referred to as a suspense, follow-up, or tickler file (Fig. 3–9). The term "tickler" came into existence because it tickles or jogs the memory at certain future dates.

Claims are usually filed by date of service, although they may be separated by insurance carrier, then filed by date of service if there are a lot of claims sent to a particular insurance company. This allows for all inquiries to be included in a single telephone call or insurance tracer (follow-up) letter. Filing by date of service allows for timely tracking at 30-, 60-, and 90-day intervals. In a computer system, billed claims can be sorted by date of service, insurance carrier, and time intervals as mentioned above. A report is then printed and used for following delinquent accounts.

Another method of tracking is an insurance claims register. As claims are billed, the date of submission, insurance company, and patient's name are recorded in a register and used for periodic follow-up. Although this method takes more time to complete, a quick glance at the register allows the insurance specialist to view all unpaid claims.

Whichever method is used, a system needs to be established to keep track of the status of each claim that has been billed. Claims are mailed in a large manila envelope to the insurance carrier. Mail claims in batches whenever possible to expedite addressing envelopes and save postage. Detailed information regarding claim follow-up for specific insurance carriers is found in Chapter 15.

Insurance Company Processing

Upon receipt at the insurance company, the claim is date-stamped and microfilmed. First, eligibility is verified by matching the patient (name and date of birth) with a policy and group number. All procedure code numbers are matched with the policy's master benefit list and cross-matched with diagnostic code numbers. A determination is made of "allowed or approved" charges and the patient's deductible amount is determined and subtracted if not met. Any coinsurance or copayment amounts are also determined and applied. An explanation of benefits (EOB) or remittance advice (RA) document is then generated, along with the insurance check, and mailed to the provider.

Insurance Payment Check and Explanation of Benefits/Remittance Advice Document

Payment from the insurance company should be received within 2 to 8 weeks accompanied by an explanation of benefits/remittance advice document. The **explanation of benefits (EOB)** document describes

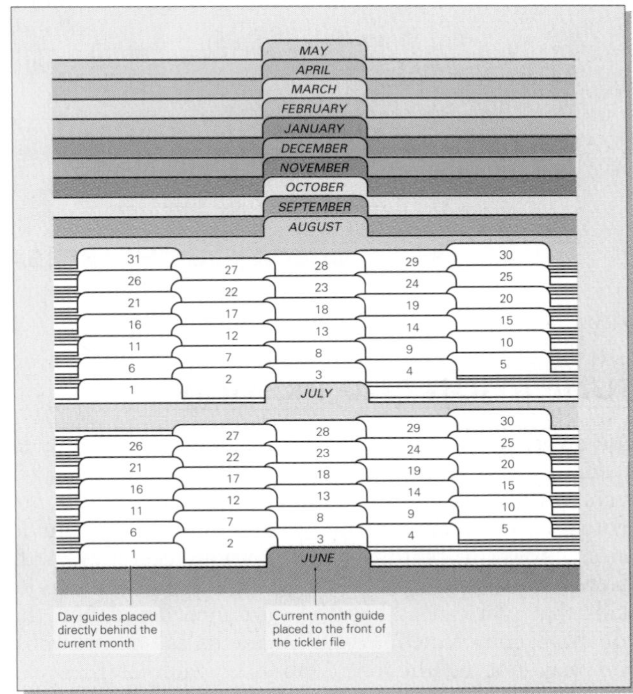

Figure 3–9. Example of a 30- to 60-day pending or tickler file used for following up on unpaid insurance claims.

services billed and includes a breakdown of how the payment was determined. In the Medicare and Medicaid programs it is called a **remittance advice (RA).** The amount received is verified against the amount billed kept either in the computer data file or the insurance pending file. The payment is posted (credited) to the patient's account/ledger and current day sheet indicating date of posting, name of insurance company, check or voucher number, amount received, and contract adjustment. The check is endorsed, entered on a bank deposit slip, and deposited in the bank.

The duplicate copy of the insurance claim is attached to the EOB/RA and filed in an annual file according to the date of payment, insurance type, or patient's name. Some practices prefer filing this information in the financial area of the patient's chart.

Patient Statement

All patients who have insurance coverage should be billed the same fee as that submitted to the insurance company. A statement should be sent within the month that the service occurred and every 30 days. It should include a note stating, "You are responsible for the entire amount; however, as a courtesy, your insurance has been billed." After the insurance plan has paid, a statement indicating the balance the patient owes should be sent immediately. Follow-up techniques for delinquent accounts are covered in Chapter 14.

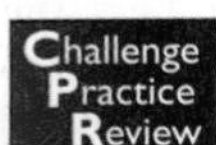

Pause and Practice CPR

REVIEW SESSIONS 3–7 THROUGH 3–13

Directions: *Complete the following questions as a review of information you have just read.*

3–7 A copy of the encounter form is used to __________ charges, payments to each patient's account.

3–8 The amount owed after all charges are recorded and payments and adjustments subtracted is called the account __________.

3–9 All transactions for patients seen in one day are recorded on a __________ or __________.

3–10 Information used on the HCFA-1500 insurance claim form is obtained from the __________, __________, __________, and/or __________.

3–11 Nurse practitioners, nurse midwives, physician assistants, and nurse anesthetists are referred to as __________.

3–12 The document that is generated to accompany the insurance check is called the __________ or __________.

3–13 The first statement should be sent __________ __________.

CHECK YOUR HEARTBEAT! Turn to the end of the chapter for answers to these review sessions.

SUMMATION AND PREVIEW

You are now familiar with most of the source documents needed to bill an insurance claim. The patient's medical record, which is another source document, will be presented in Chapter 7 along with documentation guidelines. As you work through the various exercises in the Exercise Exchange section, you will be practicing job skills that you can add to the insurance foundation that you have constructed. As an insurance billing specialist, you may not be the one who does each of these job tasks; however, you need to know what is required at each step along the reimbursement path so that you can act as a team member when this information is used in the reimbursement process.

As outlined in this chapter, there are many pieces of information that appear on the insurance claim in coded form. Next, you will learn how to code diagnoses. Diagnostic codes represent *why* the procedure or service was done. The more accurate the code, the higher the level of reimbursement.

GOLDEN RULE

Data are only as reliable as the source document.

Chapter 3 Review and Practice

Study Session

Directions: Review the objectives, key terms, and chapter information before completing the following questions.

3–1 What is another name for the patient registration form?

____

3–2 Why is it important that all blanks are filled in or marked N/A on the patient registration form?

____

3–3 How often should patient information and insurance information be verified?

____

3–4 List in what blocks the following items are recorded on the HCFA-1500 insurance claim form:

(1) Block ________ Assignment of benefits for private insurance

(2) Block ________ Assignment of benefits for government programs

(3) Block ________ Authorization to release medical information for private patients

(4) Block ________ Authorization to release medical information for government programs

3–5 How often should the diagnostic and procedure code sections on the encounter form be reviewed and updated? ______________________________

3–6 View the encounter form in Figure 3–6 and answer the following questions:

(1) List the two diagnostic codes checked on the form. ____________ and ____________

(2) List the three procedure codes checked on the form and the fees for each.

code ____________ fee ____________

code ____________ fee ____________

code ____________ fee ____________

(3) When is the patient's next appointment to be made? ____________

(4) What is the amount the patient paid? ______________

(5) What method of payment was used? ______________

(6) Who is the patient's insurance carrier? ____________________

(7) What is the type of insurance plan? ______________

3–7 Three methods of payment are ____________, ____________, and

______________________.

3–8 Another word for an adjustment made on an account is a/an ____________________.

3–9 An individual account, kept on a pegboard bookkeeping system, is referred to as a/an

____________________.

3–10 View Figure 3–7 (ledger card) and answer the following questions. Note: refer to the abbreviation key at the bottom of the ledger when needed.

(1) What did the patient have done to incur a charge of $120.80? ______________________

____

(2) How many services did the patient have on 4/6/XX? ______________________

(3) What day was the patient discharged from the hospital? ______________________

(4) What insurance company paid on the account? ______________________

(5) How much was written off of the books as an insurance contract adjustment?

____

3–11 The total amount of money owed to a medical practice for professional services is called the ______________________.

3–12 One who provides healthcare services is called a/an ______________________.

3–13 After insurance claims are sent to the insurance company, they are usually filed by ______________________.

3–14 Payment from the insurance company is typically received in ______ to ______ weeks.

3–15 When should the first statement be sent to the patient? ______________________

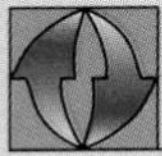

Exercise Exchange

3–1 Complete a Patient Registration Form

Directions

1. Use the College Clinic patient registration form (Form 05 in Appendix F).
2. Refer to instructions under "Patient Registration Form" in the worktext and the example shown in Figure 3–3.
3. Interview another person (e.g., classmate or relative) that has insurance coverage and fill in the patient registration form. Be sure to address all items as directed in the worktext.
4. Make up an account number. Use the current date. The patient is assigning benefits to Dr. Gerald Practon.

3–2 Abstract Information from an Insurance Identification Card

Scenario: A new patient, Eunice Young, has an appointment with Dr. Practon. The copy machine is broken at College Clinic so you are not able to copy the insurance card. She needs help filling out the patient registration form because of an injured right wrist. She has given you the information to complete the form, except for the insurance information which you will be abstracting from the insurance identification card.

Directions

1. Refer to the insurance identification card shown below and abstract the information to complete the *primary insurance section* of the patient registration form found in Appendix F (Form 06).
2. Mr. Young, the patient's husband, is the subscriber. His birth date is 6/16/66 and his Social Security number is 564-XX-3059.
3. The health insurance carrier's address is 1000 Pacific Coast Parkway, La Buena Vista, XY 12345-0001.

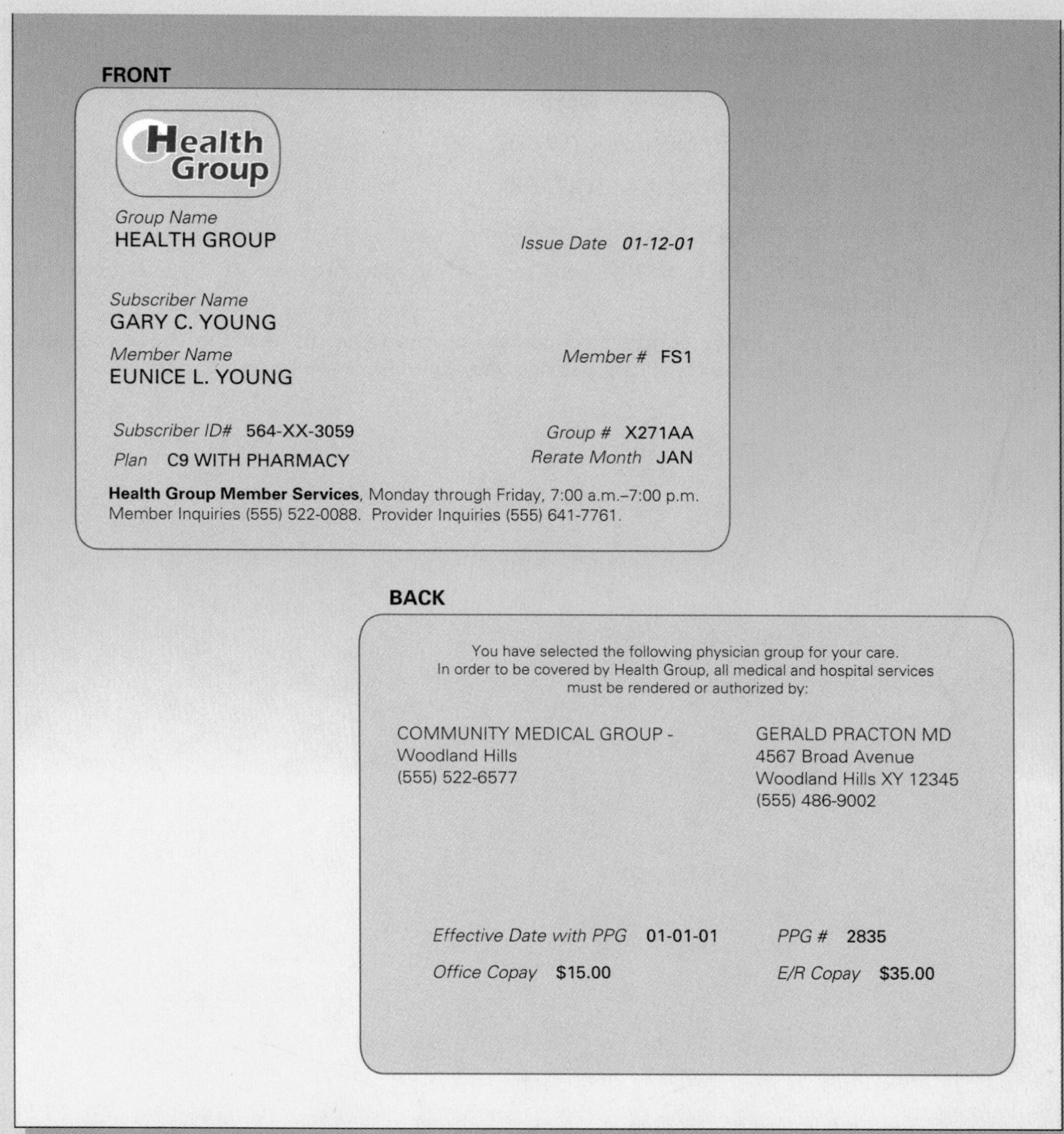
FRONT

Health Group

Group Name
HEALTH GROUP

Issue Date 01-12-01

Subscriber Name
GARY C. YOUNG

Member Name
EUNICE L. YOUNG

Member # FS1

Subscriber ID# 564-XX-3059

Group # X271AA

Plan C9 WITH PHARMACY

Rerate Month JAN

Health Group Member Services, Monday through Friday, 7:00 a.m.–7:00 p.m.
Member Inquiries (555) 522-0088. Provider Inquiries (555) 641-7761.

BACK

You have selected the following physician group for your care.
In order to be covered by Health Group, all medical and hospital services
must be rendered or authorized by:

COMMUNITY MEDICAL GROUP -
Woodland Hills
(555) 522-6577

GERALD PRACTON MD
4567 Broad Avenue
Woodland Hills XY 12345
(555) 486-9002

Effective Date with PPG 01-01-01

PPG # 2835

Office Copay $15.00

E/R Copay $35.00

3–3 **Post Transactions on a Ledger Card**

Scenario: Eunice Young, the patient in the previous exercise, comes in to see Dr. Practon for her injured right wrist. She hurt it when she fell while skating in the parkway at the beach yesterday.

Directions

1. Use the blank ledger card (Form 07) found in Appendix F.
2. Refer to information about ledger transactions under "Patient Account/Ledger" in the worktext.
3. Study the example of a completed ledger shown in Figure 3–7.
4. Follow instructions on how to record various entries to each column on the ledger card found in Table 3–1.
5. Set up the ledger card for patient Eunice Young. Her patient information may be found on Form 06 (Appendix F) used in the previous exercise.
6. Use the procedure or service code number listed under "Data to Record" below and locate the fee in the "mock fee" column of the Mock Fee Schedule located in Appendix B.

7. Add all charges and subtract all payments and adjustments to obtain a running balance for the right "current balance" column.

Data to Record on Ledger Card

1. New patient (NP) office visit (99203)
2. X-ray (two views) right wrist (73100)
3. Insurance company was billed on 8/6/XX.
4. On 9/1/XX check #5309 was received in the amount of $84.12 from Health Net Insurance Company.
5. Post the insurance contract adjustment on the same day that the check was received. The amount to adjust will be the remaining balance after the insurance payment is applied.

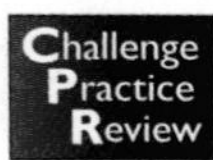

CPR Session: Answers

REVIEW SESSIONS 3–1 THROUGH 3–3

3–1 (1) Preregister during initial telephone call.
(2) Designated staff member contacts patient prior to first appointment.
(3) Patient is sent a registration form to fill out.
(4) Patient arrives early at the office to fill out the registration form.

3–2 (1) Name.
(2) Address.
(3) Telephone number.

3–3 (1) Set up a medical and financial record.
(2) Complete the health insurance claim form.
(3) Communicate with the patient.
(4) Collect on the account.

REVIEW SESSIONS 3–4 THROUGH 3–6

3–4 A copy produces error-free data.

3–5 (b) (assignment of benefits)
(c) (financial agreement)
(a) (release of medical information)

3–6 (1) Combination bill.
(2) Insurance form.
(3) Routing document.

REVIEW SESSIONS 3–7 THROUGH 3–13

3–7 post

3–8 balance

3–9 day sheet or daily log

3–10 patient registration form, insurance card, encounter form, and/or patient record

3–11 physician extenders

3–12 explanation of benefits or remittance advice

3–13 within the month that the service occurred

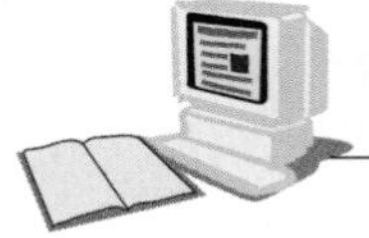

Resources

All of the source documents, such as the patient registration form, encounter form, patient ledger, pegboard accessories, insurance claim form, and patient statement, are available from medical stationery companies. They also carry office stationery, envelopes, appointment cards, appointment books, message books, file folders, chart labels, business checks, and many other types of forms and supplies used in a medical office. Custom forms, such as patient instruction forms, history forms, report forms, patient reminder cards, and others may be designed by office staff and ordered, or designed by the supply company after obtaining the necessary information. Some of these forms may be available over the Internet from the supplier's web site.

Internet Sites

Bibbero Systems, Inc.
Web site: http://www.bibbero.com

Histacount Medical Practice
Web site: http://www.histacount.com

Medical Arts Press
Web site: http://www.medicalartspress.com

Objectives

After reading this chapter and completing the exercise sessions, you should be able to:

Learning Objectives:

- ✔ Explain the purpose and importance of coding diagnoses.
- ✔ Name the basic steps in coding a diagnosis, using ICD-9-CM Volumes 1 and 2.
- ✔ State the meaning of basic abbreviations, punctuation, and symbols in the diagnostic codebook.
- ✔ Define diagnostic code terminology.
- ✔ Compare primary, secondary, admitting, and principal diagnoses.
- ✔ Explain sequencing rules for reporting diagnostic codes.
- ✔ State when signs, symptoms, and ill-defined conditions may be coded.

Performance Objectives:

- ✔ Select the main term in a diagnostic statement and locate it in the diagnostic codebook.
- ✔ Use the diagnostic codebook properly and obtain accurate codes.
- ✔ Cite the names of various tables that appear in Volume 2 of ICD-9-CM and demonstrate their use.
- ✔ Name two supplementary classifications in ICD-9-CM, state circumstances in which they are used, and select correct V and E codes.

Key Terms

acute
adverse effect
benign tumor
carcinoma in situ
chief complaint (CC)
chronic
combination code
concurrent condition
diagnosis
E codes
eponym
etiology
International Classification of Diseases, 9th Revision, Clinical Modification (ICD-9-CM)
late effects
main term
malignant tumor
manifestation
neoplasm
poisoning
primary diagnosis
principal diagnosis
secondary diagnosis
symptom
V codes

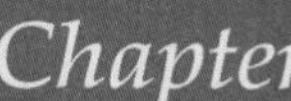

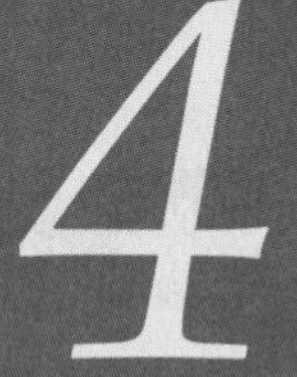

Chapter 4

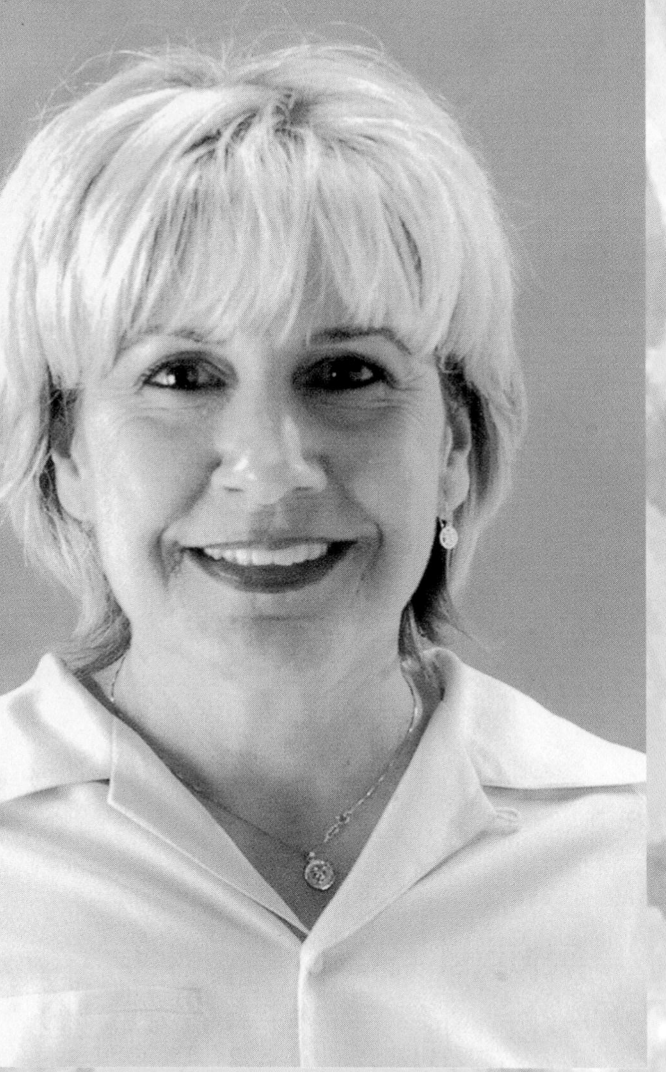

I decided to go back to school when my children left home. I graduated from a vocational insurance billing course at a local adult school and was fortunate to get a job right away. I work for a medical billing company coding diagnoses for radiology and pathology.

The patient's symptoms listed on the charge sheet need to be correlated with the final diagnoses. Sometimes I can follow a patient's progress from beginning to end. For example, a patient has a chest x-ray for shortness of breath and the radiology report indicates a lung nodule. A biopsy is then performed and the result indicates a benign mass. I code the shortness of breath for the radiologist and the benign mass for the pathologist. I work in tandem with coworkers who select the procedures/services and post charges. I code the diagnoses and try to stay ahead of them so they can submit the claim in a timely manner.

Elizabeth (Betty) Palace
Diagnostic Coder
Medical Billing Company

Coding Diagnoses

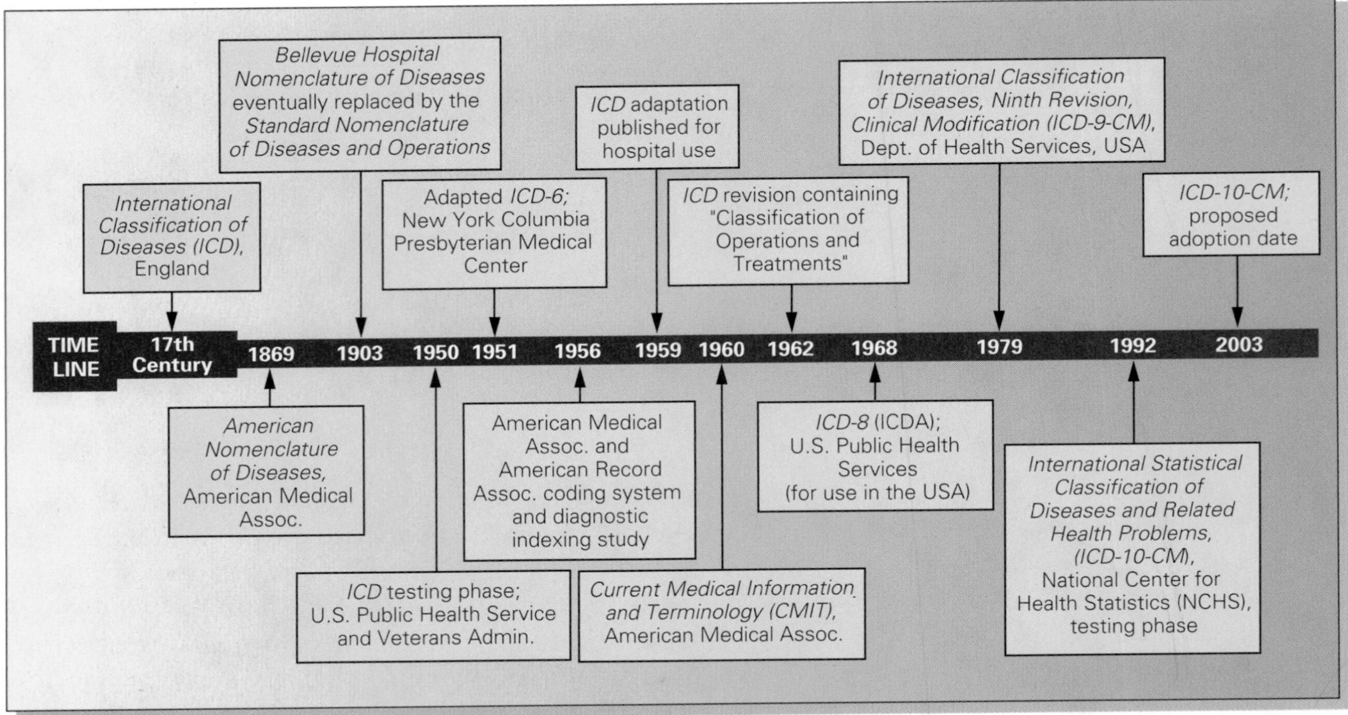

THE DIAGNOSTIC CODING SYSTEM

Several sets of codes are used on the claim form for various purposes instead of writing out information. By coding data, less space is taken up and standardized descriptions of information are provided. This chapter deals with coding diagnoses for outpatient professional services. In the next two chapters, you will learn how to code the professional services and procedures which link to diagnostic codes on the insurance claim form. Medical insurance billing specialists and coders must convert the *reasons* for the procedures and services performed, or supplies that are issued, from written diagnostic statements into ICD-9-CM diagnostic codes. There is a direct relationship between proper coding and the financial success or failure of a medical practice. A working knowledge of medical terminology, including a basic course in anatomy and physiology, is essential to becoming a topnotch diagnostic coder. The coding must be accurate because with many insurance programs the payment for services may be based on the diagnosis. Diagnostic coding was developed for the following reasons:

1. Classifying morbidity (sickness)
2. Classifying causes of mortality (death)
3. Evaluating hospital service utilization
4. Medical research

Insurance companies mandate that diagnostic codes be used on insurance claim forms instead of written diagnostic descriptions. If codes are not used, it affects the physician's level of reimbursement, and claims can be denied, fines or penalties can be levied, and sanctions can be imposed. When claims are coded correctly, payments are accurate and prompt.

Official coding and reporting guidelines have been developed and approved by the following organizations:

- American Hospital Association (AHA)
- American Health Information Management Association (AHIMA)
- Health Care Financing Administration (HCFA), now known as Centers for Medicare and Medicaid Services (CMS)
- National Center for Health Statistics (NCHS)

Resource information regarding the official coding and reporting guidelines is found at the end of this chapter.

Diagnosis-Related Procedures

Some insurance companies have a list of specific diagnoses that are linked to diagnostic procedures and will only pay for such procedures if a diagnosis from the list appears on the claim form. If a diagnosis from the list is not evident on a claim, the insurance company will reply, stating, "This procedure/item is not payable for the diagnosis as reported." An example of this would be a patient who has had magnetic resonance imaging (MRI) of the brain with the diagnosis listed as transient ischemic attack (TIA) or Alzheimer's disease. Medicare will not pay for MRIs with these diagnoses; however, they would pay if the listed diagnosis was cerebral insufficiency.

Procedures that are diagnosis related may include:

- Cardiovascular services (echocardiography, electrocardiography, Doppler studies, exercise stress testing, Holter monitors)

- Imaging services (computed tomography [CTs], MRIs, x-ray films)
- Laboratory services
- Neurologic services (electroencephalography, noninvasive ultrasonography)
- Vitamin B_{12} injections

It is important to verify all diagnoses and relate them to the procedure being billed. First, you must know the procedures that are diagnosis related. Unfortunately, all insurance companies do not disclose this information, which is referred to as *code linkage.* A reference book may be helpful in this situation, such as *St. Anthony's Medicare National Correct Coding Guide* or *St. Anthony's Medicare Correct Coding and Payment Manual for Procedures and Services.* Refer to Resources at the end of this chapter for information regarding these publications.

INTERNATIONAL CLASSIFICATION OF DISEASES, 9TH REVISION, CLINICAL MODIFICATION

Organization and Format

The ***International Classification of Diseases, 9th Revision, Clinical Modification*** **(ICD-9-CM)** is a diagnostic codebook which uses a system for classifying diseases and operations to facilitate collection of uniform and comparable health information. It has three volumes, described and used by healthcare providers as follows:

- Volume 1 — *Diseases: Tabular List*
  Used by physicians and providers for coding diagnoses for outpatient services
- Volume 2 — *Diseases: Alphabetic Index*
  Used by physicians and providers for coding diagnoses for outpatient services
- Volume 3 — *Procedures: Tabular and Alphabetic Index*
  Used by hospitals for coding inpatient procedures

It is updated annually, each October. The changes appear in three publications: *Coding Clinic, American Health Information Management Association Journal,* and the *Federal Register.* Refer to Resources at the end of this chapter for information regarding these publications. Coding from an out-of-date manual can delay payment or cause costly mistakes that can lead to financial disaster. Many insurance companies do not use the new codes until they have a chance to update their computer systems, so it is important to verify with each carrier when new codes are implemented.

Volume 1, a tabular list of diseases, is a numeric listing organized by chapters. Volume 2, an alphabetical index of diseases, lists diagnoses in alphabetical order according to main terms and includes a hypertension table and a neoplasm table located within the *Alphabetic Index.* Volume 3, a tabular list and alphabetical index of procedures, is used primarily in the hospital setting. The systematized arrangement of ICD-9-CM makes it possible to encode, computerize, store, and retrieve large volumes of information from the patient's medical record. ICD-9-CM is used by hospitals and outpatient healthcare providers to code and report clinical information required to participate in and submit medical claims to various government programs, private insurance companies, managed care organizations, and professional review organizations.

Contents

Only Volumes 1 and 2 of ICD-9-CM will be discussed in this chapter. Refer to Table 4–1 for an outline of Volumes 1 and 2, which are used in physicians' offices and other outpatient settings to complete insurance claim forms. Volume 1 lists chapter headings with

Table 4–1 Outline of Volumes 1 and 2 of ICD-9-CM

Volume 1 Chapter Headings	Codes
1 Infectious and Parasitic Diseases	001–139
2 Neoplasms	140–239
3 Endocrine, Nutritional, and Metabolic Diseases and Immunity Disorders	240–279
4 Disease of the Blood and Blood-Forming Organs	280–289
5 Mental Disorders	290–319
6 Diseases of the Nervous System and Sense Organs	320–389
7 Diseases of the Circulatory System	390–459
8 Diseases of the Respiratory System	460–519
9 Diseases of the Digestive System	520–579
10 Diseases of the Genitourinary System	580–629
11 Complications of Pregnancy, Childbirth, and the Puerperium	630–676
12 Diseases of the Skin and Subcutaneous Tissue	680–709
13 Diseases of the Musculoskeletal System and Connective Tissue	710–739
14 Congenital Anomalies	740–759
15 Certain Conditions Originating in the Perinatal Period	760–779
16 Symptoms, Signs, and Ill-Defined Conditions	780–799
17 Injury and Poisoning	800–999
Supplementary Classification	
Classification of Factors Influencing Health Status and Contact with Health Service	V01–V83
Classification of External Causes of Injury and Poisoning	E800–E999
Appendices	
A Morphology of Neoplasms	
B Glossary of Mental Disorders	
C Classification of Drugs by American Hospital Formulary Service List Number and Their ICD-9-CM Equivalents	
D Classification of Industrial Accidents According to Agency	
E List of Three-Digit Categories	
Volume 2	
Section 1: Index to Diseases and Injuries, alphabetic	
Section 2: Table of Drugs and Chemicals	
Section 3: Index of External Causes of Injuries and Poisonings	

associated code ranges. The supplemental classification consists of V and E codes, which are discussed later in this chapter. Sections A, B, C, and D of the Appendices are not used in physician outpatient billing. Section E lists three-digit code categories, under which all four- and five-digit codes are found. Volume 2 contains three sections: an alphabetical index for diseases and injuries, a table of drugs and chemicals, and an alphabetical index to external causes of injuries and poisonings (E codes).

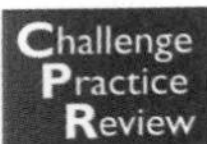

Pause and Practice CPR

REVIEW SESSIONS 4–1 THROUGH 4–6

Directions: *Complete the following questions as a review of information you have just read.*

4–1 Why do medical practices use diagnostic codes on insurance claim forms?

____

____

4–2 Name four reasons diagnostic coding was developed.

(a) ______________________________

(b) ______________________________

(c) ______________________________

(d) ______________________________

4–3 Name five categories of diagnosis-related procedures.

(a) ____________________

(b) ____________________

(c) ____________________

(d) ____________________

(e) ____________________

4–4 How many volumes are in ICD-9-CM? __________

4–5 How often is ICD-9-CM updated? ______________________________

4–6 Name two tables that appear in the *Alphabetic Index,* Volume 2.

(a) ____________________

(b) ____________________

CHECK YOUR HEARTBEAT! Turn to the end of the chapter for answers to these review sessions.

USING THE DIAGNOSTIC CODEBOOK

To become a proficient coder it is important to develop an understanding of the conventions and terminology of ICD-9-CM. Before getting started, read all of the information at the beginning of Volumes 1 and 2.

Abbreviations, Punctuation, and Symbols

Refer to Table 4–2 to become familiar with various abbreviations, punctuations, and symbols used in ICD-9-CM.

Other Conventions

Boldface type is used for all codes and code titles in Volume 1, *Tabular List. Italic type* is used for all code numbers that may not be placed in the primary position and for all exclusion notes.

Diagnostic codes must match the age and gender of the patient. Some codes only apply to newborn infants, such as code 775.10 for neonatal diabetes mellitus. Such codes may be marked with a symbol indicating their exclusive use.

Instructional Notations

A variety of instructional notes are given throughout ICD-9-CM and should be carefully observed and

Table 4–2 ICD-9-CM Code Conventions

ABBREVIATIONS

NEC — **Not Elsewhere Classifiable** (in the codebook). All codes with this listing are to be used with *ill-defined terms.* Use only when a separate code describing the disease or injury is not listed in the code manual.

Example: Fibrosclerosis
710.8 Other specified diffuse diseases of connective tissue
Multifocal fibrosclerosis (idopathic) **NEC**

NOS — **Not Otherwise Specified** (by the physician). This abbreviation is the equivalent of "unspecified." It refers to a lack of sufficient detail in the physician's diagnostic statement to be able to assign a specific code.

Example: Malignant neoplasm of colon
153.9 Malignant neoplasm of colon, unspecified
Large intestine **NOS**

Note: The malignant portion of the colon needs to be stated in the medical record. Avoid using nonspecific codes, if possible. Ask the physician for more information so that a specific code may be used.

PUNCTUATION

[ ] — **Brackets** are used in the *Tabular List* to enclose synonyms, alternative wordings, or explanatory phrases.

Example: 426.13 Other second-degree atrioventricular block
Mobitz (type) I [**Wenckebach's**]

( ) — **Parentheses,** found in the *Tabular List* and *Alphabetic Index,* are used to enclose supplementary, descriptive words that do not affect the code assignment; referred to as *nonessential modifiers.*

Example: 287.1 Qualitative platelet defects
Thrombasthenia (**hemorrhagic**) (**hereditary**)

: — **Colons** are used in the *Tabular List* after an incomplete term that needs one or more of the modifiers that follow to make it assignable to a given category.

Example: 112 Candidiasis
Includes: infection by *Candida* species
Moniliasis

} — **Braces** are used to enclose a series of terms, each of which is modified by the statement appearing at the right of the brace.

Example: 103.0 Pinta, primary lesions
Chancre (primary) }
Papule (primary) } **of pinta** [carate]
Pintid }

OFFICIAL GOVERNMENT SYMBOLS (may not be used in all texts)

□ — The **lozenge symbol** printed in the left margin of the *Tabular List,* preceding a disease code in ICD-9-CM indicates that the content of a four-digit code has been modified from the original ICD-9.

Example: 016.1 Tuberculosis of genitourinary system,
Bladder

§ — The **section mark symbol,** printed in the left margin preceding a code, denotes the placement of a footnote at the bottom of the page that is applicable to all subdivisions of that code.

Example: § 364.6 Cysts of iris, ciliary body, and anterior chamber

OTHER SYMBOLS—may change from publisher to publisher and are shown to illustrate various types of symbols that may be encountered.

[code] — **Italicized (slanted) brackets** enclosing a code, used in Volume 2, the *Alphabetic Index,* indicates the need for another code. Record both codes in the order as indicated in the index.

Example: Microaneurysm, retina 362.14
Diabetic 250.5 ***[362.01]***

• — **Black circle** may signal a code is new to this revision.

⊏ — **Large bracket** may signal a new or revised code.

▲ — **Black triangle** may signal a revised code.

④ ⑤ / ☑ 4th ☑ 5th — Either of these symbols signal that a *fourth or fifth digit is required* for coding to indicate the highest level of specificity.

Note: Other symbols may indicate: male diagnosis only, female diagnosis only, newborn diagnosis only, pediatric diagnosis only, or adult diagnosis only.

obeyed. Following are definitions and examples of some of the instructional notes:

- *Notes*—are given throughout ICD-9-CM to define terms and give coding instructions. Be aware of fifth-digit subclassification notes.
- *See*, *See Also*, and *See Category*—serves as a cross-reference and directs the coder to look elsewhere for closely related terms, code categories, and synonyms (Fig. 4–1). Always follow these references.
- *Inclusion and exclusion*—terms are used to define what is, or what is not, included in a code category

See, See Also, and See Category

Inflammation, inflamed, inflammatory
(with exudation)-*continued*

spinal
cord (*see also* Encephalitis) 323.9
late effect—*see* category 326
membrane—*see* Meningitis
nerve—*see* Disorder, nerve

Figure 4–1. Illustration of cross-referencing synonyms, closely related terms, and code categories. (From *International Classification of Diseases, 9th Revision, Clinical Modification*, Volume 2, *Diseases: Alphabetic Index*.)

or subcategory. An "exclusion" box may appear indicating (1) the condition may have to be coded elsewhere, (2) the code cannot be assigned if the associated condition is present, or (3) additional codes may be required to fully explain the condition (Fig. 4–2).

- *Code First*—appearing in Volume 1, directs the coder to another code to be used as the primary code and alerts the coder that this code may not be coded in the first position (Fig. 4–3).
- *Use Additional Code*—appearing in Volume 1, provides the coder with suggestions for the use of additional codes that may give a more complete picture of the diagnosis (Fig. 4–4).
- *And*—is to be interpreted as "and/or" when it appears in a code description (Fig. 4–5).
- *With*—used in a title indicates that there are two conditions and both conditions mentioned must be present in the diagnostic statement. The first condition represents the primary disorder and the second condition represents a complication (Fig. 4–6).

Inclusion and Exclusion Notes

255 Disorders of adrenal glands
Includes: the listed conditions whether the basic disorder is in the adrenals or is pituitary-induced

255.0 Cushing's syndrome
Adrenal hyperplasia due to excess ACTH
Cushing's syndrome:
NOS
iatrogenic
idiopathic
pituitary-dependent
Ectopic ACTH syndrome
Iatrogenic syndrome of excess cortisol
Overproduction of cortisol

Use additional E code to identify cause, if drug induced

Excludes: *congenital adrenal hyperplasia (255.2)*

Figure 4–2. Illustration of Inclusion and Exclusion Notes. (From *International Classification of Diseases, 9th Revision, Clinical Modification*, Volume 1, *Diseases: Tabular List*.)

Code First

713.1 Arthropathy associated with gastrointestinal conditions other than infections
Code first underlying disease as:
regional enteritis (555.0–555.9)
ulcerative colitis (556)

Figure 4–3. Illustration of etiology note which states "code first underlying disease . . . " (From *International Classification of Diseases, 9th Revision, Clinical Modification*, Volume 1, *Diseases: Tabular List*.)

Coding Vocabulary and Instructions

Code only the conditions or problems that the physician is actively managing at the time of the visit and all diagnoses that *affect* the current status of the patient. This may include conditions that existed at the time of the patient's initial contact with the physician, as well as conditions that develop subsequently that affect the treatment received. A physician's diagnosis is usually checked off or listed on an encounter form. In the medical record it is often listed under *impression*, or the abbreviations *imp*, or *Dx*. Diagnoses that relate to a patient's previous medical problem(s) that has no bearing on the patient's present condition are not coded.

For example, a patient presents with a stuffy head, deep cough, and wheezing. The patient has a history of a musculoskeletal disorder. The physician diagnoses bronchial asthma and prescribes a decongestant and inhaler. Code only the bronchial asthma (493.9) because the musculoskeletal disorder has no effect on the present condition.

If the same patient had a history of benign hypertension instead of a musculoskeletal disorder, and the physician evaluated the patient's blood pressure and antihypertensive medication before choosing a decongestant, you would include the benign hypertension code in the second position (401.1). This is because many decongestant medications affect the blood pressure and

Use Additional Code

⑤250.8 Diabetes with other specified manifestations
Diabetic hypoglycemia
Hypoglycemic shock

Use additional code to identify manifestation, as:
any associated ulceration (707.10–707.9)
diabetic bone changes (731.8)

Use additional E code to identify cause, if drug-induced

Figure 4–4. Illustration of coding note directing the coder to use an additional code. (From *International Classification of Diseases, 9th Revision, Clinical Modification*, Volume 1, *Diseases: Tabular List*.)

And/Or

194 Malignant neoplasm of other endocrine glands and related structures
Use additional code, if desired, to identify any functional activity

Excludes: *islets of Langerhans (157.4)*
ovary (183.0)
testis (186.0-186.9)
thymus (164.0)

194.0 Adrenal gland
Adrenal cortex
Adrenal medulla
Suprarenal gland

194.1 Parathyroid gland

194.3 Pituitary gland and craniopharyngeal duct
Craniobuccal pouch
Hypophysis
Rathke's pouch
Sella turcica

194.4 Pineal gland

194.5 Carotid body

194.6 Aortic body and other paraganglia
Coccygeal body
Glomus jugulare
Para-aortic body

Figure 4–5. Illustration of the word "and" appearing in a code description that is interpreted as "and/or." (From *International Classification of Diseases, 9th Revision, Clinical Modification,* Volume 1, *Diseases: Tabular List.*)

the physician would need to take this into consideration when managing the patient's asthma.

Chief Complaint and Primary Diagnosis

In an office setting the main reason for a patient's encounter is called the **chief complaint (CC).** This is usually a **symptom** that has brought the patient to the doctor's office (e.g., "I feel tired all of the time, my arm hurts, this runny nose won't go away"). The chief complaint typically becomes the **primary diagnosis** listed on the insurance claim form and is sometimes a symptom (e.g., headache—784.0), but is preferably stated as a **diagnosis** (e.g., migraine headache—346.90). Code symptoms only if a diagnosis is not documented. After the patient encounter, the physician may be able to make a more specific diagnosis (e.g., intractable cluster migraine headache—346.21). The more specific the diagnosis, the better the chance for maximum payment from the insurance carrier.

Another example would be a patient that presents in the office complaining of low back pain and the physician is not able to formulate a reason for the pain. The primary diagnosis would be the symptom, *low back pain* (724.2). If, however, the physician determines that the reason for the low back pain is muscle strain, then the primary diagnosis would be *lumbar strain* (847.2), and low back pain would not be coded.

Secondary Diagnosis

Up to three additional or concurrent conditions can be listed on the claim form, sequenced after the primary diagnosis. A **concurrent condition** (comorbidity) is one that coexists with the primary condition, complicating the treatment and management of the primary disorder. The **secondary diagnosis** is that which may contribute to the condition, treatment, or recovery from the condition shown as the primary diagnosis. It also may define the need for a higher level of care, but is not the underlying cause.

Etiology and Manifestation

The underlying cause of a disease is referred to as the **etiology** and is sequenced in the first position. Certain conditions are classified according to etiology (cause) and in these cases you should follow the instructions "Code first underlying disease. . ." (see Fig. 4–3). Code the etiology in the first position and the manifestation in the second position. The **manifestation** is the sign or symptom associated with the disease.

Words to look for in the diagnostic statement that may indicate there is an underlying cause include "acquired," "associated with," "congenital," "obstetric,"

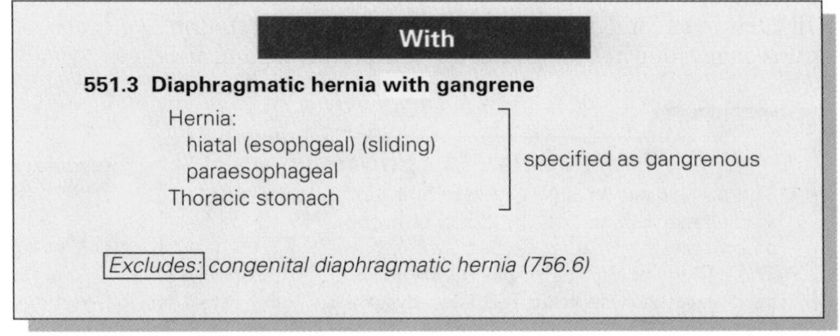
With

551.3 Diaphragmatic hernia with gangrene
Hernia:
hiatal (esophgeal) (sliding)
paraesophageal
Thoracic stomach
} specified as gangrenous

Excludes: *congenital diaphragmatic hernia (756.6)*

Figure 4–6. Illustration of the word "with" appearing in a title indicating that two separate conditions (primary disorder and secondary complication) must be present to use this code. (From *International Classification of Diseases, 9th Revision, Clinical Modification,* Volume 1, *Diseases: Tabular List.*)

"nonobstetric," "transmissible," "not transmissible," "traumatic," and "nontraumatic."

Admitting Diagnosis

When a patient is admitted to a hospital facility, he or she is assigned an *admitting diagnosis*, which is similar to the chief complaint. The inpatient admission diagnosis may be expressed as one of the following.

1. One or more significant findings (signs or symptoms) representing patient distress
2. One or more abnormal findings on examination
3. A diagnosis that has been previously established (during ambulatory care or on a previous hospital admission)
4. An injury
5. A poisoning
6. A reason or condition not classifiable as an illness or injury (e.g., pregnant—in labor, follow-up inpatient diagnostic tests).

Principal Diagnosis

The **principal diagnosis** is the diagnosis obtained after study that prompted the hospitalization. It is possible that the primary and the admitting or principal diagnosis codes may be the same, but not in all cases. It is important to note that the concept of a "principal diagnosis" is only applicable to *inpatient* hospital coding.

When your physician employer makes hospital visits, code the reason for the visit, which may *not* necessarily be the reason the patient was admitted to the hospital.

Signs, Symptoms, and Ill-Defined Conditions

In outpatient coding, *do not code* diagnoses documented as "likely," "probable," "questionable," "rule out," "suspected," or "suspicion of," as if they existed or were established. Instead, code the chief complaint, sign, symptom, abnormal test result, or other reasons for the visit to the highest degree of certainty. A qualified diagnosis is considered a *working diagnosis* that is not yet proven and may be ruled out after study. It is not considered an *active diagnosis*. For example, a patient presents complaining of respiratory difficulty. The physician takes a chest x-ray and documents lung mass, *probable* abscess. Assign code 786.6, mass in chest, which is an abnormal test result, instead of abscess of lung (513.0), because the abscess has not been established and cannot be used as a definitive diagnosis.

Chapter 16 of ICD-9-CM, Symptoms, Signs, and Ill-Defined Conditions (code category 780–799), contains many but not all codes for symptoms. Again, it is preferable not to code from this chapter; however, there are certain situations when it cannot be avoided. The following are instances in which sign and symptom codes may be used.

- No precise diagnosis can be made (see Example 4–1).
- Signs or symptoms are transient, and a specific diagnosis was not made (see Example 4–2).
- Provisional diagnosis for a patient who does not return for further care (see Example 4–3).
- A patient is referred to a specialist before a definite diagnosis is made (see Example 4–4).

Example 4–1

No Precise Diagnosis

- The patient has an enlarged liver, and further diagnostic studies may or may not be done. Use code 789.10 for hepatomegaly.
- The patient complains of painful urination, and the urinalysis is negative. Use code 788.1 for dysuria.

Example 4–2

Transient Symptoms

The patient complains of chest pain on deep inspiration. On examination, the physician finds nothing abnormal and tells the patient to return in 1 week. When the patient returns, the pain has ceased. Use code 786.52 for painful respiration.

Impending or Threatened Condition

Impending or threatened conditions are not the same as conditions that are being ruled out. When the diagnostic statement includes the words "impending or threatened," search for a code that accurately describes the situation (see Example 4–5).

Combination Code

There are instances when two diagnoses are stated within a single code description, referred to as a **combination code** (see Fig. 4–6). Often this occurs when the etiology (cause) and manifestation (symptom) are both recorded in the diagnostic statement. When two diagnoses or a diagnosis with an associated secondary process (manifestation) or complication is present, always search for one code including both. Wording in the combination code description must fully identify both conditions and may include the words "with," "due to," and "in."

Multiple Coding

There are times when it may be necessary to use two or more separate codes to completely describe a given diagnosis. The two conditions listed in the diagnostic statement may or may not be interrelated. Instructions

Example 4–3

Provisional Diagnosis

On examination, the physician documents abnormal percussion of the chest. The patient is sent for a chest x-ray and asked to return for a recheck. The patient does not have the x-ray taken and fails to return. Use code 786.7 for abnormal chest sounds.

Example 4–4

Symptoms

A patient complains of nausea and vomiting and is referred to a gastroenterologist. Use code 787.01 for nausea with vomiting.

Example 4–5

Impending or Threatened Condition

- The patient presents in the emergency department complaining of chest pain, nausea, and diaphoresis. It is suspected that the patient is about to have a myocardial infarction. Use code 411.1 for intermediate coronary syndrome; *impending infarction.*
- A pregnant patient presents in the obstetrician's office complaining of abdominal cramping. She is not sure if she is having contractions. She is 26 weeks' gestation. Use code 644.03 for *threatened premature labor;* antepartum condition.

in the *Tabular List* indicating a separate code may be necessary; include the terms "code also," "use additional code. . .," and "note. . ." Remember, do not code the patient's complaints (symptoms or signs) when a confirmed diagnosis has been made (see Fig. 4–4).

Code Sequencing

To ensure maximum reimbursement, diagnostic codes must be selected and recorded accurately, linked to the proper service or procedure, and listed in the correct order (code sequencing) on the insurance claim form. Codes must be sequenced correctly so that the chronology of patient care events and severity of

Table 4–3 **Sequencing of Diagnostic Codes**

Primary Code	• ICD-9-CM code that defines the most important reason for the encounter; physician must be actively managing condition or problem. • *Italicized codes* that appear in the *Tabular List* may never be sequenced as primary. • Codes in slanted brackets *[ ]* must be sequenced in the order specified in the *Alphabetic Index.*
Secondary Code	• All codes listed after the primary code that describe factors important to the current episode of care. • Any *coexisting* condition complicating the treatment and management of the primary condition.
Acute/Chronic	• Code *acute condition* in the first position. • Code *chronic condition* in the second position.
Etiology and Manifestation	• Code the *etiology* (underlying condition) in the first position. • Code the *manifestation* (sign or symptom) in the second position.
Routine Health Examinations	• Health exams (e.g., V70.1 and V70.3–V70.7) are sequenced in the first position.
Ancillary Diagnostic Services	• Sequence first the problem for which the services are being performed (e.g., V72.5 Radiological exam). The results may be used to determine the diagnosis.
Sterilization	• Encounters for elective sterilization only; sequence V code in the first position (e.g., V25.2). • Patients sterilized subsequent to other services (e.g., after OB delivery); sequence other service first and V code for sterilization second. • Sterilization that occurs as an incidental result from another procedure; only code the condition or disease process that caused the sterilization.
E Codes	• Never sequence an E code in the first position. (Note: E codes are not used on claim forms in outpatient billing.)
Burns	• Code first the site and degree. • Code second the percent of body surface involved. • Sequence the highest degree of burn first.
Surgery	• The postoperative diagnosis becomes the primary diagnosis used for the surgical code.
Preoperative Evaluations	• Patient seen with no specific health problems except surgical diagnosis: use V Code first (V72.8) and surgical diagnosis second. • Patient seen for specific health problem (e.g., cardiac history): code health problem first, and surgical diagnosis second.
Surgery Complications	• Code the complication in the first position. • If the complication can be classified to the 996–999 category (Complications of Surgical and Medical Care, Not Elsewhere Classified), list a code specifying the complication in the second position.
Neoplasm	• Treatment directed at the malignancy: code first. • Mention of invasion, extension, or metastasis to another site: code in second position unless the primary site is unknown, then code in the first position. • Admission for managing a problem associated with a malignancy (e.g., anemia, and the treatment ONLY involved treatment of the anemia): code the problem (anemia) in the first position (principal diagnosis), and the malignancy in the second position. • Encounter or admission for chemotherapy or radiotherapy: use V code first (V58.1, V58.0) and code malignancy second.
Pregnancy, Delivery, Abortion, and the Puerperium	• List codes in Chapter 11 (630–677) first; they have sequencing priority over codes listed from other chapters. Additional codes that further specify conditions may be listed in the second position. • For cesarean deliveries, code first the reason indicating the need for the cesarean section.
Late Effects	• Code the late effect (the reason the patient is seeing the physician) as the primary diagnosis and the cause of the late effect (original injury or illness) in the second position.

disease can be understood. On the insurance claim form there are four possible locations for placement of diagnostic codes referred to as the first, second, third, and fourth positions. Rules and discussion regarding the proper sequencing of diagnostic codes is presented throughout this chapter. Refer to Table 4–3 for a summary of these rules.

Acute/Chronic

The word **acute** means that something has changed in an otherwise stable condition. It usually refers to a condition that runs a short but relatively severe course. The word **chronic** means a condition persisting over a long period of time—a "recurrent" condition. When the terms "acute" or "chronic" are listed in the diagnostic statement, always search for these terms in the code description. When a condition is stated in the diagnosis as both acute (or subacute) and chronic, and separate codes are available for each, use both codes sequencing the acute code in the first position. Only code chronic conditions when the patient receives treatment or when the condition affects current decision making (Fig. 4–7).

Certain diseases need the term "acute" documented to support the medical necessity for hospital admission (e.g., pericarditis, respiratory failure, appendicitis). When a patient is admitted and the physician has not used the term "acute," ask for this additional documentation. Other terms are used with certain diseases to designate change and need for acute hospital admission, such as out-of-control diabetes, unstable angina, or decompensated congestive heart failure. When acute versus chronic is an issue, make sure the documentation makes it clear that the patient is sick *now*.

Acute, Subacute, and Chronic

245 Thyroiditis
245.0 Acute thyroiditis
Abscess of thyroid
Thyroiditis:
nonsuppurative, acute
pyogenic
suppurative
Use additional code to identify organism
245.1 Subacute thyroiditis
Thyroiditis:
deQuervain's
giant cell
Thyroiditis:
granulomatous
viral
245.2 Chronic lymphocytic thyroiditis
Hashimoto's disease
Struma lymphomatosa
Thyroiditis:
autoimmune
lymphocytic (chronic)

Figure 4–7. Illustration of acute, subacute, and chronic code descriptions. (From *International Classification of Diseases, 9th Revision, Clinical Modification,* Volume 1, *Diseases: Tabular List.*)

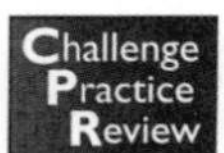

Pause and Practice CPR

REVIEW SESSIONS 4–7 THROUGH 4–15

Directions: *Complete the following questions as a review of information you have just read.*

4–7 NEC stands for (a) ______________________ and is to be used when a separate code describing the disease or injury is (b) ______________________.

4–8 NOS stands for (a) ______________________ and is to be used when (b) ______________________.

4–9 Circle the correct answer. Synonyms are found in the *Tabular List:*

(a) after a colon (:)

(b) enclosed in parentheses ()

(c) enclosed in brackets []

4–10 The main reason for the patient's encounter is referred to as the ______________ ______________ and is sometimes used as the primary diagnosis.

4–11 If a precise diagnosis cannot be made or is not documented, you would code the patient's ______________________.

4–12 How many additional or concurrent conditions may be listed on the insurance claim form?

_______________.

4–13 The etiology (cause) of a disease is sequenced in the _______________ position.

4–14 In which chapter are sign and symptom codes found in ICD-9-CM?

_______________.

4–15 When two diagnoses are stated within a single code description, this is referred to as a/an

_______________ code.

CHECK YOUR HEARTBEAT! Turn to the end of the chapter for answers to these review sessions.

The Coding Process

Diagnostic coders always double-check their work by using both Volume 1 (*Tabular List*) and Volume 2 (*Alphabetic Index*) before assigning a code. Never use just one volume. Begin with the *Alphabetic Index* to locate the main term of the diagnosis, then turn to the code number in the numeric index to verify the code. Some may think that ICD-9-CM is put together backward since you turn to the *Alphabetic Index*—Volume 2—first, then go to the numeric index—Volume 1. Think of ICD-9-CM like any other reference book where you would first look in the index to locate the place in the text where the information is listed and then you would go to the page number to find the information. In ICD-9-CM, you use the index (Volume 2) and then go to the *code number* (instead of the page number) in the numeric listing (Volume 1). Some codebooks show the *Alphabetic Index* first and the *Tabular List* second. You will note, however, that the volume numbers remain the same regardless of where they are located.

Many times you locate a diagnostic code in Volume 2 only to find that the code is the same when verified in Volume 1. As a timesaver, indicate these codes in Volume 2 with a colored highlighter pen to remind you that this code has been verified and is correct as described in Volume 2.

Volume 2—Alphabetic Index

The *Alphabetic Index* has three sections:

- *Section 1* is the index to diseases and injuries and is used most often. This section also contains a table for indexing hypertension codes found under the letter "H," and a table for indexing neoplasm codes found under the letter "N."
- *Section 2* is a table of drugs and chemicals, listed in alphabetical order, which will be discussed later in this chapter.
- *Section 3* is the alphabetical index for E codes which represent the external causes of injury and poisoning. A tab placed in this section will prove useful, not only for locating E codes quickly but also so that you do not end up in this alphabetical listing thinking that you are in the alpha listing for Section 1. Section 3 will also be discussed later in this chapter.

Section 1 of Volume 2

The primary arrangement of Volume 2, Section 1, the alphabetical index of diseases, is by *condition*, referred to as the **main term** of the diagnosis. Volume 2 is structured as follows (Fig. 4–8*A* and *B*):

- *Main terms* are classifications of diseases and injuries and appear as headings in **boldface** type.
- *Subterms* describe differences in etiology, clinical status, and location. They are listed under main terms, indented two spaces to the right.
- *Sub-subterms* are additional listings under subterms and are indented an additional two spaces to the right.
- *Carryover lines* continue the text and are indented more than two spaces from the level of the preceding line.
- *Nonessential modifiers* are enclosed in parentheses and provide additional description. They do not affect the code assignment.

First you must decide what the main term (condition) is for a diagnosis. Table 4–4 shows examples of diagnostic statements with main terms.

Occasionally there is a diagnostic statement where the main term or subterm cannot be found in the *Alphabetic Index*. It may then be necessary to try looking under another term, using a synonym, or looking in a medical dictionary to research unfamiliar terminology. An example of this would be the diagnostic statement "*tear;* capsular portion of the spleen." The main term or condition is the tear; however, if you look in the index you will not find the subterm, spleen, located under the main term, tear. You can locate this code using several methods. Even though the term capsular is an adjective describing the part of the spleen that is torn, it can also be an adjective *describing the tear* (capsular tear). If you look under tear, then capsule, you will find the word spleen, and a note that directs you to look under *laceration*, spleen, capsule. You could also have used injury, another synonym for the word tear, and then looked for the subterm, spleen, and the sub-subterm, tear, capsular; this would have led you to the same code.

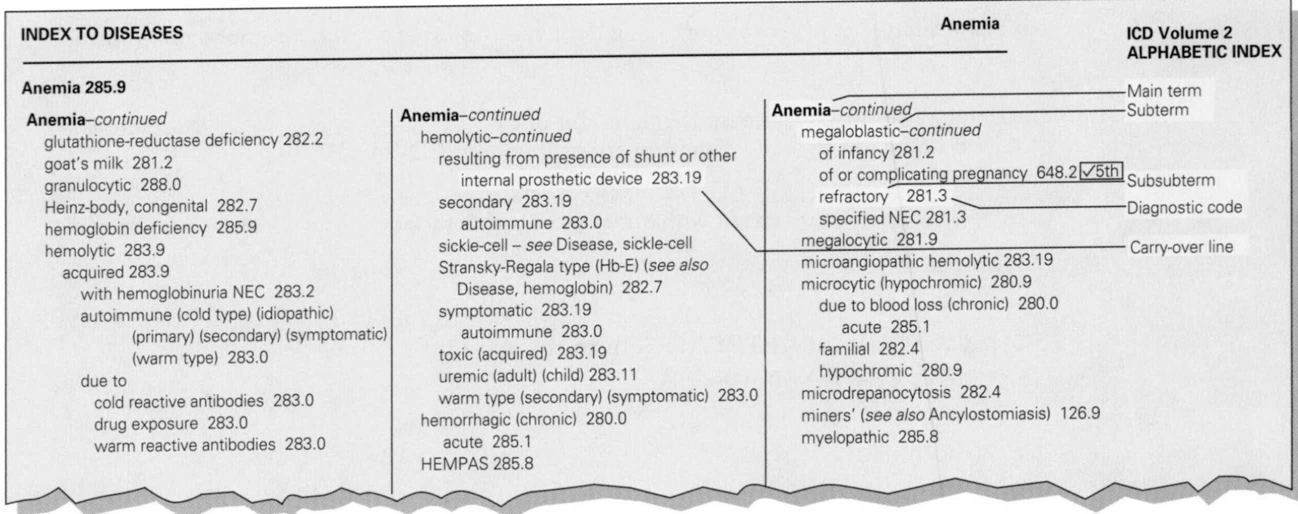
INDEX TO DISEASES

Anemia

ICD Volume 2
ALPHABETIC INDEX

Anemia 285.9

Anemia–*continued*
glutathione-reductase deficiency 282.2
goat's milk 281.2
granulocytic 288.0
Heinz-body, congenital 282.7
hemoglobin deficiency 285.9
hemolytic 283.9
acquired 283.9
with hemoglobinuria NEC 283.2
autoimmune (cold type) (idiopathic) (primary) (secondary) (symptomatic) (warm type) 283.0
due to
cold reactive antibodies 283.0
drug exposure 283.0
warm reactive antibodies 283.0

Anemia–*continued*
hemolytic–*continued*
resulting from presence of shunt or other internal prosthetic device 283.19
secondary 283.19
autoimmune 283.0
sickle-cell – *see* Disease, sickle-cell
Stransky-Regala type (Hb-E) (*see also* Disease, hemoglobin) 282.7
symptomatic 283.19
autoimmune 283.0
toxic (acquired) 283.19
uremic (adult) (child) 283.11
warm type (secondary) (symptomatic) 283.0
hemorrhagic (chronic) 280.0
acute 285.1
HEMPAS 285.8

Anemia–*continued*
megaloblastic–*continued*
of infancy 281.2
of or complicating pregnancy 648.2 ✓5th
refractory 281.3
specified NEC 281.3
megalocytic 281.9
microangiopathic hemolytic 283.19
microcytic (hypochromic) 280.9
due to blood loss (chronic) 280.0
acute 285.1
familial 282.4
hypochromic 280.9
microdrepanocytosis 282.4
miners' (*see also* Ancylostomiasis) 126.9
myelopathic 285.8

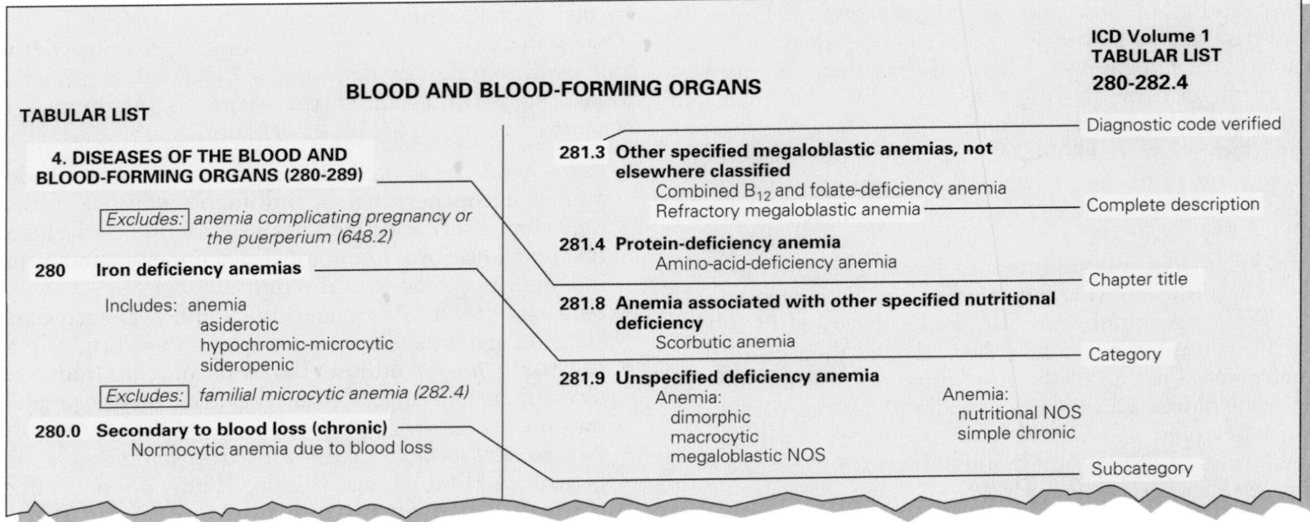
TABULAR LIST

BLOOD AND BLOOD-FORMING ORGANS

ICD Volume 1
TABULAR LIST
280-282.4

4. DISEASES OF THE BLOOD AND BLOOD-FORMING ORGANS (280-289)

Excludes: *anemia complicating pregnancy or the puerperium (648.2)*

280 Iron deficiency anemias
Includes: anemia
asiderotic
hypochromic-microcytic
sideropenic

Excludes: *familial microcytic anemia (282.4)*

280.0 Secondary to blood loss (chronic)
Normocytic anemia due to blood loss

281.3 Other specified megaloblastic anemias, not elsewhere classified
Combined B_{12} and folate-deficiency anemia
Refractory megaloblastic anemia

281.4 Protein-deficiency anemia
Amino-acid-deficiency anemia

281.8 Anemia associated with other specified nutritional deficiency
Scorbutic anemia

281.9 Unspecified deficiency anemia
Anemia:
dimorphic
macrocytic
megaloblastic NOS
Anemia:
nutritional NOS
simple chronic

Figure 4–8. *A* and *B*, Excerpts from *International Classification of Diseases, 9th Revision, Clinical Modification*, Volume 1, *Diseases: Tabular List* and Volume 2: *Diseases: Alphabetic Index.*

Note in Volume 2 that eponyms appear as both main term entries and modifiers under main terms such as "disease" or "syndrome" and "operation." An **eponym** is the name of a disease, structure, operation, or procedure, usually derived from the name of a place or the person(s) who discovered it or described it first.

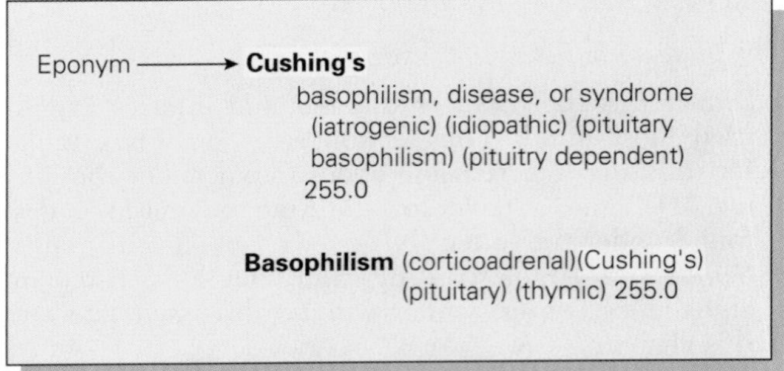

Figure 4–9. Illustration of coding a diagnosis associated with an eponym. (From *International Classification of Diseases, 9th Revision, Clinical Modification*, Volume 2, *Diseases: Alphabetic Index.*)

Table 4–4 Main Terms Found in Diagnostic Statements

Diagnostic Statement	Main Term
Left upper quadrant breast *mass*	mass
Closed *fracture* of the right ulna bone	fracture
Seborrheic infantile *dermatitis*	dermatitis
Vitamin B_{12} *deficiency*	deficiency
Newborn; *perforation* of the intestine	perforation

Three-Digit Code

430 Subarachnoid hemorrage
Meningeal hemorrhage
Ruptured:
berry aneurysm
(congenital) cerebral aneurysm NOS

Excludes: *syphilitic ruptured cerebral aneurysm (094.87)*

Figure 4–10. Illustration of a three-digit code. (From *International Classification of Diseases, 9th Revision, Clinical Modification*, Volume 2, *Diseases: Alphabetic Index*.)

Refer to Figure 4–9 and look at all of the nonessential modifiers (sublisted terms in parentheses) that are associated with the eponym Cushing's.

Occasionally, when the *Alphabetic Index* lists a term that is used in the diagnostic statement (e.g., pericarditis; chronic) and directs you to a code in the *Tabular List* (423.8), the medical term (pericarditis) will not be included in the code description (e.g., 423.8—Other specified diseases of pericardium; calcification/fistula of pericardium). In such cases you have to "trust the index."

Sometimes you have to be a word detective and look under several different locations. In order to keep your frustration level down while learning the common main terms that appear in the index, keep a trail of all the locations that you go to and review which trail led you to the correct code the fastest. This will also help when asked, "How did you find the code?" You will be able to name the signposts on the trail that led you in the right direction. It is easy to get lost in the word forest, so remember to always mark your trail. If a repeat trip is necessary, it will be easier for you to commit the trail to memory and find the right path. A Diagnostic Code Worksheet is available in Appendix F (Form 08). Copy this form and use it each time you code to help document the diagnostic trail.

Volume 1—Tabular List

After locating the code in Volume 2, turn to Volume 1 to verify the code and make sure that you have assigned the highest level of code available. Diagnostic codes can be three, four, or five digits. The more specific the description, the more digits the code has. Always code to the highest degree of specificity. The arrangement of codes in Volume 1 is as follows. Refer to Figure 4–8*B* as you read the descriptions:

- *Chapters*—(17) organized by disease types (many relating to specific body systems) and printed in boldface, uppercase letters followed by a range of codes, listed in parentheses.
- *Sections*—major topic divisions representing a group of related conditions within the chapter, with section title and code ranges for groups of three-digit codes.
- *Categories*—major topics, further divided into three-digit code numbers representing a single condition or disease.
- *Subcategories*—four-digit code numbers representing specific code descriptions that further describe three-digit topics.
- *Fifth-digit subclassifications*—five-digit code numbers representing the most specified code descriptions.

Digit Assignments

A three-digit code may be used only when there are no four-digit codes within the category (Fig. 4–10). When a three-digit code has subdivisions, the appropriate subdivision must be coded. The same is true of four-digit codes. A four-digit code may only be used when there are no five-digit codes within the category. Some insurance carrier computer systems kick out lower-level codes (three-digit codes) and hold the claim forms for medical review, thereby delaying payment or denying such claims altogether. A decimal point is placed after the third digit before adding a fourth or fifth digit; however, this decimal is not included on the insurance claim form. Figure 4–11 illustrates three-, four-, and five-digit codes with descriptions.

Fifth-Digit Locations

The use of five digits is NOT optional; therefore, select a codebook that has the categories clearly marked with references indicating "4th digit needed," or "5th digit needed." Such cross-references may be symbols which are color-coded so fifth digits will not be overlooked. There are several ways that the fifth digit appears in Volume 1. Following is a list describing where in ICD-9-CM this may happen and examples of each:

- At the beginning of a chapter (Fig. 4–12).
- At the beginning of a section (Fig. 4–13).

Three-, Four-, and Five-Digit Code

DISEASES OF THE EAR AND MASTOID PROCESS (380-389)

Three-digit → **380 Disorders of external ear**
Four-digit → ⑤**380.0 Perichondritis of pinna**
Perichondritis of auricle
Five-digit → **380.00 Perichondritis of pinna, unspecified**
380.01 Acute perichondritis of pinna
380.02 Chronic perichondritis of pinna

Figure 4–11. Illustration of three-, four-, and five-digit codes. (From *International Classification of Diseases, 9th Revision, Clinical Modification*, Volume 1, *Diseases: Tabular List*.)

5th Digit At Beginning of Chapter

MUSCULOSKELETAL SYSTEM AND CONNECTIVE TISSUE

13. DISEASES OF THE MUSCULOSKELETAL SYSTEM AND CONNECTIVE TISSUE (710-739)

The following fifth-digit subclassification is for use with categories 711-712, 715-716, 718-719, and 730:

0 site unspecified

1 shoulder region

Acromioclavicular, Glenohumeral, Sternoclavicular, Clavicle, Scapula — joint(s)

2 upper arm

Elbow joint	Humerus

3 forearm

Radius	Wrist joint
Ulna	

4 hand

Carpus	Phalanges (fingers)
Metacarpus	

5 pelvic region and thigh

Buttock	Hip (joint)
Femur	

6 lower leg

Fibula	Patella
Knee joint	Tibia

7 ankle and foot

Ankle joint	Phalanges, foot
digits (toes)	Tarsus
Metatarsus	Other joints in foot

8 other specified sites

Head	Skull
Neck	Trunk
Ribs	Vertebral column

9 multiple sites

Figure 4–12. Illustration of fifth-digit subclassification found at beginning of chapter in *International Classification of Diseases, 9th Revision, Clinical Modification*, Volume 1, *Diseases: Tabular List.*

5th Digit At Beginning of Section

OTHER CONDITIONS ORIGINATING IN THE PERINATAL PERIOD (764-779)

The following fifth-digit subclassification is for use with categories 764-765 to denote birthweight:

0 unspecified (weight)
1 less than 500 grams
2 500-749 grams
3 750-999 grams
4 1,000-1,249 grams
5 1,250-1,499 grams
6 1,500-1,749 grams
7 1,750-1,999 grams
8 2,000-2,499 grams
9 2,500 grams and over

⑤ 764 Slow fetal growth and fetal malnutrtion

Figure 4–13. Illustration of fifth-digit subclassification found at beginning of section in *International Classification of Diseases, 9th Revision, Clinical Modification*, Volume 1, *Diseases: Tabular List.*

5th Digit At Beginning of Three-Digit Category

789 Other Symptoms involving abdomen and pelvis

The following fifth-digit subclassification is to be used or codes 789.0, 789.3, 789.4, 789.6

- **0 unspecified site**
- **1 right upper quadrant**
- **2 left upper quadrant**
- **3 right lower quadrant**
- **4 left lower quadrant**
- **5 periumbilic**
- **6 epigastric**
- **7 generalized**
- **9 other specified site**
  multiple sites

Excludes: symptoms referable to genital organs:
female (625.0-625.9)
male (607.0-608.9)
psychogenic (302.70-302.79)

Figure 4–14. Illustration of fifth-digit subclassification found at beginning of three-digit category in *International Classification of Diseases, 9th Revision, Clinical Modification*, Volume 1, *Diseases: Tabular List.*

- At the beginning of a three-digit category (Fig. 4–14).
- In a four-digit subcategory (Fig. 4–15).

Do not arbitrarily use a zero as a filler character when typing a diagnostic code number. The addition of a zero to a code number that does not require an additional digit can cause a claim to be denied (see Example 4–6).

Example 4–6

Adding an Invalid Digit

Invalid code due to zero added	Valid code
373.20	373.2
496.0	496

Fourth-Digit Subcategories

It should be noted that four-digit subcategories .8 and .9 are usually, but not always, reserved for "other specified" and "unspecified" conditions, respectively (Fig. 4–16). "Other specified (NEC)" and "unspecified (NOS)" subcategories are referred to as *residual subcategories.* As previously described in Table 4–2, residual categories are used for (1) conditions that are specifically named in the medical record but not specifically listed under a code description (NEC), and (2) a diagnostic statement that lacks detail in describing a specific condition (NOS). Be alert when using such fourth-digit subcategories.

Occasionally, a fourth-digit subdivision will appear similar to a fifth-digit subclassification at the beginning of a section (Fig. 4–17). These should be flagged so that they do not go unnoticed.

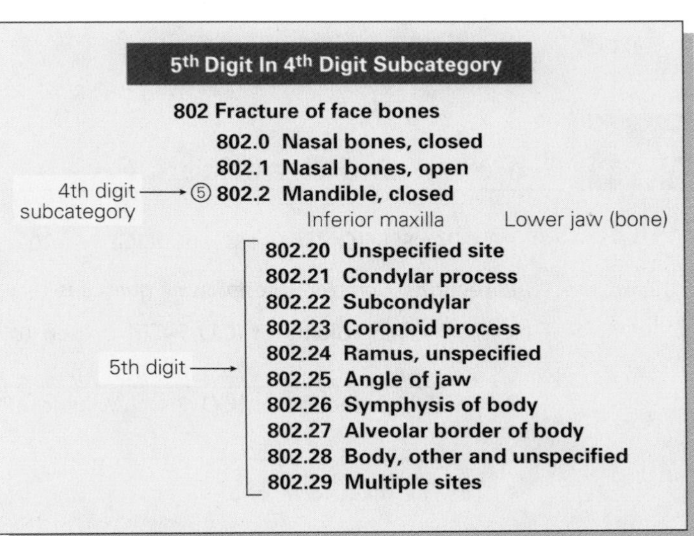

5th Digit In 4th Digit Subcategory

802 Fracture of face bones

802.0 Nasal bones, closed
802.1 Nasal bones, open
4th digit subcategory → ⑤ **802.2 Mandible, closed**
Inferior maxilla Lower jaw (bone)

5th digit →
802.20 Unspecified site
802.21 Condylar process
802.22 Subcondylar
802.23 Coronoid process
802.24 Ramus, unspecified
802.25 Angle of jaw
802.26 Symphysis of body
802.27 Alveolar border of body
802.28 Body, other and unspecified
802.29 Multiple sites

Figure 4–15. Illustration of fifth-digit subclassification found within four-digit subcategory in *International Classification of Diseases, 9th Revision, Clinical Modification*, Volume 1, *Diseases: Tabular List.*

710.4 Polymyositis ← Specified

710.5 Eosinophilia myalgia syndrome ← Specified
Toxic oil syndrome
Use additional E code to identify drug if drug induced

710.8 Other specified difuse diseses of connective tissue ← Other specified
Multifocal firosclerosis (idiopathic) NEC
Systemic fibrosclerosing syndrome

710.9 Unspecified diffuse connective tissue disease ← Unspecified
Collagen disease NOS

Figure 4–16. Illustration of fourth-digit residual subcategories (.8 and .9) representing "other specified," and "unspecified" disease conditions. (From *International Classification of Diseases, 9th Revision, Clinical Modification,* Volume 1, *Diseases: Tabular List.*)

Fourth-Digit Subdivision

OTHER PREGNANCY WITH ABORTIVE OUTCOME (634-639)
Note: Use the following fifth-digit subclassification with categories 634-637:
0 Unspecified
1 Incomplete
2 Complete

The following fourth-digit subdivisions are for use with categories 634-638:

.0 Complicated by genital tract and pelvic infection
Endometriosis
Salpingo-oophoritis
Sepsis NOS
Septicemia NOS
Any condition classifiable to 639.0, with condition classifiable to 634-638
Excludes: *urinary tract infection (634-638 with .7)*

.1 Complicated by delayed or excessive hemorrhage
Afibrinogenemia
Defibrination syndrome
Intravascular hemolysis
Any condition classifiable to 639.1, with condition classifiable to 634-638

.2 Complicated by damage to pelvic organs and tissue
Laceration, performation, or tear of:
bladder
uterus
Any condition classifiable to 639.2, with condition classifiable to 634-638

Figure 4–17. Illustration of fourth-digit subdivision occurring at beginning of section in *International Classification of Diseases, 9th Revision, Clinical Modification,* Volume 1, *Diseases: Tabular List.*

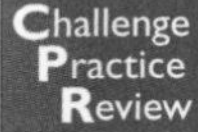

Pause and Practice CPR

REVIEW SESSIONS 4–16 THROUGH 4–20

Directions: *Complete the following questions as a review of information you have just read.*

4–16 Which volume of ICD-9-CM is used to look up the main term of the diagnosis?

____

4–17 Which section of ICD-9-CM, Volume 2 is used most often?

____

4–18 The main term of a diagnosis is the ______________________________.

4–19 When is it acceptable to use a three-digit code? ______________________________

____.

4–20 Which code is most specific?

(a) three-digit

(b) four-digit

(c) five-digit

PRACTICE SESSION 4–21

Directions: *Complete this exercise to develop and enhance your diagnostic coding skills by identifying main terms.*

4–21 Underline the main term in the following diagnostic statements.

(a) peritoneal adhesions

(b) paralytic strabismus

(c) irritable bowel syndrome

(d) iron deficiency anemia

(e) malignant neoplasm of cervical lymph node

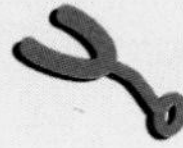

CHECK YOUR HEARTBEAT! Turn to the end of the chapter for answers to these review and practice sessions.

BASIC STEPS IN CODING

Use a standard method and establish a routine for locating diagnostic codes. Refer to Figure 4–10*A* and *B* while following these recommended steps for coding the first diagnosis, *refractory megaloblastic anemia*.

1. Determine the diagnosis, which may be listed on an encounter form or hidden within the patient's medical record and identify the main term (*refractory megaloblastic* **anemia**).
2. Locate the main term in the *Alphabetic Index*, Volume 2 *(anemia)*.
   a. Refer to any notes under the main term *(none shown)*.
   b. Read any nonessential modifiers (notes enclosed in parentheses) following the main term *(none shown)*.
   c. Look for the appropriate subterm and *do not* skip over any subterms indented under the main term *(megaloblastic)*.
   d. Look for the appropriate sub-subterm *(refractory)*.
   e. Follow any cross-reference instructions *(none given)*.
   f. Write down the code *(281.3)*.
3. Verify the code number in the *Tabular List*, Volume 1 *(281.3)*.
   a. Look to see if you are in the correct chapter for the disease being coded *(Diseases of the Blood and Blood-Forming Organs)*.
   b. Read and be guided by all notes and instructional terms that appear by the chapter heading, three-

Example 4–7

Coding Chronic Alcoholic Liver Disease

Step 1. Determine the diagnosis, *chronic alcoholic liver disease,* and identify the main term, *disease.*

Step 2. Look under main term, *disease* (the condition) in Volume 2.
   a. A note states "see also Syndrome" and would be followed if you cannot locate the code.
   b. There are no nonessential modifiers to read.
   c. Find the subterm *liver.*
   d. Locate the sub-subterm *chronic.*
   e. There are no cross-references listed.
   f. Write down the code number 571.3.

Step 3. Verify the code number—not the page number in Volume 1.
   a. Verify you are in the correct chapter, Diseases of the Digestive System.
   b. The three-digit code category is *Chronic liver disease and cirrhosis* (571).
   c. Note, there are no 5th-digit code requirements.
   d. The complete description reads "571.3 Alcoholic liver damage, unspecified." The code and its title refer to any liver damage caused by alcoholism, without specification as to the nature of the disorder. Because there are no exclusion notes, this is the correct code.

Step 4. Assign and record the correct code, 571.3.

digit code category *(281)*, and four-digit code *(281.3)* that may apply to the code you are assigning *(none listed)*.

c. Note fourth- and fifth-digit requirements *(fourth digit required)*.
d. Read complete description of the code you are assigning *(Other specified megaloblastic anemias not elsewhere classified; refractory megaloblastic anemia)*.

4. Assign the diagnostic code and record it on the insurance claim form, proofreading all numbers. The location on the insurance claim form will be covered in Chapter 8 *(281.3)*.

There are no shortcuts. Always consult the code description in the *Tabular List* before assigning a code because additional notes may be included which are not in the *Alphabetic Index*. For each subsequent diagnosis in a patient's medical record, repeat these steps. Let's try one more before you begin your practice session. Refer to Example 4–7 and follow the steps while coding *chronic alcoholic liver disease*.

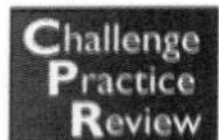

Pause and Practice CPR

REVIEW SESSION 4–22

Directions: *Complete this exercise to review the basic steps in diagnostic coding.*

4–22 Name the four basic steps in diagnostic coding.

1. ______________________
2. ______________________
3. ______________________
4. ______________________

PRACTICE SESSIONS 4–23 THROUGH 4–28

Directions: *Underline the main term and code the following diagnostic statements using your diagnostic codebook.*

4–23 sudden infant death syndrome (SIDS) ____________

4–24 intestinal hernia ____________

4–25 Japanese river fever ____________

Directions: *Code the following diagnostic statements using your diagnostic codebook and assign the correct fifth digit.*

4–26 laceration of spleen with hematoma (without rupture of capsule) ____________

4–27 closed fracture of mandible; multiple sites ____________

4–28 arthralgia of pelvis ____________

CHECK YOUR HEARTBEAT! Turn to the end of the chapter for answers to these review and practice sessions.

Tables

Tables are listed in the *Alphabetic Index*. They help simplify locating codes and expedite the coding process to ensure accuracy in assignment of codes that are similar in nature. Tables are arranged as follows:

- *Main term* is the name of the table under which all subterms and sub-subterms are listed (e.g., Hypertension Table, Neoplasm Table).
- *Subterms* are listed in the first column.
- *Sub-subterms* are listed in successive columns and will contain a code if they apply to the subterm.

Read the forward at the beginning of all tables. Even though these tables make it easier to locate codes, all codes found in tables need to be verified in the *Tabular List*, Volume 1.

Hypertension Table

The medical term *hypertension* is used for the lay term "high blood pressure" (HBP). Elevated blood pressure without the mention of hypertension is coded as a symptom (796.2). See category 642 for coding hypertension in pregnancy.

The Hypertension Table (Fig. 4–18) is a brief table found in the *Alphabetic Index* under the main term "Hypertension." It contains a complete listing of all conditions that are *due to* or *associated with* hypertension. The three headings at the top of the table are defined as:

- *Malignant*—presenting a high risk; considered severe or life-threatening; out of control.
- *Benign*—presenting a low risk; considered mild or non-life-threatening; under control.
- *Unspecified*—indicating the status of malignant or benign is not documented in the diagnostic statement or medical record.

Note the many nonessential modifiers (terms listed in parentheses) found at the beginning of and within this table. Remember that they do not change the meaning of the code, but help the coder locate various terms. The first column lists the subterms of hypertension, such as "accelerated," "antepartum," "cardiorenal," and so forth. The first subterm "with" indicates a second disease process and two codes may be necessary to completely define the diagnosis. Under the subterms you will find sub-subterms with many listings. The remaining three columns serve as a subdivision further defining the type of hypertension as "malignant," "benign," or "unspecified."

Two common forms of hypertension are secondary hypertension, which indicates the hypertension was caused by another primary condition, and essential hypertension, which is benign hypertension for which no cause can be found.

Hypertension can cause various forms of heart and vascular disease as well as other conditions. Hypertensive heart disease refers to the secondary effects on the heart of prolonged hypertension. When the diagnostic

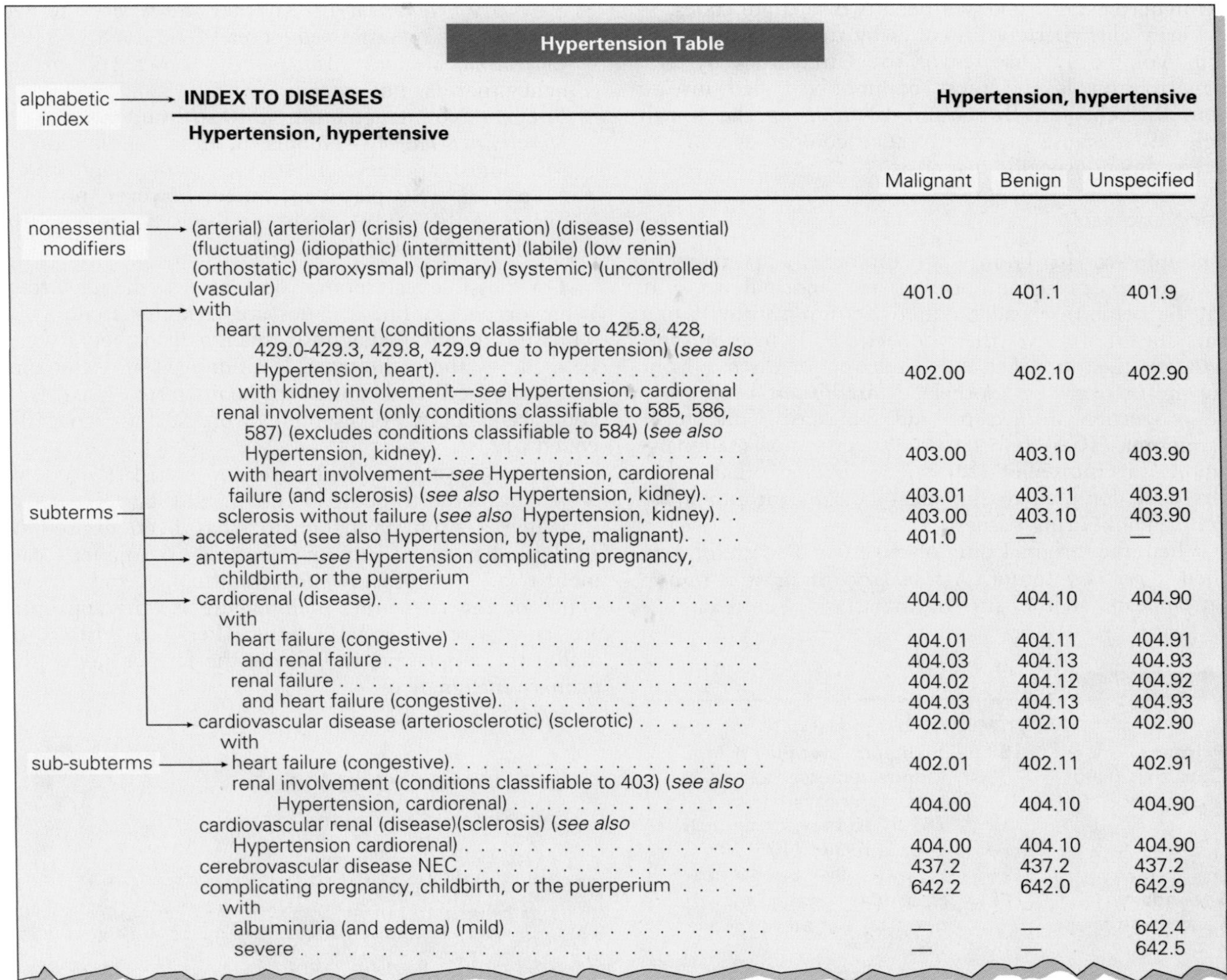

INDEX TO DISEASES — **Hypertension, hypertensive**

Hypertension, hypertensive	Malignant	Benign	Unspecified
(arterial) (arteriolar) (crisis) (degeneration) (disease) (essential) (fluctuating) (idiopathic) (intermittent) (labile) (low renin) (orthostatic) (paroxysmal) (primary) (systemic) (uncontrolled) (vascular)	401.0	401.1	401.9
with			
heart involvement (conditions classifiable to 425.8, 428, 429.0-429.3, 429.8, 429.9 due to hypertension) (*see also* Hypertension, heart)	402.00	402.10	402.90
with kidney involvement—*see* Hypertension, cardiorenal			
renal involvement (only conditions classifiable to 585, 586, 587) (excludes conditions classifiable to 584) (*see also* Hypertension, kidney)	403.00	403.10	403.90
with heart involvement—*see* Hypertension, cardiorenal			
failure (and sclerosis) (*see also* Hypertension, kidney)	403.01	403.11	403.91
sclerosis without failure (*see also* Hypertension, kidney)	403.00	403.10	403.90
accelerated (see also Hypertension, by type, malignant)	401.0	—	—
antepartum—*see* Hypertension complicating pregnancy, childbirth, or the puerperium			
cardiorenal (disease)	404.00	404.10	404.90
with			
heart failure (congestive)	404.01	404.11	404.91
and renal failure	404.03	404.13	404.93
renal failure	404.02	404.12	404.92
and heart failure (congestive)	404.03	404.13	404.93
cardiovascular disease (arteriosclerotic) (sclerotic)	402.00	402.10	402.90
with			
heart failure (congestive)	402.01	402.11	402.91
renal involvement (conditions classifiable to 403) (*see also* Hypertension, cardiorenal)	404.00	404.10	404.90
cardiovascular renal (disease)(sclerosis) (*see also* Hypertension cardiorenal)	404.00	404.10	404.90
cerebrovascular disease NEC	437.2	437.2	437.2
complicating pregnancy, childbirth, or the puerperium	642.2	642.0	642.9
with			
albuminuria (and edema) (mild)	—	—	642.4
severe	—	—	642.5

Figure 4–18. Illustration of hypertension table. (From *International Classification of Diseases, 9th Revision, Clinical Modification*, Volume 2, *Diseases: Alphabetic Index*.)

Expressions from Experience

The work I do is very satisfying. Providing a code to communicate the correct diagnosis is essential and is a large contribution toward the billing service's reimbursement. I also like knowing that I am helping to keep our company in compliance with Medicare by accurately coding services and procedures.

Elizabeth (Betty) Palace
Diagnostic Coder
Medical Billing Company

statement indicates a cause by stating "heart condition *due to* hypertension" or "hypertensive heart disease," use codes 402.0X through 402.9X. If the diagnostic statement reads "*with* hypertension" or "cardiomegaly *and* hypertension," you will need two separate codes.

Verify all hypertension codes by turning to Chapter 7 in Volume 1, Diseases of the Circulatory System. Hypertension is the most commonly coded disease from this chapter. Be careful when using the fourth digit ".9" because many insurance companies will not accept this nonspecific diagnosis.

Neoplasm Table

A **neoplasm,** also known as a tumor, is a spontaneous new growth of tissue forming an abnormal mass. It may be benign or malignant. A **benign tumor** is one that does not have the properties of invasion and *metastasis* (i.e., transfer and spreading of disease from one site or organ to another). A **malignant tumor** has the properties of invasion and metastasis. The term "carcinoma" (CA) refers to a cancerous or malignant tumor. **Carcinoma in situ** refers to cancer that is localized or confined to the site of origin without invasion of neighboring tissues.

When the original site of a tumor is stated, it is called a *primary* tumor. A *secondary* tumor is a tumor that appears at the site of metastasis (see Example 4–8). A diagnostic statement including the words "metastatic from . . . " indicates the site of the primary tumor, whereas "metastatic to . . . " indicates the site of the secondary tumor. If the diagnosis does not mention metastasis, then code a primary tumor. If the diagnostic statement indicates "malignant neoplasm spread to," code the primary site in the first position and the secondary site in the second position. When the phrase "recurrent malignancy" is used in the diagnostic statement, code a primary neoplasm.

Note that lesions are not neoplasms. A lesion is any visible abnormality of tissue such as a boil, rash, sore, or wound. These may be benign or malignant. A cyst is a type of lesion in which a closed sac in or under the skin contains fluid or semisolid material.

The Neoplasm Table includes a comprehensive listing, by anatomic site, found in the *Alphabetic Index* under the main term "Neoplasm" (Table 4–5). The column headings include:

- *Primary (Malignancy)*—Original site of tumor.
- *Secondary (Malignancy)*—Another site where the malignancy has metastasized (spread).
- *Carcinoma in Situ (Malignancy)*—Localized malignancy that has not spread.
- *Benign*—Nonmalignant, noninvasive tumor.
- *Uncertain Behavior*—Neoplasm, after examination by pathologist, appears neither benign nor malignant.
- *Unspecified*—Neoplasm identified; however, no indication of the nature of the tumor is documented in the diagnostic statement.

For possible carcinoma, do not use the uncertain behavior codes. These codes are used for tumors for which no definitive diagnosis (malignant or benign) can be made by the pathologist. If a tumor is suspected and not confirmed, look under the main term "mass" and code accordingly. For example, a breast mass would be coded 611.72.

Anatomic sites marked with an asterisk (*) are always considered to be neoplasms of the skin.

When a primary malignancy has been excised or eradicated from its site, and there is no adjunct treatment (e.g., chemotherapy or radiotherapy) and no evidence of any remaining malignancy, use the appropriate code from the V10 series (Personal history of malignant neoplasms) to indicate the former site of the primary malignancy.

Example 4–8

Primary/Secondary Tumor

Primary Cancerous tumor	**189**	**Malignant neoplasm of kidney** and other and unspecified urinary organs **189.0 Kidney,** except pelvis Kidney NOS Kidney parenchyma
Secondary Cancerous tumor	**198**	**Secondary malignant neoplasm** of other specified sites Excludes: lymph node metastasis (196.0–196.9) **198.0 Kidney**

Expressions from Experience

I wasn't sure that I would secure a job in this field and be able to do what I am now doing. By taking the insurance course it has opened up a whole new world for me; it can happen for you too!

Elizabeth (Betty) Palace
Diagnostic Coder
Medical Billing Company

Table 4–5 Coding Neoplasms

	Malignant				Uncertain	
	Primary	Secondary	Ca in situ	**Benign**	**Behavior**	**Unspecified**
Neoplasm, neoplastic	199.1	199.1	234.9	229.9	238.9	239.9

Note—1 The list below gives the code numbers for neoplasms by anatomic site. For each site there are six possible code numbers according to whether the neoplasm in question is malignant, benign, in situ, of uncertain behavior, or of unspecified nature. The description of the neoplasm will often indicate which of the six columns is appropriate; e.g., malignant melanoma of skin, benign fibroadenoma of breast, carcinoma in situ of cervix uteri.

Where such descriptors are not present, the remainder of the Index should be consulted where guidance is given to the appropriate column for each morphologic (histologic) variety listed; e.g., Mesonephroma—see Neoplasm, malignant; Embryoma—see also Neoplasm, uncertain behavior; Disease, Bowen's—see Neoplasm, skin, in situ. However, the guidance in the Index can be overridden if one of the descriptors mentioned above is present, e.g., malignant adenoma of colon is coded to 153.9 and not to 211.3 as the adjective "malignant" overrides the Index entry "Adenoma—see also Neoplasm, benign."

Note—2 Sites marked with the sign * (e.g., face NEC*) should be classified to malignant neoplasm of skin of these sites if the variety of neoplasm is a squamous cell carcinoma or an epidermoid carcinoma, and to benign neoplasm of skin of these sites if the variety of neoplasm is a papilloma (any type).

	Primary	Secondary	Ca in situ	Benign	Uncertain Behavior	Unspecified
abdomen, abdominal	195.2	198.89	234.8	229.8	238.8	239.8
cavity	195.2	198.89	234.8	229.8	238.8	238.8
organ	195.2	198.89	234.8	229.8	238.8	238.8
viscera	195.2	198.89	234.8	229.8	238.8	239.8
wall	173.5	198.2	232.5	216.5	238.2	239.2
connective tissue	171.5	198.89	—	215.5	238.1	239.2
abdominopelvic	195.8	198.89	234.8	229.8	238.8	239.8

Table of Drugs and Chemicals

The Table of Drugs and Chemicals is found in Section 2 of the *Alphabetic Index* (Table 4–6). It contains a classification of drugs and other chemical substances listed in alphabetical order in column 1. Corresponding codes, listed under the heading "Poisoning" in column 2, are used when there is a state of poisoning, overdose, wrong substance given or taken, or intoxication. The remaining five columns categorize associated E codes used to indicate the external causes of adverse effects.

Adverse effects are unfavorable, detrimental, or pathologic reactions to a drug that occur when appropriate doses are given to humans for prophylaxis (prevention of disease), diagnosis, or therapy (Example 4–9). When an adverse reaction occurs (i.e., drug reaction, hypersensitivity, drug intolerance), a code is assigned (from the Index to Diseases—Volume 2) to the diagnosis that classifies the specific reaction or symptom (e.g., dermatitis, syncope, tachycardia, urticaria). An E code, identifying the chemical substance involved, is selected from the Therapeutic Use column.

The headings at the top of the table are defined as:

- *Poisoning*—indicates a condition resulting from an intentional overdose of drugs or chemical substances or from the wrong drug or agent given or taken in error. Refer to Example 4–10 for poisoning examples and coding a poisoning case scenario.

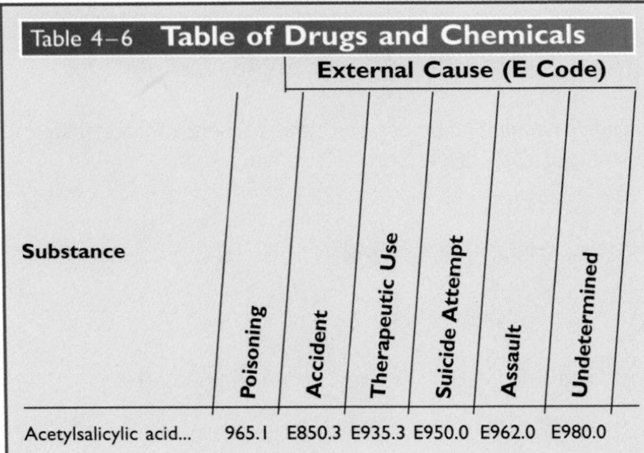

Table 4–6 Table of Drugs and Chemicals

		External Cause (E Code)				
Substance	**Poisoning**	**Accident**	**Therapeutic Use**	**Suicide Attempt**	**Assault**	**Undetermined**
Acetylsalicylic acid...	965.1	E850.3	E935.3	E950.0	E962.0	E980.0

Example 4–9

Coding an Adverse Effect

The patient had an adverse effect (ventricular fibrillation) to the medication digoxin, which was prescribed by her physician and taken correctly.

Step 1.	Refer to the Table of Drugs and Chemicals in Volume 2 and look up *digoxin.*
Step 2.	Because this medication was for *therapeutic use,* locate the correct E code number under that column.
Step 3.	The correct number is *E942.1.*
Step 4.	Locate the main term *fibrillation* in the Index to Diseases.
Step 5.	Find the subterm *ventricular.*
Step 6.	The correct code number is *427.41.*
Step 7.	*Verify* the code number 427.41 in Volume 1, *Tabular Listing.*

Sequencing: 427.41 Ventricular fibrillation (chief complaint)
E942.1 Therapeutic use, Digoxin

Note: For outpatient billing, the E code would not be listed.

Example 4–10

Poisoning Examples

- Taking the wrong medication
- Receiving the wrong medication
- Taking the wrong dose of the right medication
- Receiving the wrong dose of the right medication
- Ingesting a chemical substance not intended for human consumption
- Overdose of a chemical substance (drug)
- Prescription drug taken with alcohol
- Mixing prescription drugs and over-the-counter medications without the physician's advice or consent

Coding a Poisoning

Scenario: Baby Kathy got into the kitchen cabinet and ingested liquid household ammonia.

Step 1.	Refer to the Table of Drugs and Chemicals in Volume 2 and look up *ammonia.*
Step 2.	Find the subterm *liquid (household).*
Step 3.	Since this is a case of ingesting a chemical substance not intended for human use, locate the code number under the *Poisoning* column.
Step 4.	Write down the code number *983.2.*
Step 5.	Since this was an accident, locate the E code in the *Accident* column (*E861.4*).

Sequencing: 983.2 Poisoning, ammonia
E861.4 Poisoning, accidental, ammonia

Note: The manifestation (outcome of the poisoning, e.g., nausea and vomiting) would be coded in the first position if documented in the medical record. For outpatient billing, the E code would not be listed.

The following headings represent external causes in which E codes are used:

- *Accident (External Cause)*—indicates accidental overdose, wrong substance given or taken, and to show external causes of poisonings. Unless the medical record clearly states otherwise, use a code from this column.
- *Therapeutic Use (External Cause)*—indicates the correct substance given or taken that caused an adverse effect. This may be documented in the medical record as *intoxication* when a drug, such as digitalis, reaches a toxic level in the patient's bloodstream and causes an adverse reaction.
- *Suicide Attempt (External Cause)*—indicates a self-inflicted poisoning.
- *Assault (External Cause)*—indicates a poisoning that has been inflicted by another person intending to harm or kill.
- *Undetermined (External Cause)*—indicates that the medical record does not state whether the poisoning was accidental or intentional.

Never use a poisoning code with a code from the Therapeutic Use column and never sequence an E code in the first position.

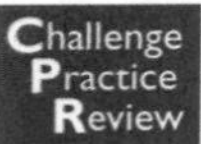

Pause and Practice CPR

PRACTICE SESSIONS 4–29 THROUGH 4–34

Directions: *Use your diagnostic codebook and code the following scenarios using the tables listed in Volume 2, the Alphabetic Index.*

4–29 Benign hypertension. ____________

4–30 Benign hypertension complicating pregnancy with chronic preeclampsia. ____________

4–31 Malignant neoplasm of the urinary bladder; anterior wall. ____________

4–32 Primary liver cancer. ____________

For the next two problems, find the code for the type of "poisoning" that occurred and sequence in the first position. Locate the code for the external cause (E code) and code in the second position.

4–33 Accidental overdose of Valium. (1) ____________ (2) ____________

4–34 Toxic level of Dilantin in patient's blood; patient took correct dosage. (1) ____________ (2) ____________

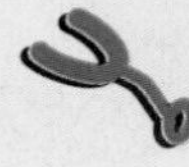

CHECK YOUR HEARTBEAT! Turn to the end of the chapter for answers to these practice sessions.

CODING SPECIAL CONDITIONS

For additional instruction and practice coding special conditions such as: (1) diabetes mellitus, (2) diseases of the circulatory system (myocardial infarction, arteriosclerotic cardiovascular disease, and arteriosclerotic heart disease), (3) pregnancy, delivery, abortion, and the puerperium, (4) injury and poisoning, (5) late effects, and (6) burns, go to the web site http://www.wbsaunders.com/merlin/fordney/insurance/.

SUPPLEMENTARY CLASSIFICATIONS

V Codes

V codes are supplementary classifications of codes located in a separate section at the end of Volume 1, *Tabular List.* In Volume 2, the V codes are included in the major section of the *Alphabetic Index* and are used for the following circumstances:

1. When a person who is not currently sick encounters health services for some specific purpose (e.g., vaccination).
2. When a patient presents for a specific treatment of a known condition or disease (e.g., chemotherapy, cast change, dialysis).
3. When a patient's health status is influenced by some circumstance which is not in itself a current injury or illness (e.g., family history of coronary artery disease, personal history of tobacco use).

Following is a list of common encounters, with main terms italicized, to help you become familiar with key terms and locate codes which fall into this category:

- *admission* for elective surgery (e.g., breast augmentation, face-lift)
- *circumcision*
- *consultation* or *counseling* regarding a problem that is not in itself a disease or injury
- *family* planning
- *history* of disorder or disease (personal or family)
- nursing home *evaluation*
- *observation* of a suspected disease (e.g., cardiovascular, mental, neoplasm)
- occupational health *examination*
- preoperative *examination*
- *problem* (e.g., marital, occupational, thumb-sucking)
- routine annual physical *examination*
- *screening* for cholesterol
- sterilization (*contraception*)
- *supervision of* normal *pregnancy*
- tissue or organ *donor*
- *vaccination*
- well-baby *checkup*

In the above examples, the V code would be sequenced in the first position as long as the patient was not seen for an active illness or injury. Be cautious when using V codes as second or third diagnoses because the claim will be automatically rejected by Medicare and possibly other insurance companies that adopt Medicare policies.

Preoperative Evaluations

For patients receiving preoperative clearance who have no known health problems besides the surgical diagnosis, use a code from subcategory V72.8 to describe the preoperative (pre-op) consultation, sequenced in the first position. Use the surgical diagnostic code in the second position (see Scenario A in Example 4–11).

For patients receiving preoperative clearance because of a known health problem (besides the surgical diagnosis), code the known health problem in the first position and use the surgical diagnostic code in the second position (see Scenario B in Example 4–11).

E Codes

A second, supplementary classification contains E codes which are located in a separate section of Volume 1, *Tabular List* following V codes. In Volume 2, at the very end of the text, a separate E code index entitled Index to External Causes of Injury and Poisoning is located following the regular *Alphabetic Index.*

E codes are used to code the reason for an injury or poisoning. This is referred to as the external cause. Their use provides data for research and prevention of injuries and poisonings. The *cause, intent,* and *place* where the injury or poisoning occurred are provided in code descriptions. E codes are not used to describe the

Example 4–11

Preoperative Clearance

Scenario A: Dr. Practon sends Mr. Montoya to Dr. Cardi for cardiac clearance before his gallbladder surgery. Mr. Montoya has no known health problems other than cholelithiasis with cholecystitis. Dr. Cardi would code Mr. Montoya's visit as follows:

V72.81	Preoperative cardiovascular examination (type of clearance)
574.10	Cholelithiasis with cholecystitis (reason for surgery)

Scenario B: Dr. Caesar sends Mrs. Genovese to Dr. Coccidioides for pulmonary clearance before her hysterectomy which is being performed due to bleeding uterine fibroids. She has a history of late-onset asthma and has been experiencing an active cough with some difficulty breathing for the past 2 months. Dr. Caesar would code Mrs. Genovese's visit as follows:

493.10	Intrinsic (late-onset) asthma (current health problem which is being evaluated prior to surgery)
218.9	Leiomyoma (fibroid) of uterus, unspecified (reason for surgery)

Note: V72.82 (preoperative respiratory examination would not be used in Scenario B because the patient has a known health problem).

primary reason for the patient's visit. The use of an E code after the primary or other acute secondary diagnosis explains the mechanism of the injury or poisoning. By doing this, it provides a more descriptive clinical picture for the insurance carrier. Some states and insurance companies do not accept E codes and generally E codes are not used for insurance claims submitted by physicians' offices. They are considered optional and do not affect third party payment; however, some physicians may decide to use them for thoroughness when documenting a case, especially workers' compensation and personal injury cases. The use of E codes for coding adverse effects of drugs and chemicals has already been discussed along with the Table of Drugs and Chemicals earlier in this chapter. Instructions are included here for additional knowledge about the classification system.

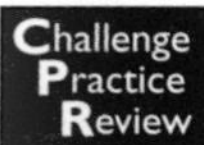

Pause and Practice CPR

PRACTICE SESSIONS 4–35 THROUGH 4–39

Directions: *Use your diagnostic codebook and code the following supplementary classification problems.*

4–35 Family history of schizophrenia ____________

4–36 MMR vaccination (mumps, measles, and rubella) ____________

4–37 Fall from balcony ____________

4–38 Child abused by stepfather ____________

4–39 Circular saw accident ____________

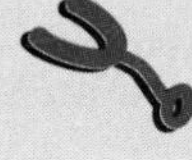

CHECK YOUR HEARTBEAT! Turn to the end of the chapter for answers to these practice sessions.

ICD-10-CM DIAGNOSIS AND PROCEDURE CODES

Now that you have learned the basics of ICD-9-CM coding, let's take a brief look at the revolutionary new system (ICD-10-CM) which will eventually replace ICD-9-CM.

For the past 20 years the ICD-9-CM diagnostic coding system has been used. Although it has been updated, the system has outlived its usefulness due to advances in technology, discovery of new diseases, development of new procedures, and the need to report more details for statistical purposes. The time is fast approaching to adopt another system. Actually, there are two systems:

1. *International Classification of Diseases, 10th Revision, Clinical Modification*, ICD-10-CM (will replace ICD-9-CM, Volumes 1 and 2—diagnostic codes)
2. *International Classification of Diseases, 10th Revision, Procedure Coding System*, ICD-10-PCS (will replace ICD-9-CM, Volume 3—hospital procedure codes; will not replace CPT)

Both outpatient and hospital insurance billers need to be concerned with the new diagnosis codes, but only hospital billers need to concern themselves with the procedure codes. Changes in ICD-10-CM include:

1. Organization overhaul
2. Expansion of codes (50% more codes than ICD-9-CM)
3. New chapters (V and E codes are featured in separate chapters)
4. New categories
5. Six-digit alphanumeric codes with greater specificity of site (see Example 4–12)

Example 4–12

ICD-9-CM

Fracture of Upper Limb (810–819)

810 Fracture of clavicle

Includes: collar bone
interligamentous part of clavicle

The following fifth-digit subclassification is for use with category 810:

0 unspecified part
Clavicle NOS
1 sternal end of clavicle
2 shaft of clavicle
3 acromial end of clavicle

✓5th **810.0 Closed**

ICD-10-CM

S42.00 Closed Fracture of Clavicle
S42.001 Closed Fracture of Right Clavicle
S42.002 Closed Fracture of Left Clavicle
S42.009 Closed Fracture of Clavicle, Unspecified Side

6. Expansion of notes and instruction
7. Room for expansion as new codes are assigned

This new system allows more code choices and requires more documentation in the medical record. A coder must have a higher level of clinical knowledge to work with ICD-10-CM. It would be wise to attend an anatomy and physiology course, if you have not done so, to prepare for the new coding manual.

As of the publication of this worktext, ICD-10-CM is to be implemented before 2003. ICD-10-PCS will follow after that. The Centers for Medicare and Medicaid Services (CMS) must give 2 years' notice before changing any code set. The next edition of this worktext will feature how to code using ICD-10-CM.

SUMMATION AND PREVIEW

Diagnostic coding affects the payment process by giving the insurance carrier a clear picture of what the patient has been seen and treated for. The financial status of the physician's office is also affected by employing an experienced, accurate coder. The best way to learn how to code is to practice. Refer to the coding conventions that were presented in this chapter, as well as the figures, examples, and tables, to help in future coding. As you develop as a coder, your goal is to be accurate, meticulous, and as specific as possible.

In the next chapter, you will learn how to code procedures and services that will eventually link on the insurance claim form to the diagnostic codes that represent the reason the patient was seen.

GOLDEN RULE

Code to the highest level of specificity.

Chapter 4 Review and Practice

Study Session

Directions: Review the objectives, key terms, and chapter information before completing the following questions. Fill in the blank or circle the correct answer. Refer to your diagnostic codebook when necessary.

4–1 Name four consequences if diagnostic codes are not used on physician claim forms.

(a) ______________________________

(b) ______________________________

(c) ______________________________

(d) ______________________________

4–2 Relating and connecting a diagnosis to a procedure is referred to as ____________________ ____________________.

4–3 Name the two volumes of ICD-9-CM that are used in the physician's office for coding diagnoses.

(a) ______________________________

(b) ______________________________

4–4 When the physician's statement lacks sufficient detail to assign a specific code, which of the following type of codes must be used?

a. NOS code

b. NEC code

c. Nonessential modifier

4–5 Parentheses found in the *Tabular List* and *Alphabetic Index* are used to enclose supplementary, descriptive words that do not affect the code assignment and are referred to as ______________________________.

4–6 Maximum payment from an insurance carrier is dependent on a ____________________ diagnosis.

4–7 A condition that coexists with the primary condition, complicating the treatment and management of the primary disorder, is referred to as a/an ______________________________.

4–8 A disorder that may contribute to the condition, treatment, or recovery from the condition shown as the primary diagnosis is called the ______________________________.

4–9 The underlying *cause* of a disease is referred to as the ______________________________.

4–10 The sign or symptom associated with a disease is also referred to as the ____________________ of the disease.

4–11 When a patient is admitted to a hospital facility, he or she is first assigned a/an ____________________ diagnosis, which is similar to the chief complaint in an outpatient setting.

4–12 A diagnosis, obtained after study, that prompted a patient's hospitalization is referred to as a/an ______________________________ diagnosis.

4–13 List some terms that precede a qualified diagnosis that is not yet proven.

(a) ______________________________

(b) ______________________________

(c) ______________________________

(d) ______________________________

(e) ______________________________

4–14 How many locations are provided on the insurance claim form to list diagnostic codes?

____

4–15 Diagnoses are found in the *Alphabetic Index* of ICD-9-CM under the ______________________ ______________________ in the diagnostic statement.

4–16 Define an eponym. ____

____

____

4–17 The use of five digits is not optional.

(a) true

(b) false

4–18 All fifth-digit categories appear at the beginning of the chapter.

(a) true

(b) false

4–19 NEC and NOS categories are referred to as ______________________________ subcategories.

4–20 Which volume contains the Hypertension Table, Neoplasm Table, and the Table of Drugs and Chemicals? ____

4–21 List the three reasons why a V code is used.

(1) ____

____

(2) ____

____

(3) ____

____

4–22 Describe what the supplementary classification of E codes are used for.

____

4–23 Name the new diagnostic coding system that will eventually replace ICD-9-CM in the physician's office. ____

4–24 What course is suggested to help a coder prepare for ICD-10-CM?

____

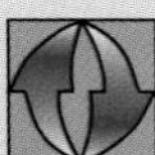

Exercise Exchange

Directions: *Use the diagnostic codebook to locate the correct code(s) for the following exercises. A Diagnostic Code Worksheet is found in Appendix F (Form 08) to assist in writing down the main term and recording the trail that you take to select a code. After scoring the exercises, use the Assignment Score Sheet found in Appendix F (Form 10) to weigh your success. Perform an examination to review areas of deficiency, clarify coding rules, and rehearse new skills when needed.*

4–1 abnormal blood level of iron 790.6

4–2 missed abortion 632

4–3 cornea abrasion 918.1

4–4 abscess in left axilla region 682.3

4–5 congenital stenosis of cervical canal 752.49

4–6 acute cerebrovascular accident (CVA) ______

4–7 erythematosa acne 695.3

4–8 Bell's palsy facial paralysis 351.0

4–9 calcification of shoulder joint 719.81

4–10 tension headache 307.81

4–11 cleft lip with cleft palate 749.20

4–12 Christmas disease 286.1

4–13 dysplasia of cervix (uteri) 621.6

4–14 pitting edema of bilateral ankles ______

4–15 gastrojejunocolic fistula ______

4–16 abnormal weight loss ______

4–17 primary malignant neoplasm of ovary ______

4–18 fetal eye damage caused by forceps delivery ______

4–19 kyphosis due to tuberculosis of spine ______

4–20 familial cardiomyopathy due to Chagas' disease ______

V CODES

4–21 special screening examination for heavy metal (chemical) poisoning ______

4–22 special screening for sickle cell anemia ______

4–23 routine infant well-baby health checkup ______

4–24 antenatal screening ______

4–25 routine laboratory examination (adult) ______

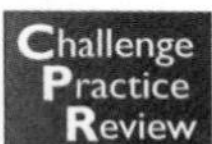

CPR Session: Answers

REVIEW SESSIONS 4–1 THROUGH 4–6

4–1 Takes up less space and provides standardized descriptions of information
4–2 (a) classifying morbidity (sickness)
(b) classifying causes of mortality (death)
(c) evaluating hospital service utilization
(d) medical research
4–3 (a) cardiovascular services
(b) imaging services
(c) laboratory services
(d) neurologic services
(e) vitamin B_{12} injections
4–4 three
4–5 yearly, each October
4–6 (a) Hypertension Table
(b) Neoplasm Table

REVIEW SESSIONS 4–7 THROUGH 4–15

4–7 (a) not elsewhere classifiable
(b) not listed in the code manual
4–8 (a) not otherwise specified
(b) the physician's diagnostic statement lacks sufficient detail to be able to assign a code
(c) NOS (not otherwise specified) code
4–9 (c) brackets [ ]
4–10 chief complaint
4–11 chief complaint, sign, symptom, abnormal test result
4–12 up to three
4–13 first
4–14 Chapter 16
4–15 combination

REVIEW SESSIONS 4–16 THROUGH 4–20

4–16 Volume 2, *Alphabetic Index*
4–17 Section 1, Index to Diseases and Injuries
4–18 condition
4–19 When there is no four-digit code available within the category
4–20 (c) five-digit

PRACTICE SESSION 4–21

4–21 (a) peritoneal *adhesions*
(b) paralytic *strabismus*
(c) irritable bowel *syndrome*
(d) iron deficiency *anemia*
(e) malignant *neoplasm* of cervical lymph node

REVIEW SESSION 4–22

4–22 (1) Determine the diagnosis and identify the main term
(2) Locate term in the *Alphabetic Index*, Volume 2
(3) Verify code in the *Tabular List*, Volume 1
(4) Assign and record the diagnostic code on the insurance claim form

PRACTICE SESSIONS 4–23 THROUGH 4–28

4–23 death (condition), syndrome (condition) 798.0
4–24 hernia (condition) 553.9
4–25 fever (condition), Japanese (eponym) 081.2
4–26 laceration (condition) 865.01 *Note: Since there was no mention of open wound into cavity, the fourth digit would be "0"*
4–27 fracture (condition) 802.29
4–28 arthralgia (condition—note sends you to Pain, joint) 719.45 *Note: the fifth digit determines the anatomic site (location).*

PRACTICE SESSIONS 4–29 THROUGH 4–34

4–29 401.1
4–30 642.7
4–31 188.3
4–32 155.0
4–33 (1) 969.4 [accidental overdose—poisoning]
(2) E853.2 [accident]
4–34 (1) 966.1 [poisoning by receiving toxic level]
(2) E936.1 [therapeutic use]

PRACTICE SESSIONS 4–35 THROUGH 4–39

4–35V17.0
4–36 V06.4
4–37 E882
4–38 E967.0
4–39 E919.4

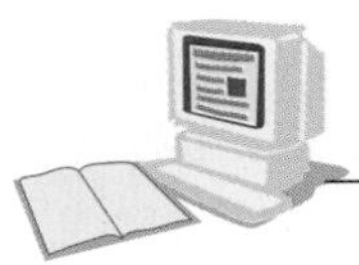

Resources

You may want to research a career as a diagnostic coder. A reference for self-employment coding is:

- *Independent Medical Coding,* Donna Avila-Weil and Rhonda Regan, 1999, Rayve Productions, Inc., Windsor, CA (800) 852-4890.

A diagnostic coder relies on resource material for coding guidelines, updates, and code linkage references. Coding questions can be answered by using the following instructions and diagnostic code web sites:

(1) Match your question with the query language for the site you are using. The information that details the language for the site usually precedes the search button. A common mistake is the use of quotations and words such as "and," "or," or "the."
(2) Query several databases.
(3) After locating an answer, be sure there is no contradictory authority with greater weight, e.g., CMS may have issued a regulation that supersedes the insurance carrier's manual.

Diagnostic Code Web Sites

- Central Office for ICD-9-CM
  Web Site: http://www.icd-9-cm.org/
- Federal Register
  Web Site: http://www.nara.gov/fedreg

Coding Questions

- Listserv (subscribe and communicate via e-mail)
  Web address:
  PARTB-L@USALNET
- ICD-9-CM Coding Handbook with Answers, Faye Brown, American Hospital Association, Chicago, IL (800) 242-2626
- Medicare Coding Questions
  Web Site:
  http://www.partbnews.com/enroll

Coding Guidelines

- Central Office on ICD-9-CM of the American Hospital Association (312) 422-3000

Newsletters

- *Coding Clinic,* American Hospital Association, 1 North Franklin, Chicago, IL 60606 (800) 242-2626
- *American Health Information Management Association Journal,* American Health Information Management Association, 233 North Michigan Avenue, Suite 2150, Chicago, IL 60601-5519 (800) 335-5535

Reference Books

- *St. Anthony's Medicare National Correct Coding Guide,* St. Anthony/Ingenix Publishing Group, P.O. Box 96561, Washington, DC 20090 (800) 632-0123
- *St. Anthony's Medicare Correct Coding and Payment Manual for Procedures and Services* St. Anthony/Ingenix Publishing Group, P.O. Box 96561, Washington, DC 20090 (800) 632-0123

Diagnostic Code Book

ICD-9-CM—available from a variety of publishers including the following:

- Channel Publishing Ltd., 4750 Longley Lane, Suite 110, Reno, NV 89502 (800) 248-2882
- Practice Management Information Corporation (PMIC), 4727 Wilshire Blvd., Suite 300, Los Angeles, CA 90010, (800) MED-SHOP
- St. Anthony/Ingenix Publishing Group, P.O. Box 96561, Washington, DC 20090 (800) 632-0123

NOTES

Objectives

After reading this chapter and completing the exercise sessions, you should be able to:

Learning Objectives:

- ✔ Explain the purpose of coding professional services.
- ✔ List the sections of CPT.
- ✔ Write a definition for evaluation and management services.
- ✔ Name the key components of evaluation and management services.
- ✔ State when a modifier should be applied to a CPT code.
- ✔ Explain the difference between consultation and counseling services.
- ✔ Define critical care and emergency care.
- ✔ Indicate reasons a patient would be seen for preventive medicine.

Performance Objectives:

- ✔ Demonstrate how to determine the level of service for evaluation and management encounters.
- ✔ Code evaluation and management services.

Key Terms

consultation
counseling
critical care
Current Procedural Terminology (CPT)
emergency
emergency care
established patient
Evaluation and Management (E/M) services
Health Care Financing Common Procedure Coding System (HCPCS)
inpatient
key components
modifier
National Drug Code (NDC)
new patient
observation status
outpatient
preventive medicine
procedure coding
Prolonged Services
referral

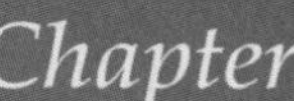

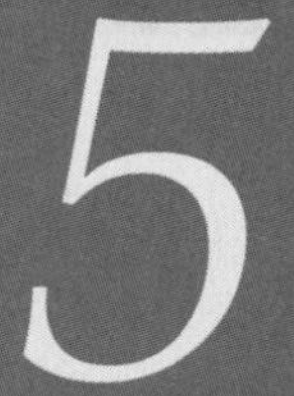

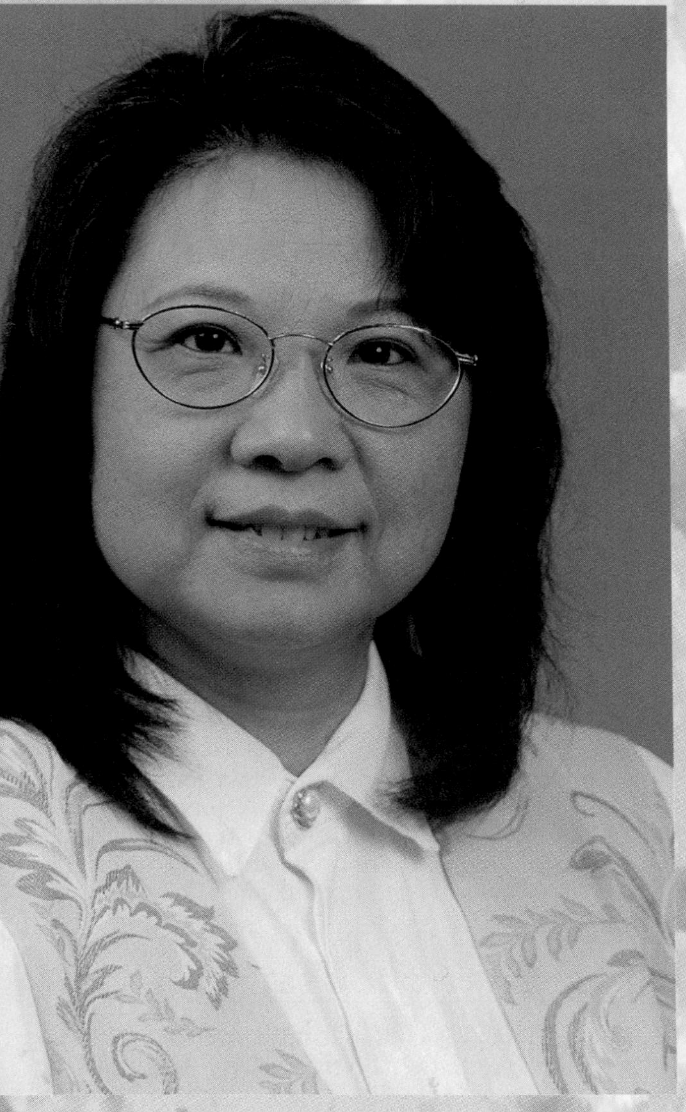

I came to this country as a foreign student from Hong Kong and when my husband became ill I realized I didn't have any employment skills. I enrolled at an occupational center to learn a trade and chose the medical field because everyone gets sick, so there would always be a need for workers. I work as a ward clerk/transcriptionist in the emergency room of an HMO hospital.

One day the manager asked me to help with the non-member billing. Staff physicians were struggling with a new "encounter coding record" and I wanted to learn more about it, so I enrolled in a medical insurance billing class. I soon began verifying the encounter coding record to make sure all entries were correct. Medical coding is really fun, just like solving a puzzle! I'm glad that I had an opportunity to apply what I learned at my workplace.

Katrina Ginn
Ward Clerk/Transcriptionist
Hospital Emergency Room

Coding Procedures Part I:

Introduction and Evaluation and Management Services

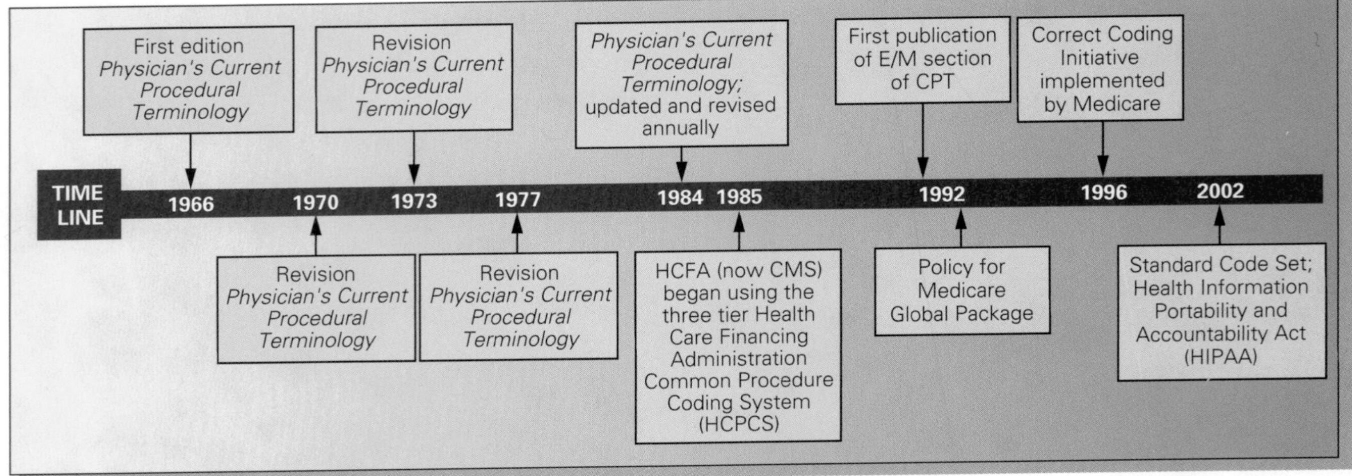

THE IMPORTANCE OF PROCEDURE CODING

Now that you have learned some insurance terminology and the basics of diagnostic coding, the next step is to learn how to code procedures. **Procedure coding** is a standardized method used to transform written descriptions of procedures and professional services into numeric designations (code numbers). Procedure code descriptions precisely define services provided by physicians and allied health professionals. The code numbers are inserted on an insurance claim form which is optically scanned by insurance companies. The general acceptance of the codes by insurance carriers and government agencies assures the physician who uses a standardized coding system that the services and procedures he or she performs can be objectively identified and priced. Even though coding is standardized, it is an art, not an exact science. Because individual viewpoints differ, interpretation of the medical record varies and conclusions regarding coding choices may not always be the same.

The coding rules presented in this chapter and Chapter 6 will deal with physicians billing for outpatient and inpatient services. An **outpatient** is a patient who receives services in a healthcare facility such as a physician's office, clinic, urgent care center, emergency department, or ambulatory surgery center. In an outpatient setting, routine procedures and services are usually listed on an encounter form. The physician rendering medical care indicates which procedures and services were performed by checking them on the encounter form. Unusual services or rarely performed procedures may be written in.

An **inpatient** is a patient who has been formally admitted to a hospital or other healthcare facility for an overnight stay. Hospital services, nursing home services, and surgical procedures are commonly indicated on another type of tracking form.

After completing the encounter form (or other tracking form), an accurate accounting of all procedures and services are either written into the patient's medical record, dictated into a recording machine and transcribed into the record, or keyed directly into a computerized medical record. The insurance billing specialist either obtains procedure code numbers from the encounter form, or abstracts pertinent information from the medical record or operative report and assigns procedure codes.

Every procedure or service must be assigned correct and complete code numbers to be paid promptly and at the highest level possible. Because of the complexity of procedure coding, a working knowledge of medical terminology, including anatomy and physiology, is essential.

THE STANDARD CODE SET

The **Health Care Financing Administration Common Procedure Coding System (HCPCS)** (pronounced "hick-picks") was developed by the Centers for Medicare and Medicaid Services (CMS), formerly known as the Health Care Financing Administration (HCFA), for the Medicare program. There are three levels of codes and modifiers in the HCPCS, as illustrated in Figure 5-1.

Because different rules have been used by various insurance programs regarding which codes they accept, it has complicated the job of the medical insurance billing specialist. A standard code set has been introduced to ensure that all Medicare, Medicaid, and commercial payers will accept the same codes. The approved code set is to be in place by October 2003 for all providers and by October 2004 for small healthcare plans and includes the following:

1. ICD-9-CM diagnostic codes
2. *Current Procedural Terminology (CPT)* (HCPCS Level I)
3. Current Dental Terminology (CDT)
4. Health Care Financing Administration Common Procedure Coding System (HCPCS Level II)
5. National Drug Code (NDC)

When this system is in place, HCPCS Level III (local) codes will be phased out. During the phase-out pe-

Health Care Financing Administration Common Procedure Coding Systems (HCPCS)

LEVEL	DEVELOPED BY	USED	TYPE OF CODE	EXAMPLES	MODIFIERS	EXAMPLES
I	American Medical Association (AMA)	Nationally	Current Procedural Terminology (CPT)	99203	2 or 5-digits	-57 or 09957
II	Centers for Medicare and Medicaid Services—CMS (formerly Health Care Financing Administration—HCFA)	Nationally	(1) HCPCS (A—V Codes) (2) National Drug Codes (NDC)	(1) A6215 (2) 00314062270	(1) 1-alpha digit 2-alpha digits 2-alpha-numeric digits (2) none	(1) -N -GA -F1 (2) none
III	State Fiscal Intermediaries	Regionally	HCPCS (W—Z Codes)	W1000	Unique to individual regions	

Figure 5–1. An overview of the Health Care Financing Administration Common Procedure Coding Systems (HCPCS), currently referred to as Healthcare Common Procedure Coding System, three levels of codes indicating who they were developed by, where they are used, types of codes and modifiers, and examples.

riod, carriers should be contacted to identify which codes they are accepting. Following is an explanation of the three-tier HCPCS coding system and the new NDC codes.

Level I Codes—*Current Procedural Terminology (CPT)*

Level I codes are the predominant codes used in most states for assignment of physician or provider services and procedures. They are found in ***Current Procedural Terminology (CPT)***.* CPT uses a basic five-digit numeric system for coding services rendered by physicians. Procedure code numbers represent evaluation and management services and diagnostic and therapeutic procedures and services on medical billing statements and insurance claim forms, as seen in Example 5–1.*

Code Modifiers

In some billing cases, it is necessary to use a two-digit **modifier** or a separate five-digit code to give a more accurate description of the services rendered. Modifiers do not change the definition of the code; they are used

**Current Procedural Terminology* was formerly known as *Physician's Current Procedural Terminology.*

*Examples shown in this chapter reflect wording pertinent to coding specific procedures and may be missing complete code descriptions and chart entries; therefore, there may be a gap of information for the reader.

Example 5–1

Procedure Code Numbers Representing an Evaluation and Management Service, Diagnostic Service, and Therapeutic Service

A 45-year-old woman is seen for an *initial office visit* for evaluation of recurrent right shoulder pain. The exam required a detailed history and detailed physical examination (D HX and D PX) with low-complexity medical decision making (L MDM). Patient complains of pain radiating down right arm. *Complete x-ray films of the right shoulder* were taken in the office and read by the physician. A corticosteroid solution was *injected into the shoulder joint.*

CPT Code	Description of Services
99203	Office visit, new patient **(Evaluation and management [E/M] service)**
73030	Radiologic exam, shoulder; two views **(Diagnostic service)**
20610	Arthrocentesis injection; major joint, shoulder **(Therapeutic service)**

Expressions from Experience

Presently, all physicians treating patients in the emergency room are responsible for coding emergency room services; but for the future I am hoping that the hospital will open a coding position so that I can do all of the coding for the emergency room. I know this would increase the percentage of cases that are coded correctly and help the compliance rate and reimbursement.

Katrina Ginn
Ward Clerk/Transcriptionist
Hospital Emergency Room

Example 5–3

Multiple Modifier

A physician sees a patient who is grossly obese. The operative report documents that a *bilateral* sliding-type *inguinal herniorrhaphy* was performed; the procedure took *2 hours and 15 minutes.*

Code	Description of Services
49525-**99**	*Bilateral* repair sliding inguinal hernia *requiring*
-50	*2 hours 15 minutes*
-22	
	OR
49525	Repair sliding inguinal hernia
09999	**Multiple modifier**
09950	Bilateral procedure
09922	Unusual services requiring increased time (2 hours 15 minutes)

in addition to the procedure code. Modifiers permit the physician to indicate circumstances in which a procedure as performed differs in some way from that described by its usual five-digit code. A modifier can indicate:

- A service or procedure has either a professional or technical component.
- A service or procedure was performed by more than one physician and/or in more than one location.
- A service or procedure has been increased or reduced.
- A service or procedure was provided more than once.
- Only part of a service was performed.
- An adjunctive service was performed.
- A bilateral procedure was performed.
- Unusual events occurred during a service or procedure.

In most cases the two-digit add-on modifiers are accepted. However, if an insurance company's input system accepts only five digits, such as with electronic claims, then it is necessary to use five-digit modifiers. If in doubt, ask the insurance company to express its desire for one form (two digits) or the other (five digits), as shown in Example 5–2.

When coding services or procedures, modifiers should be considered as an exception. The majority of professional services or procedures rendered are performed exactly as described by the CPT code.

Example 5–2

Modifiers

2-digit	27590-**80** Amputation, thigh; Assistant surgeon
	or
	27590 Amputation, thigh
5-digit	**09980 Assistant surgeon**

Modifiers will be presented throughout this chapter and Chapter 6 as they apply to each section of CPT. Refer to Appendix C for a complete list of CPT modifiers with brief descriptions.

Multiple Modifiers (-99)

If a procedure requires more than one modifier, use the two-digit modifier -99 after the usual five-digit code number, all typed on one line. An alternate method is to use the separate five-digit code 09999 in addition to the basic five-digit procedure code number, each typed on separate lines. Many insurance companies require -99 with a separate note in Block 19 of the HCFA-1500 claim form. When submitting electronic claims, indicate which two or more modifiers are being used in the freeform area. Remember to ask the insurance company which format is preferred when submitting claims that reflect modifier -99 (Example 5–3).

Symbols Representing Code Changes

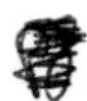

CPT is updated and revised annually. As new procedures are developed or existing procedures modified, descriptions may change making existing codes obsolete. Therefore, code descriptions are modified and code numbers are added and deleted each year. A complete listing of such changes is found in Appendices B and C of CPT. These changes are shown in each edition by the use of symbols, as seen in Figure 5–2.

It is important to become familiar with the new codes and any description changes for the specialized areas that will be used. When using a new code marked with a bullet (●), remember that it may take as long as 6 months before an insurance carrier has a mandatory value assignment; therefore, reimbursements will be received in varying amounts during that time. For a revised procedure descriptor marked with a triangle (▲), or for new or revised text listed between

New code
- • 54163 Repair incomplete circumcision

Revised procedure descriptor
- ▲ 57022 Incision and drainage of vaginal hematoma; obstetrical/postpartum

New or revised text
- ►◄ 36532 Removal of implantable intravenous infusion pump ► (if imaging guidance is performed, use 76000) ◄

Figure 5–2. Symbols indicating new codes, revised procedure descriptors, and new or revised text (including deleted codes) that appear in *Current Procedural Terminology* codebook. (CPT codes, descriptions, and material only are copyright 2001 American Medical Association. All rights reserved.)

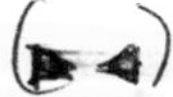

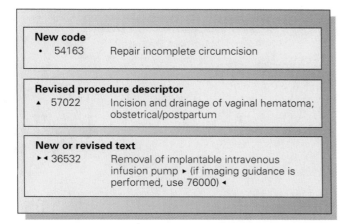

the triangular symbols (◄ ►), highlight what is new or revised. This will save time in trying to figure out what was changed and will prevent using these codes incorrectly.

Level II—National HCPCS Codes

Level II codes, commonly referred to as HCPCS codes, are used by Medicare and, in some states, Medicaid, TRICARE, and many private carriers for the assignment of the following services:

- Chemotherapy
- Chiropractic services
- Dental procedures
- Drugs (other than oral—to be replaced with NDC codes)
- Durable medical equipment (DME)
- Enteral and parenteral therapy
- Orthotic and prosthetic procedures
- Selected diagnostic radiology, vision, and hearing services
- Supplies (medical and surgical)
- Transportation services
- Unique procedures and professional services

You may find that one case may be coded at two or possibly three different coding levels. When both CPT and Level II codes have the same description, the CPT code should be used. If the descriptions are not identical (e.g., the CPT code narrative is generic and the HCPCS Level II code is specific), the Level II code should be used.

Refer to Appendix C for a partial list of HCPCS Level II codes with brief descriptions.

National Drug Codes

Eleven-digit **National Drug Codes (NDCs)** will be used instead of HCPCS Level II codes for reporting the use of drugs for Medicare and other federal and private payer electronic claims submissions, effective October 2002. The standard code set of NDCs is currently used as the universal product identifier for human drugs and is listed in reference manuals (see *Red Book Annual* and *Red Book Updates* under Resources at end of chapter) with the manufacturer's name and the average wholesale price (AWP).

By using NDCs a better description of the drug used in the treatment of patients will be communicated to the insurance company. For ease in locating NDCs, a crosswalk may be available from your local Medicare carrier that lists the previously used HCPCS Level II drug code (e.g., J3420, injection, vitamin B_{12} cyanocobalamin, up to 1000 μg) and the new NDC code (00302808982, vitamin B_{12} cyanocobalamin, 1000 μg/mL, vial injection, Genetco). After the phase-in period, penalties of $100 per violation up to $25,000 per year for each requirement will be applied for noncompliance.

It is always wise to check the private carrier's provider manual or telephone the carrier to verify usage of Level II codes and NDC codes before sending in claims for medications, DME, and other mentioned services. HCPCS is updated each spring. Refer to Chapter 11 for additional information on coding for Medicare cases.

Level III—Regional or Local HCPCS Codes

Level III codes have been used to identify new procedures or specific supplies and drugs for which there is no national code. These are five-digit alphanumeric codes that use the letters S and W through Z. When the standard code set is implemented, these codes are to be phased out.

HCPCS Modifiers

Besides CPT modifiers, HCPCS Level II modifiers may be used by some commercial carriers and Medicare.

Expressions from Experience

I like the freedom my job gives because I do it at my own pace. I also like the challenge of being involved in the major process of assigning codes so that claims are coded accurately.

Katrina Ginn
Ward Clerk/Transcriptionist
Hospital Emergency Room

Example 5–4

HCPCS Level II Two-Digit Alpha Modifiers

When taking x-ray films of both feet, the billing portion of the insurance claim would appear as follows:

05/06/XX	73620 RT	Radiologic examination, foot—right
05/06/XX	73620 LT	Radiologic examination, foot—left

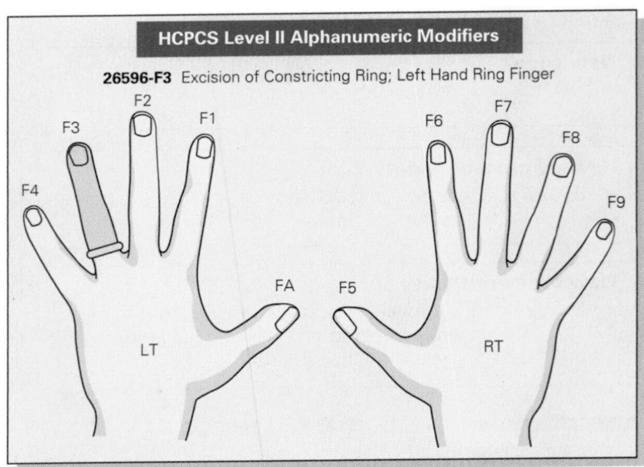

Figure 5–3. HCPCS level II alpha modifiers (LT and RT) used to identify right and left hands and alphanumeric modifiers (FA through F9) used to identify digits (fingers) of right and left hands.

Level III modifiers are also used by Medicare in local regions to help further describe the services provided.

Level II modifiers have one or two letter characters (see Example 5–4), or two alphanumeric characters (Fig. 5–3). A brief list of these modifiers may be found in Appendix C of the CPT codebook. A comprehensive list may be found in an HCPCS national Level II codebook.

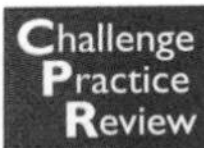

Pause and Practice CPR

REVIEW SESSIONS 5–1 THROUGH 5–5

Directions: *Complete these exercises to enhance your knowledge about the types of patients seen in the physician's office and the CPT coding system.*

5–1 A patient who receives services in a physician's office, clinic, urgent care center, emergency department, or ambulatory surgery center is referred to as a/an ____________________.

5–2 A patient who has been formally admitted to a hospital or other healthcare facility for an overnight stay is referred to as a/an ____________________.

5–3 What is the acronym for the organization that developed the three-tier coding system?

____________________.

5–4 State the two ways to list modifiers when completing an insurance claim.

(a) ____________________

(b) ____________________

5–5 What two-digit number represents a multiple modifier? ____________________

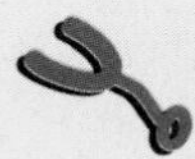

CHECK YOUR HEARTBEAT! Turn to the end of the chapter for the answers to these review sessions.

INTRODUCTION TO THE CPT CODEBOOK

The CPT codebook is a systematic listing of five-digit code numbers with no decimals. It is divided into seven code sections and appendices, as shown in Figure 5–4. Within each of the main sections are subsections and categories divided according to anatomic body system, organ, or site; procedure or service; condition; and specialty. Each digit of a CPT code indicates the section in which it is found, type of code, and level of service, as indicated in Example 5–5.

Category I, II, and III Codes

To improve the existing CPT Code system, a CPT-5 Project was implemented, which includes two new code sets: category II codes, intended for performance

Current Procedural Terminology (CPT)	
SECTIONS	**CONTENTS**
Evaluation and Management (E/M)	99201 to 99499
Anesthesia	00100 to 01999
Surgery	10021 to 69990
Radiology, Nuclear Medicine and Diagnostic Ultrasound	70010 to 79999
Pathology and Laboratory	80048 to 89399
Medicine	90281 to 99569
Category II Codes	0001T to 0026T
APPENDICES	
Appendix A	Modifiers
Appendix B	Summary of Additions, Deletions, and Revisions
Appendix C	Update to Short Descriptors
Appendix D	Clinical Examples (E/M)
Appendix E	Summary of CPT Add-on Codes
Appendix F	Summary of CPT Codes Exempt from Modifier -51
Index	Organized by main terms

Figure 5–4. *Current Procedural Terminology* contents listing code sections, appendices, and index. (CPT codes, descriptions, and material only are copyright 2001 American Medical Association. All rights reserved.)

measurement, and category III codes, intended for new and emerging technology. Existing CPT codes are considered category I.

Category II codes are being tested and as of the date of this publication, have not been released for use. They will be assigned an alphanumeric identifier with a letter in the last field (e.g., 1234F) to distinguish them from category I CPT codes. Use of these codes is optional and not required for correct coding.

Category III codes are a temporary set of tracking codes used for new emerging technologies. They are intended to expedite data collection and assessment of new services and procedures to substantiate widespread use and clinical effectiveness. Category III codes can take the place of temporary local codes (HCPCS Level III) that are being phased out and eliminated under the Health Insurance Portability and Accountability Act (HIPAA). These codes appear in CPT 2002 in a separate section following the Medicine section. They also have an alphanumeric identifier with a letter in the last field (e.g., 0025T, determination of corneal thickness with interpretation and report, bilateral) to distinguish them from category I codes.

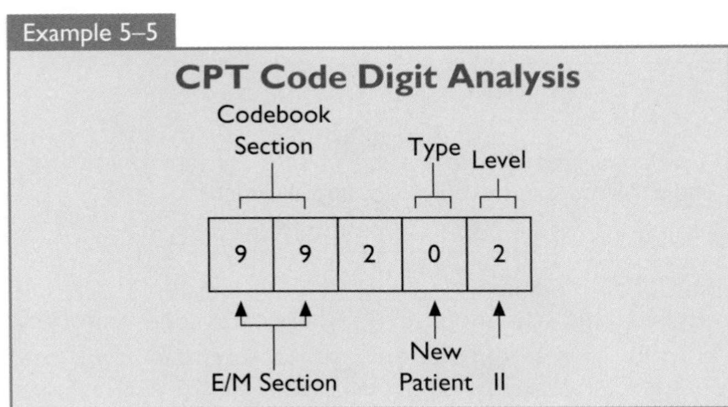

CODING EVALUATION AND MANAGEMENT SERVICES

Evaluation and Management Section

Directions for use of the CPT differ when coding **Evaluation and Management (E/M) services** and services from other sections; therefore, only the use of CPT for E/M services will be defined here. Evaluation and Management services are services the physician provides to evaluate patients that were previously referred to as office, hospital, or home visits. These services are provided in a variety of locations and also involve the physician's management of the patient's condition. Note that the E/M section is located first in the manual and that code numbers (99201–99499) are out of numeric sequence with the rest of the text (00100–99569). Also note, that in the Medicine section, there are a few code numbers that also start with "99" listed under Special Services, Procedures, and Reports, in the Miscellaneous category, that may be used in addition to or in lieu of E/M codes. These will be discussed later in this chapter.

Table 5–1 **Evaluation and Management Subsections**
Office or Other Outpatient Services
Hospital Observation Services
Hospital Inpatient Services
Consultations
Patient Transport
Emergency Department Services
Critical Care Services
Neonatal Intensive Care
Nursing Facility Services
Domiciliary, Rest Home, or Custodial Care Services
Home Services
Prolonged Services
Case Management Services
Care Plan Oversight Services
Preventive Medicine Services
Newborn Care
Special Evaluation and Management Services
Other Evaluation and Management Services

Subsections, Categories, and Subcategories

The E/M section of CPT has subsections, as seen in Table 5–1.

To begin the E/M coding process, the insurance billing specialist must identify the correct subsection. Instead of using the index to locate codes in the E/M section, turn to the Table of Contents at the beginning of CPT and read the list of subsections. Then turn to the E/M section of CPT and examine the various subsections which are either the place of service (POS) (e.g., office, hospital, nursing facility) or type of service (TOS) (e.g., consultation, preventive medicine, or newborn care).

Next, select the correct category and/or subcategory which is either the patient status (e.g., new patient or established patient), or time factor (e.g., time spent providing critical care, prolonged services, preventive medicine counseling services, care plan oversight services, or discharge of a patient). See Example 5–6 for an illustration of a section, subsection, category, and subcategory. Note that not all subsections have a category listed. Some headings start with a subcategory (e.g., Office and Other Outpatient Services [subsection], New Patient [subcategory]). Pay careful attention to the size of the title to determine what area you are in. Some codebooks have titles color-coded, making this determination easier.

Example 5–6

E/M Section, Subsection, Category, and Subcategory

Section → **Evaluation and Management**
Subsection → **Consultations**
Category → Office and other outpatient consultations
Subcategory → New or established patient

Patient Status

In procedure coding, two categories of patient status are considered: the new patient and the established patient. A **new patient** (NP) is one who *has not* received any professional services from the physician, or another physician of the same specialty who belongs to the same group practice, *within the past 3 years.* The first time a patient is seen in the office or the first time a patient is seen in the hospital for each admission, it is referred to as an *initial visit.*

An **established patient** is one who *has received* professional services from the physician, or another physician of the same specialty who belongs to the same group practice, *within the past 3 years.* When a patient returns to an outpatient setting after an initial visit, it is called a return or follow-up visit. When a patient is seen in the hospital after the initial visit, it is referred to as subsequent care.

Some insurance policies allow only two moderate- or high-complexity office visits per patient, per year. Therefore, it is important to contact the insurance company prior to the patient's first visit to learn whether there are any limitations. It is also important that a physician's practice have a system in place to track this.

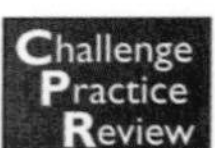

Pause and Practice CPR

REVIEW SESSIONS 5–6 THROUGH 5–10

Directions: *Complete these exercises by filling in or marking the correct answers to enhance your knowledge about the organization of the CPT manual and E/M codes. Use your procedure codebook.*

5–6 How many sections is the CPT manual divided into? ______________

5–7 Which appendix contains a full description of all modifiers? ______________

5–8 Which digit(s) of the CPT code determines the section of CPT where the code may be found? ______________________________

5–9 When looking for a consultation code, the consultation category would be considered a:

(a) place of service.

(b) type of service.

(c) location of service.

5–10 What category would you look under to find a code for services provided to a patient admitted to a hospital? ______________________

CHALLENGE SESSION 5–11

Directions: *Use critical thinking skills to complete this exercise.*

5–11 A patient is seen in the office by Dr. Practon on April 10, 2001. When reviewing the medical record it is noted that the patient's last visit was on March 12, 1998.

(a) Select the correct term used to indicate the status of this patient when coding E/M services.

(1) New patient

(2) Established patient

(b) Give the rationale used to determine your answer.

____

____

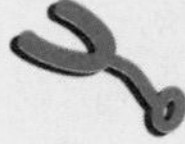

CHECK YOUR HEARTBEAT! Turn to the end of the chapter for the answers to these review and challenge sessions.

Level of Service

After the correct category and subcategory have been located, you are ready to identify the correct level of service and assign a code. There are three to five levels of service used for reporting purposes. These levels, represented by the last digit, are based on the following **key components:**

- History (family, personal, and social)
- Examination (physical exam)
- Medical decision making (judgment about complexity of establishing the diagnosis and selection of treatment options)

Contributory factors, such as counseling, coordination of care, nature of the presenting problem, and face-to-face time with the patient and/or family, are also considered. Contributory factors help the physician determine the extent of the history, examination, and medical decision making required to treat the patient. It is not necessary to document counseling and coordination of care for every patient. Review Figure 5–5 for a quick glance of the major subsections, categories, and levels of service found in the E/M section. Note the definitions used for the abbreviations of the key components.

Key components are clinical in nature and reflect the information in the patient record. It is important that the physician state elements regarding these factors and document them in the patient's record to assist in coding each case. A brief description of the requirements for all levels of the three key components are found in Figure 5–6. *Three* out of *three* key components need to be present at a specific level to assign a code to a *new* patient encounter. *Established* outpatient visits and subsequent hospital visits only require that *two* out of the *three* key components be met. Read through the clinical examples presented in Appendix D of CPT to become familiar with some of the case scenarios that commonly occur for the codes that appear in the E/M section. Review the sample in Figure 5–7 illustrating an E/M code for a new patient seen in the office or in an outpatient setting.

In a case in which counseling and coordination of care dominate the face-to-face physician/patient encounter (more than 50%), then *time* is considered the key component to qualify for a particular level of E/M service (see Example 5–7). It may be necessary to remind the physician that reimbursement is made according to services and procedures, not time, unless the above criteria are met.

Established Patient/Physician's Presence Not Required

E/M code 99211, listed for an established patient in an outpatient setting, does not require a physician in attendance. This, however, is one of the most abused codes according to CMS. In order to report CPT code

Evaluation and Management Services

Key Components			
History (HX) & Physical Examination (PX)		**Medical Decision Making (MDM)**	
PF	Problem Focus	**SF**	Straight Forward
EPF	Expanded Problem Focus	**L**	Low Complexity
D	Detailed	**M**	Moderate Complexity
C	Comprehensive	**H**	High Complexity

Office/Outpatient

New Patient Office Visit (3 out of 3)

Level	History	Exam	Decision Making	Time
99201	PF	PF	SF	10
99202	EPF	EPF	SF	20
99203	D	D	L	30
99204	C	C	M	45
99205	C	C	H	60

Established Office Visits (2 out of 3)

Level	History	Exam	Decision Making	Time
99211	Physician presence not required			5
99212	PF	PF	SF	10
99213	EPF	EPF	L	15
99214	D	D	M	25
99215	C	C	H	40

Hospital Care

Initial Hospital Care (3 out of 3)

Level	History	Exam	Decision Making	Time
99221	D	D	SF/L	30
99222	C	C	M	50
99223	C	C	H	70

Subsequent Hospital Care (2 out of 3)

Level	History	Exam	Decision Making	Time
99231	PF	PF	S/L	15
99232	EPF	EPF	M	25
99233	D	D	H	35
99238	Discharge Day Management			<30
99239	Discharge Day Management			>30

Emergency Room (3 out of 3)

Level	History	Exam	Decision Making
99281	PF	PF	SF
99282	EPF	EPF	L
99283	EPF	EPF	M
99284	D	D	M
99285	C	C	H

Observation Care (2 out of 3)

Level	History	Exam	Decision Making
99218	D/C	D/C	SF/L
99219	C	C	M
99220	C	C	H
99217	Observation Care Discharge		

Critical Care

99291	First Hour
99292	Each Additional 30 minutes

Codes that can be used with critical care codes: 36000, 36410, 36415, 36600, 71010,71020, 91105, 92953, 93561, 93562, 94656, 94657, 94660, 94662, 99090

Observation for Inpatient Care (Inc. Admin & Discharge)

Level	History	Exam	Decision Making	Problem
99234	D/C	D/C	SF/L	L
99235	C	C	M	M
99236	C	C	H	H

Preventive Medicine Services (New)

Level	History	Exam	Age
99381	C	C	<1 yr
99382	C	C	1-4 yrs
99383	C	C	5-11 yrs
99384	C	C	12-17 yrs
99385	C	C	18-39 yrs
99386	C	C	40-64 yrs
99387	C	C	65+ yrs

Preventive Medicine Services (Established)

Level	History	Exam	Age
99391	C	C	<1 yr
99392	C	C	1-4 yrs
99393	C	C	5-11 yrs
99394	C	C	12-17 yrs
99395	C	C	18-39 yrs
99396	C	C	40-64 yrs
99397	C	C	65+ yrs

Consultation

Office Consultation (3 out of 3)

Level	History	Exam	Decision Making	Time
99241	PF	PF	SF	15
99242	EPF	EPF	SF	30
99243	D	D	L	40
99244	C	C	M	60
99245	C	C	H	80

Inpatient Consultation (3 out of 3)

Level	History	Exam	Decision Making	Time
99251	PF	PF	SF	20
99252	EPF	EPF	SF	40
99253	D	D	L	55
99254	C	C	M	80
99255	C	C	H	110

Confirmatory Consultation (3 out of 3)

Level	History	Exam	Decision Making
99271	PF	PF	SF
99272	EPF	EPF	SF
99273	D	D	L
99274	C	C	M
99275	C	C	H

Follow-Up Inpatient Consultation

Level	History	Exam	Decision Making	Time
99261	PF	PF	SF/L	10
99262	EPF	EPF	M	20
99263	D	D	H	30

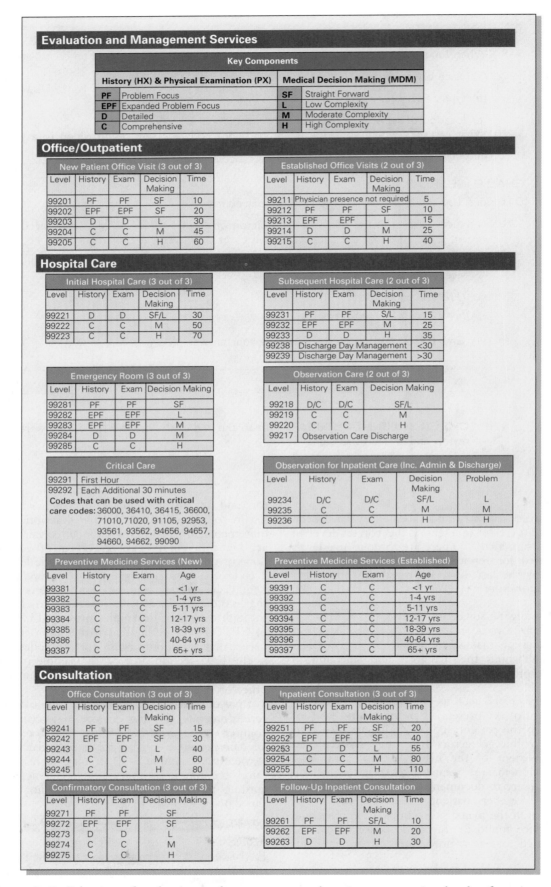

Figure 5–5. Selection of evaluation and management subsections, categories, levels of service, and key components. (CPT codes, descriptions, and material only are copyright 2001 American Medical Association. All rights reserved.)

Required Component For Documentation

History Component

History Type (level)	Chief Complaint	Present Problem	System Review	Past family and social history
Problem focused	✓	Brief	None	None
Expanded problem focused	✓	Brief	Problem Pertinent	None
Detailed	✓	Extended	Extended	Pertinent
Comprehensive	✓	Extended	Complete	Complete

Examination Component

Type/Level	Body Area or System to be Examined
Problem focused	Affected body system only
Expanded problem focused	Affected body system only; other related system
Detailed	Extended exam of affected body system and other symptomatic or related organ system(s)
Comprehensive	Complete single system or multi-system examination

Medical Decision Making Component (Must meet or exceed 2 of 3 in one column)

Level	Straight Forward	Low Complexity	Moderate Complexity	High Complexity
Number of diagnoses/management options	Minimal	Limited	Multiple	Extensive
Amount/complexity of data to be reviewed	None/ Minimal	Limited	Moderate	Extensive
Risk of complications and/or morbidity or mortality	Minimal	Low	Moderate	High

Figure 5–6. Required key components used for documentation purposes indicating factors that must be present to qualify for a specific level of history, physical examination, and medical decision making. This information is abstracted from the evaluation and management standards found in the 2001 *Current Procedural Terminology*, published by the American Medical Association.

99211 when the physician is not providing the service, the following criteria have to be met:

- Medical assistant, nurse, or other practitioner must have face-to-face contact with the patient.
- Physician must be in the office.
- Separate service (in addition to an injection) must be provided.
- Documentation must include date of service, reason for visit, medical necessity, patient encounter information, and signature of practitioner.

Remember, if an injection is given but no E/M service is provided, use only the injection code.

Special E/M Services

When a patient applies for life or disability insurance and an evaluation is requested by the insurance company, code 99450 should be assigned. For a work-related or medical disability evaluation requested by the insurer, codes 99455 and 99456 apply.

Example 5–7

Counseling and Coordination of Care

Lyndsay White, a 15-year-old new patient, came to the dermatologist's office with a long history of severe cystic acne. *Typically, this visit would be a Level 3 E/M service taking 30 minutes and the correct code assignment would be as follows:*

CPT Code	Description of Services
99203	• Office or other outpatient visit • detailed history (D HX) • detailed physical examination (D PX) • low-complexity medical decision making (L MDM) *(30 minutes' time spent face-to-face with patient)*

However, the physician spent *45 minutes* with the patient and *25 minutes was spent counseling* the patient regarding her low self-esteem that resulted from the acne scars. **Since more than 50% of the total time was spent on counseling and coordination of care, the next level of code, 99204 (which carries a 45-minute time allotment) is assigned.** Note that a "V" code from the section V65.4 (other counseling) would be used for such cases.

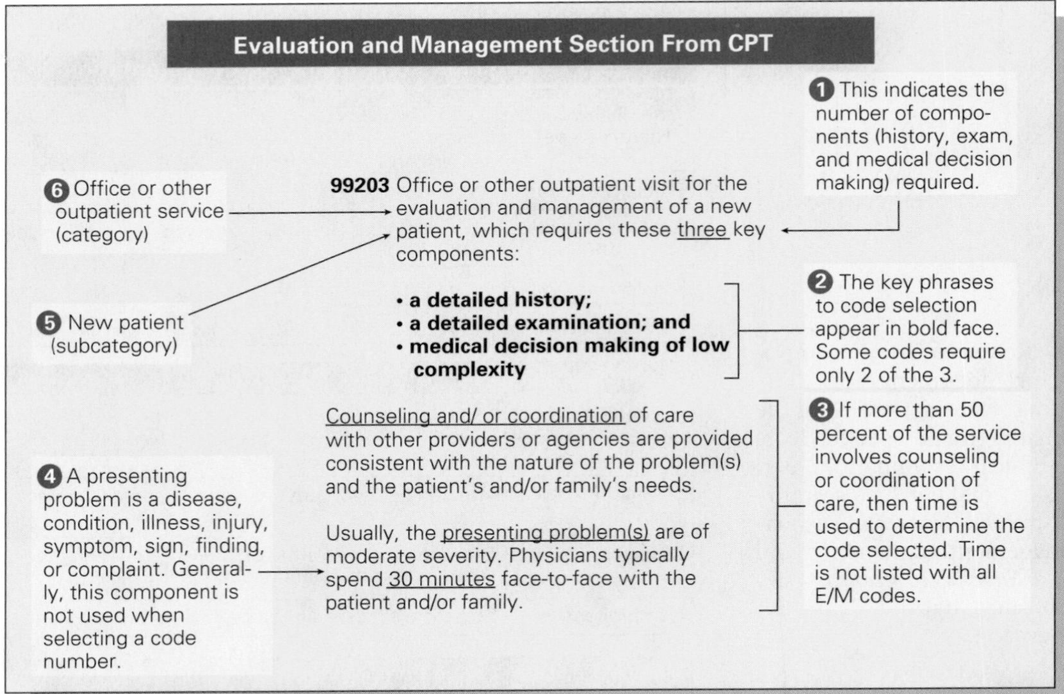

Figure 5–7. Evaluation and management code 99203 defining main words and phrases. This code is used for a new patient seen in the office or in an outpatient or ambulatory setting. (CPT codes, descriptions, and material only are copyright 2001 American Medical Association. All rights reserved.)

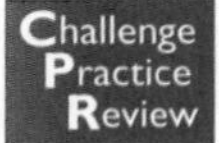

Pause and Practice CPR

REVIEW SESSIONS 5–12 THROUGH 5–17

Directions: *Complete these exercises to enhance your knowledge about the types of patients seen in the physician's office and the CPT coding system. Refer to Figure 5–6 for questions 5–15 through 5–17.*

5–12 How many key components are in an Evaluation and Management code? ________________

5–13 How many key components must be present to assign an E/M code for a/an:

(a) established patient ________________

(b) new patient ________________

5–14 List the definitions for the following abbreviations used to describe key components.

(a) HX ________________

(b) PX ________________

(c) MDM ________________

(d) C ________________

(e) PF ________________

(f) SF ________________

(g) L ________________

(h) EPF ________________

(i) H ________________

(j) D ________________

5–15 List the type of *system review* that the physician would need to perform for a problem-focused history. ____________________

5–16 If the physician performed a complete single-system examination, what *type/level of examination* would it be? ____________________

5–17 What level of *decision making* would the physician select if there were multiple diagnostic/management options, uncomplicated minimal data to be reviewed, and a moderate risk of complications? ____________________

PRACTICE SESSIONS 5–18 THROUGH 5–20

Directions: *Complete these exercises to develop and enhance your E/M procedure coding skills. Use your procedure codebook.*

5–18 A patient presents in the physician's office and the clinical medical assistant takes the patient's blood pressure and temperature, and changes a dressing. What established patient E/M code would be assigned? ____________________

5–19 List the level of E/M service for the following codes:

(a) 99254 ____________________

(b) 99211 ____________________

(c) 99275 ____________________

(d) 99283 ____________________

5–20 Refer to Figure 5–5 or your CPT manual and list the correct codes for the following E/M services.

(a) Subsequent hospital care with an expanded problem-focused history and examination (EPF HX PX); moderate medical decision making (M MDM). ____________

(b) New patient office visit (NP OV) with a comprehensive history and examination (C HX PX); moderate medical decision making (M MDM). ____________

(c) Preventive medicine service on a 12-year-old established patient. ____________

CHECK YOUR HEARTBEAT! Turn to the end of the chapter for the answers to these review and practice sessions.

Consultation

When services are rendered by a physician whose opinion or advice is requested by another physician or agency in the evaluation or treatment of a patient's illness or a suspected problem, it is referred to as a **consultation.** The opinion is often requested to assist the primary care physician in diagnosing the patient. The request must be documented and the consulting physician must submit a written report to the requesting physician. Diagnostic and/or therapeutic services needed to formulate an opinion may be ordered by the consultant. Categories for consultations are as follows:

- Office or other outpatient consultation (new or established patient).
- Initial new patient consultation (new or established patient).
- Follow-up inpatient consultation (established patient).
- Confirmatory consultation (new or established patient). This type of consultation calls for an opinion about the necessity or appropriate nature of the patient treatment plan, after a diagnosis has been made. If a second opinion is required by the insurance company, modifier -32 (mandated services) is added to the consultation code.

If after a consultation is completed, the consulting physician assumes responsibility for management of all of the patient's condition(s), do not use the follow-up consultation codes. In the office setting, use the appropriate initial consultation code for the initial encounter, then the appropriate code for an established patient. In a hospital setting, use the appropriate inpatient hospital consultation code, and then subsequent hospital care codes.

Referral

The term "referral" can be used in several different ways. A referral can be the transfer of specific or total care of a patient from one physician to another for *known problems.* For example, a patient is sent to an orthopedist for care of a fracture. It is not the same as a consultation because a second opinion is not being requested.

When dealing with managed care patients, the term "referral" is used when requesting an authorization for the patient to receive services, for example, requesting authorization for the patient to have surgery, an x-ray, diagnostic tests, or to see a specialist. When a referral is obtained for services outside of the medical practice, the receiving physician may send a thank-you letter to the referring physician as a courtesy, with comments about the patient's condition.

Emergency Care

An **emergency** is a sudden, unexpected medical condition, or the worsening of a condition, that poses a threat to life, limb, or sight and requires immediate treatment (e.g., shortness of breath, chest pain, drug overdose). **Emergency care** is the care given to prevent serious impairment of bodily functions or serious dysfunction to any body part or organ. Advanced life support may be required. Not all care provided in an emergency department of a hospital can be termed "emergency care." Emergency care provided by the patient's physician in an office setting or emergency department or care provided by the emergency room physician may occur as described in the following situations:

- *Patient's physician provides care in the office*—Code 99058, found in the Medicine section, may be used when billing private insurance carriers in addition to a code from the E/M section. Note that Medicare does not pay for code 99058 and other carriers may also deny this code. If a patient comes into the office requiring emergency care for a wound trauma, and you bill for the office visit, suturing of the laceration, and the surgical tray, most insurance carriers will pay only for the suturing. The office visit and tray are considered bundled (services grouped together that are related to a procedure) with the surgical code and may not be paid separately. However, if you code the claim for office services provided on an emergency basis (E/M code and 99058), most carriers will reimburse for the office visit and for the emergent nature of the service (see Example 5–8).
- *Patient's physician is called to the emergency room to provide care*—If the emergency room physician does not treat the patient, but instead calls the patient's physician to come and care for the patient, codes from the Emergency Department Services subsection may be used.
- *Emergency room physician provides care in the emergency room*—Codes from the Emergency Department Services subsection are used.

Example 5–8

Office Emergency

Incorrect Coding

99212	Office visit, level 2, established patient
12005	Simple repair of scalp laceration, 12.6 cm
99070	Surgical tray (itemized)

Correct Coding

99212	Office visit, level 2, established patient
99058	*Office services provided on an emergency basis*
12005	Simple repair of scalp laceration, 12.6 cm

- *Emergency room physician calls the patient's physician to the emergency room to consult, treat, or admit the patient*—If both physicians treat the patient in the emergency room, it is important to clarify to the insurance company how the care has been distributed. The emergency room physician would use codes from the Emergency Department Services subsection. The patient's physician would do one of the following: (1) use an Office Outpatient Consultation code (new or established) if the physician merely examines and offers an opinion, (2) use an Outpatient (established patient) code if the physician treats the patient in the emergency room, or (3) use an Inpatient Hospital Care code if the patient is examined by the physician and is also admitted.

Critical Care

Critical care is intensive care provided in a variety of acute life-threatening conditions requiring constant bedside attention by a physician. Critical care can take place in various departments—the coronary care unit (CCU), intensive care unit (ICU), respiratory care unit (RCU), or emergency department (ED), also called the emergency room (ER). When critical care is performed in any one of these departments, code 99291 is used to report the first hour on any given date. Code 99292 is used to report each additional 30 minutes. The time spent on a given date should always be recorded in the patient's chart but does not have to be continuous. Time spent engaged in work directly related to the individual patient's care, whether that time was spent at the immediate bedside or elsewhere on the floor or unit, may be reported as critical care. Activities that occur outside the unit or floor (e.g., telephone calls) may not be reported since the physician is not immediately available to the patient. Refer to the Critical Care Service guidelines preceding the critical care codes in CPT to determine what services are included in the critical care codes. All other services should be reported separately. The key to obtaining the highest level of reimbursement lies in selecting diagnostic codes that convey the critical nature of the patient's condition.

There is a separate section for neonatal intensive care codes. Although the definitions for critical care are the same for adult, child, and neonate, the neonate critical care codes are not reported as hourly services. They are 24-hour global codes. The definition of a neonate is an infant who is 30 days old or less at the time of admission to an ICU. For critically ill infants older than 1 month of age at the time of admission to an ICU, report using codes 99291 and 99292.

Preventive Medicine

Preventive medicine services are provided to prevent the occurrence of illness, injury, and disease. Such services include counseling, guiding the patient, advising him or her regarding risk factor reduction interventions, and ordering appropriate laboratory, radiology, or diagnostic procedures at the initial or periodic preventive medicine exam. Preventive medicine service codes are categorized according to the patient's age. The comprehensive nature of the examination is *not* the same as the comprehensive examination reported with E/M codes.

Counseling

Counseling is a discussion that may take place during an office visit or in a separate encounter between the physician and the patient or family, or both. Codes from the Preventive Medicine category include counseling which is provided at the time of the initial or periodic comprehensive preventive medicine examination (new or established patient).

When counseling takes place at a separate encounter for the purpose of promoting health and preventing injury or illness (e.g., family problems, diet, or substance abuse), codes from the Counseling and/or Risk Factor Reduction Intervention category apply.

A separate subcategory is listed for preventive medicine group counseling. For group counseling of patients with symptoms or established illness, use code 99078 from the Medicine section.

When counseling occurs for patients with symptoms or established illness, discussions may take place regarding one or more of the following:

- Diagnosis
- Recommended studies or tests
- Treatment options
- Risks and benefits of treatment
- Prognosis

For these patients, the counseling service is bundled with the appropriate level of E/M service and should not be billed separately.

Hospital Observation Services

When a patient is designated as admitted to **"observation status"** the patient is not formally admitted to the hospital. The patient is more or less kept on hold while his or her condition is being observed while a decision is being made regarding admittance or discharge. The patient need not be in a separate observation area of the hospital in order to use codes from the Hospital Observation Services subsection as long as he or she meets the observation criteria. Observation codes include the initiation of observation, supervision of the care plan, and periodic reassessments made by the physician. The observation discharge code is used when the patient is discharged from observation status.

Nursing Facility Service

E/M services provided to patients in Nursing Facilities (formerly called Skilled Nursing Facilities [SNFs], Intermediate Care Facilities [ICFs], or Long-Term Care Facilities [LTCFs], have two categories for new and established patients. The Comprehensive Nursing Facility Assessments category is used to report comprehensive evaluations at one or more sites in the assessment process (e.g., patient's home, office, hospital, and so forth). The second category, Subsequent Nursing Home Facility Care, is used to report services for patients who do not need a comprehensive evaluation and who have not had a major, permanent change of status. Discharge codes, reflecting the time it took for the physician to perform the discharge examination, discuss the nursing facility stay, order medications, and prepare referral forms and discharge records, are listed under a separate category and should also be utilized.

Codes listed under Nursing Facility Services are also used to report services for psychiatric residential treatment centers.

Domiciliary, Rest Home, or Custodial Care Services

Codes in this subsection are used to report E/M services for patients seen in a facility that provides room, board, and other personal assistance services on a long-term basis.

Prolonged Services

Services that go beyond the usual services provided in either inpatient or outpatient settings are found under the E/M subsection **Prolonged Services.** First, you must determine whether the service provided required face-to-face contact with the patient, or did not require face-to-face contact. There are four codes for face-to-face contact, two for office or other outpatient settings, and two for inpatient settings. These services are reported in addition to all other services, including any level of E/M service. Prolonged service that is less than 30 minutes should not be billed using these codes because the time is included in the total work of the E/M codes. The prolonged time that is counted to determine which code is applied starts after the time allotted for the E/M service. For example, if a physician performs a level 3 E/M service on a new patient (99203), the typical time allotted is 30 minutes. If the physician spends an additional 30 minutes or less the time is not counted; however, if the physician spends an additional 60 minutes the code for the first hour of prolonged service (99354) may be used. The prolonged time spent with the patient need not be continuous (see Example 5–9).

When reporting prolonged services, there is also modifier -21 (Prolonged Evaluation and Management Services) that may be appended to an E/M code to report a face-to-face or floor/unit service longer than or greater than that described in the *highest*-level E/M service code (i.e., 99205, 99215, 99223). Always include documentation to accompany the claim and contact

Example 5–9

Prolonged Evaluation and Management Service

A 56-year-old new patient with multiple sclerosis and a multitude of other problems is seen and evaluated in the physician's office. The patient's history is taken and the patient is lifted, with assistance, onto the exam table and an examination is performed. After the visit the physician requires extensive time to talk with the patient's husband, sister, and daughter. The physician also reviews complex medical records and determines a comprehensive treatment plan. The physician contacts the local home health agency, occupational therapist, and physical therapist. *A total of* **60 minutes** *is spent on the history and examination of the patient and an additional* **120 minutes** *is spent conversing with the family and making arrangements for the patient's care at home.*

CPT Code	Description of Services
99205	New patient, level 5; office/outpatient visit, comprehensive history (C HX), comprehensive examination (C PX), high-complexity medical decision making (H MDM), *typical time spent face-to-face;* **60 minutes**
99358	*Prolonged evaluation and management service before and/or after face-to-face contact with patient;* **first hour**
99359 X 2	*Prolonged evaluation and management service* **each additional 30 minutes (60 additional minutes)**

individual carriers to inquire which method they prefer when reporting prolonged services.

Standby Services

There is one code provided to bill for physician standby services. The charge is based on what the physician feels is the value of his or her time. The physician must be available to give the care; however, the physician may not actually provide any care. Some insurance programs (e.g., Medicare) do not pay for operative standby, so be sure to check before billing the carrier.

Unlisted Service or Procedure

Code 99499 is an unlisted code and should be used only when an E/M service is provided that is not described in CPT. All unlisted codes end in "99" and appear at the end of each section. A report should always accompany an unlisted code to obtain reimbursement.

Adjunct Codes

There are several codes found at the end of CPT in the Medicine section; Special Services, Procedures and Reports under Miscellaneous Services which may be used in addition to or in lieu of an E/M code. Read these code descriptions carefully. They represent:

- Postoperative follow-up care included in global services
- New patient visit when starred (*) procedure constitutes major service
- Services requested after hours
- Services provided at locations other than physician's office
- Services provided on emergency basis
- Educational services provided in a group setting

Further use of these codes will be discussed in the next chapter. It should be noted that the Medicare-approved charge for physician's services is not increased or decreased due to the time of day or the day of the week that care is provided. Medicare and other insurance companies may not recognize other codes from this section, so a tracking system is necessary to evaluate their usefulness.

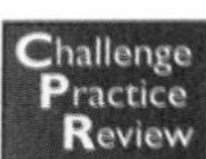

Pause and Practice CPR

REVIEW SESSIONS 5–21 THROUGH 5–26

Directions: *Complete these exercises to enhance your knowledge of terms that relate to procedure coding.*

5–21 Care that requires constant bedside attention by a physician is referred to as

______________________________.

5–22 When a patient is seen for a physical examination in the absence of illness, injury, or disease, the visit is coded as a/an ______________________________ service.

5–23 When a physician requests the opinion of another physician to assist in the diagnosis of a patient, the service is referred to as a/an ______________________________.

5–24 What is the status of a patient called when a patient is "held" in a hospital setting without being formally admitted so that a decision can be made regarding admittance or discharge?

____

5–25 Care given to prevent serious impairment of bodily functions or serious dysfunction to any body part or organ is called ______________________________.

5–26 When a discussion takes place during an office visit or in a separate encounter between the physician and patient, family, or both, this is referred to as ______________________________.

CHECK YOUR HEARTBEAT! Turn to the end of the chapter for the answers to these review sessions.

SUMMATION AND PREVIEW

In conclusion, it is best to remember that the physician is the one who assigns the value of an E/M code by documenting the level of service. As a medical insurance billing specialist, you will provide information and interpretation regarding the American Medical Association CPT guidelines and offer coding solutions. In the next chapter, you will continue learning procedure coding for the remaining sections of CPT.

GOLDEN RULE

Coding is an art, not an exact science.

Chapter 5 Review and Practice

Study Session

Directions: *Review the objectives, key terms, and chapter information before completing the following questions. Refer to your CPT codebook when necessary.*

5–1 How many levels of codes are in the HCPCS system? ________________

5–2 How often is CPT revised and updated? ________________

5–3 How many digits are in a CPT code? ________________

5–4 Which digit(s) indicates the level of service? ________________

5–5 Which digit(s) indicates the section of CPT? ________________

5–6 How many sections is CPT divided into? ________________

5–7 Refer to Figure 5–4 or your CPT manual and list the *section* in which the following codes may be found.

(a) 61550 ________________________________

(b) 99058 ________________________________

(c) 99201 ________________________________

(d) 78600 ________________________________

(e) 85007 ________________________________

5–8 Use your CPT codebook and determine the name of the E/M *subsection* you would look in to find codes for the following scenarios.

(a) An established patient of Dr. Practon presents in his office with a complaint of gastrointestinal pain. ________________________

(b) Dr. Practon goes to the home of a housebound patient he has been treating for 10 years to evaluate the patient's status. ________________________

(c) Dr. Antrum provides a consultation on a patient she has never seen at College Hospital at the request of Dr. Practon. ________________________

5–9 List what *categories* or *subcategories* of E/M subsections you would look in to find codes for the above scenarios. Note: Not all subsections have categories listed; some have only subcategories listed right after the subsection title (e.g., Emergency Department Services [subsection], New or Established Patient [subcategory]). Look at the size of the title to determine if it is a subsection, category, or subcategory (look at the title color if your CPT is color-coded).

(a) ________________________

(b) ________________________

(c) ________________________

5–10 Use your CPT book to locate the *category* and *subcategory* in which the following E/M codes are found. Note: Be careful not to list the section or subsection titles.

Code	Category	Subcategory
(a) **99252**	**Initial Inpatient Consultation**	**New/Established Patient**
(b) 99219	______________	______________
(c) 99274	______________	______________
(d) 99242	______________	______________
(e) 99301	______________	______________

5–11 Services that go beyond the usual services provided in either inpatient or outpatient settings are found under the E/M subsection: ______________

5–12 Write the code for an unlisted E/M procedure. ______________

5–13 Write the definition that is used to describe a neonate when assigning neonatal intensive care codes. ______________

____

5–14 Codes from the Nursing Facility Services category are used to report services for various types of nursing facilities and ______________

____

Exercise Exchange

Directions: *Select the correct CPT code(s) from the Evaluation and Management section for the following exercises. Use your procedure codebook or refer to Figure 5–5.*

5–1 Preventive medicine services for a:

(a) 31-year-old new patient ______________

(b) 6-year-old established patient ______________

5–2 Dr. Practon called Dr. Gaston Input requesting he do a gastrointestinal consultation at College Hospital on a patient in room 304. Dr. Input took a detailed history (D HX) and performed a detailed physical examination (D PX). The medical decision making was of low complexity (L MDM). ______________

5–3 Two days later all of the tests that Dr. Input ordered on the patient in room 304 were completed. The patient's condition was deteriorating so Dr. Practon called Dr. Input again to see the patient, evaluate the test results, and make a recommendation. An expanded problem-focused interval history and examination took place (EPF HX PX) with moderate-complexity decision making (M MDM). ______________

5–4 A patient was sent for consultation to Dr. Gene Ulibarri's office by Dr. Brady Coccidioidis, the patient's primary care physician. The patient had a long history of urinary and kidney problems which required a comprehensive history and physical examination (C HX PX); however, the medical decision making was of moderate complexity (M MDM). ______________

5–5 Dr. Raymond Skeleton, an orthopedic surgeon, saw Dr. Practon's patient in his office for a consultation regarding the patient's amputated leg. The patient's prosthesis had fallen off of the patient's right leg when the patient stepped off of a curb, causing the patient to fall. There was a stress fracture in the tibial plateau. A cast was applied, but the fracture was not healing well due to the patient's osteoporosis. Surgery was inevitable. Dr. Skeleton sent the patient to Dr. Carpenter for another opinion regarding the type of surgery to be performed. Dr. Carpenter took a comprehensive history (C HX), performed a comprehensive examination (C PX), and used high-complexity medical decision making (H MDM) skills to evaluate the patient. He sent a report to Dr. Skeleton stating the type of surgery he recommended. Code Dr. Carpenter's claim. ________________

5–6 An established patient presents in Dr. Practon's office without an appointment stating she has an *emergency*. The patient is having difficulty breathing and is taken back to the treatment room immediately. Dr. Practon takes a detailed history (D HX), performs a detailed examination (D PX) and makes a low-complexity medical decision (L MDM) regarding the patient's condition.

____

____

5–7 Dr. Skeleton is called to the emergency room at College Hospital by the ER physician to evaluate and treat one of his patients with a broken collar bone. He takes an expanded problem-focused history (EPF HX), performs an expanded problem-focused examination (EPF PX), and makes a medical decision of low complexity (L MDM). ________________

5–8 An established patient of Dr. Cardi arrives in the emergency room complaining of chest pain. He is evaluated and treated by the ER physician who takes a comprehensive history (C HX), performs a comprehensive examination (C PX), and makes a high-complexity medical decision (H MDM). ________________

5–9 An established patient of Dr. Cardi arrives in the emergency room of College Hospital complaining of chest pain, shortness of breath, and fatigue. The ER physician evaluates the patient (D HX PX, M MDM) and then calls Dr. Cardi because of the patient's grave condition. Dr. Cardi comes to the emergency room and also evaluates the patient (C HX PX, H MDM) and decides to admit the patient. Select the correct CPT codes for the ER physician's claim and Dr. Cardi's claim.

ER physician ________________

Dr. Cardi ________________

5–10 Dr. Gaston Input saw a critically ill established patient in the intensive care unit of College Hospital and provided constant bedside care for 45 minutes. ________________

5–11 Dr. Perry Cardi saw a critically ill new patient in the morning of July 10 in the cardiac care unit of College Hospital. He provided constant bedside care for 1 hour 12 minutes. That afternoon Dr. Cardi returned to the hospital and spent an additional 1 hour 10 minutes.

______________ × ______

______________ × ______

5–12 Dr. Caesar's patient delivered a low-birth-weight infant at College Hospital on March 15. The infant needed cardiac and respiratory support and was admitted to the neonatal intensive care unit. Dr. Pedro Atrics, a pediatrician, followed the child and on March 18 the child's condition was upgraded to stable. On March 19 Dr. Atrics saw the infant in the neonatal intensive care unit. Select the correct code for services provided on March 19 by Dr. Atrics.

____

5–13 A 19-year-old established female patient presented in Dr. Practon's office for a yearly physical examination. A comprehensive history and physical exam was performed and Dr. Practon discussed disease transmission during sexual activity, various birth control methods, and risks of using drugs and/or alcohol. ________________

5–14 A 4-year-old new patient came in to Dr. Practon's office with his mother for a pre-kindergarten examination. ________________

5–15 Mrs. Robertson was concerned about her 16-year-old daughter losing weight and constantly working out at the gym. The daughter refused to be examined by her primary care physician, Dr. Practon, but finally agreed to talk with him. Mrs. Robertson scheduled an appointment for her daughter to discuss diet and exercise which took 45 minutes. ________________

5–16 Mrs. Robertson's daughter agreed to return to a group counseling session the following week. About eight individuals attended the group session on eating disorders which lasted 60 minutes.

____

5–17 An established patient of Dr. Langerhans was diagnosed with diabetes mellitus. Dr. Langerhans recommended that the patient attend a group session the following month where a diabetologist would discuss diet, monitoring blood sugar, and insulin control. What CPT code would the diabetologist use on his claim form? ________________

5–18 A pregnant patient (28 weeks' gestation) with a long history of premature labor began having contractions and called Dr. Caesar, her obstetrician. Dr. Caesar recommended that the patient be placed in an observation unit in College Hospital. Dr. Caesar's care included a C HX PX, L MDM. The patient was monitored, given IV fluids, and discharged the same day.

____

5–19 Mrs. McDougall was a patient at College Hospital and Dr. Practon discharged her to College Heights Nursing Facility on March 13. Dr. Practon performed the nursing facility assessment which involved the following: D interval HX, C PX, M MDM.

____

____

5–20 Dr. Ulibarri went to the Meadow Lark Rest Home to see a patient of his with chronic urinary problems and an occluded catheter. His assessment included the following: EPF HX, D PX, M MDM.

____

5–21 Prolonged service in the office with face-to-face patient contact; 1 hour 23 minutes.

______________ × ______

______________ × ______

5–22 Prolonged service without direct face-to-face patient contact; 1 hour 50 minutes

______________ × ______

______________ × ______

5–23 Dr. Practon saw an established patient in his office and took a D HX PX, H MDM. Besides the typical 25 minutes that would usually be spent for such an encounter, he spent an additional 45 minutes in the treatment room answering patient questions, reassuring the patient, and going over treatment options.

____

______________ × ______

5–24 Dr. Atrics, the pediatrician, spent 2 hours standing by for a high-risk cesarean delivery.

______________ × ______

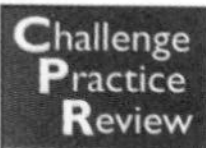

CPR Session: Answers

REVIEW SESSIONS 5–1 THROUGH 5–5

5–1 outpatient
5–2 inpatient
5–3 CMS (formerly HCFA)
5–4 (a) Two-digit add-on code
(b) Five-digit modifier code
5–5 -99

REVIEW SESSIONS 5–6 THROUGH 5–10

5–6 Seven
5–7 Appendix A
5–8 First two digits
5–9 B (type of service)
5–10 Inpatient hospital care

CHALLENGE SESSION 5–11

5–11 (a) (1) New patient.
(b) It has been over 3 years since the patient was seen by Dr. Practon.

REVIEW SESSIONS 5–12 THROUGH 5–17

5–12 Three
5–13 (a) Two out of three
(b) Three out of three
5–14 (a) history
(b) physical examination
(c) medical decision making
(d) comprehensive
(e) problem-focused
(f) straightforward
(g) low complexity
(h) expanded problem-focused
(i) high complexity
(j) detailed
5–15 none
5–16 comprehensive
5–17 moderate complexity

PRACTICE SESSIONS 5–18 THROUGH 5–20

5–18 99211
5–19 (a) level 4
(b) level 1
(c) level 5
(d) level 3
5–20 (a) 99232
(b) 99204
(c) 99394

REVIEW SESSIONS 5–21 THROUGH 5–26

5–21 critical care
5–22 preventive medicine
5–23 consultation
5–24 observation status
5–25 emergency care
5–26 counseling

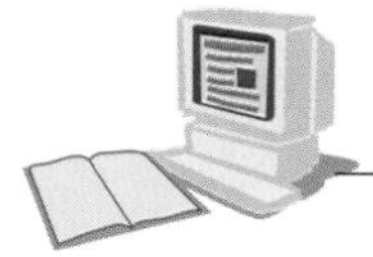

Resources

Insurance billing specialists need current comprehensive coding reference materials to code evaluation and management services appropriately. Answers to coding questions can be researched in reference books that are easy to use and provide additional coding information. Attending seminars is also a method for keeping up-to-date on coding issues. Seminars often offer sessions on coding Evaluation and Management Services and cover documentation guidelines and problems specific to different specialties. Coding hotlines, accessed through subscriptions, offer an opportunity to network with other coders and ask specific coding questions. Following is a suggested list of coding resources.

Reference Books

- *E/M Coding Made Easy* 3rd edition, 1998, Practice Management Information Corporation (PMI), 4727 Wilshire Boulevard, Los Angeles, CA 90010 (800) MED-SHOP (800) 633-7467.
- *E/M Fast Finder, 2001* (updated annually), Medicode/Ingenix Publishing Group, 5225 Wiley Post Way, Suite 500 (84116-2889), P.O. Box 27116, Salt Lake City, UT 84152-6180 (800) 999-4600.
- *Evaluation and Management Coding and Documentation Guide,* St. Anthony/Ingenix Publishing Group, P.O. Box 96561, Washington, DC 20090 (800) 632-0123.
- *Evaluation and Management Documentation Guidelines* and *Evaluation and Management Chart Auditing 2001* (updated annually), Medical Management Institute, 11405 Old Roswell Road, Alpharetta, GA 30004 (800) 334-5724.

Codebooks

- *Current Procedural Terminology* (published annually), American Medical Association, Order Department, AAMA, P.O. Box 930876, Atlanta, GA 31193-0878 Telephone (800) 621-8335.
- *HCPCS Level II Codes,* American Medical Association, Order Department, AAMA, P.O. Box 930876, Atlanta, GA 31193-0878 Telephone (800) 621-8335.
- *Red Book Annual* and *Red Book Updates* (12 issues) available from Medical Economics Company, 5 Paragon Drive, Montvale, NJ 07645-1742 (800) 232-7379.

Objectives

After reading this chapter and completing the exercise sessions, you should be able to:

Learning Objectives:

- ✔ Define procedure code terminology.
- ✔ Explain the purpose of coding for professional services.
- ✔ Name the classifications of anesthesia that may be billed separately from the surgical procedure.
- ✔ List all subsections of the Surgery section.
- ✔ Compare comprehensive codes and component codes.
- ✔ Define the meaning of the star symbol (*) in the Surgery section.
- ✔ Distinguish between surgical package and Medicare global package rules.
- ✔ Describe two ways to code for multiple procedures.
- ✔ Demonstrate an understanding of surgical terminology.
- ✔ Explain situations in which modifiers are applied to surgical codes.

Performance Objectives:

- ✔ Locate a code in the Surgery section by using the index.
- ✔ Calculate anesthesia time and compute the unit value.
- ✔ Code scenarios presented in the worktext from all sections of CPT.
- ✔ Apply CPT and HCPCS Level II modifiers when appropriate.

Key Terms

add-on code
anesthesia
bilateral procedure
bundled code
closed fracture
closed treatment
component code
comprehensive code
downcoding
elective surgery
endoscopy
fixation
fracture manipulation
global surgery policy
indented code
open fracture
open treatment
percutaneous treatment
professional component (PC)
qualitative analysis
quantitative analysis
separate procedure
stand-alone codes
star procedure
surgical package
technical component (TC)
test panel
unbundling
upcoding

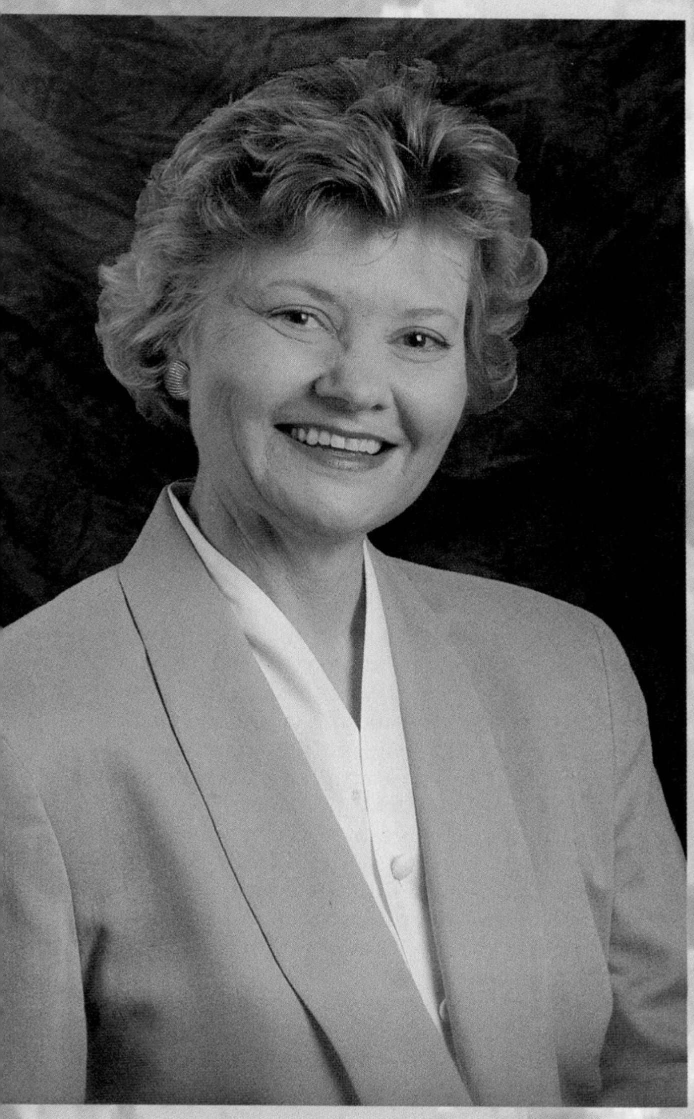

Chapter

6

I was a stay-at-home mom and did genealogy research, which required general computer knowledge. I quickly developed a love for research, history, and working on the computer. When our youngest son was preparing to go to college I began looking for a way to use my skills to earn money. I finally settled on the idea of starting my own medical billing company.

For a year I attended courses related to medical billing and worked as an intern at a local billing company. After taking a marketing course I went out and secured my first client. Instead of concentrating on marketing and building the business quickly, I focused on upholding a higher standard for my business. My husband became a part of the business; he likes managing the business side while I love coding. Together, we have made our business a success.

Charline Rambaud, CPC
Owner–Coding Specialist
Medical Billing Service

Coding Procedures Part II:

Anesthesia, Surgery, Radiology, Pathology/Laboratory, and Medicine

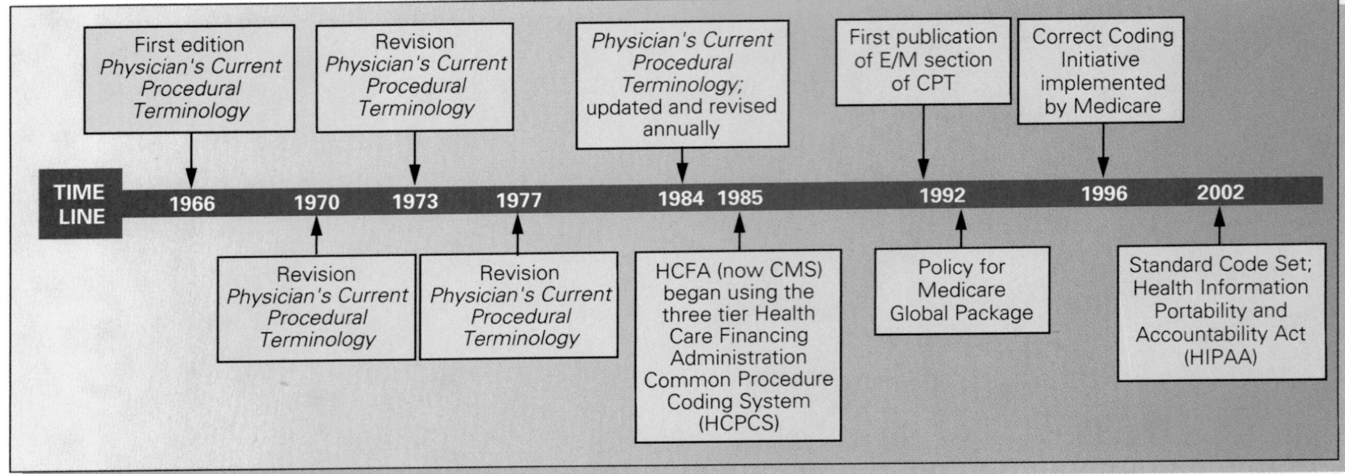

CODING PROCEDURES AND SERVICES

In the previous chapter you learned the basics of coding Evaluation and Management Services. In this chapter you will learn how to code procedures and services from the remaining sections of CPT; namely Anesthesia, Surgery, Radiology, Pathology/Laboratory, and Medicine. Before assigning codes from any of these sections, read the CPT guidelines that appear at the beginning of each section. The index at the end of CPT is recommended for locating codes in these sections, and directions will be given on its use throughout this chapter.

Anesthesia Section

Anesthesia is the partial or complete absence of normal sensation. An anesthesiologist, nurse anesthetist, or other physician provides anesthesia during a surgical procedure by introducing a pharmaceutical substance to depress the nervous system so that the patient will not feel pain. The Anesthesia section is a specialized section used to report the services of anesthesia, usually during surgery. Different types of anesthesia are classified according to the effect they have on the body. Anesthesia induced for medical or surgical purposes may be classified as topical, local, regional, or general, as seen in Table 6–1. Only the classifications of *regional* and *general* anesthesia may be billed separate from the surgical procedure and are included in this section.

Subsections in the Anesthesia section are divided by anatomic site, except for the last three subsections, Radiological Procedures, Burn Excisions or Debridement, and Other Procedures. The Radiological Procedure subsection is used when anesthesia is provided during a diagnostic or therapeutic radiologic service. The Burn subsection is arranged according to percent of body surface area treated and used when surgery is performed to excise or debride a burn.

The Anesthesia section is arranged so that the majority of anesthesia services are found under the

Table 6–1 Anesthesia Classifications

Classification	Description of Anesthetic Agent	Billing Guidelines	Example
Topical	A solution, gel, or ointment applied to the skin, mucous membrane, or cornea to reduce or eliminate sensation in a surface area (also known as surface anesthesia)	*Included* in the surgical procedure; *may not be billed separately* (surgical package rule)	Gel applied to the urethra for dilation of urethra
Local	A substance (usually injected) to reduce or eliminate sensation in one spot or part of the body	*Included* in the surgical procedure; *may not be billed separately* (surgical package rule)	Subcutaneous injection to remove a nevus (mole)
Regional	A substance used to reduce or eliminate sensation in an area or region of the body by blocking a group of nerve fibers	**Not included in the surgical procedure; may be billed separately** (Medicare does not pay for regional anesthesia by surgeon)	Epidural injection used during labor and delivery
General	A substance used to produce loss of sensation and consciousness; given primarily by inhalation or intravenous injection (including four types of nerve blocks)	**Not included in the surgical procedure; may be billed separately** (Medicare does not pay for general anesthesia by surgeon)	Inhalation of a substance during tonsillectomy to render the patient totally unconscious

Example 6–1

Anesthesia Code Assignment

Procedure	Simple bunionectomy; right foot
Diagnosis	Hallux valgus; right foot
Type of anesthesia	General—monitored anesthesia care (MAC)
Provider of anesthesia	Certified registered nurse anesthetist (CRNA), not medically directed

TYPE OF CODE	**CODE**	**DESCRIPTION**
Surgical procedure	28290	Correction, hallux valgus (bunion); simple
Diagnosis	735.0	Hallux valgus
Anesthesia	**01480-QZ-QS**	**Anesthesia for open procedures on bones of lower leg, ankle, and foot** **QZ** = CRNA service; without medical direction by physician **QS** = Monitored anesthesia care service
Optional Anesthesia reporting	28290-QZ-QS	

anatomic site where the surgery is performed. After locating the correct site you will find a list of codes that represent the type of procedure performed. Following are questions to ask when searching for an anesthesia code:

1. Where was the surgery performed (anatomic site)?
2. What type of anesthesia was administered (regional, general)?
3. Who provided the anesthesia (anesthesiologist, anesthetist, other physician)?

The type of provider and number of cases the anesthesiologist performed or supervised at one time may need to be identified by use of a modifier appended to the code. See CPT modifier -47 (anesthesia by surgeon) and HCPCS Level II modifiers in Appendix C of this worktext.

Instead of using codes from the Anesthesia section, some insurance carriers require the anesthesiologist to bill by reporting the surgical procedure with a modifier indicating who performed the anesthesia. Example 6–1 shows two ways of billing anesthesia provided during bunionectomy. To find the bunionectomy procedure code, look in the index under Repair, then bunion (type of repair); a range of codes will be listed. To find the anesthesia code, look in the index under Anesthesia, then foot (anatomic part); a range of codes will be listed.

For all cases, an anesthesiologist determines the physical status of a patient and documents this information

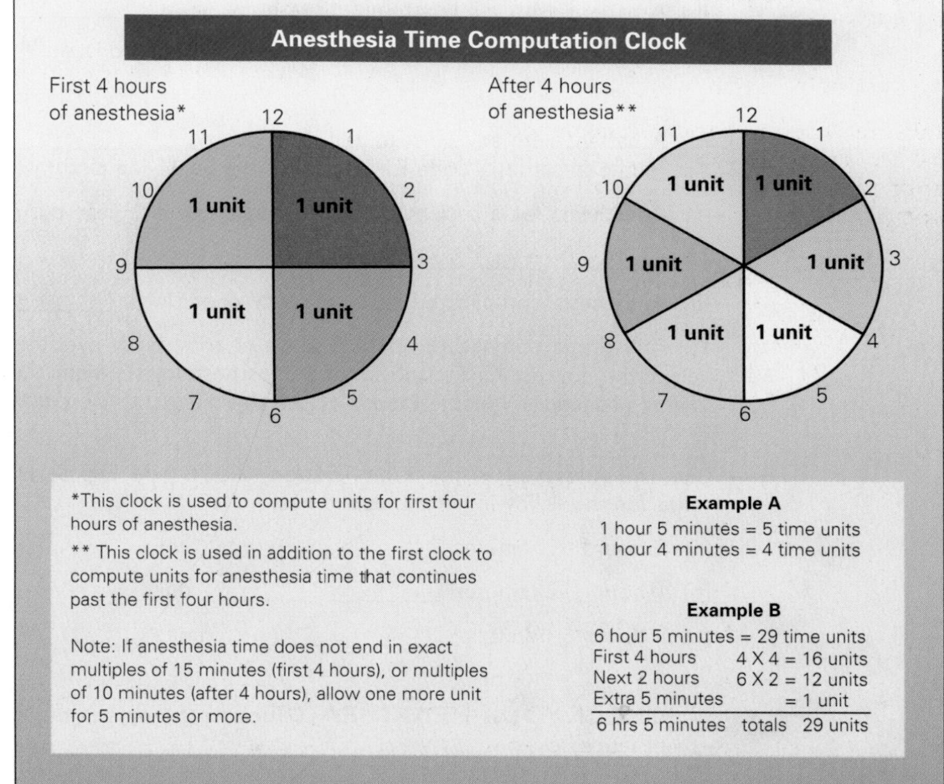

Anesthesia Time Computation Clock
First 4 hours of anesthesia*
After 4 hours of anesthesia**
1 unit
*This clock is used to compute units for first four hours of anesthesia.
** This clock is used in addition to the first clock to compute units for anesthesia time that continues past the first four hours.
Note: If anesthesia time does not end in exact multiples of 15 minutes (first 4 hours), or multiples of 10 minutes (after 4 hours), allow one more unit for 5 minutes or more.
Example A
1 hour 5 minutes = 5 time units
1 hour 4 minutes = 4 time units
Example B
6 hour 5 minutes = 29 time units
First 4 hours 4 X 4 = 16 units
Next 2 hours 6 X 2 = 12 units
Extra 5 minutes = 1 unit
6 hrs 5 minutes totals 29 units

Figure 6–1. Clock guide used to compute anesthesia time in units.

in the anesthesia record. The coder must choose a physical status modifier (P1–P6), found at the end of the Anesthesia Guidelines to append all anesthesia codes.

In some situations, qualifying circumstances may be present during anesthesia, for example, anesthesia for a patient less than 1 year of age. When any qualifying circumstances apply, assign the correct five-digit add-on procedure code found either at the end of the Anesthesia Guidelines or near the end of the Medicine section under Qualifying Circumstances for Anesthesia.

A useful tool when coding anesthesia for procedures is the American Society of Anesthesiologists (ASA) *2000 Crosswalk* (see Resources at the end of this chapter). This text will direct you from the CPT procedure code to the correct anesthesia code.

Calculating Anesthesia Time

A unique feature used when processing claims with codes from the Anesthesia section is the determination of the service based on the amount of time the anesthesia was administered. The hours and minutes of service are recorded in the patient's anesthesia record and a basic unit value is assigned to each procedure code in the Anesthesia section. Time is typically billed in 15-minute units; however, each insurance carrier or managed care plan may have criteria that vary from this. A quick way to compute units of anesthesia time is by using a guide such as that shown in Figure 6–1.

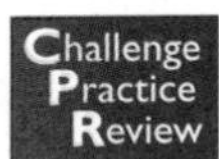

Pause and Practice CPR

PRACTICE SESSIONS 6–1 THROUGH 6–4

Directions: *Complete these exercises to develop and enhance your anesthesia procedure coding skills. Use your procedure codebook.*

6–1 List the physical status modifier for the following descriptions:

(a) A moribund patient who is not expected to survive without the operation.

____

(b) A patient with mild systemic disease. _______________

(c) A patient with severe systemic disease that is a constant threat to life.

____

(d) A patient with severe systemic disease. _______________

6–2 Assign the anesthesia code for the following qualifying circumstances:

(a) Anesthesia for a patient of extreme age, under 1 year old and over 70 years old.

____

(b) Anesthesia complicated by emergency conditions. _______________

(c) Anesthesia complicated by utilization of total body hypothermia. _______________

6–3 Select the correct CPT code for the anesthesiologist (from the Anesthesia section) for the following procedure. Needle biopsy of the thyroid gland (percutaneous core needle).

____

6–4 Use the Anesthesia Time Computation Clock (see Fig. 6–1) and calculate the correct unit value for the following anesthesia times.

(a) 2 hours 45 minutes: _______________ units

(b) 1 hours 12 minutes: _______________ units

(c) 5 hours 5 minutes: _______________ units

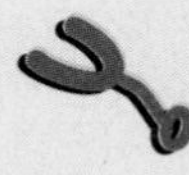

CHECK YOUR HEARTBEAT! Turn to the end of the chapter for answers to these practice sessions.

Introduction to the Surgery Section

The Surgery section is the largest section in the CPT codebook. It has 16 subsections divided according to body systems such as the Integumentary System, Musculoskeletal System, Respiratory System, and so on. Surgery guidelines for all subsections are found at the beginning of the Surgery section. Each subsection is further divided into categories that are usually based on anatomic site, for example, head, neck, back, and so on. Within each category are subcategories listed according to type of procedure (excision, repair, destruction, graft), or condition (burn, fracture, septal defect).

Before attempting to code, let's become familiar with all subsections of the Surgery section.

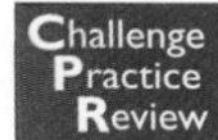

Pause and Practice CPR

PRACTICE SESSION 6–5

Directions: *Complete these exercises to become familiar with all subsections of the Surgery section and various divisions in the CPT codebook. Use your procedure codebook.*

6–5 List all subsections in the Surgery section.

(a) ______________________

(b) ______________________

(c) ______________________

(d) ______________________

(e) ______________________

(f) ______________________

(g) ______________________

(h) ______________________

(i) ______________________

(j) ______________________

(k) ______________________

(l) ______________________

(m) ______________________

(n) ______________________

(o) ______________________

(p) ______________________

(q) ______________________

(r) ______________________

CHECK YOUR HEARTBEAT! Turn to the end of the chapter for answers to these practice sessions.

How to Code Effectively

You must be able to analyze a procedure description and identify various terms that will direct you to the correct code. To do this you must know the main categories under which services and procedures are listed according to their main term in the index (Table 6–2).

After the procedure, service, or condition is identified in the index according to its main term, search for a subterm and a sub-subterm that further defines the procedure. When a code range is found, turn to the correct section and read all descriptions listed under the code range before selecting a code (Fig. 6–2).

Table 6–2 Surgery Section Main Term Categories

Main Term	Example
Procedure	abortion, arthroplasty, cystectomy, fracture repair, graft
Service	blood typing, cardiography, injection, ultrasound, x-ray
Organ	gallbladder, heart, kidney, liver, lung, stomach
Anatomic site	abdomen, arm, artery, head, leg, neck
Condition	abscess, blood clot, dislocation, fibrillation, hernia
Synonym	defibrillation = cardioversion, encephalon = brain, laceration = wound, removal = excision
Eponym	Colles' fracture, Epstein-Barr virus, Gasserian ganglion, Heller's operation
Abbreviation	CABG = coronary artery bypass graft TURP = transurethral resection of prostate VDRL = Venereal Disease Research Laboratory

Procedure descriptions are given after each code number in all sections. To understand how the definitions are interpreted and to properly read the descriptions, you must first understand the two types of codes: stand-alone codes and indented codes.

Stand-Alone and Indented Codes

Stand-alone codes have a full description. To read a description of an **indented code,** you must first read the portion of the description of the stand-alone code that comes before the semicolon (;). Any terminology after the semicolon has a dependent status, as do the subsequent indented entries. The words following the semicolon can change the code selection completely because they may change the extent of the procedure, represent an alternative anatomic site, or represent an alternative procedure (Fig. 6–3). Subsequent codes (after the semicolon) are arranged in ascending order according to resource consumption. Each code represents a more complicated procedure and has an increased dollar value.

Use Of Semicolon In CPT Descriptions

STAND-ALONE CODE	DESCRIPTION OF SERVICE
24900 $	**Amputation, arm through humerus;** with primary closure
INDENTED CODES	
24920 $	open, circular (guillotine)
24925 $$$	secondary closure or scar revision
24930 $$$$	re-amputation
24931 $$$$$	with implant

Figure 6–3. Use of semicolon in surgery section of *Current Procedural Terminology* indicating stand-alone code (24900) and indented codes (24920, 24925, 24930, and 24931). (CPT codes, descriptions, and material only are copyright 2001 American Medical Association. All rights reserved.)

Integral Code Descriptions

Surgical code descriptions may define a correct coding relationship where one code is part of another based on the language used in the description. Refer to Example 6–2 for definitions of partial and complete, partial and total, unilateral and bilateral, and single and multiple.

Parentheses

Parentheses, (), further define the code and tell where other services are located (Fig. 6–4).

Measurements

Measurements throughout the codebook are based on the metric system (e.g., cm for centimeters).

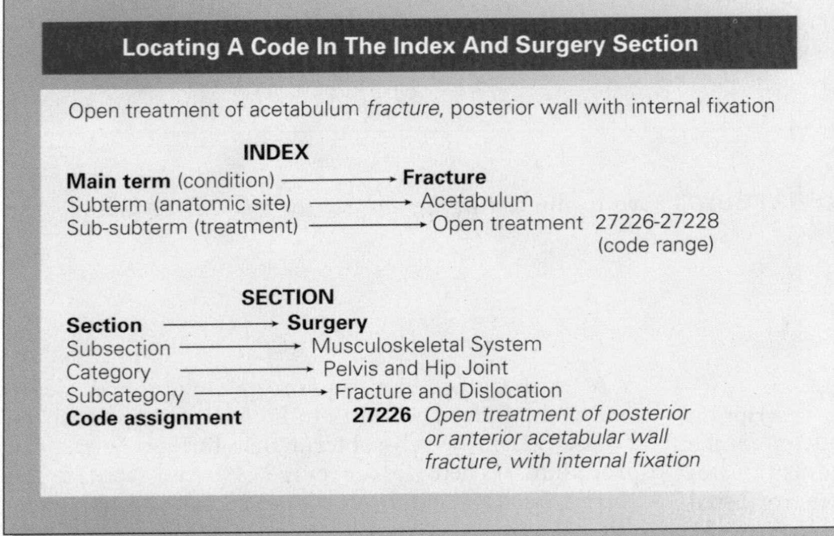

Figure 6–2. Locating the code (27226) for *open treatment of acetabulum fracture* in the index and surgery section of *Current Procedural Terminology.* (CPT codes, descriptions, and material only are copyright 2001 American Medical Association. All rights reserved.)

PROCEDURE

Coding Steps

To code effectively, follow these steps:

1. Read the *Introduction* section at the beginning of the codebook. This changes annually with each addition.
2. Use the index at the back of the book to locate the *main term* for a specific service or procedure by generalized code numbers, not by page numbers.
3. Search under the main term for subterms indicating the name of the procedure or service you are coding.
4. Turn to the beginning of the section in which the code is located and read the *Guidelines*. All sections have guidelines located at the beginning, which define commonly used terms, list subsections with code ranges, and give instructions specific to each section.
5. Read the *notes* within all sections that precede the category or subcategory where the code is located. Notes include additional definitions and instructions specific to the category or subcategory within the subsection.
6. Locate the code number and read through the narrative description to verify the correct code.
7. Determine if modifier usage is needed to give a more accurate description of the services rendered.
8. Transfer the five-digit code number (and modifier if applicable) to the claim form exactly as given for each procedure or service. Be careful not to transpose numbers.

Coding from the Operative Report

When coding surgery, obtain a copy of the patient's operative report from the hospital or surgical center. Make a photocopy and use a ruler as you scan the report line by line. Highlight words that may indicate that the procedure performed may be altered by specific circumstances and qualifies for modifier usage. Look up any unfamiliar terms and write the definitions in the margin. Beware of terms that look similar but have different meanings that could lead to coding errors.

Do not code using only the name of the procedure given in the heading of the report. Read the operative report thoroughly and code only the operations that were actually documented in the report. Determine whether procedures performed were part of the main procedure (bundled), performed independently (unbundled), or unrelated. Some cases may need two codes to describe a complete procedure while other cases may have several procedures included in one code description.

Because of liability issues, never code procedures or circumstances that the physician relays to you verbally. If the physician says the codes do not encompass all that was done, the physician may need to dictate an addendum to describe the additional procedure(s). The insurance carrier assumes that any procedure or service that is not documented in the patient's medical record was not performed. Remember the rule: Not documented, not done! Information on how to code multiple procedures that are not inherent to a major procedure may be found later in this chapter under Multiple Procedure Modifier -51.

When billing a complex surgical procedure, either include an operative report or give a brief explanation in the proper block of the insurance claim form so that the claims adjuster clearly understands the case and maximum payment is generated. If there were extensive complications, be sure the words "extensive complications" are in the report.

By reading the report you can be certain that all procedural and diagnostic codes have been identified and are properly linked. Compare the report content with the codes you include on the insurance claim.

Example 6–2

Integral Code Descriptions

Partial and complete, which means the partial procedure is included in the complete procedure.

56620 Vulvectomy simple; partial
56625 *complete*

Partial and total, which means the partial procedure is included in the total procedure.

58940 Oophorectomy, partial or total, unilateral or bilateral

Unilateral and bilateral, which means the unilateral procedure is included in the bilateral procedure.

58900 Biopsy of ovary, unilateral or bilateral

Single and multiple, which means the single procedure is included in the multiple procedure.

49321 Laparoscopy, surgical; with biopsy (single or multiple)

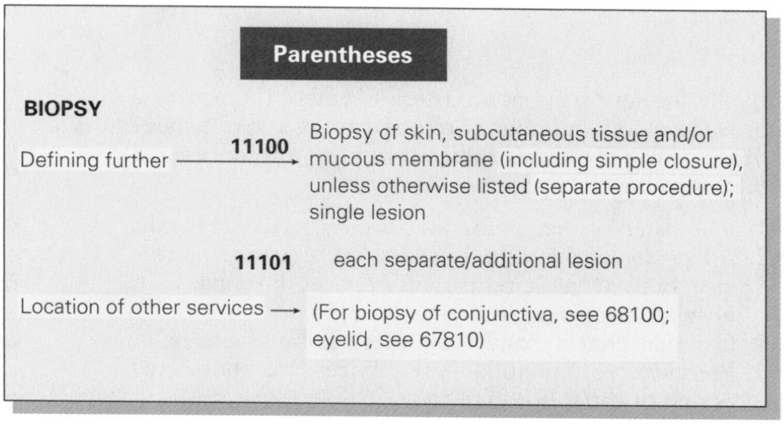

Parentheses

BIOPSY

Defining further → **11100** Biopsy of skin, subcutaneous tissue and/or mucous membrane (including simple closure), unless otherwise listed (separate procedure); single lesion

11101 each separate/additional lesion

Location of other services → (For biopsy of conjunctiva, see 68100; eyelid, see 67810)

Figure 6–4. Use of parentheses in the surgery section of *Current Procedural Terminology.* (CPT codes, descriptions, and material only are copyright 2001 American Medical Association. All rights reserved.)

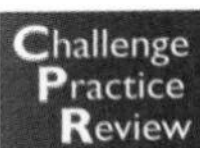

Pause and Practice CPR

REVIEW SESSIONS 6–6 THROUGH 6–8

Directions: *Complete these exercises to enhance your knowledge about the organization of, and types of codes found in, the CPT manual. Use your procedure codebook.*

6–6 Name the section of CPT where the following codes are found.

(a) 85576 ______

(b) 33600 ______

(c) 99342 ______

(d) 11010 ______

(e) 92340 ______

(f) 76090 ______

(g) 60000 ______

6–7 Refer to the main term categories listed in Table 6–2 and write the *category* of the main term for the following, as illustrated in the first example.

(a) **Kelikian procedure** **eponym**

(b) Circumcision ______

(c) ICCE ______

(d) Pelvic ______

(e) Abscess ______

(f) House call ______

(g) Lung ______

6–8 Determine and label the following codes as "stand-alone" codes or "indented" codes.

(a) 31201 ______

(b) 20200 ______

(c) 32650 ______

(d) 32662 ______

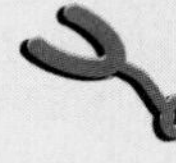

CHECK YOUR HEARTBEAT! Turn to the end of the chapter for answers to these review sessions.

Star Symbol

In the Surgery section, an asterisk symbol (*) next to a procedure code number is referred to as a **star procedure.** Star procedures indicate minor procedures and the following rules apply:

1. The listed service is for the surgical procedure only.
2. All postoperative care is added on a service-by-service basis (e.g., a return office visit, hospital visit, hospital discharge, suture removal).
3. Complications are added on a service-by-service basis.
4. Preoperative and follow-up services are considered as one of the following:

a. When a star procedure is carried out at the time of the initial (new patient) office visit and constitutes the *major* service provided at that visit, identify the procedure by listing the surgical procedure code and use Medicine code number 99025 in lieu of an E/M code for the new patient visit (refer to Example 6–3).

b. When the star procedure is carried out at the time of the initial or other patient visit involving *significant identifiable services* (e.g., removal of a *small* skin lesion at the time of a *comprehensive* history and physical examination), list the appropriate E/M service applying modifier -25, the star

Example 6–3

Medicine Section Code 99025 and Star Procedure

A new patient (NP) presents in the physician's office complaining of a skin abscess. The physician takes a problem-focused history, performs a problem-focused physical examination (PF HX PX), and decides to make an incision and drain the abscess; straightforward decision making (SF MDM).

99025	Initial new patient visit (used in lieu of E/M code)
10060*	Incision and drainage of abscess (star procedure)

This scenario indicates that the star surgical procedure, performed on a new patient, constitutes the major service. *All three requirements have been met to use code 99025.*

procedure, and all follow-up care (e.g., postoperative E/M services, suture removals, and so forth).

c. When the star procedure is carried out at the time of a follow-up (established patient) visit and this procedure constitutes the major service at that visit, the visit is usually not listed; therefore an E/M service is not coded.

d. When the star procedure requires hospitalization, both the hospital visit and the star procedure should be listed, as well as all follow-up care.

Decision for Surgery

When a decision is made for surgery during an office visit, consult, or hospital admission, and the surgery is performed that day or the next, a common question asked is whether a charge may be made for the E/M service. To understand how to bill for the preoperative service when a decision is made for surgery, refer to Figure 6–5 which lists three choices. When reviewing the criteria in Figure 6–5, questions to ask include:

- Is the patient new or established?
- Is the code number starred or nonstarred?

Example 6–4

Decision for Surgery

A new patient is seen in the office complaining of a great deal of pain. Cholangiography is done and reveals blocked bile ducts. A decision is made to operate and the patient is scheduled for surgery the next day.

8-1-20XX	99204-57	New patient office visit; decision for surgery
8-2-20XX	47600	Cholecystectomy

- Is the E/M service significant and separately identifiable from the procedure?
- What is the time lapse from the time the decision is made for surgery to the time when the procedure is performed?

The following should be noted regarding the three choices:

- 99025—This code is found in the Medicine section under Special Services and Reports; Miscellaneous Services. It is used in lieu of an E/M code *only* for a new patient having a star procedure that constitutes the major service at the visit (refer to Example 6–3).
- -57—This modifier is used strictly to report an E/M service that resulted in the initial decision to perform a major surgical procedure (i.e., those with a 90-day follow-up period) within 24 hours of the patient encounter. Modifier -57 tells the insurance company that a new or established patient office visit, an inpatient hospital visit, or an in- or outpatient consult that occurred the day of or day prior to surgery is not part of the global fee (Example 6–4).
- -25—Modifier -25 is defined as "Significant, separately identifiable evaluation and management service by same physician on the same day of the procedure or other service." In some cases you may be confused whether to assign modifier -25 or -57. The industry standard is to use -25 when a diagnostic

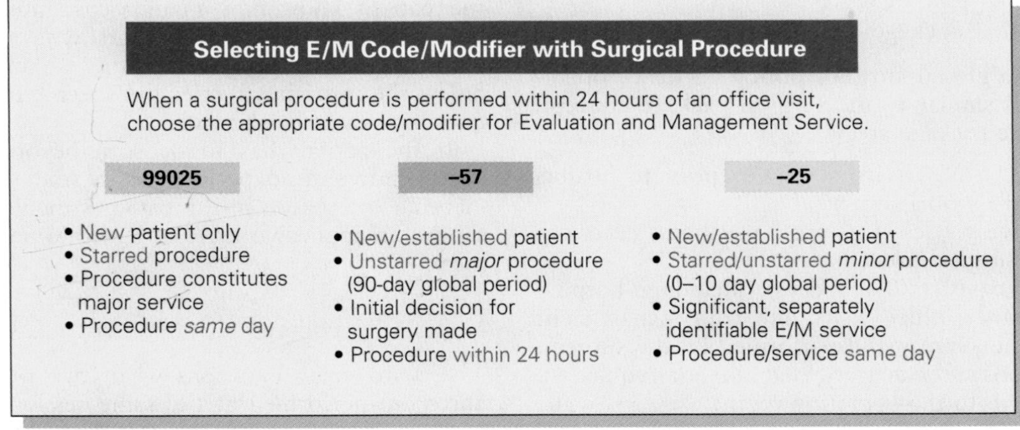

Figure 6–5. Three selections, with criteria to evaluate, when choosing the appropriate code/modifier for evaluation and management services when a surgical procedure is performed within 24 hours of an office visit.

procedure or minor procedure is involved (i.e., those with 0- to 10-day follow-up period).

There is also confusion because the CPT codebook states, "This modifier is not used to report an E/M service that resulted in a decision to perform surgery." To simplify the decision-making process, follow the criteria in Figure 6–5 when you are coding an E/M service and there is a surgical procedure performed within 24 hours.

Surgical Package

Surgical package is a phrase commonly encountered when coding operative procedures from the Surgery section. Procedures not followed by a star (*) include the "package" concept and one fee covers accompanying services. Some carriers refer to this as a global package. The majority of surgical procedures, including fracture care, are handled in this manner.

The package usually includes:

1. Surgical procedure (operation)
2. Anesthesia (local infiltration, digital block, or topical)
3. One related E/M encounter (subsequent to the decision for surgery) on the day of or day immediately prior to the procedure, including history and physical
4. Postoperative care (normal, uncomplicated follow-up hospital visits, discharge, and/or follow-up office visits)

Care should be taken when billing preoperative services separately. It is necessary to check with private carriers because many have an individual policy regarding what is included. Plans may include office visits 1 week prior to surgery or they may include only visits which occur 24 hours before surgery. Some include preoperative services for **elective surgery** but do not include those for emergency surgery. An elective surgery is scheduled in advance, recommended by the physician, done by choice of the patient, and is not an emergency.

Medicare Global Package

Medicare has a **global surgery policy** for major operations, which is similar to the surgical package concept. Included in the package are:

- Preoperative E/M service (24 hours prior to [major] or on day of [minor] surgery)
- Intraoperative services that are a usual and necessary part of the surgical procedure
- Postoperative visits (0–90 days), including hospital visits, discharge, office visits, and pain management related to the surgery and performed by the surgeon
- Complications after surgery that do not require an additional trip to the operating room
- Anesthesia by surgeon (local infiltration, digital block, topical, regional, or general)
- Supplies that are necessary for the performance of the procedure

Services provided for a Medicare patient *not included* in the global surgery package are:

- Initial consultation or evaluation (regardless of when or where it occurs)
- Diagnostic tests and procedures
- Treatment required to stabilize a seriously ill patient before surgery
- Postoperative visits unrelated to the diagnosis for which the surgical procedure was performed (modifier -24 would apply)
- Related procedure for postoperative complications that requires a return trip to the operating room (modifier -78 would apply)
- Immunosuppressive therapy after transplant surgery
- For services performed in a physician's office, separate payment may be made for splints and casting supplies, and a surgical tray (A4550) for *certain* procedures

Follow-Up Days

The number of follow-up days that are allowed after surgery for no additional fee varies. Minor surgeries may carry a 0-day or 10-day follow-up and major surgeries a 45-day or 90-day follow-up. The CPT code book does not specify how many days are included, so an additional reference manual is needed. Most states use a Relative Value Studies fee schedule for workers' compensation cases, which will list the follow-up days allowed for most surgical procedures. Another source is the *Federal Register*, which is published at the end of each year and lists follow-up days for Medicare services. Refer to the far right column of the fee schedule in Appendix C to locate the follow-up days that will be used for exercises in the worktext.

CPT code 99024, found in the Medicine section under Special Services and Reports, is available to use when documenting a postoperative visit within the global period. It has no value and is used for tracking purposes. It may be used on billing statements to let the patient know how many visits, after surgery, are being billed at no charge. Generally, it is not necessary to list this code when completing an insurance claim unless the insurance carrier has specific instructions requesting that it be shown.

If the patient has to be seen beyond the normal postoperative time period, justify the visit by documenting the reason in the patient's medical record and submit an applicable E/M code with a fee on the claim form.

Multiple Procedures

There are many occasions when two or more procedures are performed at the same session by the same provider. There are two choices when billing for more than one procedure. First, you must decide if the code is an *add-on code* or a code eligible to use modifier -51 (multiple procedure).

Multiple Procedure Modifier -51

Modifier -51 may be used to identify:

- Multiple medical procedures performed at the same session by the same provider
- A combination of multiple medical and surgical procedures
- Multiple procedures performed through separate incisions

DO NOT use modifier -51 in the following situations:

- With add-on codes (description to follow)
- When a code is marked by a symbol (Ø) indicating it is exempt from use with modifier -51
- When notes advise otherwise within a section (see note under "Arthrodesis" before code 22548).
- With E/M codes or Pathology/Laboratory codes

When modifier -51 applies, report the primary service or procedure, which can easily be determined by highest dollar value, as listed. Identify all additional services or procedures by appending code(s) with modifier -51 or use the separate five-digit modifier 09951 (see Example 6–5).

Usually, payment for the primary code is 100% of the allowable charge; second code, 50%; third code, 25%; fourth and remaining codes, 10%. However, Medicare pays 50% of the allowable charge for two to five secondary procedures and does not require the assignment of modifier -51. Always bill the full amount and let the insurance carrier make the payment adjustments for percentage consideration.

Add-on Code

An **add-on code** is noted in CPT by a cross (+) symbol. It is a code that represents an additional procedure done with a primary procedure. It cannot be billed without the primary procedure code, referred to as the *parent code.* Its description starts with "in addition," "list separately," or "second lesion" and may often be billed several times (see Example 6–6). Add-on codes are exempt from modifier -51. To cross-check refer to the list of add-on codes, which may be found in Appendix E of CPT, or refer to the list of codes exempt from modifier -51, which may be found in Appendix F of CPT.

Bilateral Procedures

A **bilateral procedure** is one performed on two sides. When a bilateral procedure is performed it is necessary to first determine if the code description defines the procedure as bilateral. For example, vasectomy, unilateral or bilateral (55250) clearly states bilateral and you would bill using the code once, without the need of a modifier. If the code does not include a bilateral description, modifier -50 would be used. There are two ways to bill for a bilateral procedure, as shown in Example 6–7. Medicare pays 150% of the entire bilateral procedure and in most regions it is not necessary to report using modifier -50.

Example 6–5

Multiple Procedure Modifier -51

Excision of 2.0 cm benign lesion on the nose and at the same session a biopsy of the skin and subcutaneous tissue of the forearm.

CODE	FEE	DESCRIPTION OF SERVICES
11442	$$	Excision, benign lesion, nose
11100-**51**	$	Biopsy of skin, forearm ***(second; multiple procedure)***

Example 6–6

Add-On Code

An abrasion procedure is done on two lesions to remove scarring.

15786	*(parent code)*	Abrasion; single lesion
+ 15787	**(add-on code)**	each additional four lesions or less (list separately in addition to code for primary procedure)

Note: In this scenario, the parent code is used to bill the first lesion and the add-on code is used to bill the second lesion.

Assistant at Surgery

Surgical procedures often need an assistant surgeon in addition to the primary surgeon. When billing for the assistant, indicate this by adding modifier -80 (assistant surgeon) to the same procedure code that the surgeon used to bill for the surgery, as shown in Example 6–8. You may need to call the office of the primary surgeon to obtain this information. If more than one surgeon is involved, clarify for whom you are billing by using two-digit modifiers (assistant surgeon, -80; minimum assistant surgeon, -81; assistant surgeon when a qualified resident surgeon is not available, -82; co-surgeon, -62; or team surgeon, -66).

The surgeon who assists is usually paid a fee of 16% to 30% of the allowed fee the primary surgeon

Example 6–7

Bilateral Procedure

Bilateral, total knee replacement

Choice 1. List the code once with *modifier* **-50** and double the fee in the charge column

27447-**50** $4000.00

Choice 2. List the code twice using the single fee, and *append the second listing with modifier* **-50**

27447 $2000.00
27447-**50** $2000.00

Note: *Modifier* -51 (multiple procedure) would also be appended to the second procedure in choice 2, thereby requiring the multiple modifier -99 to be used and the modifiers it represents described on the claim form

27447 $2000.00
27447-99 $2000.00 (99-50 51)

Example 6–8

Assistant at Surgery

Code reporting for primary and assistant surgeon, both operating to close an intestinal cutaneous fistula

CODE	DESCRIPTION OF SERVICES
44640	Closure of intestinal cutaneous fistula; *primary surgeon*
44640-**80**	Closure of intestinal cutaneous fistula; **assistant surgeon**

received. Most of the time the percentage reduction is calculated prior to claim submission and the reduced fee is listed. However, some insurance carriers may prefer having the full fee listed and calculating the reduction. Under Medicare guidelines, there may be some surgical procedures that restrict payment for an assistant surgeon, so refer to the provider manual or contact the fiscal intermediary for information.

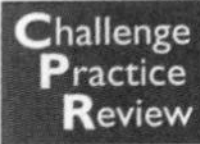

Pause and Practice CPR

REVIEW SESSIONS 6–9 THROUGH 6–14

Directions: *Complete these exercises to develop and enhance your procedure coding skills. Use your procedure codebook.*

6–9 Which procedure code numbers in the Surgery section include the surgical package concept?

____

6–10 Is an initial consultation (regardless of when it occurs) included in the Medicare global package concept? ____________

6–11 Are postoperative complications related to the surgery included in the Medicare global package concept? ____________

6–12 When billing for surgery, what are the maximum number of postoperative days allowed in the package concept? ____________

6–13 What code number is used when documenting a visit that occurs during the postoperative period? ____________

6–14 When billing for more than one procedure, what is the modifier listed to append the second and all additional procedures? ____________

CHALLENGE SESSION 6–15

Directions: *Use critical thinking skills to complete this exercise.*

6–15 A procedure is being performed on the same day as the office visit. When trying to decide between applying modifier -25 and -57, what are the main criteria to determine?

____

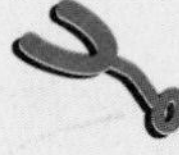

CHECK YOUR HEARTBEAT! Turn to the end of the chapter for answers to these review and challenge sessions.

Surgery Section

Integumentary System

The integumentary system is the first subsection listed in the Surgery section. It contains procedures performed on the skin (subcutaneous and accessory structures). Occasionally, a patient has a procedure performed that is described according to a category or subcategory in this subsection, but, the insurance coder gets lost looking for it in another subsection. It is important to remember that when a patient has a procedure performed that involves the *skin,* you will probably end up in the Integumentary subsection. For example: A patient presents in the office with a superficial cyst behind the left ear. The physician decides to perform a simple incision and drain the sebaceous cyst. You may think that the code would appear in the Auditory System (ear) subsection. Instead, because this type of cyst (sebaceous) grows in the layers of the skin, you will find the code in the Integumentary System subsection. Refer to Example 6–9 to locate the code for this scenario.

Example 6–9

Locating a Code in the Surgery Section

Incision and drainage of sebaceous cyst behind left ear.

INDEX	
Body system/Integumentary Skin	
Procedure	Incision and drainage
Code range	10040–10180
	INTEGUMENTARY
SUBSECTION	**SYSTEM**
Category (organ)	Skin, Subcutaneous and Accessory Structures
Subcategory (procedure)	Incision and Drainage
Type of condition	Cyst
Type of incision and drainage	Simple
Code assignment	**10060**

Careful consideration needs to be made regarding the type of cyst as well as the site where it occurs. For example, excision of a bone cyst in the hip (27065) would be found in the Musculoskeletal System subsection.

Benign versus Malignant

When coding a neoplasm, it is important to know if the specimen is benign or malignant. This will affect the procedure code, diagnostic code, and reimbursement. It is recommended to delay submission of the insurance claim and to review the pathology report and obtain the correct diagnosis.

A lesion is any discontinuity of the skin. A biopsy of a lesion performed for the purpose of determining the morphology (shape, form, and structure) is reported separately. A biopsy of a lesion followed by excision would be included in the excision procedure code, and not reported separately.

Note the following when coding removal of lesions:

- Anatomic site
- Size, measured in centimeters
- Number of lesions removed
- Process used to remove the lesions (excision, destruction, paring, shaving)
- Morphology (appearance of specimen's shape and structure used to determine benign or malignant status)

Expressions from Experience

The greatest satisfaction in my job comes through a successful argument with an insurance carrier who has inappropriately denied a claim. With knowledge and the confidence it brings, we are able to obtain the highest ethical reimbursement for our clients.

Charline Rambaud, CPC
Owner—Coding Specialist
Medical Billing Service

Measurements of a lesion should be taken from the physician's report, not the pathology report.

Repair of Lacerations

Laceration repairs, also known as wound repairs, may be classified as simple, intermediate, or complex, as described in notes preceding Repair (Closure), which is a category of the Integumentary System subsection. A brief descriptive summary follows:

- *Simple Closure*—Superficial; involving the epidermis, dermis, or subcutaneous tissue. No involvement of deeper structures; *one layered* closure/suturing.
- *Intermediate Closure*—Requires *layered closure* of deeper subcutaneous tissue in addition to the simple closure. Also included are heavily contaminated wounds that require extensive cleaning and *simple* closure.
- *Complex Closure*—Requires *more than one layered closure;* debridement, scar revision, extensive undermining, stents, or retention sutures.

If multiple lacerations are repaired with the same technique and are in the same anatomic category, the insurance billing specialist should add up the total length of all the lacerations and report one code.

PROCEDURE

Coding Repair of Mulitple Lacerations

Follow these steps to code repair of multiple lacerations:

1. Locate the type of repair (simple, intermediate, complex).
2. Locate the anatomic category (e.g., scalp, neck, axillae).
3. Add the length of all the wounds that fit into the repair type and anatomic category and report with one code.

Refer to Example 6–10 which shows a patient with three lacerations (2.5 cm, 2.7 cm, and 3.0 cm) on the right and left sides of the face. The lengths total 8.2 cm so the correct code (12015) is assigned. No modifier is needed to indicate right and left sides.

Multiple Lesions

When coding multiple lesions, watch for "add-on" (+) codes versus codes eligible for the application of modifier -51, and indented codes. Carefully read code descriptions, looking for terms such as *complex, complicated,*

Example 6–10

Repair of Multiple Lacerations

Three lacerations of the face totaling 8.2 cm

INCORRECT CODING	
12011	Repair 2.5 cm laceration of face
12013	Repair 2.7 cm laceration of face
12013	Repair 3 cm laceration of face
CORRECT CODING	
12015	Repair 8.2 cm laceration of face

Example 6–11

Paring of Seven Corns

INCORRECT CODE	DESCRIPTION OF SERVICES
11055	Paring; single lesion
11056-51	two to four lesions
11057-51	more than four lesions
OR	
11055 × 7	Paring; single lesion (×7 corns)
CORRECT CODE	**DESCRIPTION OF SERVICES**
11057	**Paring; *more than* 4 lesions** (7 corns)

extensive, more than, and *list separately in addition* to. Refer to Example 6–11 as a guide to obtain maximum reimbursement for paring of seven corns. Note in this example, the correct code is an indented code, which describes the service without the need of an additional code.

Surgical Supplies

When billing for office surgery, the routine supplies required for the surgery are bundled into the surgical code. Code 99070, found in the Medicine section; Special Services and Reports, or a HCPCS Level II code is chosen when supplies are over and above the routine supplies used, or atypical for the type of surgery being coded.

Breast Category

The breasts are considered accessory organs of the female genital system; however, various procedures involving the breast are included within the integumentary system because of the type of tissue involved. Biopsy, mastotomy, and mastectomy procedures are all found within this category. Each breast is considered separate, therefore modifier -50 (bilateral) would need to be included if procedures occurred on both sides. If a placement wire is needed to locate a lesion prior to biopsy, code(s) 19290–19291 should be used. For excision of a lesion identified by the marker, assign code 19125.

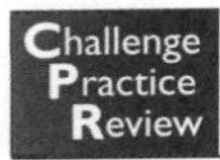

Pause and Practice CPR

PRACTICE SESSIONS 6–16 THROUGH 6–21

Directions: *Complete these exercises to develop and enhance your procedure coding skills in the Integumentary System. Use your procedure codebook.*

6–16 Incision and removal of foreign body in subcutaneous tissue. ____________

6–17 Repair of complex wound of the scalp; 5 cm. ____________

6–18 Excision of benign lesion from the neck; 0.4 cm. ____________

6–19 Simple repair of superficial wound of the lip; 2.3 cm. ____________

6–20 Initial local treatment of first-degree burn. ____________

6–21 Breast biopsy; open incisional. ____________

CHALLENGE SESSION 6–22

Directions: *Use critical thinking skills and CPT rules to code multiple wound repairs in this exercise. Use your procedure codebook.*

6–22 Simple repair of two neck wounds measuring 2.4 cm and 2.3 cm, an intermediate repair of a wound on the eyelid measuring 1.7 cm, an intermediate repair of a wound on the nose measuring 5.1 cm, and complex repair of a wound on the forehead measuring 3.1 cm.

____

____________ ____

____________ ____

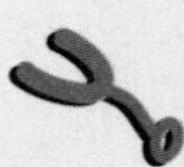

CHECK YOUR HEARTBEAT! Turn to the end of the chapter for answers to these practice and challenge sessions.

Musculoskeletal System

Most categories within the Musculoskeletal System subsection are arranged according to anatomic site. The first category (General) contains procedures that apply to many different anatomic sites. Within the General Category is the subcategory Introduction/Removal, which contains codes for injections in many anatomic regions. It is within this subcategory that arthrocentesis (surgical puncture to remove fluid) is found. Arthrocentesis is categorized according to the type of joint entered, as seen in Example 6–12.

Following the General Category, the remaining categories start with the head and continue down the body, concluding with the foot and toes. Under each anatomic category, there are subcategories that include:

- Incision
- Excision
- Introduction/Removal
- Repair/Revision/Reconstruction
- Fracture/Dislocation
- Arthrodesis
- Amputation
- Unlisted procedures

Fractures

Fractures are either open or closed. The term **open fracture** refers to the skin being broken by the fragmented bone. This is also called a *compound fracture*. A **closed fracture** would be one in which the skin is not broken. If the medical record does not state whether a fracture is open or closed, it is presumed closed and a diagnostic code indicating this may be chosen.

When coding treatment of a fracture, first locate the anatomic site and find the subcategory Fracture and/or Dislocation. Fractures are then listed by treatment as follows:

- **Open treatment**—fracture site surgically opened to align bone
- **Closed treatment**—fracture site not surgically opened to align bone
- **Percutaneous treatment**—fracture site neither open or closed; fracture not visualized so x-ray is used to place fixation across the fracture site

Example 6–12

Arthrocenteses of Small, Intermediate, and Major Joints

Section	→	Surgery
Subsection	→	Musculoskeletal
Category	→	General
Subcategory	→	Introduction/Removal
Procedure	→	**Arthrocentesis**

CODE	**DESCRIPTION OF SERVICES**
20600*	***Arthrocentesis,*** aspiration and/or injection; **small joint,** bursa or ganglion cyst
20605*	**intermediate joint,** bursa or ganglion cyst
20610*	**major joint** or bursa

Example 6–13

Fracture Treatment

A new patient comes to the office after sustaining a fall while in-line skating. She is in distress, complaining of right wrist pain and swelling of the joint. The injury is evaluated (1) with use of an x-ray film (2). It is determined that the patient has a Smith fracture and manipulation is performed. A long-arm cast is applied **(3)** using plaster material **(4).**

(1) 99203-**57**	Initial office evaluation (level 3) **with decision for surgery**
(2) 73100-RT	Radiologic examination, right wrist, AP and lateral views
(3) 25605	Closed treatment of distal radial fracture (e.g., Colles or *Smith type*), *with manipulation*
(4) 99070	Supplies: Casting material (private carrier) Medicine Section code
or	
Q4009	Supplies: Plaster material (Medicare carrier) HCPCS Level II temporary code

The patient returns in 4 weeks for follow-up care **(1).** The wrist is x-rayed again **(2),** the long-arm cast is removed **(3),** and a short-arm cast is applied **(4)** using fiberglass (Hexcelite) material **(5).**

(1) No code	Follow-up care included in global fee
(2) 73100-RT	Radiologic examination, right wrist, AP and lateral views
(3) No code	*Cast removal included in original fracture care (25605)*
(4) 29075-**58**	Application, fiberglass, elbow to finger (short arm) **staged procedure**
(5) 99070	Supplies: Casting material (private carrier) Medicine Section code
or	
Q4010	Supplies: Hexcelite material (Medicare carrier) HCPCS Level II temporary code

The open versus closed treatment should not be confused with the previously mentioned open and closed fracture.

When reading descriptions of fractures, either the phrase "with manipulation" or "without manipulation" is used. **Fracture manipulation** is the manual stretching or applying pressure or traction to realign the broken (fractured) bone. This is also referred to as a *reduction.*

Other common terms found in this subcategory are *internal* and *external* fixation. **Fixation** is the use of hardware (instrumentation) to keep a bone in place. It can either be applied internally (e.g., plate, rod, pin) or externally (e.g., pins that come through the skin to the outside to keep the fractured bone from moving).

As mentioned earlier, all fracture codes carry a 90-day follow-up period so the surgical package rule applies. When coding fractures, the initial cast application is included in the fracture care. Refer to Example 6–13 for an illustration of coding an initial fracture, and coding an application of a second cast 4 weeks later.

Note the E/M service is coded using modifier -57 to indicate that a decision was made for a major surgical procedure performed on the same day. Fracture care is considered surgery because it is located in the Surgery section of CPT. Often carriers will pay for the casting material used to prepare the cast so either code 99070 from the Medicine section or HCPCS Level II codes should be billed.

When the patient returns to the office and a short-arm cast is applied, the second cast application code should be chosen from codes 29000–29590. Modifier -58 is applied because this is considered a staged procedure. The second cast application occurred during the postoperative period and was planned at the time of the initial procedure. Cast application codes may also be used for an initial service for the following reasons as long as restorative treatment or procedures are not provided:

- Stabilizing an injury
- Protecting a fracture, injury, or dislocation
- Providing comfort to the patient

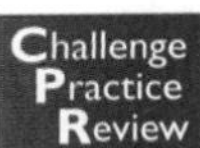

Pause and Practice CPR

REVIEW SESSIONS 6–23 AND 6–24

Directions: *Complete the statements in these exercises to review basic terms used in the musculoskeletal system.*

6–23 Define the following terms:

(a) open fracture ______________________

(b) closed fracture ______________________

(c) open treatment ______________________

(d) closed treatment ______________________

6–24 What is the term used when a surgeon performs an open treatment of a fractured tibia and fibula and uses a plate with screws to hold the fractured ends of the tibia in place?

______________ ______________

CHALLENGE SESSIONS 6–25 AND 6–26

Directions: *Use critical thinking skills and the coding concepts presented in the Musculoskeletal subsection to complete this challenge session. Use your procedure codebook.*

6–25 Chevron bunionectomy, right first metatarsal with 0.062 K-wire fixation and application of cast. Select the correct CPT code(s).

(a) 28296

(b) 28299

(c) 28296, 29425

6–26 A patient presents with chronic knee pain, anteriorly and laterally, with catching. Magnetic resonance imaging (MRI) of the right knee documents a tear in the lateral meniscus. An arthroscopic procedure is performed and the findings include a horizontal tear extending from the anterior horn to the posterior horn (parrot-beak tear) with the base at the posterior horn. Through the scope a lateral meniscectomy is performed. Assign the correct CPT code(s) with modifier. ______________ ______

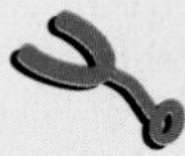

CHECK YOUR HEARTBEAT! Turn to the end of the chapter for answers to these review and challenge sessions.

Respiratory System

The Surgery subsection, Respiratory System, is organized by anatomic site, then by type of procedure. It includes procedures of the nose, sinuses, larynx (voice box), trachea (windpipe), bronchial tubes, lungs, and pleura (membrane that surrounds the lung). Be cautious when using codes in this subsection that are frequently used for cosmetic surgery such as 30400, primary rhinoplasty. If there is medical necessity for the procedure, a diagnostic code and medical record documentation need to be included with the insurance claim to substantiate the need for surgery.

There are several types of endoscopic procedures listed throughout the Respiratory System subsection. An **endoscopy** is the insertion of a flexible fiberoptic tube, referred to as a scope, into a natural body orifice (opening) such as the ears, nose, mouth, vagina, urethra, or anus. The scope may also be placed through a small incision into a body cavity. A diagnostic endoscopy is done for the purpose of visualization and determination of the disease process. It may involve biopsy, scraping, injection, and so forth. A surgical endoscopy may also include biopsy; however, it often includes procedures such as incision, repair, and/or excision. As the tube is inserted it may follow through from one site (e.g., nose) to another site (e.g., larynx). Although visualization may take place as the scope passes through several sites, it is important to select a code that reflects the full extent of the procedure. The farther the scope is passed into the body, the more complex the procedure. The CPT code should reflect the farthest area of visualization or all areas where procedures are performed.

Endoscopies are named for the body area that is being explored. For example, endoscopy of the bronchial tubes would be called bronchoscopy. The index lists such procedures under endoscopy, then the site, and also under the name of the endoscopy (e.g., bronchoscopy). It is important to select either a diagnostic or surgical endoscopy code. A diagnostic endoscopy is always included in a surgical endoscopy and may not be billed separately, as shown in Example 6–14.

Cardiovascular System

The Surgery subsection, Cardiovascular System, is organized by anatomic site, then by type of procedure. It includes procedures of the heart and blood vessels, including pacemaker implantation and coronary artery bypass graft (CABG). Refer to the Medicine section, Cardiovascular, for additional studies such as therapeutic services, cardiography, echocardiography, cardiac catheterization, and other vascular studies.

Digestive System

The Surgery subsection, Digestive System, is organized by anatomic site starting with the lips and mouth, and continuing down the route that food would travel to

Example 6–14

Diagnostic and Surgical Endoscopy

CODE	DESCRIPTION OF SERVICES
31235	Nasal/sinus *endoscopy*, **diagnostic** with sphenoid sinusoscopy
31237	Nasal/sinus *endoscopy*, **surgical**; with biopsy, polypectomy, or debridement (*separate procedure*)

Note: The diagnostic procedure code 31235 would be bundled with the surgical procedure code 31237 when billing a surgical endoscopy.

the rectum and anus. Major organs are included as follows and may be referred to using their medical term (combining form) as listed:

- Stomach (gastr/o)
- Intestines/small (enter/o); including the duodenum, jejunum, and ileum
- Intestines/large (col/o); including the cecum, ascending colon, transverse colon, descending colon, and sigmoid colon

The following accessory organs that aid in the digestive process are also included in this subsection:

- Liver (hepat/o)
- Pancreas (pancreat/o)
- Gallbladder (cholecyst/o)

Endoscopic procedures are listed throughout this subsection and are coded according to the anatomic site examined. Notes defining proctosigmoidoscopy, sigmoidoscopy, and colonoscopy are included under Rectum; Endoscopy.

When surgical entrance is made through the abdominal wall, one of two approaches may be used. The less invasive is a *laparoscopy* in which a small incision is made and a laparoscope is passed through several layers of skin and tissue to enter the abdominal cavity. If the surgeon needs a larger opening to perform a procedure, a large incision may be made referred to as a *laparotomy*. When a laparotomy is used as an approach for another surgical procedure (e.g., gastrectomy) it may never be coded separately.

Urinary System

Categories within the Urinary System subsection are arranged according to anatomic site and type of procedure. The kidney, ureters (tubes leading from the kidney to the bladder), bladder, and urethra (tube leading from the bladder to the outside) are included. Endoscopies include the following:

- *Renal endoscopy*—visualization of the kidney through an established stoma (mouth) that has been surgically created
- *Ureteral endoscopy*—visualization of the ureters through an established stoma (mouth) that has been surgically created
- *Cystoscopy*—visualization of the bladder
- *Urethroscopy*—visualization of the urethra
- *Cystourethroscopy*—visualization of urethra and bladder

A number of different types of procedures may be performed through the scope and are listed following the type of endoscopy.

Urodynamics is a separate subcategory found under Bladder. Urodynamic procedures measure how well the bladder stores and holds urine as well as the rate at which urine moves out of the bladder. These procedures are often performed in the physician's office and are done by or under direct supervision of the physician. They include all necessary supplies.

Example 6–15

Lesion Codes Found in the Male Genital System

CODE	DESCRIPTION OF SERVICES
54050	**Destruction of lesion(s), penis** (e.g., *condyloma, papilloma, molluscum contagiosum, herpetic vesicle*), *simple;* chemical
54055	electrodesiccation
54056	cryosurgery
54057	laser surgery
54060	surgical excision
54512	**Excision of extraparenchymal lesion of testis**

Male Genital System

The Male Genital System is divided by the anatomic categories of Penis, Testis, Epididymis, Tunica Vaginalis, Vas Deferens, Spermatic Cord, Seminal Vesicles, and Prostate. Lesions found on organs within this system may have specific codes assigned, and if so, use these codes instead of codes from the Integumentary System, as shown in Example 6–15.

Following the Male Genital System is a subsection entitled Intersex Surgery consisting of only two codes.

Female Genital System (Maternity Care and Delivery)

The Female Genital System codes are used mainly by general practitioners, family practitioners, and OB-GYN specialists. Codes are arranged by anatomic site and represent many procedures performed in the physician's office, as well as surgical procedures performed in an outpatient surgical center or hospital setting. This subsection starts with the external genitalia (vulva, perineum, introitus, and vagina) and progresses upward through the female genital system to the uterus (cervix uteri and corpus uteri), oviduct, which is also known as fallopian and uterine tubes (including the ends called fimbriae), and concludes with the ovary. The last category is In Vitro Fertilization.

Some incision and drainage (I&D) codes are included in this subsection with notes directing you to the Integumentary System for specific I&D procedures. Read code descriptions carefully to determine the surgical approach: vaginal or abdominal.

Many codes include bilateral descriptions as well as a variety of procedures bundled together and routinely performed at the same operative session, as shown in Example 6–16.

The procedure dilation and curettage (D&C) is described as nonobstetric for the gynecology patient. Although the D&C procedure (58120) does not have the phrase "separate procedure" included in the description, it is considered an integral part of many pelvic surgeries and may not be reimbursed by third party payers when performed at the same operative session as other procedures.

Example 6–16

Hysterectomy Code, Including Bundled Procedures

CODE	DESCRIPTION OF SERVICES
58150	**Total abdominal hysterectomy** (corpus and cervix), **with or without** removal of tube(s), **with or without** removal of ovary(s);

One code includes all of the following possibilities:

- Removal of uterus only
- Removal of uterus and one tube
- Removal of uterus and both tubes (bilateral)
- Removal of uterus and one ovary
- Removal of uterus and both ovaries (bilateral)
- Removal of uterus, including one tube and one ovary
- Removal of uterus, including both tubes and both ovaries (bilateral)

Following the Female Genital System is a short subsection on Maternity Care and Delivery. This subsection includes Antepartum Services such as amniocentesis, Vaginal Delivery, and Cesarean Delivery. Example 6–17 illustrates the correct way to code for the delivery of twins, delivered vaginally or by cesarean section.

Following Cesarean Delivery is the category Delivery After Previous Cesarean Delivery, commonly referred to as VBAC, or vaginal birth after cesarean. These codes are to be used with all patients who have previously had a cesarean section and have the expectation of delivering vaginally. Concluding this subsection is the category Abortion, which includes various types of abortions, as described in Table 6–3.

Nervous System

Codes found in the Nervous System subsection deal with both the central nervous system and peripheral nervous system. They include procedures of the brain, spinal cord, and all types of nerves, which are organized by anatomic site, then procedure. There are

Example 6–17

Coding a Twin Delivery

VAGINAL DELIVERY	CODE	DESCRIPTION OF SERVICES
Twin A	59400	Routine obstetric care, including antepartum care; vaginal delivery and postpartum care
Twin B	59409	Vaginal delivery only
C-SECTION DELIVERY	**CODE**	**DESCRIPTION OF SERVICES**
Twin A and B	59510	Routine obstetric care, including antepartum care; cesarean delivery, and postpartum care

Table 6–3 Types of Abortion

Code	Type	Definition
59812	Incomplete abortion	The uterus contains parts of the products of conception
59820, 59821	Missed abortion	The embryo or fetus has died and the products of conception have been retained
59830	Septic abortion	An infection of the products of conception is present in the endometrial lining of the uterus
59840–59857	Induced abortion	Intentional; also known as artificial and therapeutic abortion (TAB)

many injection, drainage, and aspiration codes that fall under either the Skull, Meninges, and Brain category or under Spine and Spinal Cord.

One of the first subcategories encountered in this subsection involves Twist Drill, Burr Hole(s), or Trephine. These are methods used to enter the brain cavity by making a small opening (hole) through the skull for one of the following purposes:

- Drainage of hemorrhage
- Injection of contrast material
- Insertion of monitoring device
- Placement of tubing
- Relief of pressure

Neuroplasty, which is the freeing or decompression of nerves from scar tissue, is found within the code range 64702–64727.

Eye and Ocular Adnexa/Auditory System

The subsection Eye and Ocular Adnexa includes surgical codes of the eye and related visual structures. Modifier -50 (bilateral procedure) needs to be appended to all procedures that are done on both eyes. Extensive notes are found throughout this subsection and indicate such things as "previous eye surgery" (e.g., 67331), "List separately in addition to code for primary procedure" (e.g., 67320), and directions leading the coder to other specific codes (e.g., 65775).

The subsection Auditory System is divided into the categories of External Ear, Middle Ear, Inner Ear; and Temporal Bone, Middle Fossa Approach.

Operating Microscope

The last subsection of the Surgical section, Operating Microscope, has only one code (69990). A special note directs the coder to use code 69990 for the use of an operating microscope when the surgical code does not contain the microscope as an inclusive component. This code is used with *all* Surgery subsections where the microscope needs to be coded (e.g., 19364, breast reconstruction, or 68530, removal of foreign body, lacrimal passage).

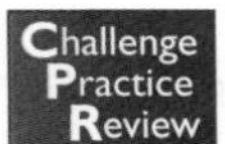

Pause and Practice CPR

PRACTICE SESSIONS 6–27 THROUGH 6–33

Directions: *Complete these exercises to develop and enhance your procedure coding skills in the Surgical section. Use your procedure codebook and circle or write in the correct CPT code(s).*

6–27 A patient presents for total ethmoidectomy with nasal endoscopy, bilateral.

(a) 31255-50

(b) 31255, 31231

(c) 31032, 31255, 31231

6–28 Esophagogastroduodenoscopy with dilation of the esophagus over a guidewire at the same operative episode.

(a) 43453, 43235

(b) 43226

(c) 43248

6–29 A patient presents in the urologist's office for a cystoscopy with transurethral fulguration of a 2.5 cm bladder tumor.

(a) 52235

(b) 52000, 52500

(c) 52000-22

6–30 Destruction of bilateral turbinates (cauterization method) was performed by the surgeon.

____

6–31 The cardiovascular surgeon performed valvuloplasty on the tricuspid valve with ring insertion. ____________

6–32 A 14-year-old girl has a tonsillectomy and adenoidectomy. ____________.

6–33 A simple cystometrogram was performed in the urologist's office. ____________

CHECK YOUR HEARTBEAT! Turn to the end of the chapter for answers to these practice sessions.

Radiology Section

The Radiology section includes nuclear medicine and diagnostic ultrasound. Subsections and index references are as follows:

- Diagnostic Radiology—X-ray (index)
- Diagnostic Ultrasound—Ultrasound (index)
- Radiation Oncology—Radiation Therapy (index)
- Nuclear Medicine—Nuclear Medicine (index)

Knowledge of medical terminology is useful when coding from this section because planes of the body (e.g., coronal and sagittal) and directional terms (e.g., anterior, posterior, lateral) are used to describe radiographic views. Number of views are also indicated in descriptions.

Professional and Technical Components

Certain procedures are a combination of a professional (physician) component and a technical (facility and operator) component. These are usually seen in the Radiology and Pathology/Laboratory sections; however, they may appear in other sections. The **professional component** refers to a portion of a test or procedure that the physician performs, that is, interpreting an electrocardiogram (ECG), reading an x-ray, or making an observation and determination using a microscope. The **technical component** refers to the use of the equipment and its operator that perform the test or procedure, that is, the ECG machine and technician, radiography machine and technician, and microscope and technician. When the physician performs both the professional and technical components there is no need to modify the code. Also, do not modify procedures that are either 100% technical or 100% professional.

Modifier -26 represents the professional element and is used when the physician performs *only* the professional component. Modifier -TC represents the technical element and is used when billing *only* for the technical component. Use of either modifier alerts the insurance company to expect a separate claim from another provider or facility for the other component.

In Example 6–18, the physician is performing only one of the two parts of the service—he or she is interpreting the results of bilateral hip x-rays and reports the service using modifier -26. The facility where the patient went to have the x-rays would bill for the technical component separately by modifying the same code with -TC. If the physician owned the equipment and read the x-rays, there would be no need to modify the x-ray code. Note: Medicare does not cover the technical component of any service rendered in a hospital inpatient or outpatient department.

Example 6–18

Professional and Technical Components

Code	Description	Fee
73520-26 or 73520 and 09926	Professional component *only* for an x-ray of both hips. *Use to bill physician's fee for interpretation of x-ray*	$
73520-TC	Technical component *only* for an x-ray of both hips. *Use to bill facility fee that owns equipment and employs technician.*	$
		=
73520	Radiologic examination (x-ray), hips, bilateral. *Use to bill complete fee when physician owns equipment, employs technician, and interprets x-ray.*	$$

Combination Coding

A coding practice commonly seen in the Radiology section is referred to as combination coding. This means that a code from this section is combined with a code from another section to completely describe the procedure performed. Following is a list of some services performed by the radiologist that may be combined with procedures found in other sections of CPT:

- Injection of contrast materials
- Placement of catheters
- Placement of guidewires
- Placement of stents

When a radiology procedure is performed that requires any of the above procedures, a code from the Radiology section describing the procedure and a code from the Surgery section describing the combination procedure (listed above) must be used. Refer to Example 6–19 for an illustration of a combination code on a patient receiving an injection for arthrography, and the arthrography procedure.

Example 6–19

Combination Coding

CODE	SECTION	DESCRIPTION OF SERVICES
27648	**Surgery**	**Injection procedure** for ankle arthrography *(billed by radiologist or surgeon)*
73615	**Radiology**	**Radiologic examination,** ankle, arthrography, radiologic supervision and interpretation *(billed by radiologist)*

Pathology and Laboratory Section

In the Pathology and Laboratory section, codes are listed in subsections according to the *type of test* performed; for example, chemistry tests, hematology tests, and immunology tests are different types of tests.

Throughout this section careful attention must be paid to select a code according to its proper description. Many tests (e.g., pregnancy test) may be performed on a blood or urine sample. Tests may be performed manually or automated. Automated multichannel tests allow several different tests to be run at the same time, on one specimen, by automated equipment. A microbiology culture identifies organisms and may involve counting the number of organisms that are growing.

Test Panels

The first subsection (Organ or Disease Oriented Panels) found in this section has a number of tests referenced by individual codes that are usually performed together, grouped together, and listed under one CPT code, which is referred to as a **test panel.** The most common tests done to investigate a specific disease or organ have been included in these panels. To use one of the panel codes, all tests listed within the panel *must be* performed. Some insurance companies require that each test in a panel also have a diagnosis that can be linked to it. If other tests are performed that are not included in the panel, they must be coded separately.

Qualitative/Quantitative Analysis

A test may be a **qualitative analysis,** which determines the presence of an agent within the body, or a **quantitative analysis,** which measures how much of the agent is within the body. For example, a *drug assay test* screens (qualitative) and looks for a specific drug within the body system. A quantitative test may be performed to measure how much of the drug is in the body.

Surgical Pathology

The subsection Surgical Pathology (88300–88309) is arranged according to levels. Level I is for *gross examination* only, which means the way the specimen looks to the naked eye before it is prepared for microscopic study. Level II is for *gross and microscopic identification* of tissue in the absence of disease. Levels III through VI are for *gross and microscopic examination of diseased tissue* and each level requires additional work of the pathologist. Various types of tissue are found under each level, in alphabetical order. Each specimen that is separately identifiable may be billed separately.

Medicine Section

The Medicine section lists codes that may be used by physicians of different specialties and in conjunction with codes from all different sections of CPT. Diagnostic and therapeutic services that are generally not surgically invasive (entering a body cavity) are listed in this section, including many types of specialized testing. Notes are found throughout the Medicine section and should be carefully read before coding from a particular subsection, category, or subcategory. Documentation may be included on the claim form to justify the use of these codes.

The following practice session will offer an opportunity to locate code ranges in several subsections of the Medicine Section.

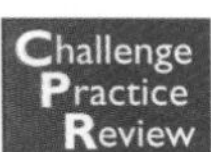

Pause and Practice CPR

PRACTICE SESSION 6–34

Directions: *Use your procedure codebook to look up the major subsections within the Medicine section. Read the description summaries for each subsection listed below and record all code ranges.*

6–34

Immune Globulins—Codes represent products used to boost the immune system (use separate codes for administration).

Code range ________ **to** ________

Vaccine, Toxoids—Codes represent vaccine products to prevent disease (use separate codes for administration).

Code range ________ **to** ________

Psychiatry—This category may be used by physicians of any specialty and has two subcategories. Read notes carefully as some of these services may not be used in conjunction with E/M services.

Code range ________ **to** ________

Dialysis—Codes include End Stage Renal Disease Services, Hemodialysis, and Miscellaneous Dialysis Procedures.

Code range ________ **to** ________

Gastroenterology—Codes include various esophageal and gastric intubation.

Code range ________ **to** ________

CHECK YOUR HEARTBEAT! Turn to the end of the chapter for answers to this practice session.

Continue to locate and read the remaining subsection headings to familiarize yourself with the Medicine Section.

Drugs and Injections

There are only five codes found in the subsection Therapeutic, Prophylactic or Diagnostic Injections, which are used to represent all subcutaneous, intramuscular, intra-arterial, and intravenous injections. The insurance company may require additional information regarding the substance being injected and this may be communicated in three different ways: (1) The material injected may be listed in the description area (Block 19) of the HCFA-1500 claim form listing the name, amount, and strength of the medication. Invoices should be sent for all experimental or expensive (e.g., chemotherapy) drugs. (2) An NDC code may be used to specify the drug, dosage, and the manufacturer. (3) An HCPCS Level II code may be used to specify the injected drug, for example, J9014, gamma globulin, 1 mL. Verify with each insurance company the preferred method on claim forms.

Special Services, Procedures, and Reports

Adjunct codes are found in the Medicine section under a subsection entitled Special Services, Procedures, and Reports, and fall under the category Miscellaneous Services. They are important to consider when billing because these codes provide the reporting physician with a means of identifying special services and reports that are an adjunct to the basic service provided. The circumstances that are covered under these codes include handling of laboratory specimens, telephone calls, seeing patients at odd hours, office emergency services, supplies and materials, special reports, travel, and educational services rendered to patients. Two commonly used codes are described as follows:

- 99000—*Handling and/or conveyance of specimen* for transfer from the physician's office to a laboratory. When a specimen (blood sample, culture, biopsy) is collected in the physician's office and then sent to an outside laboratory, use this code to bill for handling the specimen.
- 99070—*Supplies and materials* (except spectacles) provided by the physician *over and above* those usually included with the office visit or other services rendered (list drugs, trays, supplies, or materials provided). The key to this description is the phrase *over and above.* Remember, most surgical codes include the supplies that are routinely needed to perform the procedure, so this code can only be used if excess supplies are needed or if the code (such as a code from the medicine section) does not include the supplies.

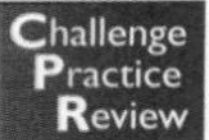

Pause and Practice CPR

PRACTICE SESSIONS 6–35 THROUGH 6–39

Directions: *Complete these exercises to develop and enhance your procedure coding skills in the Radiology and Pathology/Laboratory sections. Use your procedure codebook to select and circle or write in the correct code.*

6–35 A complete hip radiograph was taken at College Hospital and was interpreted by the orthopedic surgeon. List the code the surgeon would bill with for the professional component.

(a) 73500-TC

(b) 73525

(c) 73510-26

6–36 An electrolyte panel is performed at College Hospital Laboratory, including measurement of carbon dioxide, chloride, sodium, and potassium levels.

(a) 80051, 82374, 82435, 84295, 84132

(b) 80051

(c) 82664

6–37 A pathologist receives a specimen from Dr. Practon's office. It is a superficial muscle biopsy taken from the arm of a Mr. Alan Wang. The pathologist performs a microscopic examination with review and interpretation. (1) First, select the correct CPT codes that Dr. Practon would use to bill for the biopsy, then (2) select the correct code that the pathologist would use to bill for his services.

(1) Dr. Practon's bill

(a) 20200

(b) 20205

(c) 20206

(2) Pathologist's bill

(a) 20200

(b) 88302

(c) 88305

6–38 An upper GI series with air contrast and small bowel followthrough was done by the radiologist. ____________

6–39 Mr. and Mrs. Jerald Lehman's newborn baby boy had a circumcision performed by Dr. Atrics in the office. A bell device was used. ________________

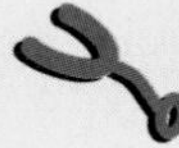

CHECK YOUR HEARTBEAT! Turn to the end of the chapter for answers to these practice sessions.

CODING TERMINOLOGY

In order to thoroughly understand how to bill using the CPT manual, it is important to understand various terms used by insurance companies that are related to coding. The following terms are used by private payers, Medicare, Medicaid, TRICARE, and workers' compensation carriers.

Bundled Code

When more than one component (service/procedure) is included in one CPT code, this is referred to as a **bundled code.** For example, in a surgical package the topical anesthesia, surgery, and follow-up care are all bundled into the surgery code. Another example would be a treadmill test, also referred to as a cardiovascular stress test. All treadmill tests include a resting ECG. Therefore, an ECG is bundled into the treadmill code and it would be incorrect to bill separately for an ECG, even if it were performed independently on the same date of service. For evaluation and management services, the cost of some services and most supplies are bundled into the code, for example, telephone services and reading of test results.

When trying to decide what procedures are combined in one code, use an unbundling book as a reference guide (see Resources at end of chapter). First, look up the code for the primary procedure, then check through the listing of all other codes to see if the additional procedure you would like to bill for is included.

Unbundling

Unbundling is the practice of coding and billing for multiple services when a single code should be used that describes the service or procedure. It is also known as *itemizing, exploding charges, fragmented billing or surgery*, or *à la carte medicine*. Some practices do this

Example 6–20

Unbundling (Fragmenting)

INCORRECT CODING	
43235	Upper GI endoscopy
43600	Biopsy of stomach
CORRECT CODING	
43239	Upper GI endoscopy; with biopsy of stomach

unknowingly, but if it is done intentionally to gain increased reimbursement, it is considered fraud. Unbundling can lead to downward payment, adjustments, and possible audit of claims.

Following are Examples 6–20, 6–21, 6–22, and 6–23 illustrating various types of unbundling:

- Fragmenting one service into component parts and coding each component as if it were a separate service.
- Reporting separate codes for related services when one comprehensive code includes all related services.
- Coding bilateral procedures as two codes when one code is inclusive.
- Separating a surgical approach from a major surgical service that includes the same approach.

The use of outdated codes often inadvertently results in unbundling. When a new technique or technology is developed, the procedure may be assigned its own code, but as it becomes common it may be bundled with another service and code.

Downcoding

Approximately 35 different procedural coding systems are used across the United States. Generally, only three to five procedural coding systems are in use in any given region at the same time. CPT codes have been emphasized in this chapter because they are the most commonly accepted. **Downcoding** occurs when the coding system used by the physician's office does not match the coding system used by the insurance company receiving the claim. The computer system converts the code submitted to the closest code in use, which is usually down one level from the submitted code; therefore, decreased payment is generated. An example of this is when a claims examiner must convert the CPT code submitted to an RVS code being used by the carrier. When there is a choice between two or three similar codes, the claim's examiner will choose the lowest-paying code.

Example 6–22

Unbundling (Bilateral)

INCORRECT CODING	
76090-RT	Mammography; unilateral
76090-LT	Mammography; unilateral
CORRECT CODING	
76091	Mammography; **bilateral**

Example 6–23

Unbundling (Surgical Approach)

INCORRECT CODING	
49000	Exploratory laparotomy
44150	Colectomy, total, abdominal
CORRECT CODING	
44150	Colectomy, total, abdominal (correct since it *includes* exploration of the surgical field)

To prevent downcoding, always monitor reimbursements and note codes that are affected by downcoding. Then call the insurance carrier and find out which code system is in use and obtain a reference list so you can code using the appropriate system (see Example 6–24).

Downcoding may also occur when a claim's examiner compares the code submitted with a written description of the procedure on an attached document. If these two do not match, the carrier will reimburse according to the lowest-paying code that fits the documented description.

Upcoding

The term **upcoding** is used to describe deliberate manipulation of CPT codes for increased payment. This practice can be spotted by Medicare fiscal intermediaries and insurance carriers using prepayment and postpayment screens or "stop alerts," which are built

Example 6–24

Downcoding

INCORRECT CODING	
20010	Incision of abscess with suction irrigation (Note: 20010 has been deleted from CPT and would result in downcoding.)
CORRECT CODING	
20005	Incision of abscess, complicated

Example 6–21

Unbundling (Comprehensive Code)

UNBUNDLED CLAIM (Incorrect)		BUNDLED CLAIM (Correct)	
58150	Total abdominal hysterectomy, with/without removal of tube(s), with/without removal of ovary(s) [$1200]	**58150**	Total abdominal hysterectomy, **with/without** removal of tube(s), **with/without** removal of ovary(s) [$1200]
58700	Salpingectomy [$650]		
58940	Oophorectomy [$685]		
Total charge	**$2535**	**Total charge**	**$1200**

Expressions from Experience

It is a full-time job just keeping up with correct coding and the best methods for obtaining ethical reimbursement. The key to being a good medical billing professional is education, education, education. Without it, success can only be an accident.

Charline Rambaud, CPC
Owner—Coding Specialist
Medical Billing Service

into most coding computer software programs. An example of intentional upcoding is when a physician selects one level of E/M service for all visits with an attitude that the costs even out. This opens the door to audits and in the end may cost the practice money. Upcoding may also occur unintentionally if the coder is not knowledgeable of coding practices or does not keep current. To keep current, join a free online list service (listserv) to make coding contacts all over the United States using e-mail. Post questions to coding experts who may know the answer to coding questions concerning a specialized practice or a current billing dilemma (see Resources at the end of chapter).

Code Edits

A Correct Coding Initiative (CCI) was implemented by Medicare and involves a code edit system consistent with Medicare policies. Its function is to eliminate improper reporting of CPT codes. When an online edit is performed, the computer software program checks codes on an insurance claim to detect improper code submissions. Such software is also used by private payers, other federal programs, and state Medicaid programs. Learning about edits is necessary because every medical practice has billing problems unique to its specialty that arise due to reduction of payment or denial of claims.

The following explanation of various code edits will help you obtain maximum reimbursement for each service rendered and avoid denials, lowered reimbursement, and possible audit.

Example 6–25

Comprehensive/Component Code

Comprehensive code	93015 Cardiovascular stress test
Component codes	93016, 93017, 93018

93015	Cardiovascular stress test using maximal or submaximal treadmill or bicycle exercise, continuous electrocardiographic monitoring, and/or pharmacologic stress; with physician supervision, with interpretation and report
93016	physician supervision only, without interpretation and report
93017	tracing only, without interpretation and report
93018	interpretation and report only

Example 6–26

Separate Procedure

Inguinal hernia repair with lesion excised from spermatic cord.

TYPE OF CODE	CODE	DESCRIPTION OF SERVICES
Comprehensive code	**49505**	Repair initial inguinal hernia, age 5 years or older, reducible
Component code:	55520	Excision of lesion of spermatic cord **(separate procedure)**

Comprehensive/Component Edits

A **comprehensive code** is a single code that describes two or more component codes that are bundled together as one unit. The comprehensive code is never indented and the basis for its description appears before the semicolon (;). Each **component code** is indented and includes the portion of the service described before the semicolon (;) in the comprehensive code, and the portion of the service described by the indented (component) code. Component codes should be used only if both portions of the service were performed (see Example 6–25).

Separate Procedure Code Edits

Another example of a component code would be a procedure code that specifies "separate procedure" in the description. A **separate procedure** is one that is an integral part of a larger procedure and does not need a separate code, unless it is performed independently and is not immediately related to other services. In other words, if a procedure has the words "separate procedure" in its description, and the surgeon performs another procedure through the same incision, you should not code the procedure listed as "separate procedure" (see Example 6–26).

Mutually Exclusive Code Edits

Procedures that meet any of the following criteria are considered mutually exclusive:

- Code combinations that are restricted by the guidelines outlined in CPT
- Procedures that cannot be reasonably done during the same session
- Procedures that represent medically impossible or improbable code combinations
- Procedures that represent two methods of performing the same service (see Example 6–27)

Example 6–27

Mutually Exclusive Code

47605	Excision, cholecystectomy; with cholangiography
47563	Laparoscopy, surgical; cholecystectomy with cholangiography

Note: *Different methods of accomplishing same procedure.*

Since both of these procedures are different methods of accomplishing removal of the gallbladder with x-ray examination of the bile ducts, they represent two methods of performing the same service and the insurance carrier would deny code 47563 as mutually exclusive of code 47605.

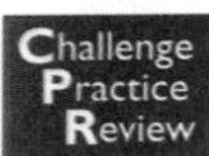

Pause and Practice CPR

REVIEW SESSIONS 6–40 THROUGH 6–43

Directions: *Fill in or circle the correct answer to review terms that apply to CPT codes. Use your procedure codebook.*

6–40 What is a single code called that describes two or more component codes, bundled together as one unit? ______________________

6–41 What is an indented code called? ______________________

6–42 Which mutually exclusive criteria apply to codes 49505 and 49650?

(a) They cannot be reasonably done during the same session.

(b) They represent a medically impossible code combinations.

(c) They represent two methods of performing the same service.

6–43 Coding all E/M services level 4 or level 5 would be considered an example of:

(a) downcoding

(b) upcoding

(c) unbundling

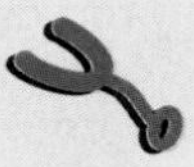

CHECK YOUR HEARTBEAT! Turn to the end of the chapter for answers to these review sessions.

ILLEGAL OR UNETHICAL CODING

It is imperative to follow basic coding guidelines and individual coding policies from various insurance carriers. Following are some examples of illegal or unethical coding that would apply to all insurance plans:

1. Coding a case differently than described in the medical record to increase reimbursement
2. Coding procedures and services for payment that were not performed
3. Coding a service in such a way that it is paid when it usually is not covered
4. Unbundling services or procedures into separate codes when one code is available
5. Failure to code a relevant condition or complication when it is documented in the medical record
6. Billing for procedures over a period of days when all treatment occurred during a single visit
7. Upcoding to increase payment when documentation does not warrant it

MODIFIERS

The most common modifiers have been presented in Chapters 5 and 6 as they relate to specific sections of CPT; however, there are other modifiers that have not yet been described. Figure 6–6*A* and *B* is a decision flow chart provided for reference when applying modifiers to multiple surgical procedures. Follow the steps by answering the questions in Figure 6–6*A* as they apply to your billing scenario, and refer to Figure 6–6*B* for key information and descriptions.

A complete list of modifiers is found in Appendix C. A comprehensive list of modifiers may be found on the worktext web site http://www.wbsaunders.com/MERLIN/Fordney/insurance/, which includes complete descriptions, clinical examples, and Medicare rules regarding modifier usage.

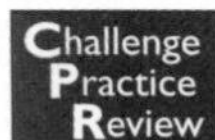

Pause and Practice CPR

PRACTICE SESSIONS 6–44 THROUGH 6–46

Directions: *Complete these exercises to develop and enhance your procedure coding skills with modifier applications. Use your procedure codebook and a HCPCS Level II codebook or Appendix C.*

6–44 A patient is sent for a chest x-ray to College Hospital (with split billing). Which modifier is assigned for the facility fee?

(a) -26

(b) -TC

(c) No modifier is needed.

6–45 Select the correct HCPCS Level II modifier to indicate left foot, second digit.

(a) -T2

(b) -T1

(c) -LT

6–46 A "midlevel provider" would use which one of the following modifiers on a billing statement?

(a) -NP

(b) -AM

(c) -AS

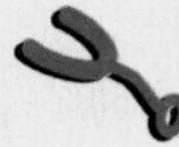

CHECK YOUR HEARTBEAT! Turn to the end of the chapter for answers to these practice sessions.

SUMMATION AND PREVIEW

This chapter has emphasized the quality of procedural coding. Productivity is also important and your coding speed will increase as you practice this skill. It is important to remember that you probably will not be coding from all sections of CPT at your worksite, nor will you be expected to memorize all coding rules. While learning it is important to be exposed to and understand the full view of all specialty areas of coding. Your focus will narrow as you apply this information to your future position. Take advantage of reference materials and coding seminars as you utilize your newly learned knowledge and coding skills.

In the next chapter you will be learning the legalities and components of a medical record, rules of medical record documentation, and how to abstract information so that it can be coded and transferred to the insurance claim form. You will have an opportunity to develop and practice the skill of medical record abstraction.

GOLDEN RULE

To be sure a surgical package is delivered correctly, check to see if it is bundled.

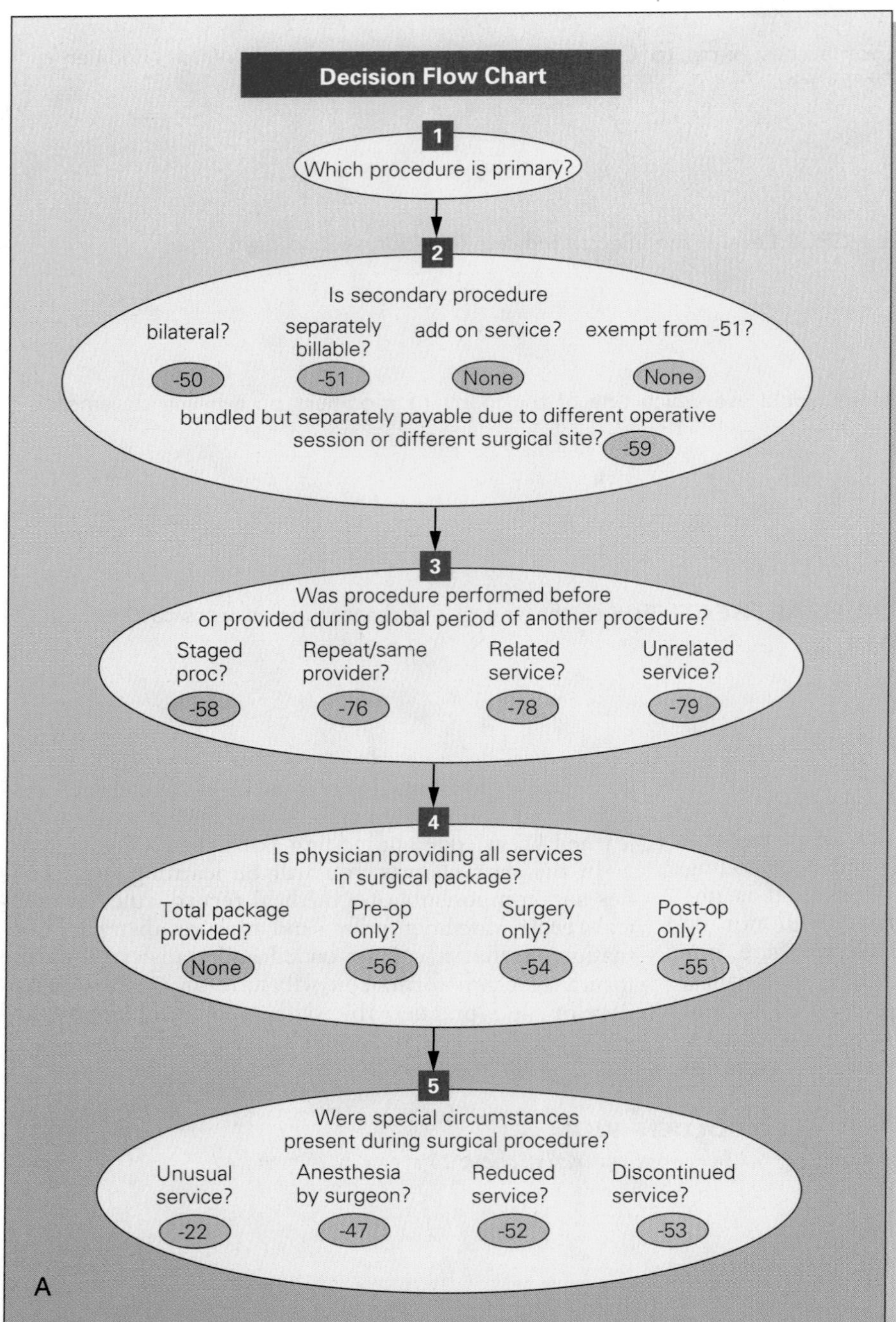

Figure 6–6. *A*, Decision flow chart for surgical procedures.

Multiple Surgical Procedures

Multiple services must be related to:
- Same patient
- Same provider
- Same date of service

1

- List all procedures in order of reimbursement, highest to lowest
- Most comprehensive service brings greatest reimbursement and is considered primary
- Check all procedures to make sure there is no unbundling, i.e., using two codes when one code describes procedure
- Decision making expands at this point. Follow numbered question to determine correct modifier usage

2

-50 bilateral procedure, not described by code
-51 not bundled, separately billable
-59 ordinarily bundled, separately payable due to special circumstance

3

- The term "primary procedure" can also refer to the first procedure initiating a global surgical period

-58 Current service was planned prospectively at time of first service
-76 Physician repeats procedure subsequent to original procedure
-78 Return to operating room for subsequent procedure, complication relating to original procedure
-79 Unrelated procedure performed during global period of previous surgery

4

- Surgical package means one fee covers the whole package, surgical procedure and postoperative care

5

-22 An extremely difficult procedure due to altered anatomy or unusual circumstances (add 10–30% to reimbursement)
-47 When the surgeon administers regional or general anesthesia
-52 Procedure/service reduced or eliminated at the discretion of the physician
-53 Procedure is discontinued due to extenuating circumstances or because of threat to the patient

B

Figure 6–6 *Continued. B,* Guidelines and description of modifiers for multiple surgical procedures flow chart.

Chapter 6 Review and Practice

Study Session

Directions: *Review the objectives, key terms, and chapter information before completing the following questions.*

6–1 List the four criteria needed to use code 99025 in lieu of an E/M code.

(a) ____________________ (c) ____________________

(b) ____________________ (d) ____________________

6–2 Refer to the right column of the mock fee schedule in Appendix B and indicate how many global follow-up days are assigned for the following procedures.

(a) 30905 __________ (c) 53240__________

(b) 59160 __________ (d) 11040__________

6–3 When billing for multiple procedures, when is modifier -51 not used?

____

6–4 What are the usual reimbursement levels for the allowable charge for multiple procedures?

1st procedure ____________________

2nd procedure ____________________

3rd procedure ____________________

4th procedure ____________________

6–5 Review the descriptions for the following code numbers and indicate with "yes" or "no" if modifier -50 is needed to indicate bilateral procedure.

(a) 69100 __________ (c) 55200__________

(b) 50045 __________ (d) 58550__________

6–6 Integumentary is another term for ____________.

6–7 Why is it important to delay billing when coding neoplasms?

____

6–8 If a biopsy is performed and a surgical excision follows, is the biopsy reported separately or bundled with the surgical code?

____

6–9 How many classifications are there for laceration repairs? ____________

6–10 The guidelines for adding up the total lengths of multiple laceration repairs state that the ____________________ of repair and the ____________________ must be the same.

6–11 Is fracture care considered surgery? ____________

6–12 How many global follow-up days does fracture care have? ____________

6–13 What modifier is used (to append the second cast code) when a physician performs fracture care and plans to remove the cast within the postoperative period and place a new cast?

____

6–14 May the physician bill for fiberglass material along with the cast application? ____________

If yes, what code(s) would be used? If no, state why not. ____________________

6–15 Other terms for *unbundling* are ____

____

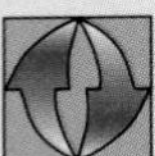

Exercise Exchange

Directions: Practice your coding skills by coding the following scenarios. Use your procedural codebooks and the coding concepts and rules presented in this chapter to code these scenarios from the Integumentary subsection.

6–1 Incision and removal of foreign body in subcutaneous tissue. ______________

6–2 Repair of complex wound of the scalp; 5 cm. ______________

6–3 Excision of benign lesion from the neck; 0.4 cm. ______________

6–4 Simple repair of superficial wound of the lip; 2.3 cm. ______________

6–5 Initial local treatment of first-degree burn. ______________

6–6 Destruction of three premalignant lesions from the face using laser treatment.

____

______________ × ______

6–7 Excision of malignant lesion from the ear (2.6 cm) requiring complex closure.

____

____

Directions: The following exercises offer practice in abstracting information from chart notes and coding procedures. Use your procedural codebook and the coding concepts and rules presented in this chapter to code these scenarios from the Surgery section.

6–8 Single-needle biopsy on Mr. McCranie's prostate gland performed in the urologist's office.

____

6–9 Dr. Caesar calls a neonatologist to College Hospital to supervise and interpret fetal monitoring and offer a second opinion on an obstetric patient who is in labor and has several high-risk factors. Select the correct CPT code for the fetal monitoring. ______________

6–10 A patient presents in the emergency room of College Hospital with severe right lower quadrant pain. Stat blood work indicates that the patient has appendicitis. A laparoscopic appendectomy was performed by Dr. Cutler, the general surgeon on staff. ______________

6–11 An ophthalmologist performs strabismus resection surgery on two horizontal muscles in the right eye of the patient. ______________

6–12 A 77-year-old grandmother presents in Dr. Lenser's office complaining that her eyes are so droopy she cannot see. Upon evaluation it is determined that she has bilateral blepharoptosis. The physician recommends surgery to repair the prolapsed eyelids. A bilateral blepharoptosis repair and internal levator resection were performed the following week. Select the CPT code and applicable modifier. ______________ – ______

6–13 A 4-year-old boy presents with his mother in the office. The mother states that the child began screaming at home while playing in the backyard. When the mother tried to find out what the problem was, the child indicated to the mother that he stuck seeds in both of his ears. The mother tried to remove them with a Q-Tip to no avail. On exam, the physician notes two distinct boluses of material, one in each ear. After an attempt to rinse the foreign bodies out, Cerumenex was tried and the ears were rinsed again after 15 minutes. Both seeds were successfully removed from the ears. Assign the correct CPT code(s) with the applicable modifier(s). _______________ – ______

6–14 Drs. Graff and Cutler were co-surgeons on a complicated skin graft procedure. What modifier would each co-surgeon use to append the procedure code? _______________

6–15 Dr. Cutler assisted Dr. Antrum with an open treatment of depressed frontal sinus fracture. Select the correct procedure code and modifier that Dr. Cutler would bill with.

_______________ – ______

6–16 Apply the correct CPT code(s) to the following radiology report:

____

____

(see report below)

College Hospital
Radiology Department
4500 Broad Avenue
Woodland Hills, XY
12345-0001

Patient Smith, Janelle	**Age** F 01-02-60	**X-ray No.** 04 22 99
Date 12/20/20XX	**Referred by** Dr. G. Practon	

COMPUTED TOMOGRAPHY OF THE ABDOMEN AND PELVIS

HISTORY: Chronic left lower extremity edema.

TECHNIQUE: Spiral scan is obtained of the abdomen through the liver without IV contrast material using spiral pitch of 1.5 and collimation of 8 mm and index of 7 mm. Spiral scans were then obtained through the abdomen and pelvis from the dome of the liver to below the symphysis during bolus injection of 100 cc of Isovue using mechanical injector.

FINDINGS: No mass is seen in the liver or spleen. There are some small calcifications layered in the dependent portion of the gallbladder consistent with small gallstones. No biliary tree dilation is seen. No mass is seen in the pancreas. Adrenal glands are unremarkable. Kidneys show no evidence of mass or hydronephrosis. No periaortic lymphadenopathy is seen. There is some calcification of the abdominal aorta.

Scans through the pelvis show calcification of the iliac arteries. No pelvic mass or lymphadenopathy is seen. No abnormal pelvic fluid collection is evident. No filling defects are seen in the common femoral veins or iliac veins.

IMPRESSION: Cholelithiasis

Coding Challenge Directions: The following scenarios contain longer chart notes and may require codes from different sections of CPT. Use your procedural codebooks, the coding concepts and rules presented in this chapter, and critical thinking skills to code the following challenge scenarios.

6–17 An orthopedic surgeon performed an ankle arthroscopy with excision of osteochondral defect of talus bone on an 83-year-old patient with mild systemic disease. Select the correct procedural codes for the anesthesiologist and the surgeon with applicable modifier(s).

Anesthesiologist ______________ – ______

Anesthesiologist ______________

Surgeon ______________

6–18 An established patient slipped while mowing the lawn and fell backward hitting his head on a sprinkler head. He was briefly unconscious but came to and went into the house and applied ice to the wound. His head was bleeding profusely and he presented at the doctor's office complaining of a severe headache, dizziness, and blurred vision. The physician worked him in as an *emergency,* provided a *full neurologic evaluation* for head trauma (Level 3), and *sutured the long 7.8 cm scalp laceration* (simple repair). Use the criteria in Figure 6–5 and assign the correct code(s) with applicable modifier(s).

______________ – ______

____

____

6–19 A 5-year-old boy presents in the Urgent Care Center with a 2.1 cm laceration of the right hand, a 1.2 cm laceration of the right index finger, and a 0.8 cm laceration of the right middle finger. He caught his hand in a piece of machinery and there were also other abrasions and contusions. All of the lacerations were repaired with 4-0 Vicryl sutures in the upper subcutaneous layers of the skin. Select the correct procedure code(s) with modifier(s) for the surgery. ______________ – ______

6–20 Ms. Croix returns to her physician's office for a monthly injection of Lupron (leuprolide acetate) for endometriosis. The nurse takes her blood pressure, pulse, and respirations and asks Ms. Croix how she has been feeling. The nurse administers the Lupron in the right dorsal gluteus muscle and the physician does not see the patient. Select the correct CPT and HCPCS Level II codes for this scenario.

____

____

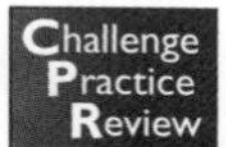

CPR Session: Answers

PRACTICE SESSIONS 6–1 THROUGH 6–4

6–1 (a) P5
(b) P2
(c) P4
(d) P3

6–2 (a) 99100
(b) 99140
(c) 99116

6–3 00322

6–4 (a) 11 units
(b) 5 units
(c) 23 units (16 units for first 4 hours, plus 6 units for next hour, plus 1 unit for extra 12 minutes)

PRACTICE SESSION 6–5

6–5 (a) General
(b) Integumentary System
(c) Musculoskeletal System
(d) Respiratory System
(e) Cardiovascular System
(f) Hemic and Lymphatic System
(g) Mediastinum and Diaphragm
(h) Digestive System
(i) Urinary System
(j) Male Genital System
(k) Intersex Surgery
(l) Female Genital System
(m) Maternity Care and Delivery
(n) Endocrine System
(o) Nervous System
(p) Eye and Ocular Adnexa
(q) Auditory System
(r) Operating Microscope

REVIEW SESSIONS 6–6 THROUGH 6–8

6–6 (a) Pathology/Laboratory
(b) Surgery
(c) Evaluation and Management
(d) Surgery
(e) Medicine
(f) Radiology
(g) Surgery

6–7 (a) eponym
(b) procedure
(c) abbreviation
(d) anatomic site
(e) condition
(f) service
(g) organ

6–8 (a) indented
(b) stand-alone
(c) stand-alone
(d) indented

REVIEW SESSIONS 6–9 THROUGH 6–14

6–9 unstarred procedure code numbers
6–10 no
6–11 yes
6–12 90
6–13 99024
6–14 –51

CHALLENGE SESSION 6–15

6–15 minor versus major procedure

PRACTICE SESSIONS 6–16 THROUGH 6–21

6–16 10121
6–17 13121
6–18 11420
6–19 12011
6–20 16000
6–21 19101

CHALLENGE SESSION 6–22

6–22 12002, 12053-51, 13132-51

REVIEW SESSIONS 6–23 AND 6–24

6–23 (a) skin broken by fragmented bone
(b) fracture with skin not broken
(c) fracture site surgically opened
(d) fracture site not surgically opened

6–24 internal fixation

CHALLENGE SESSIONS 6–25 AND 6–26

6–25 a *Rationale: Since this is the initial service and restorative treatment is provided, a separate cast application code may not be used.*

6–26 29881-RT

PRACTICE SESSIONS 6–27 THROUGH 6–33

6–27 a
6–28 c
6–29 a
6–30 30801
6–31 33464
6–32 42821
6–33 51725

PRACTICE SESSION 6–34

6–34

Subsection	**Code Range**
Immune Globulins	90281–90399
Vaccine, Toxoids	90476–90749
Psychiatry	90801–90899
Dialysis	90918–90999
Gastroenterology	91000–91299

PRACTICE SESSIONS 6–35 THROUGH 6–39

6–35 c
6–36 b
6–37 (1) Dr. Practon's bill (a)
(2) Pathologist's bill (c)
6–38 74249
6–39 54150

REVIEW SESSIONS 6–40 THROUGH 6–43

6–40 comprehensive code
6–41 component code
6–42 c
6–43 b

PRACTICE SESSIONS 6–44 THROUGH 6–46

6–44 b
6–45 b
6–46 c

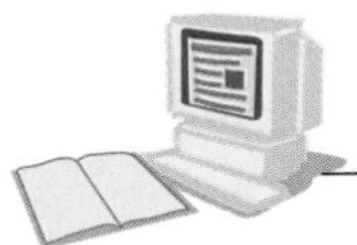

Resources

Insurance billing specialists need current comprehensive coding reference materials to code procedures appropriately. Answers to coding questions can be researched in reference books, which are easy to use and provide additional coding information. Attending seminars is also a method for keeping up-to-date on coding issues. Seminars often cover coding problems specific to different specialties and offer opportunities to obtain answers to coding problems. Following is a suggested list of coding resources.

Codebooks

- *Current Procedural Terminology (CPT)* (published annually), American Medical Association, Order Department, AAMA, P.O. Box 930876, Atlanta, GA 31193-0876 (800) 621-8335
- *Health Care Financing Administration Common Procedure Coding System (HCPCS) National Level II Medicare Codes,* published by:

  American Medical Association, (800) 621-8335

  Medicode/Ingenix Publishing Group (800) 999-4600

  Practice Management Information Corporation, (800) MED-SHOP

  St. Anthony/Ingenix Publishing Group, (800) 632-0123

  Wasserman Medical Publishers, Limited, (800) 669-3337
- *HCPCS LEVEL III* local codes are available from your local Medicare fiscal intermediary

Reference Books

- *2000 Crosswalk,* American Society of Anesthesiologists, 520 North Northwest Highway, Parkridge, IL 60068-2573, (847) 825-5586
- *Coders' Desk Reference* (published annually), Medicode/Ingenix Publishing Group, 5225 Wiley Post Way, Suite 500, Salt Lake City, UT 84116, (800) 999-4600
- *CPT Assistant* (four issues published annually), American Medical Association, Order Department, AAMA, P.O. Box 930876, Atlanta, GA 31193-0876 (800) 621-8335
- *Medicare Correct Coding and Payment Manual for Procedures and Services,* (includes unbundling information), St. Anthony/Ingenix Publishing Group P.O. Box 96561 Washington, DC 20090-4212 (800) 632-0123
- *National Correct Coding Guide* (updated annually), St. Anthony/Ingenix Publishing Group, P.O. Box 96561 Washington, DC 20090-4212 (800) 632-0123
- *National Correct Coding* manual, available by contacting NTIS, (800) 553-6487. Correct Coding Initiative (CCI) edits are also available on diskette or CD-ROM.
- *Principles of CPT Coding,* American Medical Association, Order Department, AAMA, P.O. Box 930876, Atlanta, GA 31193-0876, (800) 621-8335
- *St. Anthony's Complete RBRVS* (updated and published annually), St. Anthony/Ingenix Publishing Group, P.O. Box 96561, Washington, DC 20090-4212, (800) 632-0123
- *St. Anthony's Relative Values for Physicians* (updated and published annually), St. Anthony/Ingenix Publishing Group P.O. Box 96561, Washington, DC 20090-4212, (800) 632-0123

Coding Questions

- Listserv—subscribe, ask questions and communicate with other insurance billers via e-mail
  Web site: http://www.partbnews.com/enroll

NOTES

Objectives

After reading this chapter and completing the exercise sessions, you should be able to:

Learning Objectives:

✔ Define the term *medical record.*

✔ State the connection between the medical record and the insurance billing process.

✔ Recite principles for the release of medical information for various situations.

✔ Explain reasons for medical record documentation.

✔ Identify principles of documentation.

✔ Name various types of reports that make up a medical record.

✔ List two types of medical review and state what an audit of medical records entails.

✔ Explain techniques used to maintain confidentiality of faxed documents.

✔ Respond appropriately to the subpoena of a witness and records.

✔ Express the purpose of a compliance program and recite elements that lead to a successful program.

✔ State ways to prevent legal problems and lawsuits.

Performance Objectives:

✔ Abstract data from the medical record, including date of service, place of service, and elements of a history and physical examination (subjective information, objective information, chief complaint, symptoms, diagnosis, and procedure or service).

Key Terms

attending physician
audit
backup
comorbidity
compliance program
concurrent care
consulting physician
continuity of care
documentation
external audit
family history (FH)
facsimile (fax)
history of present illness (HPI)
internal review
medical necessity
medical record
morbidity
mortality
objective findings
ordering physician
past history (PH)
performing physician
physical examination (PE or PX)
referring physician
review of systems (ROS)
social history (SH)
subjective information
subpoena
treating physician

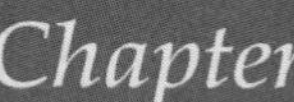

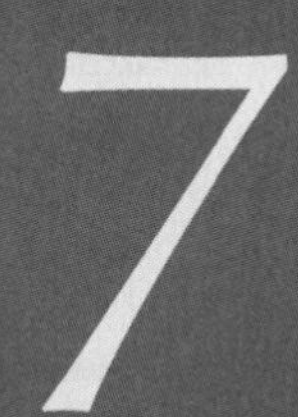

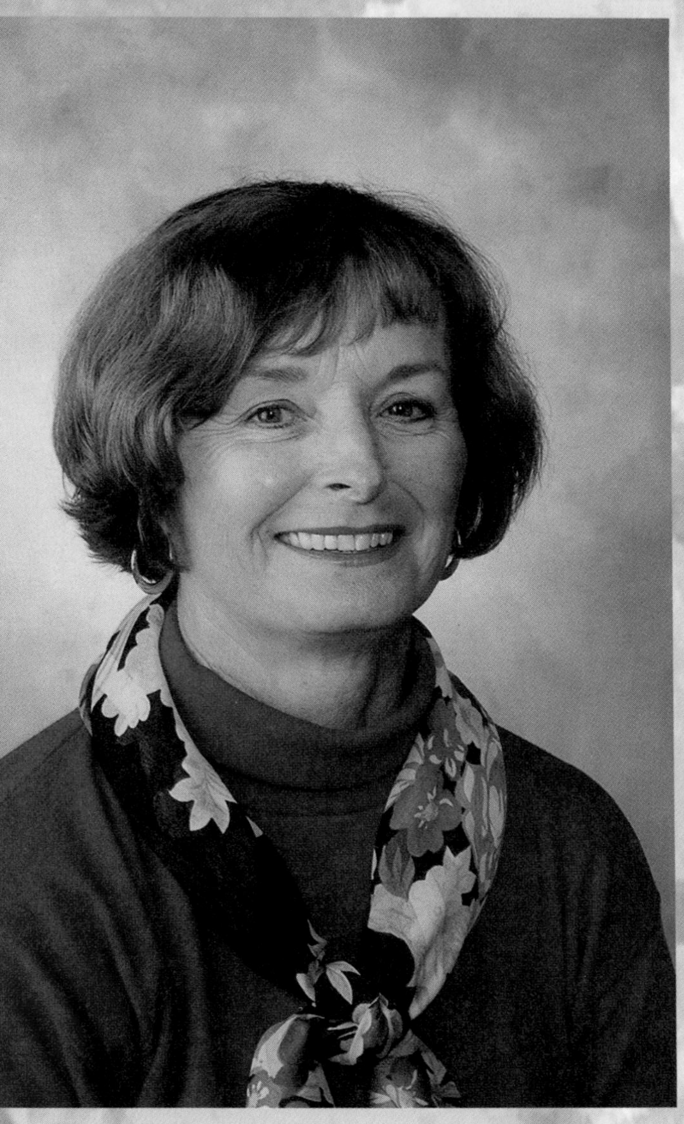

A fascination for medical terms and their meanings led me to a course in medical terminology. Following this, I studied medical transcription and learned more about the practice of medicine including symptoms, diagnoses, and the treatment of diseases. I soon became interested in applying this knowledge and trying my skills in an employment situation.

I have been fortunate to have worked for several specialties including ear, nose, and throat physicians for the past 18 years. My duties have included transcribing consultation letters, surgery billing, and coding. The combination of my varied duties has allowed me to do part of the work at my home computer.

Now I work two days a week and combine medical transcription and insurance billing. Working part-time has allowed me to be at home, raise three sons, and participate in tennis and other interests.

Sue Manion
Medical Transcriptionist/Biller
Ear, Nose, and Throat Specialty

Documentation and the Medical Record

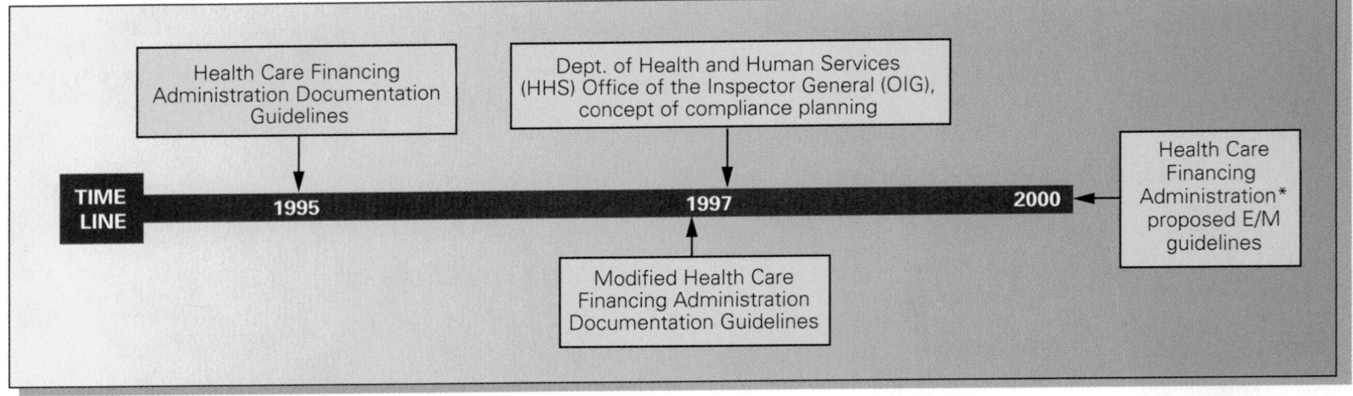

THE MEDICAL RECORD

Now that you have learned how to code diagnoses and procedures, you will be learning how to read, research, and find technical information in the patient's medical record. This process is referred to as abstracting information and most commonly occurs in one of the following three situations: (1) when completing an insurance claim form, (2) when sending a letter to justify a health insurance claim, or (3) when responding to a request from an insurance company (e.g., for additional information, clarification, or application for life, mortgage, or health insurance).

This chapter will describe the documentation process, explain various components of the medical record, and outline legal issues related to medical record keeping. The **medical record** can be defined as written or graphic information documenting facts and events during the rendering of patient care. It is a legal document and as such must be treated with utmost care.

Abstracting Information from a Medical Record

When you abstract information from the patient's record it is a matter of liability that you be extremely accurate. Be sure that you understand all medical terms and abbreviations shown in the chart, and extract only the information requested.

Information to Complete an Insurance Claim Form

A medical record provides the information the insurance billing specialist needs to complete the insurance claim form, such as the date of service (DOS), place of service (POS), type of service (TOS), diagnosis (dx or DX), and procedures or services. These data are abstracted from the medical record and transferred as codes to the claim form for interpretation by the insurance company. The key to substantiating procedure and diagnostic code selections for appropriate reimbursement is supporting documentation in the medical record. Documentation drives the coding process. Without proper documentation coding cannot be successful and maximum reimbursement cannot be obtained. Documentation needs to be accurate, legible, specific, clear, and concise, but with sufficient detail to describe the level of service provided and all procedures performed. Proper documentation can increase reimbursement and prevent penalties and refund requests should the physician's practice be reviewed or audited. It is the medical insurance billing specialist's responsibility to bring any substandard documentation to the physician's attention for improvement.

Sending a Letter to Justify a Health Insurance Claim

When submitting a health insurance claim form the medical insurance billing specialist makes a decision as to whether additional documentation is needed to substantiate the claim. Insurance companies do not like receiving additional documents unless there is a need to communicate information that cannot be included on the claim form. Attachments delay the processing of the claim and often prompt the claim to be sent to review. If additional documentation is necessary, the chart note, operative report, or discharge summary may be sent. Most of the time these documents include detailed information that can be highlighted to emphasize important data.

If an insurance claim is suspended because additional information is needed, or denied because information was not provided, it may be necessary to write a letter outlining or summarizing the treatment the patient received and stating the medical necessity. This is recommended especially if the treatment was involved and there are lengthy chart notes. Send a brief but detailed letter stating facts that are important to the case. Do not copy and send all of the medical records and expect the insurance adjuster to go through them one by one and pick out the necessary facts.

*Health Care Financing Administration is now known as Centers for Medicare and Medicaid Services.

For an insurance billing specialist to develop the skills of abstracting data and constructing a summary, it is necessary to identify and prioritize important information, abstract data, and compose a letter stating the case. The physician may be asked to do this for complicated cases and the insurance specialist can learn by reading letters sent out previously. Maximum reimbursement may be attained in difficult cases by assisting the physician with necessary documentation. Have the physician review all summary letters prior to sending them to the insurance carrier.

Request from an Insurance Company

Often, insurance companies send forms to be filled out requesting information about preexisting conditions and specific diagnoses, or because the patient is applying for some type of insurance. A narrative report dictated by the physician may be more appropriate to accompany a form, especially if there are long columns to check and no space for comments, or the chart is extremely lengthy. If you have abstracted information and filled in a form from the insurance company, place a "Please read" note on the insurance questionnaire. To avoid liability, have the physician read it to verify that the information is accurate and properly stated before he or she signs it.

The process of abstracting information is not new to you as a student. You practice this skill every time you answer CPR and Study Session questions by reading the material (the worktext) and locating specific information. This is the same skill needed when abstracting information from a medical record. This chapter explains various types of information found in a medical record and details how it is organized. With this knowledge you will be able to find information easily and abstract it for use in various situations.

Photocopying the Medical Record

It is customary for an insurance company to have a duplicating service come to the physician's office to photocopy records. A standard time is usually set aside in the physician's office for this service and you should make an appointment. Always remove the records to be copied from the chart, have the physician review the records, and be sure a consent or authorization is in place to release medical information. Advise the photocopy company of the standard fee (e.g., $25) that is to be paid prior to photocopying the records. If the information communicated in the report or form is beyond the standard, the physician can request a fee based on the length of the report or form and bill using CPT code 99080.

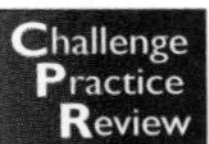

Pause and Practice CPR

REVIEW SESSIONS 7–1 THROUGH 7–3

Directions: *Complete the following questions as a review of information you have just read.*

7–1 Write the definition for the following abbreviations, which stand for the type of information abstracted from the medical record and entered on the insurance claim form.

(a) DX ______________________

(b) TOS ______________________

(c) DOS ______________________

(d) POS ______________________

7–2 If additional documentation needs to be sent with the insurance claim form, what three documents are most commonly included?

(a) ______________________

(b) ______________________

(c) ______________________

7–3 Instead of filling out a long form from the insurance company, the physician may prefer to dictate a/an ______________________

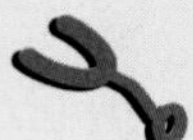

CHECK YOUR HEARTBEAT! Turn to the end of the chapter for answers to these review sessions.

THE DOCUMENTATION PROCESS

There are many approaches used to chart patient information. New charting formats are being developed to help physicians comply with documentation requirements. To abstract information from a medical record, it is necessary to distinguish between subjective and objective information.

Subjective Information

Subjective information is information that cannot be measured, typically referred to as symptoms. For example, a patient complains of tiredness, nausea, and a sore throat. To one person tiredness may mean feeling fatigued, barely being able to perform a day's work, or having difficulty lifting one foot in front of the other to walk. To another person tiredness may mean feeling sleepy and yawning all of the time, falling asleep at his or her work desk, or requiring 12 hours of sleep at night instead of the usual 8. In the same manner, to one person feeling nauseated may mean a queasy feeling in the stomach, whereas to another it may mean the feeling experienced while on a roller coaster ride right before vomiting. Regarding the third complaint (sore throat), how "sore" is a sore throat? Each person registers pain at different levels and can tolerate more or less pain. Symptoms that cannot be measured are considered subjective findings and it is then the physician's job to look closely at these to determine objective information. Subjective comments that do not relate to a medical problem should not be placed in the patient's chart, for example, "Patient is angry about her bill." Instead, record objective observations, for example, "Patient states in a loud voice that she will not pay her bill."

Objective Findings

Objective findings are information that can be determined by either seeing (visual), feeling (palpation), smelling, listening to (auscultation), or measuring, such as laboratory test results, determining size, or collecting data from a diagnostic test. In the earlier example, the "tiredness" could be measured by asking the patient how many miles he or she previously walked every day without feeling tired (e.g., 3 miles), and how many miles he or she is able to walk presently before tiredness sets in (e.g., half a mile). The severeness of "nausea" is sometimes measured by asking the patient about accompanying signs (e.g., retching, dry heaves, cold sweats, vomiting, and so forth). Objective information can be determined regarding the "sore throat" by looking at it for change in color (redness), presence of lesions (pustules), and change in contour (swelling). After all objective information is obtained, the physician assesses the subjective and objective information, puts it all together, and formulates a diagnosis and a treatment plan.

SOAP Chart Notes

For decades a popular method of charting that separates subjective and objective information was called SOAP notes. The acronym is explained in Figure 7–1.

In the above example, let's say that strep throat was the diagnosis and the physician attributed the symptoms of tiredness and nausea to a flu virus that resulted in the strep throat. The symptoms need not be

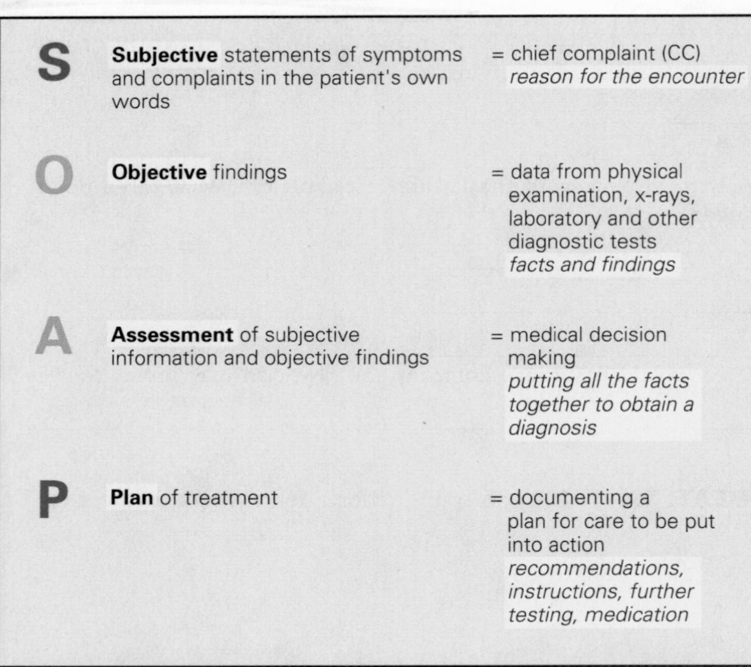

Figure 7–1. Explanation of the acronym "SOAP" used as a format for progress notes defining subjective and objective information, the assessment, and the treatment plan.

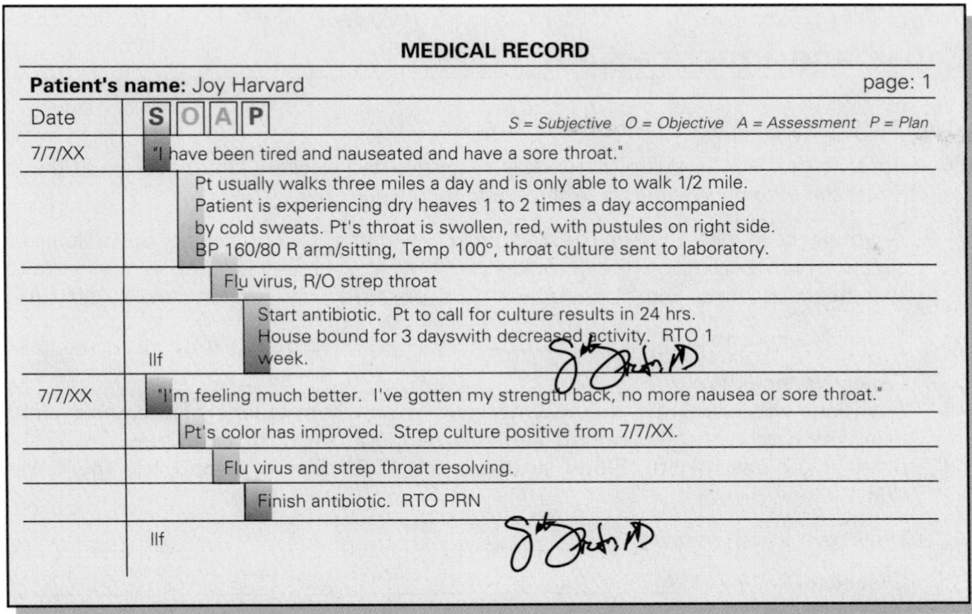

MEDICAL RECORD

Patient's name: Joy Harvard page: 1

Date	S O A P	S = Subjective O = Objective A = Assessment P = Plan
7/7/XX	S	"I have been tired and nauseated and have a sore throat."
	O	Pt usually walks three miles a day and is only able to walk 1/2 mile. Patient is experiencing dry heaves 1 to 2 times a day accompanied by cold sweats. Pt's throat is swollen, red, with pustules on right side. BP 160/80 R arm/sitting, Temp 100°, throat culture sent to laboratory.
	A	Flu virus, R/O strep throat
	P	Start antibiotic. Pt to call for culture results in 24 hrs. House bound for 3 dayswith decreased activity. RTO 1 week.
	llf	
7/7/XX	S	"I'm feeling much better. I've gotten my strength back, no more nausea or sore throat."
	O	Pt's color has improved. Strep culture positive from 7/7/XX.
	A	Flu virus and strep throat resolving.
	P	Finish antibiotic. RTO PRN
	llf	

Figure 7–2. Example of a medical record depicting SOAP-formatted chart notes.

coded because the strep throat is what the physician is treating. However, documentation of these accompanying symptoms in the medical record would warrant a higher level of evaluation and management service, because instead of a problem-focused exam looking only at the sore throat, it would qualify for an expanded problem-focused examination that included evaluating symptoms that involved different body systems.

Figure 7–2 illustrates how the previous scenario would be charted using a SOAP format in the medical record.

Record Systems

There are three basic types of record systems used by most physician's offices: the problem-oriented record, the source-oriented record, and the integrated medical record. Each system incorporates subjective and objective information, along with the assessment of the patient and the formulation of a treatment plan. Each system may also use the SOAP format to document progress notes.

Problem-Oriented Record System

The *problem-oriented record (POR)* system organizes information within the medical record according to patient problems. The four parts of this system include (1) a database, (2) problem list, (3) initial plan, and (4) progress notes. The progress notes may use the SOAP format previously described. Specialists often use the POR system because each complaint is charted from beginning to end. Physicians who treat patients over several years will have more difficulty using this system because many problems are interrelated.

Source-Oriented Record System

The *source-oriented record system (SOR)*, the most common paper-based management system, arranges information in the medical record according to its source, that is, according to the practitioners who are the source of the treatment as well as of the data collected. For example, there are sections for histories and physicals, progress notes, laboratory results, radiology reports, operative reports, and so forth. Information within each section is sequenced in chronological order with the most recent on top. The "chart order" would refer to the order of these various sections and differs from practice to practice. The advantage of an SOR is the speed at which a specific sheet of information can be located. The disadvantage is the lack of a clear picture portraying a specific patient problem because the documentation related to it is filed in different sections of the medical record.

Integrated Medical Record

The *integrated medical record* files all documents in chronological order regardless of their source. Each episode of care is clearly defined by date; however, comparing information from the same source (e.g., laboratory test results) is difficult because it is scattered throughout the medical record. Some medical practices integrate certain types of documents, like progress notes, while keeping other documents such as radiology and laboratory reports, in separate sections according to their source.

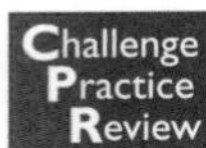

Pause and Practice CPR

PRACTICE SESSIONS 7–4 THROUGH 7–6

Directions: *To develop the skill of abstracting subjective and objective information, read the following scenarios, abstract the information, and fill in the appropriate categories.*

7–4 A young child presents in the radiology department complaining of an injured left arm. She says she was playing on the "monkey bars" at school and fell. She is crying, telling her mother that her arm hurts and "looks funny." You observe that her left arm is disfigured and swollen.

Subjective information: ____________________

Objective findings: ____________________

7–5 A patient was brought into the emergency room complaining of breathing difficulty and chest pain. Her vital signs showed an elevated temperature of 101.1°F, pulse of 90, labored respirations at 30 per minute. Blood pressure is 142/86. She is diaphoretic (perspiring) with warm skin.

Subjective information: ____________________

Objective findings: ____________________

____

7–6 A patient arrives at Dr. Practon's office complaining of an upset stomach. He states he vomited three times last night and had diarrhea. He says his stomach hurts and he feels terrible. Upon questioning, the patient states his stools are loose and watery and he had six episodes of diarrhea last night and two already this morning. Dr. Practon palpates his abdomen and finds it hard and distended. His temperature is 99.9°F, pulse 100 (fast and thready), BP 110/60.

Subjective information: ____________________

Objective findings: ____________________

____

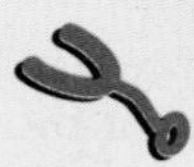

CHECK YOUR HEARTBEAT! Turn to the end of the chapter for answers to these practice sessions.

Documenters

All individuals providing healthcare services may be referred to as documenters because they record chronologically pertinent facts and observations about the patient's health. This process of recording is called **documentation,** or charting, and may be handwritten, input using a computer system, or dictated and transcribed. Many entries, such as prescription refills, telephone calls, information regarding the scheduling of diagnostic tests, and indicating when the patient is a "no-show" for an appointment, are made by medical assistants. The insurance billing specialist may also have opportunities to document facts in the medical record, such as telephone conversations with patients, authorization approval information, and other data verifying insurance status.

Documentation in the financial record (account/ledger) is frequently done by the insurance specialist as he or she records the date the insurance claim was sent for processing and the patient was billed, follow-up transactions (telephone calls or letters) with the insurance company or the patient, and the date and amount of payment received and credited (adjusted/written off) to the account.

When referring to guidelines for documentation of the medical record and completion of the insurance claim form, a physician's title may change depending on the specialty and services rendered. This can be confusing at times, so to clarify the physician's various roles, some of these titles are defined as follows:

- **Attending physician**—refers to the medical staff member who is legally responsible for the care and treatment given to a patient.
- **Consulting physician**—is a provider whose opinion or advice regarding evaluation and/or management of a specific problem is requested by another physician.
- **Ordering physician**—is the individual directing the selection, preparation, or administration of tests, medication, or treatment. The attending physician can also be the ordering physician.

- **Referring physician**—is a provider who sends the patient for testing or treatment.
- **Treating or performing physician**—is the provider who renders a service to a patient.

Medical Record Fraud

Tampering with a medical record is a fraudulent act. It is also considered a criminal offense and sanctions can include a monetary fine, serving time in prison, or both. In litigation, scientific tests can be done to determine the record's validity. Paper and ink can be analyzed, writing instruments can be determined, and indentations analyzed, all to determine if alterations to the medical record took place.

Reasons for Documentation

It is of vital importance that every patient seen by the physician have comprehensive, concise, and legible documentation regarding what occurred during the visit for the following reasons:

1. Avoidance of denied or delayed payments by insurance carriers who investigate the medical necessity of services
2. Enforcement of medical record-keeping rules by insurance carriers who require accurate documentation that supports procedure and diagnostic codes
3. Subpoena of medical records by state investigators for review by the court
4. Defense of a professional liability claim

GENERAL PRINCIPLES OF MEDICAL RECORD DOCUMENTATION

Documentation guidelines were developed by the Health Care Financing Administration (HCFA), now known as the Centers for Medicare and Medicaid Services (CMS), for *Current Procedural Terminology* (CPT) evaluation and management services in 1995, and later modified in 1997. The development of these guidelines came from auditing by Medicare of physicians' medical records and discovering that the quality of documentation needed to be improved. The medical necessity of procedures and services that had been performed were not stated clearly in the medical record. Physicians, insurance claim processors, and auditors may use either the 1995 or the 1997 guidelines. However, physicians are not required to use them, only encouraged to do so for the above-mentioned reasons. In 2000, HCFA (now CMS) proposed revised E/M guidelines which at this time have not been adopted.

Medical Necessity

Insurers may differ on the meaning of **medical necessity.** As a rule, it means that the performance of services or procedures are consistent with the diagnosis, in accordance with standards of good medical practice, performed at the proper level, and provided in the most appropriate setting. If a treatment is questioned as to whether it is medically necessary, the authorization to perform the treatment or the payment may be delayed or denied.

Documentation Guidelines

Documentation guidelines for E/M services are too detailed and lengthy to list in this worktext. They state all the elements necessary to keep a complete record on the patient, starting with how each chart entry should be dated and signed and including what each encounter should contain, which diagnoses need to be stated, the patient's health risks, the patient's progress, what role consulting physicians have in the care and treatment of the patient, how treatment plans should be written, and so forth. The essentials of these guidelines are given in the following section and the section on contents of a medical report.

Procedure and diagnostic codes reported on the health insurance claim form or billing statement should be supported by the documentation in the medical record and be at a level sufficient for a clinical peer to determine whether services have been accurately coded. The insurance specialist may be inserting entries and/or making corrections to the medical record and should be aware of how to document these.

A list of commonly used abbreviations should be compiled and posted throughout the office to ensure consistency when documenting. Chart entries should be dated and signed, including the title or position of the person signing. Write neatly and use a permanent, not water-soluble, ink pen (legal copy pen).

Corrections to a Medical Record

If a correction needs to be made to the medical record, use a legal copy pen and cross out the incorrect entry, using one single line. Write the correct information, and then date and initial the entry. If a malpractice claim is pending, never correct or amend the medical record. Never erase, white-out, or use self-adhesive paper over any information recorded on the patient record (see Example 7–1). Inaccurate computerized records also involve maintaining the original incorrect entry and adding a corrected entry. Remember the rule: Documentation should answer questions, not raise them.

Example 7–1

Correction to a Medical Record

Incorrect	BP 180/80	
	190/70	1/2/20XX mtf
Correct	BP 150/90	
	slightly	
Incorrect	right leg is ~~markedly~~ edematous...	
	slightly	
Correct	right leg is ~~markedly~~ edematous...	
		1/2/20XX mtf
Correctly typed:	right leg is slightly edematous... 1-2-20XX mtf	

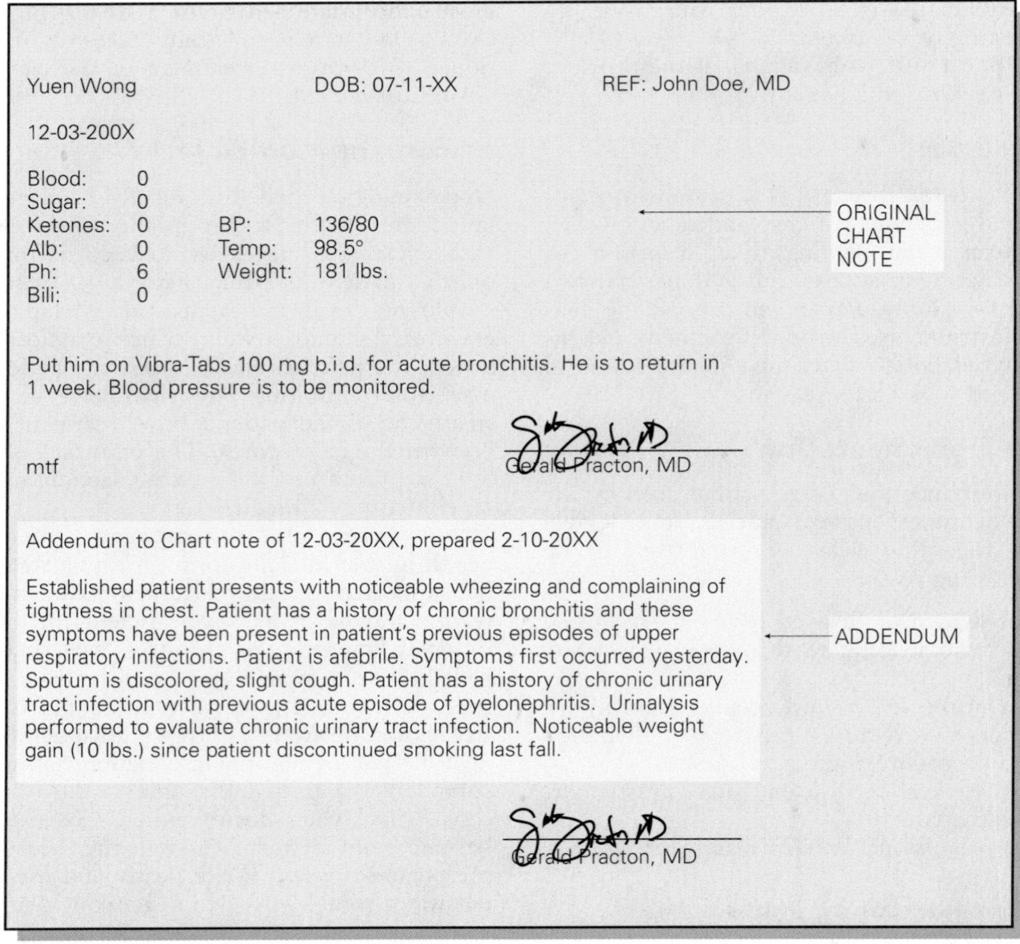
Yuen Wong DOB: 07-11-XX REF: John Doe, MD

12-03-200X

Blood:	0		
Sugar:	0		
Ketones:	0	BP:	136/80
Alb:	0	Temp:	98.5°
Ph:	6	Weight:	181 lbs.
Bili:	0		

Put him on Vibra-Tabs 100 mg b.i.d. for acute bronchitis. He is to return in 1 week. Blood pressure is to be monitored.

mtf Gerald Practon, MD

Addendum to Chart note of 12-03-20XX, prepared 2-10-20XX

Established patient presents with noticeable wheezing and complaining of tightness in chest. Patient has a history of chronic bronchitis and these symptoms have been present in patient's previous episodes of upper respiratory infections. Patient is afebrile. Symptoms first occurred yesterday. Sputum is discolored, slight cough. Patient has a history of chronic urinary tract infection with previous acute episode of pyelonephritis. Urinalysis performed to evaluate chronic urinary tract infection. Noticeable weight gain (10 lbs.) since patient discontinued smoking last fall.

Gerald Practon, MD

Figure 7–3. Example of an addendum to a patient's medical record to justify the level of service reported. The insurance carrier downcoded the services from level 99213 to 99212.

If documentation is missing from the medical record, an addendum may be preferable. The addendum to the chart note should include the date of the original chart note that is being added to, and the date it was prepared (transcribed). It needs to be signed by the physician or person who is adding additional documentation. The addendum should be entered in or attached to the chart after the last entry. If there are entries between it and the original entry, a cross-reference at the original entry should be noted (see Fig. 7–3).

Medical Terms Used in Documentation

Medical terminology is very technical and can puzzle even the most knowledgeable of insurance billing specialists. When an insurance biller is not familiar with the medical terms being used, major errors can occur. If there is a question, search for the term in a medical dictionary. If the term is not found or is still not understood, ask the physician to clarify the term and the way it is used in the medical record. Following is a brief description of selected terms that may cause confusion.

Concurrent Care

Concurrent care is the provision of similar services (e.g., hospital visits) to the same patient by more than one physician on the same day. Usually, such cases involve the presence of a separate physical disorder (e.g., heart arrhythmia) at the same time as the primary admitting diagnosis, and this disorder may alter the course of treatment or lengthen recovery time for the primary condition. For example, two internists (a general internist and a cardiologist) see the same patient in the hospital on the same day. The general internist admitted the patient for out-of-control diabetes and requested that the cardiologist also follow the patient's arrhythmia and periodic chest pain. If the second doctor is not identified in carrier records as a cardiologist, the claim may be denied because the services appear to be duplicated by physicians of the same specialty (internal medicine). When billing insurance companies, physicians providing concurrent care may be cross-referenced on the claim form. Periodically, the insurance specialist should check with the carrier's provider service representative to see if the provider has updated its subspecialty status so claims for concurrent care are not denied.

Continuity of Care

Continuity of care involves making sure that the patient's treatment is not interrupted, causing harm by a lapse in care. Every patient has the right to continuity of care. For example, if a cancer patient receives chemotherapy treatment from his or her oncologist and is then referred to a radiologist for radiology treatment, both physicians are responsible for providing arrangements for the patient's continuing care. The referring physician (oncologist) must provide records to the radiologist. The radiologist must provide an appointment within a reasonable time and follow-up to be sure records needed to perform the service are in his or her possession.

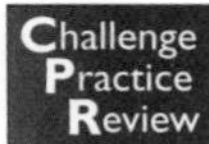

Pause and Practice CPR

REVIEW SESSIONS 7–7 THROUGH 7–9

Directions: *Complete the following questions as a review of information you have just read.*

7–7 What is the process of recording information in the medical record called?

____

7–8 Who developed documentation guidelines?

____

____

7–9 When an insurance company verifies that the performance of a procedure is consistent with the diagnosis, in accordance with standards of good medical practice, performed at the proper level, and provided in the most appropriate setting, it is said to be a/an ________________.

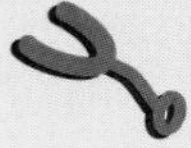

CHECK YOUR HEARTBEAT! Turn to the end of the chapter for answers to these review sessions.

COMPONENTS OF A MEDICAL RECORD

A medical record is the compilation of various types of data such as the patient's social and medical history, family history, physical examination findings, progress notes, radiology and laboratory reports, other diagnostic test results, consultation reports, correspondence related to patient care, and discharge summary if the patient receives inpatient hospital care. Operative reports, consent to perform special treatment, and consent or authorization to release records are also included in the medical record.

The physician handwrites or dictates the documentation, formulates a conclusion regarding the patient's diagnosis, and then decides on a treatment plan. All procedures and services that are used to come to this conclusion should be clearly stated in the medical record. A medical practice should have a standard policy and procedure regarding the creation, maintenance, and destruction of medical records. The order in which the data are assembled needs to be consistent. A well-organized file will save time for the physician and office staff when information needs to be retrieved. Using dividers to separate subject matter will expedite locating information. Medical personnel may refer to this record as the patient's chart, a progress note, healthcare record, medical information, or hospital record.

Contents of a Medical Report

The degree of documentation in a medical report depends on the complexity of the service and the specialty of the physician. For example, a chest examination performed by a family physician may include different elements of documentation than one performed by a cardiologist or pulmonologist.

The first time a new patient is seen, a family and social history is taken along with the patient's personal history. A chief complaint is recorded, the physical examination is performed, a medical decision-making process determines a diagnosis, and the treatment plan is formulated. On an established patient, the family and social history need not be repeated unless something new is mentioned, or unless the history pertains specifically to the patient's present problem. When a new injury or illness occurs, the documentation should also include the patient's health history, the physical examination, results from any tests that are performed, the medical decision-making process, the diagnosis, and the treatment plan.

Documentation of History

Based on Medicare's 1997 guidelines, documentation of the history should include the chief complaint (CC), history of present illness (HPI), review of symptoms (ROS), and past, family, and/or social history (PFSH). The extent of the history is dependent on clinical judgment and on the nature of the presenting problem(s) (Fig. 7–4).

As presented in Chapter 5, in the discussion of coding evaluation and management services, the history is the first key component for choosing a level of service and there are four possible histories from which to choose: (1) problem-focused—PF, (2) expanded problem-focused—EPF, (3) detailed—D, and (4) comprehensive—C. Review Figure 5–6 for various components of these history types as you refer to the following information.

Chief Complaint

As mentioned in Chapter 5, the *chief complaint* (CC) is a brief statement, in the patient's own words, describing the reason for the encounter; such as a symptom, problem, condition, or finding.

Hospital number: 00-83-06

Scott, Aimee

Gerald Practon, MD

HISTORY

CHIEF COMPLAINT: Pain and bleeding after each bowel movement for the past 3-4 months.

PRESENT ILLNESS: This 68-year old white female says she usally has three bowel movements a day in small amounts, and there has been a change in the last 3 to 4 months in frequency, size and type of bowel movement. She has slight burning pain and irritation in the rectal area after bowel movements. The pain lasts for several minutes then decreases in intensity. She has had no previous anorectal surgery or rectal infection. She denies any blood in the stool itself or associated symptoms. Bright red blood occurs after stools have passed.

PAST HISTORY:

ILNESSES: The patient had polio at age 8 from which she has made a remarkable recovery. Apparently, she was paralyzed in both lower extremities and now has adequate use of these. She has no other serious illnesses.

ALLERGIES: ALLERGIC TO PENICILLIN. She denies any other drug or food allergies.

MEDICATIONS: None.

OPERATIONS: Right inguinal herniorrhaphy, 25 years ago.

SOCIAL HISTORY: She does not smoke or drink. She lives with her husband who is an invalid and for whom she cares. She is a retired former municipal court judge.

FAMILY HISTORY: One brother died of cancer of the throat (age 59), another has cancer of the kidney (age 63).

REVIEW OF SYSTEMS:

SKIN: No rashes or jaundice.

HEENT: Head normocephalic. Normal TMs. Normal hearing. Pupils equal, round, reactive to light. Deviated septum. Oropharynx clear.

CR: No history of chest pain, shortness of breath, or pedal edema. She has had some mild hypertension in the past but is not under any medical supervision nor is she taking any medication for this.

GI: Weight is stable. See present illness.

OB-GYN: Gravida II Para II. Climacteric at age 46, no sequelae.

EXTREMITIES: No edema.

NEUROLOGIC: Unremarkable.

Gerald Practon, MD

mtf
D: 5-17-20XX
T: 5-20-20XX

Figure 7–4. Example of a medical report done in modified block format showing the six components of a history.

Expressions from Experience

Keep up with coding changes by having current diagnostic and procedure codebooks. Reference materials found in your office, such as medical dictionaries, the Physician's Desk Reference *containing drug information, the* Merck Manual *explaining diseases, and medical word books, are also of value. It is important not only to understand terms, but also spell and pronounce them correctly when communicating with other professionals.*

Sue Manion
Medical Transcriptionist/Biller
Ear, Nose, and Throat Specialty

History of Present Illness

The **history of present illness (HPI)** is a chronological description of the development of the patient's present illness from the first sign and/or symptom or from the previous encounter to the present. It includes associated signs and symptoms, their duration, location, severity, and quality, and any modifying factors. The context and timing of how, when, and where the problem presents is also noted.

Review of Systems

A **review of systems (ROS)** is an inventory of all body systems obtained through a series of questions that are used to identify signs and/or symptoms that the patient has experienced or might be experiencing. The patient usually fills out this information on a history form prior to being seen by the physician. Checklists are permitted, but if a body system is not considered, then it should be crossed out. For an ROS the following body systems are recognized: eyes; ears, mouth, nose, and throat; cardiovascular; respiratory; gastrointestinal; genitourinary; musculoskeletal; integumentary (skin and/or breast); neurologic; psychiatric; endocrine; hematologic/lymphatic; allergic/immunologic; and constitutional (e.g., fever, weight loss).

Past, Family, and Social Histories

The past, family, and social histories (PFSHs) consist of review of three areas:

1. **Past history (PH)**—patient's past experiences with illness, operations, injuries, and treatments.
2. **Family history (FH)**—review of medical events in the patient's family, including diseases that may be hereditary or place the patient at risk.
3. **Social history (SF)**—review of past and current activities depending on patient's age.

Documentation of Physical Examination

The **physical examination (PE or PX)** is objective in nature; that is, it consists of the physician's findings by examination and/or test results of organ systems or body areas. The following organ systems are recognized in single body system and general multisystem examinations: cardiovascular; ears, nose, and throat; eyes; genitourinary (including gastrointestinal for male and female); hematologic/lymphatic/immunologic; musculoskeletal; neurologic; psychiatric; respiratory; and skin. Each exam includes a constitutional component (vital signs, general appearance, nutrition).

The following body areas are included: head (including face); neck; chest (including breasts and axillae); abdomen; genitalia, groin, buttocks; back (including spine); and each extremity.

The extent of the examination, as well as what is documented, depends on clinical judgment and the nature of the presenting problem(s). It may range from limited examinations of single body areas to complete single-organ system examinations or general multisystem examinations.

As presented in Chapter 5, in Table 5–6, the PX is the second key component and the four types are identical to those used for the history (PF, EPF, D, and C).

Documentation of Medical Decision-Making Complexity

In the medical decision-making process the physician must look at the number of diagnoses and treatment options, the amount and/or complexity of data to be reviewed, and the risk of *complications* and/or morbidity or mortality. The risk of complications is based on the conditions associated with the presenting problem(s) such as diagnostic procedures, possible management options (e.g., surgery, therapy, drug management), **morbidity** (diseased condition or state), **mortality** (number of deaths in a given time or place), and **comorbidity** (underlying disease or other condition present at the time of the visit). Example 7–2 illustrates two scenarios where hospital patients have complications and comorbid conditions.

Example 7–2

Comorbid Condition and Complication

Scenario A:
A patient has had congestive heart failure for several years and is admitted to College Hospital with an admitting diagnosis of chest pain. The principal diagnosis is anterior wall myocardial infarction (MI). While hospitalized, the patient experiences atrial fibrillation.

Principal diagnosis	410.10 anterior wall myocardial infarction
Comorbid condition	428.0 congestive heart failure
Complication	427.31 atrial fibrillation

Scenario B: A patient has had chronic obstructive pulmonary disease (COPD) for the past 6 months and is admitted to College Hospital with an admitting diagnosis of chest pain. The principal diagnosis is anterior wall myocardial infarction (MI). While hospitalized, the patient experiences acute respiratory failure.

Principal diagnosis	410.10 anterior wall myocardial infarction
Comorbid condition	496 chronic obstructive pulmonary disease
Complication	518.81 acute respiratory failure

Documentation for Requesting Outpatient Services

When a physician orders outpatient services to be done at another facility, documentation on the order must include the following:

1. Date of order (service must be performed within 30 days)
2. Patient's name
3. Service ordered
4. Diagnosis or signs/symptoms
5. Physician's signature

An order not containing the the above is considered invalid. Valid orders are not only needed to perform the service but also to bill for the service. Medical staff must be compliant by checking orders to be sure that this information is complete. Diagnostic coding on orders should be done by the physician receiving the order.

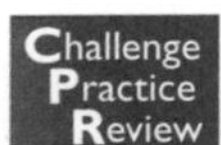

Pause and Practice CPR

REVIEW SESSIONS 7–10 THROUGH 7–14

Directions: *Complete the following questions as a review of information you have just read.*

7–10 What three types of history are taken the first time a patient is seen?

(a) ______________________

(b) ______________________

(c) ______________________

7–11 Name four elements (with abbreviations) that documentation of the patient's history should include.

(a) ______________________ __________

(b) ______________________ __________

(c) ______________________ __________

(d) ______________________ __________

7–12 When a physician takes an inventory of all body systems obtained through a series of questions that is used to identify signs and/or symptoms that the patient has experienced or might be experiencing, this is referred to as a/an:

____

7–13 How many organ systems are recognized in single body system and general multisystem examinations? __________

7–14 What three elements is the physician looking at in the medical decision-making process?

(a) ______________________

(b) ______________________

(c) ______________________

CHECK YOUR HEARTBEAT! Turn to the end of the chapter for answers to these review sessions.

LEGALITIES OF A MEDICAL RECORD

The basics of confidential communication were provided in Chapter 1 where privileged and nonprivileged information and the right to privacy were discussed along with the consent and authorization forms needed to release medical information. Principles for the release of information are shown in Table 7–1 depicting various situations when a medical record is needed, and the policy for its release. When in doubt about the release of medical or financial information, whether it be

Table 7–1 **Principles for Release of Information**

Request From or For	Policy
Physicians involved with patient care	Consent form signed by the patient.
Physician referring a patient to another doctor for consultation	Referring physician sends summary of case or copies of patient's records without signed authorization.
Patient moving to a new location or being released from medical care and transferred to another physician	Letter should be directed to the patient offering to transfer the patient's records with signed authorization to new physician.
Managed care patient seen by different physicians at each office visit	Patient records may be read by all physicians involved with the case without a separate signed authorization.
Insurance companies and others concerned from a financial point of view	Consent form signed by the patient.
Attorney in litigation case	Records may be released if subpoenaed; otherwise must have written authorization of the patient.
Any party in workers' compensation case	Insurance claims examiner can give patient copy of his or her records but physician cannot release record unless authorized by claims examiner. Authorization must be signed by employer and insurance company.
Any party via telephone	Either ask the caller to put the request in writing and to include the patient's signed authorization or obtain the name and telephone number of the caller and relationship to the patient and have the physician return the call.
Government and state agencies	Records may be reviewed without patient's consent to verify billing information and determine if services were medically necessary. Data in the records may be used only for audit and may not be released.
Employer	Written consent of patient. Special care should be exercised and the attending physician consulted before release of any information.
For psychiatric records	Consult psychiatrist or attending physician concerned with the case before records are released. If patient has threatened to harm himself or herself or someone else, the patient may lose the confidentiality privilege when he or she files litigation in which mental distress is claimed.
For publication	Written authorization of patient. Care must be exercised in release of any information for publication because this constitutes an invasion of the patient's right to privacy and can result in legal action against the physician releasing such information.
For medical information in an acquired immunodeficiency syndrome (AIDS) or human immunodeficiency virus (HIV) infection case	Seek legal counsel and/or learn the state laws before releasing any information. A specific authorization is usually required. Stamp all information released about a patient who has an HIV infection with a statement prohibiting redisclosure of the data to another party without prior consent of the patient. The party receiving the data should be requested to destroy the information after the stated need is fulfilled.
For medical information on a minor	If a minor patient is legally capable of consenting to medical treatment, only the minor patient may sign a consent form for disclosure. In all other cases, the consent must be signed by the minor's parent, guardian, or other legal representative.
For medical information on a minor who has received alcohol and/or drug abuse treatment	Where state law permits the minor to apply for and obtain alcohol or drug abuse treatment, the minor may authorize disclosure.

by mail, fax, or electronic transmission, ask the physician or office manger for guidance and make sure to obtain the patient's consent and/or authorization in writing.

Faxing Documents

A **facsimile (fax)** is the transmission of written and graphic matter by electronic means. Fax transmission is a system of sending and receiving copies of information instantly over telephone lines and has become an important communication tool. In the medical office, the insurance billing specialist may use the fax to transmit insurance claims data directly to the electronic claims processor, resubmit an unpaid insurance claim, send documentation to accompany a claim, send an authorization to request surgery or a test, and send medical reports between offices and other medical facilities. Use typewritten, computer-generated, or documents that have been handwritten with pen (not pencil) to assure clear reception. Documents received via plain paper fax machines do not deteriorate; however, to prevent deterioration of documents that have been received on a *thermal paper fax machine*, photocopy the document onto regular paper before it is filed in the medical record.

Faxing Confidential Information

From the legal standpoint, protecting the patient's confidentiality in the fax process is critical. The American Health Information Management Association (AHIMA) advises that fax machines "should not be used for routine transmission of patient information." AHIMA recommends that documents should be faxed only when (1) hand or mail delivery will not meet the needs of immediate patient care, or (2) required by a third party for ongoing certification of payment for a hospitalized patient. If, due to circumstances, medical records or a report must be faxed, you should have the patient sign an authorization to release information via facsimile equipment.

Fax machines should be located in secure or restricted access areas. To ensure protection, a cover sheet should be used for all transmissions. It should contain the following information:

- Date
- Name of sender with fax and telephone number
- Name of recipient with fax and telephone number
- Total number of pages, including the cover sheet
- Statement indicating that the communication is personal, privileged, and confidential medical information intended for the named recipient only (Fig. 7–5)

What Not to Fax

Financial information and documents containing information on sexually transmitted diseases, drug or alcohol treatment, or human immunodeficiency virus (HIV) status should not be faxed. Psychiatric records should not be faxed except for emergency requests.

Transmittal Destination

Program frequently used fax numbers into the machine to avoid misdirecting faxed communications. To ensure that a faxed document has reached the correct destination, do one of the following:

- Arrange a scheduled time for transmission with the recipient.
- Telephone the destination to verify receipt.
- Request that the authorized receiver sign and return an attached receipt form at the bottom of the cover sheet after receiving the faxed information.
- Send the fax to a coded mail box that only allows a receiver who has the code that was used to fax the information to activate the printer.

FAX TRANSMITTAL SHEET

To: College Hospital (outpatient surgery) Date 10-21-20XX

Fax Number: (555) 486 8900 Telephone Number (555) 487 6789 Time 10:00 a.m.

Number of pages (including this one): 3

From: Raymond Skeleton, MD Phone (555) 486 9002

Note: This transmittal is intended only for the use of the individual or entity to which it is addressed, and may contain information that is privileged, confidential, and exempt from disclosure under applicable law. If you are not the intended recipient, any dissemination, distribution, or photocopying of this communication is strictly prohibited. If you have received this communication in error, please notify this office immediately by telephone and return the original FAX to us at the address below by U.S. Postal Service. Thank you.

Remarks: Enclosed are Margaret Yont's radiology reports on her L. tibia/fibula and L. foot fractures

If you cannot read this FAX or if pages are missing, please contact:

College Clinic
4567 Broad Avenue
Woodland Hills, XY
12345-0001
TEL:(555) 486-9002
FAX:(555) 487-8976

INSTRUCTIONS TO THE AUTHORIZED RECEIVER: PLEASE COMPLETE THIS STATEMENT OF RECEIPT AND RETURN TO SENDER VIA THE ABOVE FAX NUMBER.

- -

I, Cheryl Watson, CMA, verify that I have received 3 (no. of pages including cover sheet)

from Raymond Skeleton, MD (sending facility's name)

Figure 7–5. Example of a fax cover sheet for medical document transmission.

- Arrange with the recipient to block out the name of the patient, and instead fax using a reference number (e.g., patient's Social Security number).

To safeguard against a fax sent to the wrong destination, include a request to destroy misdirected information and ask that the receiver advise the physician's office when this has occurred. In such an occurrence, document the incident, along with the misdialed number in the patient's medical record.

Faxing Legal Documents

Consult an attorney to make sure that documents (e.g., contracts, proposals, insurance claims) requiring signatures are legally binding if faxed. To ensure legality, do the following:

- Transmit a cover page that refers specifically to what is being sent.
- Transmit the entire document, not only the page to be signed, so the receiver has full disclosure of the agreement.
- Obtain confirmation that the receiver is in receipt of all pages sent; an incomplete document is insupportable in court and may invalidate legality.
- Insert a clause in the contract stating faxed signatures will be treated as originals, for example, "Facsimile signatures shall be sufficient unless originals are required by a third party."
- Send the original document as soon as possible and obtain the original signature in hard copy.

Subpoena

Subpoena literally means "under penalty." It is a written order, signed by a judge or an attorney, requiring the appearance of a witness at a trial or other proceeding. A *subpoena duces tecum* requires the witness to appear and to bring and/or send certain records "in his possession." Frequently only the records may be sent, and the physician is not required to appear in court.

It is possible for a state investigator to subpoena patient records to substantiate documentation of treatment provided. Medical records may also be subpoenaed as proof in a medical malpractice case. Complete documentation and well-organized patient records establish a strong defense in a medical professional liability claim.

The Subpoena Process

A subpoena must be *personally served* or handed to the prospective witness or the keeper of the medical records. The acceptance of a document by an authorized person is the equivalent of personal service. The medical office should appoint one person as keeper of the medical records designated to accept subpoenas. In some states, provision is made for substitute service by mail or through newspaper advertisements. This is permitted only after all reasonable efforts to effect personal service have failed.

Never accept a subpoena or give records to anyone without the physician's prior approval. If the subpoena is only for medical records and/or financial data, the representative for the specific doctor can then usually accept it. In such cases the physician is not usually called to court, but there is no guarantee. In the event that the physician is called to appear, he or she should be prepared to defend all documentation in the medical record. Willful disregard of a subpoena is punishable as contempt of court.

The medical office is given a prescribed time in which to produce the records. It is not necessary to show them at the time the subpoena is served unless the court order so states. After the subpoena has been served, pull the chart and place it and the subpoena on the doctor's desk for review.

The attorney usually employs a person or duplication service to photocopy records that are under subpoena. At the time the subpoena is served, a date is usually agreed upon in which the representative will return and photocopy the portion of the record that is named in the subpoena. If original records are requested, move them to a safe place, preferably under lock and key, so that they cannot be taken away or tampered with before the trial date. Often, only the portion of the medical record requested is removed from the original chart and put in a copy folder. Items such as the patient information form, encounter form, and explanation of benefit or remittance advice documents should not be included. Make photocopies of the original records being subpoenaed and number all pages. This is to prevent total loss of the records and facilitate discovery of any altering or tampering while they are out of your custody.

Prevention of Legal Problems

There are many instances in which an insurance biller must be careful in executing job duties to avoid the possibility of a lawsuit. A summary of guidelines for prevention of lawsuits is shown in Table 7–2.

Expressions from Experience

Take advantage of meetings sponsored by insurance carriers to receive the latest information and network with other professionals. Seminars and workshops can mean not only a "free lunch," but also an opportunity to ask questions and address specific problems

Sue Manion
Medical Transcriptionist/Biller
Ear, Nose, and Throat Specialty

Table 7–2 Guidelines for Prevention of Lawsuits

1. Keep information about patients strictly confidential.
2. Obtain proper instruction and carry out responsibilities according to the employer's guidelines.
3. Keep abreast of general insurance program guidelines, annual coding changes, and medical and scientific progress to help when handling insurance matters.
4. Secure proper written consent in all cases before releasing a patient's medical record.
5. Do not refer to consent or acknowledgement forms as "releases." Use the word, "consent" or "authorization" forms as required by law. This also produces a better understanding of the document to be signed.
6. Make sure documentation of patient care in the medical record corresponds with billing submitted on the insurance claim.
7. Exercise good judgment in what you write and how you word electronic mail because it does not give security against confidentiality.
8. Make every effort to reach an understanding with patients in the matter of fees by explaining what services will be received and what the "extras" may be. For hospital cases, it is advisable to explain that the fee the physician charges is for his or her services only and that charges for the bed or ward room, operating room, laboratory tests, and anesthesia will be billed separately in addition to the physician's charges.
9. Do not discuss other physicians with the patient. Patients sometimes invite criticism of the methods or results of former physicians. Remember that you are hearing only one side of the story.
10. Tell the physician immediately if you learn that a new patient is still under treatment by another physician.
11. Do not compare the respective merits of various forms of therapy and refrain from discussing patients' ailments with them. Patients come to talk to the physician about their symptoms, and you may give them incorrect information. Let the physician make the diagnosis. Otherwise, you may seriously embarrass the physician, yourself, or both of you.
12. Report a physician who is doing something illegal that you are aware of. You can be held responsible for being silent and failing to report an illegal action.
13. Say nothing to anyone except as required by the attorney of the physician or by the court if litigation is pending.
14. Be alert to hazards that may cause injury to anyone in the office and report such problems immediately.
15. Consult the physician before turning over a delinquent account to a collection agency.
16. Be courteous in dealing with patients and always act in a professional manner.

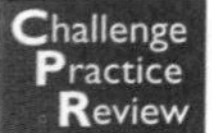

Pause and Practice CPR

CHALLENGE SESSION 7–15

Directions: *To help develop the skill of abstracting information, reread the information you have read thus far about faxing confidential information and abstracting specific data.*

7–15 Abstract and list the main points of the American Health Information Management Association's stand on using the fax machine in the physician's office.

(a) ______________________________

(b) ______________________________

(c) ______________________________

(d) ______________________________

REVIEW SESSIONS 7–16 AND 7–17

Directions: *Complete the following questions as a review of information you have just read.*

7–16 What does a *subpoena duces tecum* require? ______________________________

7–17 In a physician's office, when a subpoena is "personally served," who may receive it?

____

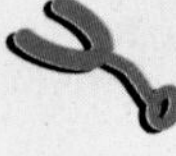

CHECK YOUR HEARTBEAT! Turn to the end of the chapter for answers to these challenge and review sessions.

DATA STORAGE

Today, most medical records are either stored in file folders containing a collection of paper documents or reside in electronic databases via computer access. Regardless of the system used, there are state and local laws that govern the retention of records.

Medical Record Retention

Preservation of medical records is governed by state and local laws. It is the policy of most physicians to retain medical records of all living patients indefinitely. Records such as x-ray films, laboratory reports, and pathologic specimens probably should also be kept indefinitely. Deceased patients' charts should be kept for at least 5 years. Calendars, appointment books, and telephone logs should be filed and stored. Recommended retention periods for paper files are shown in Table 7–3. These retention periods are a guide but because state and federal laws vary, always contact your state legislature for current information.

A paperless office requires an organized and efficient system for keeping files that have been saved to the hard drive against accidental destruction. The computer may initiate automated **backup**, or a screen prompt may appear instructing the operator to back up before quitting the program. If not, always back up files at the end of the day so information is not lost during a power outage (e.g., surge, spike, blackout, brownout, lightning, computer breakdown, or head crash). Keep financial electronic records on disks or tapes and store in an area that does not have temperature extremes or magnetic fields. Electronic health records may have different retention periods depending on state laws, as shown in Table 7–4.

A person's medical record may be of value not only to himself or herself in later years but also to the person's children. In some states a minor may file suit, several years after he or she has attained legal age, for any act performed during childhood that the person believes to be wrong or harmful. Thus, it is important to keep records until patients are 3 to 10 years beyond the age of majority, which varies from state to state.

Financial Document Retention

According to income tax regulations, the Internal Revenue Service can audit a tax return up to 3 years after it was due, or from the date the return was filed, whichever is later. If possible fraud is an issue, the audit deadline becomes 6 years. Keep tax records for 7 years and the tax return permanently. Always contact an accountant before discarding records that may determine tax liability. Suggested retention periods are included in Table 7–3.

A federal regulation mandates that assigned claims for Medicaid and Medicare be kept for 7 years; the physician is subject to auditing during that period.

Destruction of Medical Records

Shred documents that are no longer needed. Some practices prefer to use medical record storage compa-

Table 7–3 Medical/Financial Record Retention Schedule

Temporary Record	Retention Period (yr)	Permanent Record	Retained Indefinitely
Appointment sheets	1	Accounts payable records	
Bank deposit slip (duplicate)	1	Bills of sale for important purchases (or until you no longer own them)	
Bank statements and canceled checks	7	Capital asset records	
Billing records (for outside services)	7	Certified financial statements	
Cash receipt records	10	Contracts	
Contracts (expired)	7	Credit history	
Correspondence, general	1–5	Deeds	
Day sheets (balance sheets and journals)	5	Equipment guarantees and records (or until you no longer own them)	
Employee contracts	6	Income tax returns	
Employee time records	5	Insurance policies and records	
Employment applications	3	Leases	
Insurance claim forms (paid)	3	Legal correspondence	
Invoices	7	Medical records (active patients)	
Medical records (expired patients)	5	Medical records (inactive patients)	
Medicare Remittance Advice documents	7	Mortgages	
Payroll records	7	Property appraisals and records	
Petty cash vouchers	3	Telephone records	
Postal and meter records	1	X-ray films	
Tax worksheets and supporting documents	7	Year-end balance sheets and general ledgers	

Note: The above are general guidelines and may vary according to state and federal laws.

Table 7–4 Electronic Health Records: State Retention Periods

State	Routine Patients (yr)	Films X-Ray (yr)	Nursing Homes (yr)	Minors (yr)	Medicaid (yr)
Alabama	22	5	At least 5		
Alaska	7	5		At least 2	3
Arizona	10				
Arkansas	10			7	
California	7	7	1		
Colorado	10			Majority + 10	
Connecticut	25		10		
Delaware					
District of Columbia	10				
Florida	7	5	5		
Georgia	6			Until 27th birthday	
Hawaii	7	7		Majority + 7	
Idaho	3	5	7	18th birthday + 7	
Illinois	10–22		5		
Indiana	7	5			
Iowa	Statute of limitations		3		
Kansas	10			18th birthday + 1	
Kentucky	5			Majority + 3	
Louisiana	10	3			
Maine	Statute of limitations				
Maryland	5			Majority + 3	
Massachusetts	5				
Michigan			6		
Minnesota	7				
Mississippi	7–10	4		Majority + 7	
Missouri	Statute of limitations		5		
Montana	10			Majority + 10	
Nebraska	10			Majority + 3	
Nevada	5		1		
New Hampshire	7	7	7	Majority + 7	
New Jersey	10	5		At least 23rd birthday	
New Mexico	10	4			
New York	6			Majority + 3	
North Carolina	Statute of limitations				
North Dakota	25		10	Majority + 3	
Ohio					
Oklahoma	5				6
Oregon		10	7	7	
Pennsylvania	7			Majority + 7	
Rhode Island	5			23rd birthday	
South Carolina	10		10		
South Dakota	Statute of limitations				
Tennessee	10	4	10	Majority + 1	
Texas	10			20th birthday	
Utah	10				
Vermont	10		6		
Virginia	5			23rd birthday	
Washington	10			21st birthday	
West Virginia	NONE				
Wisconsin	5				
Wyoming	30	5			

From Amatayahul M, Brown L, Cavanaugh F, et al: Comprehensive Guide to Electronic Health Records Washington, DC, Eli Research, Inc., 1997.

nies, which may put records on microfilm before disposal. If records are disposed of by a professional company, be sure and obtain a document verifying the method used. Maintain a log of all destroyed records, showing the patient's name, date of birth, Social Security number, date of last visit, and date destroyed.

AUDITING A MEDICAL RECORD

An **audit** is a formal, methodical examination or review done to inspect, analyze, and scrutinize the way something is being done. Most frequently, an audit is performed on financial records to ensure that good bookkeeping practices are being followed and all monies are accounted for. In the case of an audit of medical records, the goal is to substantiate that the documentation supports the services and procedures that are being submitted to the patient or insurance carrier for payment and that proper care is being provided.

Various audit tools (e.g., worksheets) are used to break down the elements of a medical record into manageable parts. These simplify and expedite the auditing process. During the performance of an audit, a point system is used while reviewing each patient's medical record. Points are awarded only if documentation is present for elements required in the medical record. This point system is used to show where deficiencies occur in medical record documentation. It is also used to evaluate and substantiate proper use of diagnostic and procedure codes.

Managed care organizations (MCOs), government, and private insurance carriers who have a contract with a physician have the right to audit medical records and may claim refunds in the event of accidental or intentional miscoding. If improper coding patterns exist and are not corrected, then the provider of service will be penalized. Medical fiscal intermediaries have "walk-in rights" (access to a medical practice without an appointment or search warrant) that they may invoke to conduct documentation reviews, audits, and evaluations. Medicare has the power to levy fines and penalties and exclude providers from the Medicare program. Remember, insurance carriers go by the rule "not documented, not done," and they have the right to deny reimbursement.

Billing patterns that may draw attention to a medical practice for possible audit are:

- Intentional billing for unnecessary services
- Incorrect billing for services of physician extenders (e.g., nurse practitioner, midwife, physician assistant)
- Diagnostic tests billed without a separate report in the medical record
- Dates of service changed on insurance claims in order to comply with policy coverage dates
- Copayments or deductibles waived without good reason and documentation
- Discounts given illegally
- Excessive diagnostic tests ordered
- Provider identification numbers misused resulting in incorrect billing (e.g., two different provider numbers used to bill the same service for the same patient)
- Improper modifiers used to obtain financial gain
- Overpayments not returned to the Medicare program

Without complete, accurate, specific clinical documentation from the physician, correct coding cannot occur.

Internal Reviews

There are two types of **internal reviews:** the *prospective review*, which is done before billing is submitted, and the *retrospective review*, which is done after billing insurance carriers.

A prospective review is done to verify that completed encounter forms match all patients seen according to the appointment schedule, and all services/procedures have been posted on the day sheet. All procedures/services and diagnoses listed on the encounter forms are then matched with the data on the insurance claim forms.

A retrospective review is done by randomly pulling 15 to 20 medical records from the last 2 to 4 months and reviewing them to determine whether there is a lack of documentation.

External Audit

An **external audit** is a retrospective review (review done after claims have been billed) of medical and financial records by an insurance company or Medicare representative to investigate suspected fraudulent and abusive billing practices. Most insurance companies perform routine audits on unusual billing patterns.

If there is any suspicion of fraud, the insurance company will notify the medical practice, specify a date, and indicate the records they wish to audit. Investigators question the patient, look at the documentation in the medical record, and interview the staff and all physicians who have participated in the care of the patient.

Audit Terminology to Avoid

It is not only necessary for the physician to state what he or she is doing for the patient and what results have been obtained, it is also necessary to state these facts clearly and specifically, not in general terms. Following are two common phrases found in medical records that will not pass an audit.

Within Normal Limits

A commonly seen phrase or abbreviation that may not support billing of services and not pass an external audit is "within normal limits" (WNL). For example, if used to document that "all extremities are within normal limits," this statement does not indicate how many extremities or which extremities were examined. Documentation must indicate exactly which limb was examined. For example, "Front and back of both arms and legs were examined for skin irregularities and no abnormalities were found.

Negative Findings

Another phrase commonly used when an examination results in a normal finding is the term "negative." For example, "chest x-ray negative." Again, this phrase does not state what service the physician provided. The physician needs to document that there are no abnormalities in the system being examined. For example "PA and lateral chest films were reviewed and no abnormalities were seen."

Compliance

Since the concept of compliance first came about in 1997, physicians have been asked to voluntarily develop and implement compliance programs in their offices. A **compliance program** is composed of policies and procedures to accomplish uniformity, consistency, and conformity in medical record keeping that fulfill official requirements. The ultimate goals of a compliance program are to improve the quality of care to patients, control claim submissions, and reduce fraudulent insurance claims, abuse, waste, and the cost of healthcare to federal, state, and private health insurers. A manual that outlines policies and procedures helps employees know what you expect from them and what they can expect from you. It can help the office run smoothly and offers protection from a lawsuit. Benefits of a compliance program are:

- Effective internal procedures that ensure compliance with regulations, payment policies, and coding rules
- Improved medical record documentation
- Reduction of denied claims
- Reduced exposure to penalties
- Avoidance of potential liability stemming from noncompliance
- Streamlined practice operations through comprehensive policies and improved communication

If a medical practice experiences an external audit and a compliance program is in place, it may be viewed that a reasonable effort to avoid and detect misbehavior has been made. If errors are found and a determination is made as to whether there was intent to commit healthcare fraud, a compliance plan provides evidence that any errors made were inadvertent.

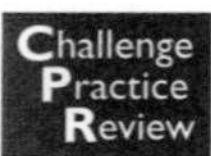

Pause and Practice CPR

REVIEW SESSIONS 7–18 THROUGH 7–20

Directions: *Complete the following questions as a review of information you have just read.*

7–18 List the record retention periods in your state for the following type of documents:

(a) Electronic patient records ________________

(b) Inactive patient records ________________

(c) Paid insurance claim forms ________________

(d) Minor children's electronic records ________________

(e) Medicare Remittance Advice documents ________________

7–19 How long should assigned claims for Medicare and Medicaid be kept? ________________

7–20 What are two common phrases found in medical records that will not pass an audit?

(a) ________________________________

(b) ________________________________

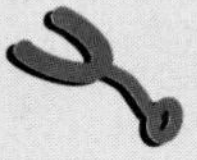

CHECK YOUR HEARTBEAT! Turn to the end of the chapter for answers to these review sessions.

SUMMATION AND PREVIEW

The flow of information between physicians, hospitals, providers, and health plans enables the patient to get the best possible care possible. Remember that documentation should answer questions, not raise them. Understanding the medical record and documentation guidelines is the foundation to learning the skill of medical record abstraction. This skill takes time to learn and improves each time it is practiced. Developing a methodical system to abstract information from a medical record is the first step in mastering this job skill after the basic foundation has been laid. You will be building this skill by doing the exercises at the end of this chapter.

In the next chapter, you will be applying all of your newly acquired skills as you learn to fill out the HCFA-1500 insurance claim form.

GOLDEN RULE

Not documented, not done!

Chapter 7 Review and Practice

Study Session

Directions: *Review the objectives, key terms, and chapter information before completing the following study questions.*

7–1 List three situations that most commonly occur when abstracting information from the medical record.

(a) ______________________________

(b) ______________________________

(c) ______________________________

7–2 What is the key to substantiating procedure and diagnostic code selections for appropriate reimbursement? ______________________________

____

7–3 Name several steps to take when arranging for records to be copied in the physician's office.

(a) ______________________________

(b) ______________________________

(c) ______________________________

(d) ______________________________

(e) ______________________________

7–4 All ____________________ that cannot be measured are considered subjective information.

7–5 Objective information can be determined by:

(a) ______________________________

(b) ______________________________

(c) ______________________________

(d) ______________________________

(e) ______________________________

7–6 Read the following definitions and write in the title of the physician.

(a) A provider whose opinion or advice is requested by another physician.

____

(b) A provider who sends the patient for testing or treatment.

____

(c) A provider who renders a service to a patient.

____

(d) The medical staff member who is legally responsible for the care and treatment given to a patient. ______________________________

(e) The physician directing the selection, preparation, or administration of tests, medication, or treatment. ______________________________

7–7 Name four reasons why comprehensive legible documentation is necessary.

(a) ______________________________

____

(b) ______________________________

____

(c) ______________________________

____

(d) ______________________________

____

7–8 When two physicians provide similar services to the same patient on the same day for separate physical disorders, this is called ______________________________.

7–9 Providing uninterrupted treatment for a patient is referred to as ______________________________ ________ ____________________.

7–10 What does the degree of documentation in the medical report depend on?

____

____

7–11 Is the physical examination subjective or objective in nature, and why?

____

____

7–12 Give some examples of a constitutional component in a physical examination.

____

7–13 Define the following three terms that are used in the medical decision-making process.

(a) morbidity ______________________________

(b) mortality ______________________________

(c) comorbidity ______________________________

7–14 Name circumstances when an insurance specialist might use a fax machine.

(a) ______________________________

(b) ______________________________

(c) ______________________________

(d) ______________________________

(e) ______________________________

7–15 To ensure that a faxed document has reached the correct destination, which one of the listed suggestions would you use, and why? ______________________________

____

7–16 To save files to the hard drive in a computer system and guard against accidental destruction, the operator should perform a ______________________________.

7–17 What is the goal of a medical record audit? ____

____

____

____

Exercise Exchange

7–1 Abstract Information from a Chart Note

Directions

1. Read the following chart note.
2. Identify the DOS, POS, all procedures, services, symptoms, and diagnoses.
3. Abstract the above information and enter it under the correct category.

Chart Note:
10/21/XX Claramae Churchill was referred to Dr. Gene Ulibarri, a urologist, for a recurring urinary tract infection (UTI). She complained of burning with urination, urinary frequency, and suprapubic pain. A PF HX was taken and the patient underwent a PF PX. A urine sample was collected and a urinalysis (UA) performed. A portion of the sample was *sent to* College Hospital Laboratory for a culture and sensitivity. Multiple bacteria and red blood cells were noted in the UA. Dr. Ulibarri started the patient on a course of antibiotic treatment for urinary tract infection; site unspecified and organism unidentified.

DOS: ______________________ **POS:** ____

Procedures and services: ____

Symptoms: ____

Diagnosis: ____

7–2 Abstract Information from a Progress Report

Directions

1. Read the following progress report.
2. Identify the DOS, POS, all procedures, services, symptoms, and diagnoses.
3. Abstract the above information and enter it under the correct category.

Progress Report
5/15/XX Bradford Buell returned to see Dr. Practon, complaining of tiredness, excessive thirst, and weight gain. An EPF HX was taken and an EPF PX performed. A fasting blood sugar (FBS) test, hematocrit (Hct), and UA test were done. The urinalysis was negative, except for positive sugar. Blood test results indicated Mr. Buell is anemic and has adult-onset diabetes mellitus (NIDDM). The patient was prescribed iron and oral glucose-lowering medication and instructed to return the following week for a follow-up FBS and to receive instructions on monitoring blood sugar levels at home.

DOS: ______________________ **POS:** ____

Procedures and services: ____

Symptoms: ____

Diagnosis: ____

Web Site: For an additional exercise on abstracting information from a medical record, visit the web site http://www.wbsaunders.com/MERLIN/Fordney/insurance/.

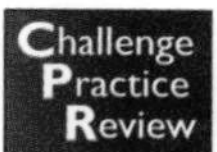

CPR Session: Answers

REVIEW SESSIONS 7–1 THROUGH 7–3

7–1 (a) diagnosis
(b) type of service
(c) date of service
(d) place of service

7–2 (a) chart notes
(b) operative report
(c) discharge summary

7–3 summary letter or narrative report

PRACTICE SESSIONS 7–4 THROUGH 7–6

7–4 Subjective: injured arm, arm hurts.

Objective: disfigured arm ("looks funny"), arm swollen. *Rationale: These are actual visual changes.*

7–5 Subjective: difficulty breathing, chest pain.

Objective: temperature (101.1), pulse (90), respirations (30), BP (142.86), diaphoresis, warm skin. *Rationale: Diaphoresis (sweating) can be seen; warm skin can be felt.*

7–6 Subjective: upset stomach, stomach hurts, feels terrible. *Rationale: Cannot measure these complaints.*

Objective: vomiting, diarrhea eight times (loose and watery), abdomen hard and distended, temperature (99.9), pulse (100), BP (110/60). *Rationale: Although the physician did not see the bowel movements, the patient was able to describe them with sufficient detail (how they visually appeared and how many times they occurred); therefore, it is an objective finding.*

REVIEW SESSIONS 7–7 THROUGH 7–9

7–7 documentation

7–8 Health Care Financing Administration (HCFA), now known as Centers for Medicare and Medicaid Services (CMS)

7–9 medical necessity

REVIEW SESSIONS 7–10 THROUGH 7–14

7–10 (a) family history
(b) social history
(c) personal history

7–11 (a) chief complaint (CC)
(b) history of present illness (HPI)
(c) review of symptoms (ROS)
(d) past, family, and/or social history (PFSH)

7–12 review of systems (ROS)

7–13 Ten: (1) cardiovascular, (2) ears, nose, and throat, (3) eyes (4) genitourinary, (5) hematologic/lymphatic/immunologic, (6) musculoskeletal, (7) neurologic, (8) psychiatric, (9) respiratory, (10) skin.

7–14 (a) number of diagnoses and treatment options
(b) amount and/or complexity of data to be reviewed
(c) risk of complications and/or morbidity or mortality

CHALLENGE SESSION 7–15

7–15 (a) Do not use the fax for routine transmission of patient information.
(b) Use when hand or mail delivery will not meet the needs of immediate patient care.
(c) Use when required by a third party for ongoing certification of payment for a hospitalized patient.
(d) Have the patient sign an authorization to release information via facsimile equipment.

REVIEW SESSIONS 7–16 AND 7–17

7–16 The witness to appear and to bring and/or send certain records "in his possession."

7–17 The prospective witness or the keeper of the medical records. *Note: The acceptance of a document by an authorized person is the equivalent of personal service.*

SESSIONS 7–18 THROUGH 7–20

7–18 (a) answers will vary (refer to Table 7–4)
(b) indefinitely (refer to Table 7–3)
(c) 3 years (refer to Table 7–4)
(d) answers will vary (refer to Table 7–4)
(e) 7 years (refer to Table 7–3)

7–19 7 years

7–20 (a) within normal limits
(b) negative findings

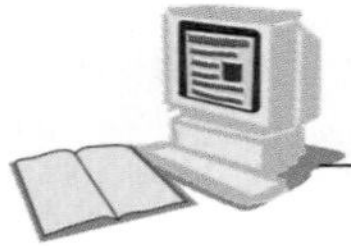

Resources

The American Health Information Management Organization (AHIMA) has been a forerunner in the development of guidelines for the use and protection of health information. Both consumers and healthcare providers use the Internet as a resource to improve the quality of health and healthcare. It is an effective tool for healthcare communication and record keeping as long as data quality and privacy are incorporated. Because the Internet can pose a risk to patient privacy, the AHIMA has developed fundamental principles and operational guidelines for consumers, healthcare providers, and e-health developers. These principles and guidelines serve as a blueprint for protecting patient privacy and improving the quality of personal health information on the web. A list of laws and regulations with which e-health sites must comply are listed under "e-health tenets." They, along with other information regarding medical record keeping and privacy issues, are found at the following addresses:

Internet Sites

- AHIMA E-health Tenets (click on "search" and use key word "e-health tenets")
  Web site: http://www.ahima.org
- Dictionary/Thesaurus for English and medical words
  Web site: http://www.yourdictionary.com
- State laws relative to patient consent
  Web site: http://www.alllaw.com/state_resources

Magazines

- ADVANCE for Health Information Professionals, biweekly (free subscription), (800) 355-1088. Information on medical record keeping, medical transcription, and diagnostic and procedure coding

Reference Books

- Wordbooks, pharmacy books, and additional medical dictionaries: Refer to the Resources listed at the end of Chapter 1

NOTES

Objectives

After reading this chapter and completing the exercise sessions, you should be able to:

Learning Objectives

- ✔ State when the universal claim form may and may not be used.
- ✔ Define two types of claim submission.
- ✔ Outline insurance claim time limit requirements.
- ✔ Explain the difference between clean, pending, rejected, incomplete, and invalid claims.
- ✔ Identify techniques required for submission of optically scanned insurance claims.
- ✔ Describe reasons why claims are rejected.
- ✔ Specify differences between manual and electronic claim submission.
- ✔ Explain the difference between carrier-direct and clearinghouse electronically submitted claims.
- ✔ State the job duties of an electronic claims processor.
- ✔ Identify blocks on the HCFA-1500 claim form used for specific purposes.

Performance Objectives

- ✔ Abstract data and complete individual blocks on the HCFA-1500 insurance claim form.
- ✔ Execute general guidelines for completing the HCFA-1500 claim form.

Key Terms

audit trail
carrier-direct system
clean claim
clearinghouse
crossover claim
digital signature
dingy claim
dirty claim
durable medical equipment (DME) number
electronic claim
electronic claims processor (ECP)
electronic claim submission (ECS)
electronic data interchange (EDI)
electronic signature
employer identification number (EIN)
facility provider number
group provider number
Health Insurance Claim Form (HCFA-1500)
incomplete claim
Internet
invalid claim
local area network (LAN)
national provider identifier (NPI)
optical character recognition (OCR)
other claim
paper claim
pending claim
provider identification number (PIN)
rejected claim
Social Security number (SSN)
state license number
supplemental insurance
unique provider identification number (UPIN)
wide area network (WAN)

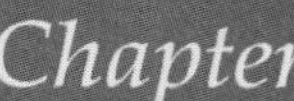

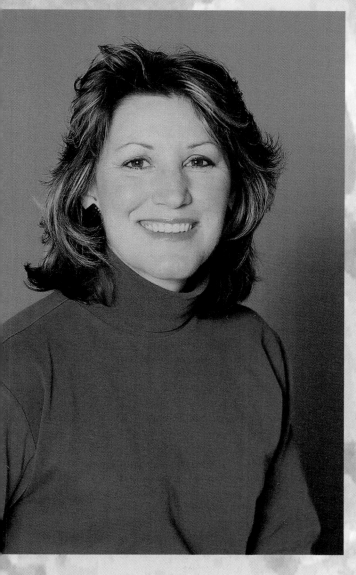

Chapter

8

My first job in the medical field was working for a surgical oncologist. I took an adult education course on medical billing to increase my knowledge, and, with the help of a friend, I learned by trial and error. I branched out and did freelance billing for an internal medicine office and then worked for a podiatrist, psychologist, and family practitioner.

I now have my own full-line medical insurance billing business that includes billling, coding, and all follow-up. I also post incoming payments and handle patient inquiries. My accounts include four surgeons and a registered nurse first assistant (RNFA).

I examine all of the charge tickets from the physician's office, editing them to locate incomplete and incorrect information. Then, I input the new patient demographics and edit changes in existing patient files. Next, I input charges into the computer system and link them with the proper diagnosis. I bill claims electronically whenever possible.

Deborah Pitts
Medical Insurance Billing Specialist
Billing Service

The Health Insurance Claim Form:
Completion and Submission

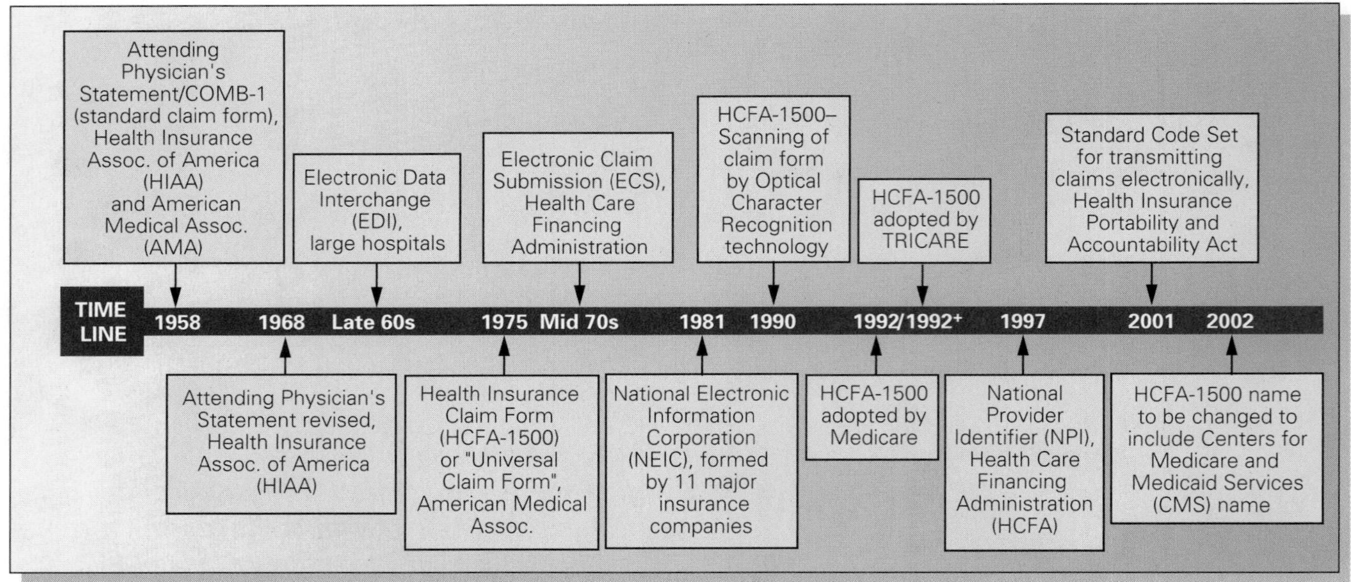

THE INSURANCE BILLING PROCESS

Now that you have acquired a foundation in medical terminology, understand the basics of medicolegal issues and medical record documentation, and have obtained the skills of coding and abstracting information from a medical record, you are ready to learn the insurance billing process.

Generally, the insurance billing specialist in the physician's office completes the insurance claim form for the following cases: (1) evaluation and management services, procedures, and testing (radiology and laboratory) done in the physician's office in which benefits are assigned to the physician; occasionally physicians choose to bill for unassigned claims; (2) hospital, emergency room, nursing facility, and home visits; and (3) surgeries, whether performed in an acute care hospital, ambulatory surgery center, or the physician's office.

There are four basic methods of creating insurance claims for processing by a medical practice: (1) generating an insurance claim form using a computer system, (2) manually preparing the insurance form using a typewriter or word processor, (3) filing the insurance data electronically using an in-office computer with modem and telecommunication lines, and (4) contracting with an outside billing agency to prepare and file claims manually or electronically. Regardless of which method is used, an understanding of the required data that are entered on the insurance claim form is necessary to file claims accurately and troubleshoot problems when they occur.

Whether using a computer system or filing claims manually, claims should be grouped according to insurance type to make completion of forms easier and to cut down on errors. If done manually, patient ledgers should be gathered so entries can be made indicating the date the insurance was billed. Patient charts may be needed for reference, depending on the type of procedures and services that are being billed. Organize your work week according to the volume of patients seen with various insurance types. For example, an internal medicine practice that sees 80% Medicare patients might require billing Medicare 3 days a week and other insurance types 2 days a week, whereas an orthopedic office that sees a lot of workers' compensation cases may bill workers' compensation 3 days a week, Medicare 1 day, and other insurance types 2 days.

Submission Time-Limit Requirements

Submit claims as soon as possible after professional services are rendered. For patients who are receiving care over an extended period of time, billing is often sent at the end of treatment, or every 15 to 30 days. Hospital and skilled nursing facility patients are usually billed after discharge, or on the 15th and 30th of each month. When the physician does surgery, the surgical bill should be sent immediately.

There are time limit requirements (30 days to $1^1/_2$ years) for filing an insurance claim, starting from the date of service (DOS). This will vary depending on the commercial carrier, managed care plan, and federal or state program. Claims filed after the time limit will be denied and it will be a lengthy process to appeal and try to receive payment. It is estimated that the cost of rebilling a claim doubles from the cost of original claim submission. Some claims are held at the insurance carrier awaiting other claims for similar services. For example, the assistant surgeon's and anesthesiologist's claims would be held until the primary surgeon's claim is received, and radiology and laboratory claims may be held until the ordering physician's claim is processed. The insurance company may pay the first bill received for a patient receiving concurrent care and the other physician may have a difficult time receiving payment if both doctors do not cross-reference each other on the claim form.

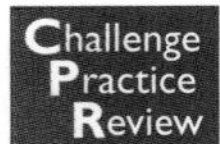

Pause and Practice CPR

REVIEW SESSIONS 8–1 THROUGH 8–3

Directions: *Complete the following questions as a review of information you have just read.*

8–1 List the three types of cases that the insurance billing specialist in the physician's office completes the insurance claim form for:

(1) ______________________________

(2) ______________________________

(3) ______________________________

8–2 List the four basic methods used to create insurance claims for processing by a medical practice:

(1) ______________________________

(2) ______________________________

(3) ______________________________

(4) ______________________________

8–3 Fill in the typical time for filing claims for the following scenarios.

(a) Office visit ______________________________

(b) Hospital patient ______________________________

(c) Surgical patient ______________________________

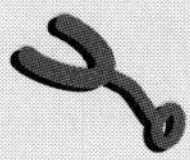

CHECK YOUR HEARTBEAT! Turn to the end of the chapter for answers to these review sessions.

THE HEALTH INSURANCE CLAIM FORM

The **Health Insurance Claim Form,** known as the **HCFA-1500,** is a universal claim form used by the Medicare and TRICARE programs. As of the publication of this worktext, it has been announced that the claim form will be renamed using the name Centers for Medicare and Medicaid Services (CMS) when supplies run out (i.e., CMS-1500). Since a date has not been announced for this change, the claim form will be referred to as the "HCFA-1500" throughout this worktext.

This form has received approval from the AMA and the National Association of Blue Shield Plans. The HIAA endorses and recommends that their members, who are private insurance companies, accept this form. In some states, the Medicaid program, as well as industrial carriers (workers' compensation), also use this form to process claims.

Types of Claims

Claims are categorized as either paper or electronic, as described below:

Electronic claim—is submitted directly to insurance carriers via personal computer by using a modem to transmit over telecommunication lines. Electronic claims are never printed on paper.

Paper claim—is submitted on paper (usually using the HCFA-1500 form) and includes computer-generated claims and optically scanned claims that are converted to electronic form by insurance carriers. Occasionally paper claims are faxed using a green HCFA-1500 form. The fax is never printed to paper at the receiving end but instead encoded by an optical code reader and transmitted into the claims processing system.

Widespread use of the HCFA-1500 form will save time and simplify processing of claims for both physicians and carriers. Following are several ways to submit a paper HCFA-1500 claim form for processing by the insurance company:

1. Complete the HCFA-1500 form using a typewriter or word processor.
2. Print out data on the HCFA-1500 form from a computer database.
3. Accept the patient's private insurance form. Verify completion of the patient's and employer's portions of the form and signatures for release of information and assignment of benefits, if applicable, and attach it to the HCFA-1500 form with the physician's portion completed.

4. Complete the patient's portion of the HCFA-1500 form and attach an encounter form that includes the physician information.

Optical Character Recognition (OCR)

It is preferable to complete the HCFA-1500 form using **optical character recognition (OCR)** or *intelligent character recognition* (ICR) guidelines so that it can be optically scanned at the insurance company which expedites payment. Such scanners are being used more frequently across the nation in processing insurance claims because of their speed and efficiency. A scanner reads the bar code in the upper left corner of the claim form and transfers printed or typed text to the insurance company's computer memory. Since most insurance carriers use scanning equipment, a photocopy of the form is not acceptable. The form has to be printed in red ink, with the bar code on the top left corner. Scanners read at such a fast speed that they reduce data entry cost and decrease processing time. Claims are read accurately and coding errors are decreased because the information is entered exactly as coded by the insurance biller. OCR guidelines are presented in this worktext and will be used for completion of all case scenarios. Since insurance carriers use various computer programs and equipment that optically scan claims, instructions on completion of the form may vary from locale to locale and program to program. Always contact local representatives of insurance carriers to find out whether the HCFA-1500 form is acceptable before submitting any claims.

Government programs and some insurance plans prefer electronic claim submission to reduce costs and expedite reimbursement. Details about electronic claim submission will be discussed later in this chapter.

Claim Payment Turnaround Time

Participating provider electronic submissions are processed within approximately 7 to 14 days of receipt. Whether the physician is a participating provider or nonparticipating provider, paper claims are not processed until at least 15 days of receipt and often take 27 days to generate a check for payment.

Claim Status

A claim can be designated as clean or pending (in suspense). A **clean claim** indicates that the claim was submitted within the program or policy time limit and contains all necessary information to be processed and paid promptly. On a *physically clean claim*, the bar code area has not been deformed and the form has not been folded, stapled, torn, wrinkled, smudged, or highlighted.

A **pending claim** is an insurance claim that has been held in *suspense* while it is being reviewed or additional information is requested. These claims may be cleared for payment or denied.

Medicare Claim Status

In the Medicare program, the definition of a clean claim has been expanded to include the following:

1. The claim has no deficiencies and passes all electronic edits.
2. The carrier does not need to investigate outside of the carrier's operation before paying the claim.
3. The claim is investigated on a postpayment basis, meaning a claim is not delayed before payment is made.
4. The claim is subject to medical review with attached information or forwarded simultaneously with electronic medical claim (EMC) records.

Besides the phrase "clean claims," Medicare uses additional terms such as dingy, dirty, incomplete, invalid, rejected, and other claims to describe various claim processing situations. These following terms may or may not be used by other insurance programs.

Dingy claim—cannot be processed due to the type of software program used to transmit the claim; it may be incompatible with the receiving system.

Dirty claim—is submitted with errors, requires manual processing to resolve problems, or is rejected for payment.

Incomplete claim—has missing information which is identified to the provider so that the claim can be corrected and resubmitted for payment.

Invalid claim—contains complete information, but the information is illogical or incorrect (e.g., listing an incorrect provider number for a referring physician). An invalid claim is identified to the provider and may be corrected and resubmitted.

Rejected claim—needs further clarification, possible investigation, and answers to questions. The carrier may indicate the situation and the provider would need to investigate and correct the claim for resubmission.

Other claim—requires investigation or development on a prepayment basis to determine if Medicare is the primary or secondary carrier.

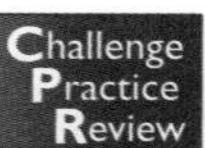

Pause and Practice CPR

REVIEW SESSIONS 8–4 THROUGH 8–8

Directions: *Complete the following questions as a review of information you have just read.*

8–4 What insurance plans and programs accept the HCFA-1500 insurance claim form? ____________

8–5 Define electronic claims. ____________

8–6 Define paper claims. ____________

8–7 List the meaning of the acronym OCR. ____________

8–8 How is an OCR form processed? ____________

CHECK YOUR HEARTBEAT! Turn to the end of the chapter for answers to these review sessions.

COMPLETION OF INSURANCE CLAIM FORMS

Use the universal claim form as often as possible. As mentioned earlier, it is accepted by nearly all private insurance carriers, as well as Medicaid, Medicare, TRICARE, and workers' compensation. Complete and submit a claim form whether asked to do so by the patient or not, even though there may be an unmet deductible. If eligibility or coverage is in question, check with the insurance carrier for precertification or eligibility status before completing a claim form.

Individual Insurance Forms

When a patient brings in a form from a private insurance plan that is not the HCFA-1500 form, have him or her sign it. In addition, have the patient sign the HCFA-1500 form in two places: (1) the release of information found in Block 12, and (2) the assignment of benefits found in Block 13. Refer to Figure 3–5 in Chapter 3 for a visual example of these areas. Make sure that the patient's portion of the private insurance form is complete and accurate. Generate a HCFA-1500 form and mail both forms to the insurance carrier. You may attach them with paper clips, but do not staple.

It is not recommended to let patients direct their own forms to insurance carriers or employers unless they paid in cash and need to bill their insurance for reimbursement purposes. Patients may lose forms, forget to send them, could alter data on documents before mailing, or mail them to an incorrect address; you would have no way of tracking the form or knowing when payment is received.

Group Insurance Forms

When a patient has group insurance through an employer and brings in a form stating that it must be used to file the claim, make sure that the employer's section is completed. If it has not been completed, send the form to the employer for completion and signature. Once the employer's section is complete, generate a HCFA-1500 form and send both forms directly to the insurance carrier.

Secondary Insurance Submission

When two private insurance policies are involved, sometimes called dual coverage, one is considered primary and the other secondary. When a patient and his or her spouse are both insured, the primary policy is the policy held by the patient, which will pay first. The secondary policy is the policy held by the patient's spouse, which will pay second. This is the rule regardless of the amounts of insurance coverage, deductibles, and copayments (see Example 8–1). Obtain the patient's signature

Example 8–1

Primary versus Secondary Insurance

Scenario: A husband and wife have insurance through their employers and each has added the spouse to their plans for secondary coverage. Following is a brief summary of their plans.

Insured Party	Insurance Plan	Copayment Amount	Coverage and Benefits
Wife	ABC Insurance	$25	70% of allowed amount
Husband	Global Insurance	$5	80% of allowed amount

Rationale: The wife is seen for treatment so the insurance plan sponsored by her employer (ABC Insurance) would be primary and her husband's plan (Global Insurance) would be secondary. The fact that the husband's copayment amount is less and his benefits are better does not affect the primary/secondary insurance determination.

for the release of information and assignment of benefits for both insurance plans at the first office visit.

After payment is made by the primary plan, then a claim is submitted to the secondary carrier with a copy of the explanation of benefits (EOB) document from the primary carrier.

If a patient has purchased a second insurance policy to cover only what the first insurance does not cover, it is considered a **supplemental insurance** policy and would always be billed second.

In the case of a patient having Medicare and Medigap coverage, or Medicare and Medicaid, the primary insurance carrier (Medicare) automatically submits the claim to the secondary carrier if the secondary insurance portion of the claim is completed correctly (Blocks 9a–d). This is referred to as a **crossover claim.** Other secondary insurance situations will be discussed within the chapters in the Insurance Programs section.

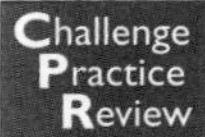

Pause and Practice CPR

REVIEW SESSIONS 8–9 THROUGH 8–11

Directions: *Complete the following questions as a review of information you have just read.*

8–9 When a patient has two private insurance plans, it is often called _______________ coverage.

8–10 When a private secondary insurance claim is being submitted, what is sent along with the claim?____

____

8–11 When a claim is sent automatically from Medicare to a Medigap or Medicaid carrier, it is referred to as a/an_______________________ claim.

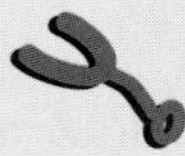

CHECK YOUR HEARTBEAT! Turn to the end of the chapter for answers to these review sessions.

CLAIM FORM REQUIREMENTS

While reading information pertaining to the HCFA-1500 form, view the private insurance template (Figure D–3) found in Appendix D and Figures 8–1 and 8–2 showing different sections of a completed claim form. Refer to the various blocks as they are being discussed. Claim form completion using OCR guidelines require that all entries inserted appear in capital letters, with no punctuation, and no comments in blocks that do not apply (leave blocks blank). The computer scanner will kick out the claim if the above guidelines are not followed. Note the OCR bar code on the top left portion of the claim (see Fig. 8–1).

If the claim form is not to be optically scanned, check with the carrier to see if they require DNA (does not apply), or N/A (not applicable) in blocks that do not require information.

Divisions of the Claim Form

The HCFA-1500 form is divided into two major sections: patient/insured information and physician/supplier information. The Patient/Insured Information section (see Fig. 8–1) is the top portion of the claim form and contains both patient information (e.g., name, address, telephone number), and insurance information (e.g., subscriber, policy and group numbers). The upper section is made up of 13 numbered blocks (1 through 13), 11 for data input and 2 signature blocks. Some of the blocks require more than one piece of information. For example, Block 3 requires both the patient's date of birth and the patient's sex (see Fig. 8–1, Block 3). Other blocks are subdivided and labeled (a, b, c, and so forth) and contain specific information related to the main block. For example, Block 9 is subdivided into a, b, c, and d which are designed to contain specific information regarding the subscriber named in Block 9 who holds a secondary insurance plan (see Fig. 8–1, Block 9a–d).

The Physician/Supplier Information section is the bottom portion of the claim form (see Fig. 8–2) and consists of 20 numbered blocks (14 through 33), 19 for data input and 1 signature block. Again, some of the blocks contain more than one piece of information and others are subdivided and labeled. Block 24 is the largest block in the lower section of the claim form and contains six lines used to report various compo-

TOP PORTION

PLEASE DO NOT STAPLE IN THIS AREA

MILLARD NATIONAL INSURANCE COMPANY
2233 HIGHLAND AVENUE
OMAHA XY 12345 0001

Insurance company name and address

Patient name and address

Patient issued through group health plan

Date of birth and gender

Insurance identification number and group number

1. MEDICARE MEDICAID CHAMPUS CHAMPVA GROUP HEALTH PLAN FECA BLK LUNG OTHER
(Medicare #) (Medicaid #) (Sponsor's SSN) (VA File #) [X] (SSN or ID) (SSN) (ID)

1a. INSURED'S I.D. NUMBER (FOR PROGRAM IN ITEM 1)
5230906A 456

2. PATIENT'S NAME (Last Name, First Name, Middle Initial)
TOMPSETT BRIAN T

3. PATIENT'S BIRTHDATE MM DD YYYY SEX
10 17 1970 M [X] F

4. INSURED'S NAME (Last Name, First Name, Middle Initial)
SAME

Patient and insured are "same" person

5. PATIENT'S ADDRESS (No, Street)
626 ALA MOANA LANE

6. PATIENT RELATIONSHIP TO INSURED
Self [X] Spouse Child Other

7. INSURED'S ADDRESS (No, Street)

CITY PAPILLIAN STATE XY

8. PATIENT STATUS
Single Married [X] Other
Employed [X] Full-Time Student Part-Time Student

CITY STATE

Patient is the insured; married and employed

ZIP CODE 12345 TELEPHONE (include Area Code) (555) 295 1031

ZIP CODE PHONE (Include Area Code) ( )

9. OTHER INSURED'S NAME (Last Name, First Name, Middle Initial)

10. IS PATIENT'S CONDITION RELATED TO:

11. INSURED'S POLICY GROUP OR FECA NUMBER

a. OTHER INSURED'S POLICY OR GROUP NUMBER

a. EMPLOYMENT? (CURRENT OR PREVIOUS)
YES [X] NO

a. INSURED'S DATE OF BIRTH MM DD YYYY SEX M F

b. OTHER INSURED'S DATE OF BIRTH MM DD YYYY SEX M F

b. AUTO ACCIDENT? PLACE (State)
YES [X] NO

b. EMPLOYER'S NAME OR SCHOOL NAME

c. EMPLOYER'S NAME OR SCHOOL NAME

c. OTHER ACCIDENT?
YES [X] NO

c. INSURANCE PLAN NAME OR PROGRAM NAME

d. INSURANCE PLAN NAME OR PROGRAM NAME

10d. RESERVED FOR LOCAL USE

d. IS THERE ANOTHER HEALTH BENEFIT PLAN?
YES [X] NO *If yes, return to and complete item 9a-d*

Patient does not have secondary insurance

PATIENT AND INSURED INFORMATION

READ BACK OF FORM BEFORE COMPLETING & SIGNING THIS FIRM
12. PATIENT'S OR AUTHORIZED PERSON'S SIGNATURE. I authorize the release of any medical or other information necessary to process this claim. I also request payment of government benefits either to myself or to the party who accepts assignment below.

SIGNED SOF DATE

13. INSURED'S OR AUTHORIZED PERSON'S SIGNATURE. I authorize payment of medical benefits to the undersigned physician or supplier for services described below.

SIGNED SOF

Patient's signature is on file in the physician's office for authorization to release medical information

Illness/injury of patient is not related to work or an accident

Patient's signature is on file in the physician's office for assignment of benefits

Figure 8–1. Top portion of HCFA-1500 claim form with labeled descriptions.

nents of a service. These are subdivided and labeled A through K. There are more than 100 places to enter specific information on the form.

Block-by-Block Instructions and Insurance Templates

Block-by-block instructions for all private insurance carriers and each major carrier (i.e., Medicaid, Medicare including Medicare/Medicaid, Medicare/Medigap, and Medicare Secondary Payer [MSP], TRICARE, CHAMPVA, and workers' compensation) are included in Appendix D along with figures that have highlighted areas illustrating completion of individual blocks. Each plan is color-coded and includes an icon so that you can quickly find information related to a particular block of a specific plan.

Insurance templates showing completed claim forms for the above programs are found at the end of Appendix D (see Figs. D–3 through D–12). Placement of information on the claim forms is given to illustrate correct entries and positioning. Screened areas on each template do not apply to the insurance program example and should be left blank.

These references should be used when completing the HCFA-1500 form and referred to each time there is a question about data that are to be entered in a specific block. By doing this repeatedly, you will be able to

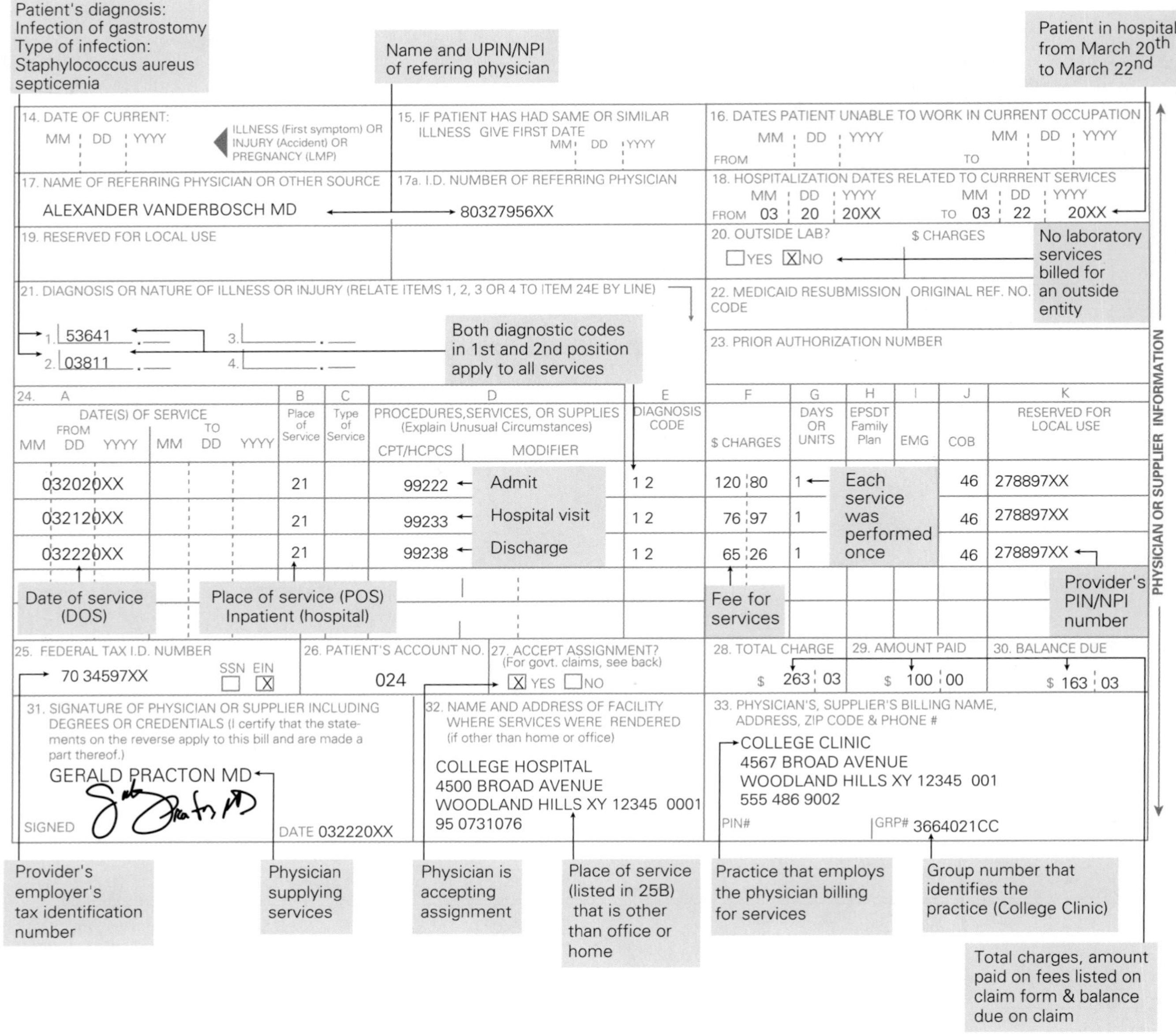
14. DATE OF CURRENT: MM DD YYYY ILLNESS (First symptom) OR INJURY (Accident) OR PREGNANCY (LMP)
15. IF PATIENT HAS HAD SAME OR SIMILAR ILLNESS GIVE FIRST DATE MM DD YYYY
16. DATES PATIENT UNABLE TO WORK IN CURRENT OCCUPATION MM DD YYYY FROM MM DD YYYY TO
17. NAME OF REFERRING PHYSICIAN OR OTHER SOURCE: ALEXANDER VANDERBOSCH MD
17a. I.D. NUMBER OF REFERRING PHYSICIAN: 80327956XX
18. HOSPITALIZATION DATES RELATED TO CURRRENT SERVICES MM DD YYYY FROM 03 20 20XX TO 03 22 20XX
19. RESERVED FOR LOCAL USE
20. OUTSIDE LAB? YES [X] NO $ CHARGES
21. DIAGNOSIS OR NATURE OF ILLNESS OR INJURY (RELATE ITEMS 1, 2, 3 OR 4 TO ITEM 24E BY LINE)
1. 53641 . 3. .
2. 03811 . 4. .
22. MEDICAID RESUBMISSION CODE ORIGINAL REF. NO.
23. PRIOR AUTHORIZATION NUMBER

24. A DATE(S) OF SERVICE FROM MM DD YYYY	TO MM DD YYYY	B Place of Service	C Type of Service	D PROCEDURES, SERVICES, OR SUPPLIES (Explain Unusual Circumstances) CPT/HCPCS	MODIFIER	E DIAGNOSIS CODE	F $ CHARGES	G DAYS OR UNITS	H EPSDT Family Plan	I EMG	J COB	K RESERVED FOR LOCAL USE
032020XX		21		99222		1 2	120 80	1			46	278897XX
032120XX		21		99233		1 2	76 97	1			46	278897XX
032220XX		21		99238		1 2	65 26	1			46	278897XX

25. FEDERAL TAX I.D. NUMBER 70 34597XX SSN EIN [X]
26. PATIENT'S ACCOUNT NO. 024
27. ACCEPT ASSIGNMENT? (For govt. claims, see back) [X] YES NO
28. TOTAL CHARGE $ 263 03
29. AMOUNT PAID $ 100 00
30. BALANCE DUE $ 163 03
31. SIGNATURE OF PHYSICIAN OR SUPPLIER INCLUDING DEGREES OR CREDENTIALS (I certify that the statements on the reverse apply to this bill and are made a part thereof.) GERALD PRACTON MD SIGNED DATE 032220XX
32. NAME AND ADDRESS OF FACILITY WHERE SERVICES WERE RENDERED (if other than home or office) COLLEGE HOSPITAL 4500 BROAD AVENUE WOODLAND HILLS XY 12345 0001 95 0731076
33. PHYSICIAN'S, SUPPLIER'S BILLING NAME, ADDRESS, ZIP CODE & PHONE # COLLEGE CLINIC 4567 BROAD AVENUE WOODLAND HILLS XY 12345 001 555 486 9002 PIN# GRP# 3664021CC

Figure 8–2. Bottom portion of HCFA-1500 claim form with labeled descriptions.

memorize block requirements for the major insurance programs.

Although instructions are straightforward and contain all pertinent information needed to complete the claim form, much information on specific coverage guidelines, program policies, and practice specialties could not be included. Consult your local intermediary or private carrier for specific instructions that may vary from state to state and locale to locale.

Block instruction numbers match numbers on the HCFA-1500 form. Italicized sections refer students to guidelines in completing the worktext billing break assignments when there are optional ways of completing a block.

The following information regarding specific blocks on the claim form are offered for emphasis and clarification.

Insurance Company Name and Address

When generating paper claims via computer, many software programs insert the insurance carrier's name and address in the top right corner of the HCFA-1500 form (see Fig. 8–1). When completing a claim form for this worktext, it is suggested that this same procedure be followed.

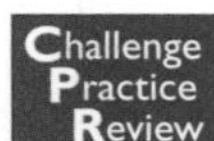

Pause and Practice CPR

PRACTICE SESSION 8–12

Directions: *Refer to the Block Instructions and Private Insurance Template (Fig. D–3) found in Appendix D, as well as Figure 8–1 while completing this practice session. This session is designed to enhance your knowledge of block requirements for the top portion of the claim form. It will also help you develop the skill of inserting information on the HCFA-1500 form.*

8–12 Use the following form and the information listed below and fill in the required data on the HCFA-1500 form.

(1) The patient is Kathryn Elizabeth Dunn.

(2) She lives at 587 Cambria Drive, Summerland, XY 12345 0001; telephone number (555) 658-2404

(3) She is the insured and has group insurance through her work. She does not have secondary coverage.

(4) The insurance is SafeNet Insurance Company, 2277 Center Street, Tarzana, XY 12345-0001; identification number 7686960; group number KED600.

(5) She is unmarried and her birth date is 5/30/1970.

(6) She is seeing Dr. Vera Cutis for a mole removal and the physician is accepting assignment. Her signature for release of medical information to the insurance carrier and assignment of benefits is on file.

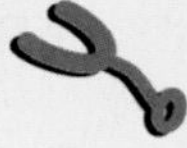

CHECK YOUR HEARTBEAT! Turn to the end of the chapter for answers to this practice session.

1. MEDICARE ☐ (Medicare #) MEDICAID ☐ (Medicaid #) CHAMPUS ☐ (Sponsor's SSN) CHAMPVA ☐ (VA File #)	GROUP HEALTH PLAN ☐ (SSN or ID) FECA BLK LUNG ☐ (SSN) OTHER ☐ (ID)	1a. INSURED'S I.D. NUMBER (FOR PROGRAM IN ITEM 1)
2. PATIENT'S NAME (Last Name, First Name, Middle Initial)	3. PATIENT'S BIRTHDATE MM | DD | YYYY SEX M☐ F☐	4. INSURED'S NAME (Last Name, First Name, Middle Initial)
5. PATIENT'S ADDRESS (No, Street)	6. PATIENT RELATIONSHIP TO INSURED Self☐ Spouse☐ Child☐ Other☐	7. INSURED'S ADDRESS (No, Street)
CITY STATE	8. PATIENT STATUS Single☐ Married☐ Other☐	CITY STATE
ZIP CODE TELEPHONE (include Area Code) ( )	Employed☐ Full-Time Student☐ Part-Time Student☐	ZIP CODE TELEPHONE (Include Area Code) ( )
9. OTHER INSURED'S NAME (Last Name, First Name, Middle Initial)	10. IS PATIENT'S CONDITION RELATED TO:	11. INSURED'S POLICY GROUP OR FECA NUMBER
a. OTHER INSURED'S POLICY OR GROUP NUMBER	a. EMPLOYMENT? (CURRENT OR PREVIOUS) ☐YES ☐NO	a. INSURED'S DATE OF BIRTH MM | DD | YYYY SEX M☐ F☐
b. OTHER INSURED'S DATE OF BIRTH MM | DD | YYYY SEX M☐ F☐	b. AUTO ACCIDENT? ☐YES ☐NO PLACE (State)	b. EMPLOYER'S NAME OR SCHOOL NAME
c. EMPLOYER'S NAME OR SCHOOL NAME	c. OTHER ACCIDENT? ☐YES ☐NO	c. INSURANCE PLAN NAME OR PROGRAM NAME
d. INSURANCE PLAN NAME OR PROGRAM NAME	10d. RESERVED FOR LOCAL USE	d. IS THERE ANOTHER HEALTH BENEFIT PLAN? ☐YES ☐NO *If yes, return to and complete item 9a-d*
READ BACK OF FORM BEFORE COMPLETING & SIGNING THIS FORM 12. PATIENT'S OR AUTHORIZED PERSON'S SIGNATURE. I authorize the release of any medical or other information necessary to process this claim. I also request payment of government benefits either to myself or to the party who accepts assignment below. SIGNED ______	DATE ______	13. INSURED'S OR AUTHORIZED PERSON'S SIGNATURE. I authorize payment of medical benefits to the undersigned physician or supplier for services described below. SIGNED ______

Expressions from Experience

I have learned not to take anything at face value, always to question it. For example, a claim can be denied for the lack of a timely submission, but when I check the patient's account I find that the primary insurance was billed in a timely manner. This information can be submitted for justification to help get the claim paid.

Deborah Pitts
Medical Insurance Billing Specialist
Billing Service

Diagnosis

In Block 21, the diagnosis field, insert all accurate diagnostic codes that affect the patient's condition, listing the primary diagnosis code first, followed by any secondary diagnostic codes. Never submit a diagnosis without supporting documentation in the medical record. Be certain that the diagnosis agrees with the treatment listed in Block 24D and is correctly linked on the claim form in Block 24E by using the indicator(s) (1, 2, 3, and/or 4) which represents the position of the diagnostic code supporting the treatment (see Fig. 8–2). If there is no formal diagnosis at the conclusion of an encounter, enter the code(s) for the patient's symptom(s).

Certain insurance companies accept more than one diagnostic code indicator in Block 24E, and, when listed, leave one space between numbers. Others only accept one code indicator per line; however, additional codes may be listed on the claim form. To avoid problems, it is best to list only one illness or injury and its treatment per claim, unless there are concurrent conditions.

Service Dates

In Block 24A, do not submit more than one date of service per line. It is unacceptable to use ditto marks to indicate the same date of service on separate lines (i.e., 24-1, 24-2, 24-3, and so forth). It is not advisable to charge for services rendered in different years on the same claim form because deductible and eligibility factors may be affected, therefore delaying payment. For OCR guidelines, fill in the "from" date in Block 24A when indicating a single date of service. The "to" date in Block 24A is used for consecutive date ranging and need not be filled in for a single date of service.

Consecutive Dates

Some carriers allow hospital and/or office visits to be grouped if the following criteria are met. Each visit needs to:

(1) Fall on consecutive dates
(2) Occur in the same month
(3) Require the same procedure code
(4) Result in the same fee

In such cases, both the "from" and "to" dates listed in Block 24A are used to record the first and last dates of consecutive services. The fee for one procedure/service is listed in Block 24F, and the number of times the procedure/service was performed is listed in Block 24G. In Figure 8–3 the same level of hospital visit (99232) occurred on October 4, 5, 6, 7, and 8; therefore, the date ranging indicates "from—10/04/20XX" "to—10/08/20XX" and five units are listed in Block 24G to indicate the number of consecutive days being billed. Never list consecutive dates for different months on the same line (e.g., consecutive services for 11/29, 11/30, 12/1, 12/2).

A calculation should be made by multiplying the number of units in Block 24G (5) times the single fee listed in Block 24F ($55.56) to determine the total fee in Block 28 ($277.80), which includes the consecutive services (see Fig. 8–3). Check with private insurance carriers because some carriers may require a total fee listed in Block 24F rather than the fee for a single procedure. If there is a difference in the procedure code used or the fee, or the dates are not consecutive, each hospital/office visit must be itemized by placing each procedure code and charge on separate lines.

Place of Service and Type of Service

Blocks 24B and C are used to insert codes which indicate the place of service (POS) and type of service (TOS) (see Fig. 8–2). Figure D–1 in Appendix D lists the various places a service may be rendered (e.g., patient's home, inpatient hospital, outpatient hospital, and so forth). This block is completed for all insurance types.

24	A		B	C	D	E	F	G	H	I	J	K
	DATE(S) OF SERVICE FROM MM DD YY	TO MM DD YY	Place of Service	Type of Service	PROCEDURES, SERVICES, OR SUPPLIES (Explain Unusual Circumstances) CPT/CPCS | MODIFIER	DIAGNOSIS CODE	$ CHARGES	DAYS OR UNITS	EPSDT Family Plan	BMG	COB	RESERVED FOR LOCAL USE
1	100420XX	100820XX	21		99232	1	55 56	5				
2												

28. TOTAL CHARGE $ 277 80

Figure 8–3. Consecutive date ranging for hospital visits.

Figure D–2 in Appendix D lists the type of service codes used for Medicaid, TRICARE, and workers' compensation carriers. These codes categorize services into groups and may vary depending on region and carrier.

No Charge

Do not submit a claim for services that have no charge unless the patient or insurance company requests you to do so. These services are documented in the patient's medical and financial records.

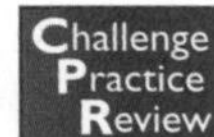

Pause and Practice CPR

PRACTICE SESSIONS 8–13 THROUGH 8–16

Directions: *Refer to the Block Instructions and Private Insurance Template (Fig. D–3) found in Appendix D, as well as Figure 8–2, while completing this practice session. This session is designed to enhance your knowledge of block requirements for the bottom portion of the claim form. It will also help you develop the skill of inserting information on the HCFA-1500 form.*

8–13 Look up the following CPT codes and list the procedure/service description. Now enter the procedure codes in Block 24D on the claim form in the order presented.

(1) 99203 ______________________________

(2) 93000 ______________________________

(3) 94010 ______________________________

(4) 81002 ______________________________

(5) 36415 ______________________________

(6) 99000 ______________________________

8–14 Look up the following diagnostic codes in the ICD-9-CM manual and write their description. Now enter the diagnostic code numbers in the order presented in Block 21 of the claim form.

(1) 786.59 ______________________________

(2) 518.4 ______________________________

(3) 780.6 ______________________________

(4) 788.1 ______________________________

8–15 Link the diagnostic codes to each procedure/service by inserting the indicator (1, 2, 3, or 4) in Block 24E on the claim form. Note: The blood work is being done because of the patient's fever.

8–16 Look up the fees for the listed procedures in the Mock Fee Schedule in Appendix B. List the mock fees in Block 24F of the claim form for each procedure/service.

21. DIAGNOSIS OR NATURE OF ILLNESS OR INJURY (RELATE ITEMS 1, 2, 3 OR 4 TO ITEM 24E BY LINE) — 22. MEDICAID RESUBMIS

1. ____ . __ 3. ____ . __ — 23. PRIOR AUTHORIZATIC

2. ____ . __ 4. ____ . __

24. A						B	C	D		E	F
DATE(S) OF SERVICE FROM MM	DD	YYYY	TO MM	DD	YYYY	Place of Service	Type of Service	PROCEDURES, SERVICES, OR SUPPLIES (Explain Unusual Circumstances) CPT/HCPCS	MODIFIER	DIAGNOSIS CODE	$ CHARGES

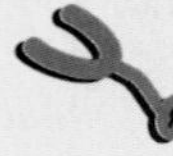

CHECK YOUR HEARTBEAT! Turn to the end of the chapter for answers to these practice sessions.

Physicians' Identification Numbers

Insurance companies, as well as federal and state programs, require certain identification numbers on claim forms submitted from individuals, groups, and facilities who provide and bill for services to patients. Because there are so many types of identification numbers, this can be confusing to the beginner as well as to someone experienced in medical insurance billing. Following are the various types of identification numbers with explanations of where they are found on the HCFA-1500 form. Refer to Figure 8–4 to locate areas for placement.

State License Number

To practice within a state, each physician must obtain a physician's **state license number.** Sometimes this number is requested on forms and used as a provider number (e.g., Block 24K).

Employer Identification Number

Each physician, whether practicing solo or in a group, must have his or her own federal tax identification number known as an **employer identification number (EIN).** This is issued by the Internal Revenue Service for income tax purposes (see Block 25).

Social Security Number

Each physician has a **Social Security number (SSN)** for personal use. A physician in solo practice may be issued a *tax identification number (TIN)* which is identical to their Social Security number (e.g., Block 25).

Provider Numbers

Claims can require three separate provider identification numbers for the (1) referring physician, (2) ordering physician, and (3) performing physician (billing entity). It is possible that the ordering physician and the performing physician are the same; for example, Dr. Practon orders an ECG and his medical assistant performs the ECG, and therefore Dr. Practon would bill for it. Depending on the circumstances of the case, the number may be the same for all three, but more frequently two or three different numbers are required.

For placement of the provider number(s) on the HCFA-1500 form, refer to the block-by-block instructions in Appendix D. Locate Blocks 17a, 24J–K, and 33 (PIN or GRP number). Keep in mind what role the physician(s) and his or her number(s) represents in relationship to the billing entity or provider listed in Block 33.

Provider Identification Number

Every physician who renders services to patients may be issued a carrier-assigned **provider identification number (PIN)** by each insurance company (see bottom left of Block 33).

Unique Provider Identification Number

The Medicare program issues each physician a **unique provider identification number (UPIN)** (see Block 17a).

Group Provider Number

The **group provider number** is used instead of the individual physician's number (PIN) for the performing provider who is a member of a group practice that submits claims to insurance companies under the group name (see bottom right of Block 33).

Performing Provider Identification Number

In the Medicare program, in addition to a group number, each member of a group is issued an eight-character *performing provider identification number (PPIN)*, which correlates to that particular group. Each physician has a separate PPIN for each group office/clinic in which he or she practices. If a doctor practices in two of the group's four offices, he or she will have two PPINs (see Example 8–2).

Example 8–2

Performing Provider Identification Number

College Clinic
4567 Broad Avenue
Woodland Hills, XY
12345-0001 — Group PIN: 3664021CC
Cosmo Graff, MD — PPIN: WA 24516B

College Clinic
20 South Main Street
Louisville, XY 12670-0341 — Group PIN: 3664021CC
Cosmo Graff, MD — PPIN: WA 01021A

National Provider Identifier

The Centers for Medicare and Medicaid Services (CMS), previously known as HCFA, began issuing each provider a Medicare lifetime 10-digit **national provider identifier (NPI)** that was originally intended to replace the provider identification number (PIN) and the unique provider identification number (UPIN). This number is recognized by Medicaid, Medicare, TRICARE, and CHAMPVA programs and may be used by private insurance carriers; however, use of the NPI is not mandatory and does not apply to physician extenders. When using this 10-digit number, it is placed in Blocks 24J and K.

Durable Medical Equipment Number

Medicare providers who charge patients a fee for durable medical equipment (e.g., urinary catheters, ostomy supplies, surgical dressings, splints, braces, and so forth) must bill Medicare using a **durable medical equipment (DME) number** (i.e., bottom of Block 33).

Facility Provider Number

Each facility (e.g., hospital, laboratory, radiology center, skilled nursing facility) is issued a **facility provider number** to be used by the performing physician to report services done at that location (see Block 32).

To assist you with claims completion, compile a reference list of all physician identification numbers. To obtain ordering and referring physicians' provider numbers, call their offices or obtain them through your Medicare carrier. *When completing worktext assignments, refer to Appendix A for College Clinic physician identification numbers and College Hospital facility identification numbers.*

14. DATE OF CURRENT: MM | DD | YYYY ◀ ILLNESS (First symptom) OR INJURY (Accident) OR PREGNANCY (LMP)

15. IF PATIENT HAS HAD SAME OR SIMILAR ILLNESS GIVE FIRST DATE MM | DD | YYYY

16. DATES PATIENT UNABLE TO WORK IN CURRENT OCCUPATION FROM MM | DD | YYYY TO MM | DD | YYYY

17. NAME OF REFERRING PHYSICIAN OR OTHER SOURCE

17a. I.D. NUMBER OF REFERRING PHYSICIAN — REFERRING PHYSICIAN UPIN/NPI

18. HOSPITALIZATION DATES RELATED TO CURRENT SERVICES FROM MM | DD | YYYY TO MM | DD | YYYY

19. RESERVED FOR LOCAL USE

20. OUTSIDE LAB? ☐ YES ☐ NO — $ CHARGES

21. DIAGNOSIS OR NATURE OF ILLNESS OR INJURY (RELATE ITEMS 1, 2, 3 OR 4 TO ITEM 24E BY LINE)

1. ___ . ___
2. ___ . ___
3. ___ . ___
4. ___ . ___

22. MEDICAID RESUBMISSION CODE — ORIGINAL REF. NO.

23. PRIOR AUTHORIZATION NUMBER

24. A DATE(S) OF SERVICE FROM MM DD YYYY	TO MM DD YYYY	B Place of Service	C Type of Service	D PROCEDURES, SERVICES, OR SUPPLIES (Explain Unusual Circumstances) CPT/HCPCS | MODIFIER	E DIAGNOSIS CODE	F $ CHARGES	G DAYS OR UNITS	H EPSDT Family Plan	I EMG	J COB	K RESERVED FOR LOCAL USE
											PERFORMING
											PHYSICIAN
											PIN/NPI
											FOR EACH LINE
											OF SERVICE
											LISTED

25. FEDERAL TAX I.D. NUMBER — EMPLOYER ID NUMBER — SSN ☐ EIN ☒

26. PATIENT'S ACCOUNT NO.

27. ACCEPT ASSIGNMENT? (For govt. claims, see back). ☐ YES ☐ NO

28. TOTAL CHARGE $

29. AMOUNT PAID $

30. BALANCE DUE $

31. SIGNATURE OF PHYSICIAN OR SUPPLIER INCLUDING DEGREES OR CREDENTIALS (I certify that the statements on the reverse apply to this bill and are made a part thereof.) SIGNED ________ DATE ________

32. NAME AND ADDRESS OF FACILITY WHERE SERVICES WERE RENDERED (If other than home or office) — FACILITY PROVIDER NUMBER (IF A SEPARATE FACILITY IS LISTED HERE OTHER THAN OFFICE OR HOME)

33. PHYSICIAN'S, SUPPLIER'S BILLING NAME, ADDRESS, ZIP CODE & PHONE # — LIST EITHER A PIN NUMBER FOR A SINGLE PRACTICE PHYSICIAN, OR A GROUP NUMBER WHEN BILLING FOR A GROUP PRACTICE — PIN# INDIVIDUAL PIN/NPI | GRP# GROUP NUMBER

Figure 8–4. Bottom portion of HCFA-1500 form illustrating location of identification numbers.

You have just completed reading a comprehensive presentation of all physician identification numbers. Before completing the next practice session, study Figure 8–4 which illustrates a visual summary of the locations of identifying numbers for blocks on the HCFA-1500 form.

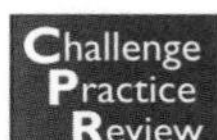

Pause and Practice CPR

PRACTICE SESSIONS 8–17 THROUGH 8–21

Directions: *Refer to Figure 8–4 as you complete this practice session. Look up block instructions in Appendix D when needed. Locate the College Clinic physician identification numbers in Appendix A. This session is designed to enhance your knowledge of physician identification numbers. It will also help you develop the skill of abstracting appropriate numbers from the College Clinic physician file and inserting them in the proper location on the HCFA-1500 form.*

8–17 What is the correct referring physician number that goes in Block 17a for Raymond Skeleton, M.D.? ________________

8–18 What is the correct facility provider number that goes in Block 32 for College Hospital? ________________

8–19 What is the correct employer tax identification number that goes in Block 25 for Bertha Caesar M.D.? ________________

8–20 What is the correct group practice number that goes in Block 33 for College Clinic? ________________

8–21 What is the correct physician number that goes in Block 24JK for Clarence Cutler, M.D.?

____

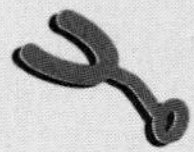

CHECK YOUR HEARTBEAT! Turn to the end of the chapter for answers to these practice sessions.

Physician's Signature

Generally, when submitting insurance claims, the provider must handwrite his or her name attesting to the document. However, check with individual insurance carriers because they may accept one of the following signature formats:

1. Handwritten by physician
2. Handwritten by physician's representative
3. Signature stamp (facsimile)
4. Electronic signature

Some carriers may not require a signature if the following requirements are met:

- Physician's name is preprinted on the form (accepted by most private insurance carriers).
- Provider has a notarized authorization on file (accepted by some insurance carriers).

Physician's Representative

If approved by the insurance carrier, a physician may give signature authorization to one person on staff to sign insurance claim forms who then becomes known as the physician's representative. A notarized document that outlines the responsibility for this person may be required. This responsibility carries with it the knowledge that if the practice is ever audited and fraud or embezzlement is discovered, the person who had signature authorization can be brought into the case as well as the physician.

Signature Stamp

If approved by the insurance carrier, a facsimile signature stamp can be used so the staff can process insurance claims and other paperwork. This eliminates interrupting the physician or waiting for his or her signature. A document of this type should also be notarized. Caution should be noted, because the use of a signature stamp can lead to problems. It is possible to stamp unauthorized checks, transcribed medical reports, prescriptions, or credit card charge slips. If such a stamp is used infrequently, then discontinue the practice. If one is used regularly, prevent problems by doing the following:

- Make only one stamp.
- Allow only authorized, bonded staff members to have access.
- Keep the stamp in a locked, secured location.

For information on state laws, contact your state legislature at your state capitol.

Electronic and Digital Signatures

There are two types of computerized signatures, electronic and digital. An **electronic signature** looks like the signer's handwritten signature. Two parties agree that the signature will show intent and approval of the document content. The signer authenticates the document by key entry or with a pen pad using a stylus to capture the live signature.

A **digital signature** may be lines of text or a text box stating the signer's name, date/time, and a statement indicating a signature has been attached from within the software application.

Check with individual insurance carrier requirements and have the physician sign, or use a method of authorized signature to sign, the completed insurance claim form above or below the typed or preprinted physician's name appearing in Block 31 (Fig. 8–5).

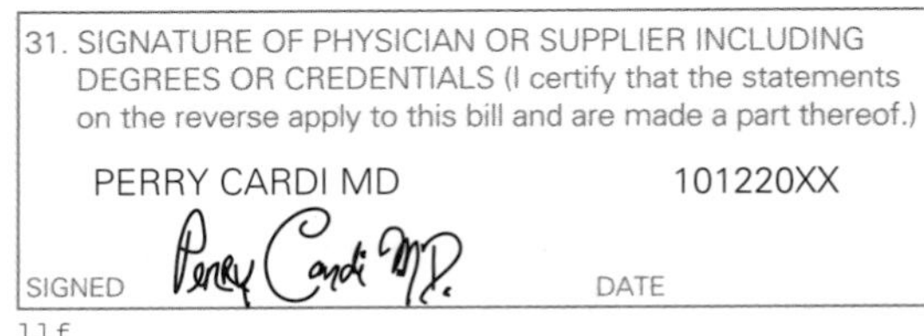

31. SIGNATURE OF PHYSICIAN OR SUPPLIER INCLUDING DEGREES OR CREDENTIALS (I certify that the statements on the reverse apply to this bill and are made a part thereof.)

PERRY CARDI MD 101220XX

SIGNED Perry Cardi M.D. DATE

llf

Figure 8–5. Block 31 of the HCFA-1500 claim form illustrating placement of physician's name and signature, date, and insurance billing specialist's initials.

Insurance Biller's Initials

The medical insurance billing specialist may place his or her initials in the bottom left or top right corner of the claim form, per office policy (see Fig. 8–5). Be consistent in placing this reference. Three good reasons to adopt this habit are:

1. To assign accountability for who prepared the claim
2. To decrease errors by learning from previous mistakes
3. To avoid being accused of someone else's error, especially if the previous biller submitted a fraudulent claim

Proofreading Claims

Proofread every claim regardless of the amount billed. Be aware of claims that involve large sums of money and may be more difficult to complete accurately. Proofread for transposition of numbers (policy, group, physician's ID, procedure and diagnostic codes), misspelled names, missing date of birth, unfilled mandatory blocks, and attachments.

Supporting Documentation

To obtain maximum reimbursement, occasionally claims require supporting documents that verify or further explain services billed. When submitting an attachment, include the patient's name, subscriber's name (if different from the patient), and insurance identification number in case the document becomes separated from the claim during processing.

If medication is expensive or experimental, send a copy of the invoice received from the supply house or pharmacy.

When a procedure is complicated, include a copy of all pertinent reports (e.g., operative, radiology, laboratory, pathology, discharge summary). For a service or procedure not listed in the procedure codebook, send in a detailed report giving the nature, extent, and medical necessity for the service. If the claim is submitted electronically, this description should be keyed in the narrative field. Select a code number for unlisted services or procedure which usually ends in "99," for example, an unlisted allergy testing procedure would be code number 95199.

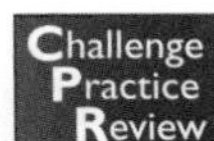

Pause and Practice CPR

REVIEW SESSIONS 8–22 THROUGH 8–24

Directions: *Complete the following questions as a review of information you have just read.*

8–22 List four common formats for physician signature requirements.

(1) ______________________________

(2) ______________________________

(3) ______________________________

(4) ______________________________

8–23 If no physician signature is required by the insurance carrier, what other requirements are usually in place?

(1) ______________________________

(2) ______________________________

8–24 List the two types of computerized signatures.

(1) ______________________________

(2) ______________________________

CHECK YOUR HEARTBEAT! Turn to the end of the chapter for answers to these review sessions.

COMPUTERS IN THE MEDICAL OFFICE

A computer in the medical office setting has many roles. It can manage the appointment schedule in a solo practice or in large practices with many locations, store diagnostic and procedural codes in its database with a search feature that allows the coder to find codes quickly, store medical records allowing easy data input and retrieval, function as a word processor producing letters and memos, and manage financial data.

Financial applications include producing payroll; handling the accounts payable and accounts receivable, including aging of A/R; controlling patient accounts and patient billing; storing insurance data; and processing electronic insurance claims. Financial reports can be created to access the productivity of the medical practice and assist the insurance billing specialist with many of his or her job functions.

Electronic Data Interchange

As stated earlier, an electronic claim is one that is submitted by means of direct wire or dial-in-telephone. Electronic claims can also be uploaded or downloaded on a personal computer using a modem or the Internet. The transmission of such claims is known as

electronic data interchange (EDI). This is the process by which understandable data are sent back and forth using computer linkages. Two or more entities function alternatively as sender and receiver.

Computer Claims Systems

The Health Insurance Portability and Accountability Act (HIPAA), passed by Congress in 1996, legislated two important actions: health insurance reform and administrative simplification. One of the administrative simplification provisions directs the federal government to adopt national electronic standards for automated transfer of certain healthcare data between healthcare payers, plans, and providers, thus eliminating all nonstandard formats currently in use.

Previously, each carrier had special electronic billing requirements and knew which systems were compatible in format to meet their criteria. A physician who planned to bill electronically had to contact all major insurers and the fiscal intermediaries for each government and/or state program for a list of vendors approved to handle **electronic claims submission (ECS).** Once HIPPA code set standards are in place, the healthcare provider will be able to submit a standard transaction for querying patient eligibility, requesting prior authorization, submitting electronic claims, sending attachments, checking claim status, and receiving remittance advice (RA/EOB) statements. The same format will be used by providers to submit claims to all payers. This will simplify many applications and reduce costs.

The standard code set is ANSI ASCX12N v4010 837 and was tentatively scheduled for implementation in October 2001 and compliance by October 2002. This electronic claim may be referred to as the Health Care Claim: Professional, and if printed on paper would take up five pages. Although several screens are used for data input in a computer system, the field data requested is almost identical to that required on the HCFA-1500 form.

Insurance carriers may add administrative monetary penalties to claims that are not submitted electronically as a negative incentive to use ECS. There are two systems that transmit insurance claims electronically (i.e., carrier-direct and clearinghouse). It is important to understand how these two systems operate to comprehend electronic claims submission.

Carrier-Direct System

Many electronic insurance claims are transmitted via a **carrier-direct system.** With this type of system, the medical practice has its own computer and software, keys in the claim data, and transmits the information directly to the insurance carrier over a dedicated telephone line. Fiscal agents for Medicaid, Medicare, TRICARE, and many private insurance carriers use this type of system. It is necessary to have a signed agreement with each carrier with whom the physician wishes to submit electronic claims.

Clearinghouse

The National Electronic Information Corporation (NEIC) provides a national network to receive, process, edit, sort, and transmit electronic claims to insurers. The NEIC system allows the physician to use one version of software to communicate with different insurers. Claims can be submitted directly to NEIC for

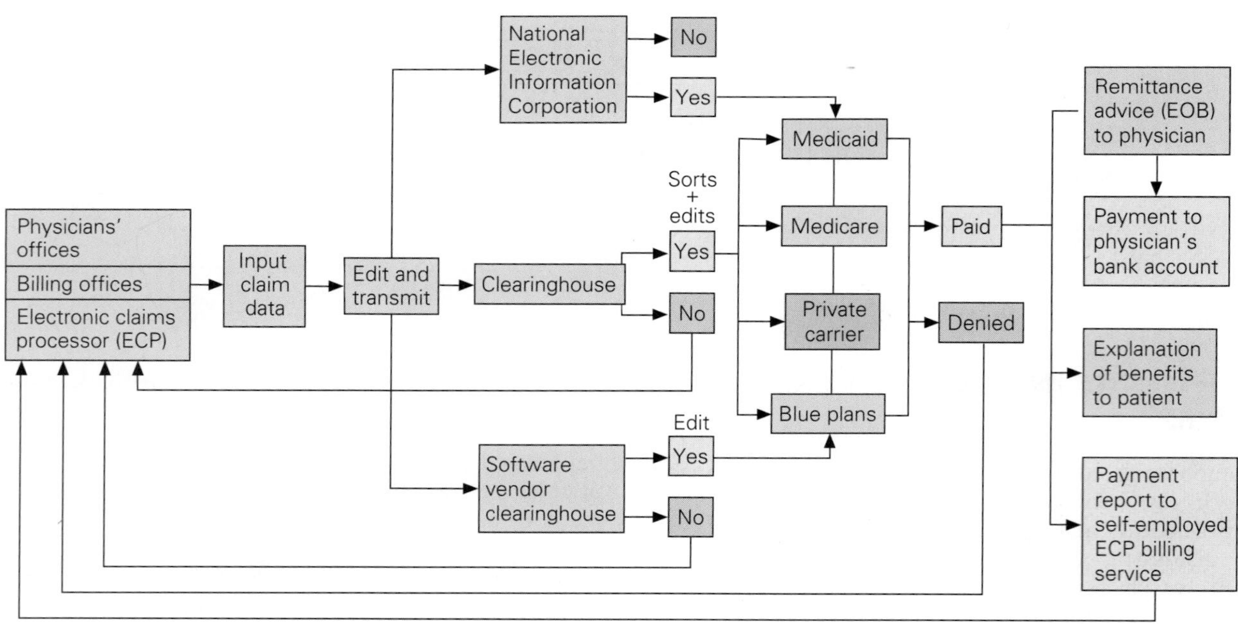

Figure 8–6. Flow sheet of electronic transmission systems showing path for claim payment via NEIC, clearinghouse, and independent software vendor. Also indicates when payment is made to physician and depicts locations where claims may not pass an edit and/or are denied.

routing, or through a network of independent software vendors, billing centers, and clearinghouses.

If the physician's system cannot be linked with the insurance carrier or the insurers do not accept claims directly from physicians' offices, then the physician may use a clearinghouse.

A **clearinghouse,** also referred to as a third party administrator (TPA), is an entity that receives transmission of claims from physicians' offices, separates claims by carrier, performs software edits on each claim to check for errors, and then forwards claims electronically to the proper insurance payer, charging the physician a fee. Some clearinghouses have additional services, such as manually processing claims to carriers that are not online. This would enable the physician's office to send all claims electronically to the clearinghouse rather than processing half electronically and printing and mailing the rest. Figure 8–6 is a flow sheet illustrating electronic claim submission via NEIC, a clearinghouse, and using a software vendor.

Electronic Claims Processor

An individual who converts insurance claims to standardized electronic format and transmits electronic claims data is known as an **electronic claims processor (ECP).** This individual can work in a physician's office, clinic setting, billing center, or be self-employed. A knowledgeable and efficient ECP can expedite payment to the physician and reduce the number of rejected claims.

As mentioned in Chapter 3, an encounter form is often used to input charges into a computer system. An abbreviated style of the encounter form (crib sheet) was designed by physicians listing key components for Evaluation and Management (E/M) services to aid the physician in determining the correct level of E/M service, ensure each component is addressed in the physician's documentation, and expedite data entry of professional services. Figure 8–7 illustrates a portion of a crib sheet. Because crib sheets are abbreviated and not in detail, they, along with other types of billing forms, cannot be used in place of documentation in the patient record and may not withstand an external audit.

Some encounter forms are designed so that they may be scanned to input procedures, charges, and diagnoses into the patient's computerized account. Figure 8–8 shows a portion of a scannable encounter form. Time is saved and fewer errors occur because no keystrokes are involved.

Crib Sheet

New Patient

✓	Code	HX	PX	MDM
	99201*	PF	PF	SF
	99202*	EPF	EPF	SF
	99203*	D	D	LC
	99204*	C	C	MC
	99205*	C	C	HC

Established patient

✓	Code	HX	PX	MDM
	99211+	May not require presence of physician		
	99212+	PF	PF	SF
	99213+	EPF	EPF	LC
	99214+	D	D	MC
	99215+	C	C	HC

Key: HX: history PX: physical examination

PF	problem focused	EPF	expanded problem focused
D	detailed	C	comprehensive

MDM: medical decision making

SF	straight forward	LC	low complexity
MC	moderate complexitiy	HC	high complexity
*	3 key components required	+	2 out of 3 key components required

Figure 8–7. Example of a partial crib sheet which uses abbreviations to assist the physician in selecting an E/M code according to the three key components: history, physical examination, and medical decision making.

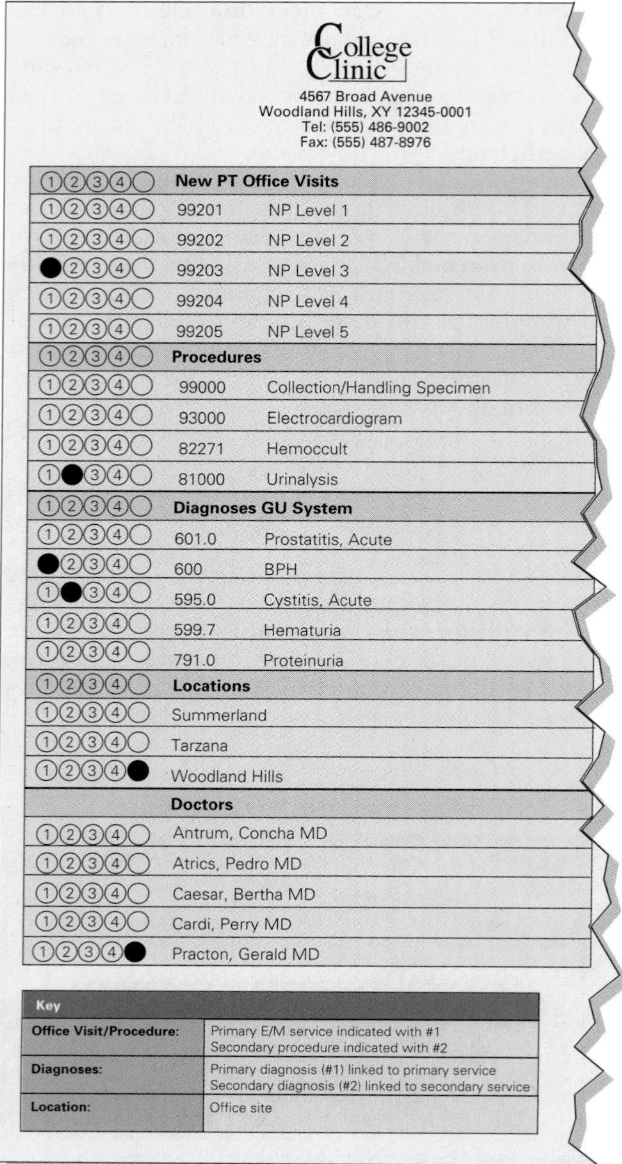

College Clinic
4567 Broad Avenue
Woodland Hills, XY 12345-0001
Tel: (555) 486-9002
Fax: (555) 487-8976

①②③④○	**New PT Office Visits**	
①②③④○	99201	NP Level 1
①②③④○	99202	NP Level 2
●②③④○	99203	NP Level 3
①②③④○	99204	NP Level 4
①②③④○	99205	NP Level 5
①②③④○	**Procedures**	
①②③④○	99000	Collection/Handling Specimen
①②③④○	93000	Electrocardiogram
①②③④○	82271	Hemoccult
①●③④○	81000	Urinalysis
①②③④○	**Diagnoses GU System**	
①②③④○	601.0	Prostatitis, Acute
●②③④○	600	BPH
①●③④○	595.0	Cystitis, Acute
①②③④○	599.7	Hematuria
①②③④○	791.0	Proteinuria
①②③④○	**Locations**	
①②③④○	Summerland	
①②③④○	Tarzana	
①②③④●	Woodland Hills	
	Doctors	
①②③④○	Antrum, Concha MD	
①②③④○	Atrics, Pedro MD	
①②③④○	Caesar, Bertha MD	
①②③④○	Cardi, Perry MD	
①②③④●	Practon, Gerald MD	

Key	
Office Visit/Procedure:	Primary E/M service indicated with #1 Secondary procedure indicated with #2
Diagnoses:	Primary diagnosis (#1) linked to primary service Secondary diagnosis (#2) linked to secondary service
Location:	Office site

Figure 8–8. Example of a partial scannable encounter form. Primary service/procedure is marked (with a #2 pencil) in the #1 location and linked to the primary diagnosis which is also marked in the #1 location. The secondary procedures are marked in the #2 location as is the secondary diagnosis. The primary linkage for all services and procedures is connected to the physician performing the service and the location in which it took place.

Advantages of Electronic Claim Submission

Claims sent electronically require no repeated keying of patient data; no searching for an insurance carrier's address, provider identification, facility address and identification number, or referring physician identification; no trips to the post office or postage fees; no filing of claim forms in a file cabinet; and no storage of claims in bins or storage facilities. They leave an **audit trail** that is a chronological record of submitted data that can be traced to their source to determine the place of origin. A proof of receipt (Fig. 8–9) is generated at the carrier's end, thus eliminating the insurance carrier's excuse, "We never received the claim, please resubmit."

Almost all insurance companies participate in electronic claims submission. Generally, less time is spent processing claims, freeing staff for other duties, thus decreasing overhead and labor costs. Human error is minimized because data go from one computer to another. One of the biggest advantages is improved cash flow. Payment from electronically submitted claims is received in 2 weeks or less. In comparison, payment from claims completed manually and sent by mail takes 4 to 6 weeks to receive.

Another important advantage of ECS is the error-edit process. This allows the person processing the claim to know of an error immediately so a correction can be made. Editing software can be incorporated by the physician's office, clearinghouse, or insurance company.

Edit Checks

Computer software programs contain edit checks that automatically screen transmitted insurance claims and electronically examine them for errors or conflicting information. Most insurance companies have edit checks that are run on incoming claims. Healthcare providers should incorporate compliance software edits to ensure correct coding and billing practices. Prebilling screens, postbilling audits, and monitoring functions can be done easily with such software.

Medical Software Programs

There are many types of medical software programs used by physician's offices. Some common programs include:

- Apex Medical Practice Management (AMPM) System
- Avanta
- CompuMedic (Data Strategies)
- Lytec
- MedAssist

Expressions from Experience

I have learned that if something looks like it is off, it may very well be. For example, when an insurance payment is decreased by 50% of the billed amount, something is wrong. This happened when I billed three surgeries totaling $450 and got paid $50. They only processed one surgery, not multiple units.

Deborah Pitts
Medical Insurance Billing Specialist
Billing Service

College Clinic
Practon, Gerald MD
4567 Broad Avenue
Woodland Hills, XY 12345-0001

12345-0001

XYZ INSURANCE COMPANY

ELECTRONIC CLAIMS ACKNOWLEDGMENT REPORT

DATE:	02-28-20XX
SUBMITTER CODE:	000002469
RECEIPT DATE:	02-28-20XX

THERE WERE NO EDIT ERRORS DETECTED AND THE CLAIMS WERE PASSED TO OUR CLAIMS PROCESSING SYSTEM.

YOU SHOULD BE INFORMED OF THE STATUS OF ALL CLAIMS ON THE NEXT OUTPUT REPORT YOU RECEIVE FROM US.

FOLLOWING ARE STATISTICS RELATED TO THE PROCESSING OF YOUR BATCH:

TOTAL CLAIMS SUBMITTED	50
TOTAL CLAIMS ACCEPTED	50
TOTAL CLAIMS REJECTED	0
TOTAL CLAIMS ACCEPTED WITH ERRORS	0
% OF ERRORS TO CLAIMS EDITED	0%
TOTAL CHARGES ACCEPTED:	$15,267.00
TOTAL ASSIGNED CHARGES:	$4,289.00
TOTAL NON ASSIGNED CHARGES:	$0.00
TOTAL CROSSOVER CHARGES:	$10,978.00
TOTAL CHARGES REJECTED:	$0.00
TOTAL BATCHES TRANSMITTED	1
TOTAL DETAIL LINES SUBMITTED	146

Figure 8–9. Electronic Claims Acknowledgment Report indicating status of all claims transmitted electronically to XYZ Insurance Company on February 28, 20XX.

- Medical Manager
- MediSoft
- MediTech
- On-Staff 2000 (Prime Clinical Systems, Inc.)

The software program represents the computer instructions required to make the computer hardware perform a specific task. Until the standard code set is implemented, it is important to use a software program that can interface with the major insurance companies the physician's office submits claims to.

Networks

Computers may be interconnected in a number of different ways to exchange information. This is referred to as networks.

Local area network (LAN)—connects computers that are contained within a room or building (e.g., clinics, large medical practices, hospitals); they share files and devices such as printers.

Wide area network (WAN)—covers a large geographical area (e.g., America Online) and is considered a communication network.

Internet—a large interconnected message-forwarding system linking academic, commercial, government, and military computer networks all over the world.

Internet applications include electronic mail (e-mail), online conversations (one-on-one or in chat rooms), information retrieval, and bulletin board systems (BBS) where messages may be posted via the *World Wide Web* which links documents between locations. Some insurers offer incentives to practitioners for using the Web to process medical claims, make referrals, and check patient eligibility, deductibles, and claim status. Incentives can consist of faster payment of claims, payment of claims transaction fees, and direct deposit of claim payments to the practice's bank account. Independent medical insurance billers working out of their home can also use the Internet to transfer claim information.

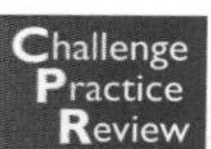

Pause and Practice CPR

REVIEW SESSIONS 8–25 THROUGH 8–27

Directions: *Complete the following questions as a review of information you have just read on computers in the medical office and electronic claim submission.*

8–25 List five basic functions of a computer in the medical office.

(1) ______

(2) ______

(3) ______

(4) ______

(5) ______

8–26 List the functions the provider will be able to do when using the new standard code set.

(1) ______

(2) ______

(3) ______

(4) ______

(5) ______

(6) ______

8–27 Name the two systems used for transmitting electronic claims.

(1) ______

(2) ______

CHECK YOUR HEARTBEAT! Turn to the end of the chapter for answers to these review sessions.

SUMMATION AND PREVIEW

You have now completed the final step and learned all of the necessary components to file an insurance claim. Each of these components—understanding medicolegal issues and insurance contracts, plans, and regulations; coding diagnoses and procedures; abstracting information from the medical record; and filling out the HCFA-1500 form—are needed to process a successful claim and receive maximum reimbursement.

In the following chapters you will learn about major insurance plans and programs (e.g., Medicaid, Medicare, TRICARE, workers' compensation) and their specific requirements for submitting claim forms. Remember that you are not expected to remember or memorize everything; however, you are required to know where to go to find the information that you will need to complete future assignments and file insurance claims.

GOLDEN RULE

Have a block party. Know the insurance carrier requirements for each block.

Chapter 8 Review and Practice

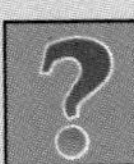

Study Session

Directions: *Review the objectives, key terms, and chapter information before completing the following study questions.*

8–1 When billing, how should claims be grouped to make completion of forms easier and to cut down on errors? Insurance Type

8–2 List four ways of creating a HCFA-1500 paper claim for submission by mail.

pg 203 & 204

(1) ______

(2) ______

(3) ______

(4) ______

8–3 List three requirements when entries are made on the HCFA-1500 form using OCR guidelines.

pg 206

(1) ______

(2) ______

(3) ______

8–4 Name the two major sections of the HCFA-1500 form.

pg 206

(1) ______

(2) ______

8–5 Which block is used in the upper portion of the claim form to obtain a signature for the release of medical information? Block 12

8–6 Which block is used in the upper portion of the claim form to obtain a signature for the assignment of benefits for a private insurance plan? Block 13

8–7 Name the blocks on the top portion of the claim form that require more than one piece of information but are not necessarily subdivided by letters.

(a) 1a. ID# & Group# (pg 507)

(b) 3

(c) 5

(d) 7

(e) 8

(f) 9b

(g) 11b

(h) 12

8–8 What is the largest block on the lower portion of the claim form and what is it used for?

Block 24 used report various components of service

8–9 Turn to Appendix D (Fig. D–1) and locate the place of service codes. Enter the correct code for the following descriptions.

(1) Nursing facility ______

(2) Emergency department ______

(3) State or local public health clinic ______

(4) Ambulatory surgical center ______

(5) Inpatient psychiatric facility ______

8–10 Turn to Appendix D (Fig. D–2) and locate the type of service codes. Enter the correct code for the following descriptions.

(1) Drugs ______

(2) Maternity ______

(3) Surgery ______

(4) Diagnostic laboratory ______

(5) Venipuncture ______

8–11 List the correct physician identification numbers for the following:

(1) Dr. Ulibarri's Social Security number ______

(2) Dr. Coccidioides' state license number ______

(3) Dr. Antrum's federal tax ID number ______

(4) Dr. Perry's UPIN ______

(5) Dr. Skeleton's state license number ______

8–12 If a facsimile signature stamp is used in the physician's office regularly, what measures should be taken to prevent problems?

(1) ______

(2) ______

(3) ______

8–13 List three reasons for inserting an insurance billing specialist's initials on the claim form.

(1) ______

(2) ______

(3) ______

8–14 List errors and omissions to look for when proofreading a claim. ______

______

______

8–15 When submitting supporting documentation with a claim form, what should be included on all attachments? ______

______

8–16 Handwriting on a claim form is only acceptable in ______ blocks.

8–17 Claim forms should be mailed in a/an ______ envelope.

8–18 The transmission of electronic claims is known as ______

pg 216

8–19 What is the name of the standard code set? ANSI ASC X12N v 4010 837

8–20 State the functions of a clearinghouse.

pg. 217

Exercise Exchange

8–1 Complete Top Portion of the HCFA-1500 Claim Form

Directions:

1. Abstract patient and insurance information from the Patient Registration form on page 224 and enter it into the correct blocks on the HCFA-1500 form using OCR guidelines.
2. Refer to block-by-block instructions and the private insurance template (Fig. D–3) in Appendix D and Figure 8–1 in this chapter.
3. Sign the claim using the date July 30, 20XX for release of medical information and assignment of benefits as if you were the patient.

1. MEDICARE ☐ (Medicare #) MEDICAID ☐ (Medicaid #) CHAMPUS ☐ (Sponsor's SSN) CHAMPVA ☐ (VA File #)	GROUP HEALTH PLAN ☐ (SSN or ID) FECA BLK LUNG ☐ (SSN) OTHER ☐ (ID)	1a. INSURED'S I.D. NUMBER (FOR PROGRAM IN ITEM 1)
2. PATIENT'S NAME (Last Name, First Name, Middle Initial)	3. PATIENT'S BIRTHDATE MM DD YYYY SEX M☐ F☐	4. INSURED'S NAME (Last Name, First Name, Middle Initial)
5. PATIENT'S ADDRESS (No, Street)	6. PATIENT RELATIONSHIP TO INSURED Self☐ Spouse☐ Child☐ Other☐	7. INSURED'S ADDRESS (No., Street)
CITY / STATE	8. PATIENT STATUS Single ☐ Married ☐ Other ☐	CITY / STATE
ZIP CODE / TELEPHONE (include Area Code) ( )	Employed ☐ Full-Time Student ☐ Part-Time Student ☐	ZIP CODE / TELEPHONE (Include Area Code) ( )
9. OTHER INSURED'S NAME (Last Name, First Name, Middle Initial)	10. IS PATIENT'S CONDITION RELATED TO:	11. INSURED'S POLICY GROUP OR FECA NUMBER
a. OTHER INSURED'S POLICY OR GROUP NUMBER	a. EMPLOYMENT? (CURRENT OR PREVIOUS) ☐YES ☐NO	a. INSURED'S DATE OF BIRTH MM DD YYYY SEX M☐ F☐
b. OTHER INSURED'S DATE OF BIRTH MM DD YYYY SEX M☐ F☐	b. AUTO ACCIDENT? ☐YES ☐NO PLACE (State)	b. EMPLOYER'S NAME OR SCHOOL NAME
c. EMPLOYER'S NAME OR SCHOOL NAME	c. OTHER ACCIDENT? ☐YES ☐NO	c. INSURANCE PLAN NAME OR PROGRAM NAME
d. INSURANCE PLAN NAME OR PROGRAM NAME	10d. RESERVED FOR LOCAL USE	d. IS THERE ANOTHER HEALTH BENEFIT PLAN? ☐YES ☐NO *If yes, return to and complete item 9a-d*
READ BACK OF FORM BEFORE COMPLETING & SIGNING THIS FORM 12. PATIENT'S OR AUTHORIZED PERSON'S SIGNATURE. I authorize the release of any medical or other information necessary to process this claim. I also request payment of government benefits either to myself or to the party who accepts assignment below. SIGNED ______ DATE ______		13. INSURED'S OR AUTHORIZED PERSON'S SIGNATURE. I authorize payment of medical benefits to the undersigned physician or supplier for services described below. SIGNED ______

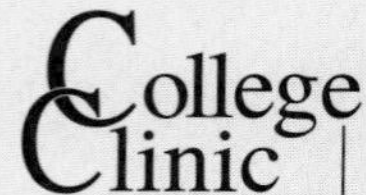

4567 Broad Avenue
Woodland Hills, XY
12345-0001
Tel (555) 486-9002
Fax (555) 487-8976

REGISTRATION
(PLEASE PRINT)

Account # 0426 Today's Date: 07/30/XX

PATIENT INFORMATION

Name Zamora (Last Name) Callie (First Name) J (Initial) Soc. Sec. # 239-XX-4631

Address 280 Cottage Place Home Phone (555) 967-4021

City Woodland Hills State XY Zip 12345

Single ✓ Married ___ Separated ___ Divorced ___ Sex M ___ F ✓ Birthdate 01/11/1980

Patient Employed by Junipero Preschool Occupation Teacher

Business Address 400 Junipero Street Business Phone (555) 972-1100

Spouse's Name N/A Employed by: ___ Occupation ___

Business Address ___ Business Phone ___

Reason for Visit pap smear/breast check If accident: ___ Auto ___ Employment ___ Other ___

By whom were you referred? mother

In case of emergency, who should be notified? Corine Zamora (Name) mother (Relation to Patient) Phone (555) 967-3925

PRIMARY INSURANCE

Insured/Subscriber Zamora (Last Name) Callie (First Name) J (Initial)

Relation to Patient same Birthdate ___ Soc. Sec.# ___

Address (if different from patient's) N/A

City ___ State ___ Zip ___

Insurance Company Union Insurance Company

Insurance Address 2121 Broadway, Westchester, XY 12345

Insurance Identification Number 239-XX-4631 Group # A45

ADDITIONAL INSURANCE

Is patient covered by additional insurance? Yes ___ No ✓

Subscriber Name N/A Relation to Patient ___ Birthdate ___

Address (if different from patient's) ___ Phone ___

City ___ State ___ Zip ___

Subscriber Employed by ___ Buisness Phone ___

Insurance Company ___ Soc. Sec. # ___

Insurance Address ___

Insurance Identification Number ___ Group # ___

ASSIGNMENT AND RELEASE

I, the undersigned, certify that I (or my dependent) have insurance coverage with Union Insurance Company (Name of Insurance Company(ies)) and assign directly to Dr. Caesar insurance benefits, if any, otherwise payable to me for services rendered. I understand that I am financially responsible for all charges whether or not paid by insurance. I hereby consent for the doctor to release all information necessary to secure the payment of benefits. I authorize the use of this signature on all insurance submissions.

Callie J. Zamora (Responsible Party Signature) self (Relationship) 07/30/XX (Date)

8–2 **Complete Bottom Portion of the HCFA-1500 Claim Form**

Directions:

1. Abstract physician information from the encounter form on page 226 and enter it into the correct blocks on the HCFA-1500 form using OCR guidelines.

2. Refer to block-by-block instructions and the private insurance template (Fig. D–3) in Appendix D, and Figure 8–2 in this chapter.

3. Obtain physician identification numbers from the clinic/physician file in Appendix A.

4. The physician is accepting assignment.

5. The claim processing date is July 31, 20XX.

6. Sign the form with the physician's name as the physician representative and initial the form.

14. DATE OF CURRENT: MM | DD | YYYY ◀ ILLNESS (First symptom) OR INJURY (Accident) OR PREGNANCY (LMP)

15. IF PATIENT HAS HAD SAME OR SIMILAR ILLNESS GIVE FIRST DATE MM | DD | YYYY

16. DATES PATIENT UNABLE TO WORK IN CURRENT OCCUPATION FROM MM | DD | YYYY TO MM | DD | YYYY

17. NAME OF REFERRING PHYSICIAN OR OTHER SOURCE

17a. I.D. NUMBER OF REFERRING PHYSICIAN

18. HOSPITALIZATION DATES RELATED TO CURRRENT SERVICES FROM MM | DD | YYYY TO MM | DD | YYYY

19. RESERVED FOR LOCAL USE

20. OUTSIDE LAB? ☐YES ☐NO $ CHARGES

21. DIAGNOSIS OR NATURE OF ILLNESS OR INJURY (RELATE ITEMS 1, 2, 3 OR 4 TO ITEM 24E BY LINE)

1. ___ . ___ 3. ___ . ___
2. ___ . ___ 4. ___ . ___

22. MEDICAID RESUBMISSION CODE | ORIGINAL REF. NO.

23. PRIOR AUTHORIZATION NUMBER

24. A						B	C	D		E	F	G	H	I	J	K
DATE(S) OF SERVICE FROM			TO			Place of Service	Type of Service	PROCEDURES, SERVICES, OR SUPPLIES (Explain Unusual Circumstances)		DIAGNOSIS CODE		DAYS OR UNITS	EPSDT Family Plan			RESERVED FOR LOCAL USE
MM	DD	YYYY	MM	DD	YYYY			CPT/HCPCS	MODIFIER		$ CHARGES			EMG	COB	

25. FEDERAL TAX I.D. NUMBER SSN ☐ EIN ☐

26. PATIENT'S ACCOUNT NO.

27. ACCEPT ASSIGNMENT? (For govt. claims, see back) ☐YES ☐NO

28. TOTAL CHARGE $

29. AMOUNT PAID $

30. BALANCE DUE $

31. SIGNATURE OF PHYSICIAN OR SUPPLIER INCLUDING DEGREES OR CREDENTIALS (I certify that the statements on the reverse apply to this bill and are made a part thereof.)

SIGNED DATE

32. NAME AND ADDRESS OF FACILITY WHERE SERVICES WERE RENDERED (if other than home or office)

33. PHYSICIAN'S, SUPPLIER'S BILLING NAME, ADDRESS, ZIP CODE & PHONE #

PIN# | GRP#

TAX ID #3664021CC
Medicaid #HSC12345F

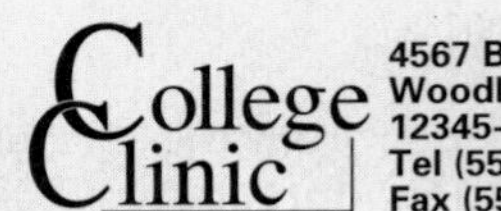

4567 Broad Avenue
Woodland Hills, XY
12345-0001
Tel (555) 486-9002
Fax (555) 487-8976

Doctor No. 3

☒ PRIVATE ☐ MANAGED CARE ☐ MEDICAID ☐ MEDICARE ☐ TRICARE ☐ W/C

ACCOUNT #	PATIENT'S LAST NAME	FIRST	INITIAL	TODAY'S DATE
0426	Zamora	Callie	J	07/ 30 / XX

ASSIGNMENT: I hereby assign payment directly to College Clinic of the surgical and/or medical benefits, if any, otherwise payable to me for his/her services as described below.
SIGNED (Patient, or Parent, if Minor) *Callie J. Zamora* DATE: 07/30/XX

✓ DESCRIPTION	CPT-4/MD	FEE	✓ DESCRIPTION	CPT-4/MD	FEE	✓ DESCRIPTION	CPT-4/MD	FEE
OFFICE VISIT–NEW PATIENT			**WELL BABY EXAM**			**LABORATORY**		
Level 1	99201		Initial	99381		Glucose Blood	82962	
Level 2	99202		Periodic	99391		Hematocrit	85013	
✓ Level 3	99203	70.92	**OFFICE PROCEDURES**			Occult Blood	82270	
Level 4	99204		Anoscopy	46600		Urine Dip	81000	
Level 5	99205		ECG 24-hr	93224		**X-RAY**		
OFFICE VISIT–ESTAB. PATIENT			Fracture Rpr Foot	28470		Foot – 2 view	73620	
Level 1	99211		I & D	10060		Forearm - 2 view	73090	
Level 2	99212		Suture Repair			Nasal Bone - 3	70160	
Level 3	99213					Spine LS - 2 view	72100	
Level 4	99214		**INJECTIONS/VACCINATIONS**					
Level 5	99215		DPT	90701		**MISCELLANEOUS**		
OFFICE CONSULT-NP/EST			IM-Antibiotic	90788		✓ Handling of Spec	99000	5.00
Level 3	99243		OPU-Poliovirus	90712		Supply	99070	
Level 4	99244		Tetanus	90703		Venipuncture	36415	
Level 5	99245							

COMMENTS:

Physician: *Bertha Caesar MD*

RETURN APPOINTMENT PRN
____ Week(s) ____ Month(s)

DIAGNOSIS:	DESCRIPTION	CODE
Primary:	Fibrocystic breast	610.1
Secondary:		

REC'D BY:
☐ BANK CARD
☐ CASH
☑ CHECK
\# 237

PREVIOUS BALANCE	-0-
TODAY'S FEE	75.92
AMOUNT REC'D/CO-PAY	10.00
BALANCE	65.92

8–3 View Insurance Video

Video: Saunders Critical Thinking Skills for Medical Assistants, Tape Six: "The HCFA-Files: A Case for Medical Billing Accuracy," is an interesting and entertaining presentation about what happens to rejected claim forms. It gives reasons why claims are denied and gives solutions to avoid such problems. It is an excellent enhancement when used at the conclusion to this chapter. This assignment is presented for completion after viewing this video.

Directions:

1. Preread the questions regarding the video tape.
2. Take notes while watching the video.
3. Use notes to answer questions.

Questions:

1. What is the difference between a generic ICD-9-CM code and a specific code?

   ____

2. On average, what percentage of claims never get paid? ______________________________

3. Give an example of a gender-specific diagnostic code. ______________________________

____

4. During the review of a claim, what is looked at most closely?

____

5. What are the long-term consequences of rejected claims?

____

6. List types of problems why a claim may be either denied or rejected after receipt by the insurance company.

   (a) ____

   (b) ____

   (c) ____

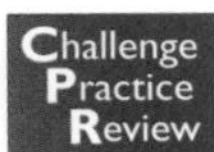

CPR Sessions: Answers

CPR REVIEW SESSIONS 8–1 THROUGH 8–3

8–1 (1) E/M services, procedures, and testing done in the physician's office in which benefits are assigned to the physician
(2) Hospital, emergency room, nursing facility, and home visits
(3) Surgeries, whether performed in an acute care hospital, ambulatory surgery center, or the physician's office

8–2 (1) Generating an insurance claim form using a computer system
(2) Manually preparing the insurance form using a typewriter or word processor
(3) Filing the insurance data electronically using an in-office computer with modem and telecommunication lines
(4) Contracting with an outside billing agency to prepare and file claims manually or electronically

8–3 (a) As soon as possible (or if extended care is received, every 15 to 30 days or at the end of treatment)
(b) After discharge
(c) Immediately

CPR REVIEW SESSIONS 8–4 THROUGH 8–8

8–4 Medicare, TRICARE, Blue Shield, private insurance carriers who are members of HIAA, and Medicaid and industrial (workers' compensation) carriers in some states

8–5 Claims submitted to insurance carriers via personal computer using a modem

8–6 Claims submitted on paper, usually using the HCFA-1500 form, including computer-generated claims, optically scanned claims, and faxed claims

8–7 Optical character recognition

8–8 Using optical scanning equipment, the insurance form is electronically scanned, transferring printed text to the insurance company's computer memory.

CPR REVIEW SESSIONS 8–9 THROUGH 8–11

8–9 Dual

8–10 Copy of the explanation of benefits (EOB) document from the primary carrier

8–11 Crossover

CPR PRACTICE SESSION 8–12

8–12 See correct form on top of page 230.

CPR PRACTICE SESSIONS 8–13 THROUGH 8–16

8–13 (1) Level 3 NP; office or other outpatient visit
(2) Electrocardiogram, routine; 12 leads with interpretation and report
(3) Spirometry
(4) Urinalysis; nonautomated without microscopy
(5) Venipuncture; routine
(6) Handling of specimen (blood from venipuncture) for transfer to an outside laboratory

8–14 (1) Chest pain, other (discomfort, pressure, tightness)
(2) Acute edema of lung, unspecified
(3) Fever
(4) Dysuria

8–13 through 8–16 See correct form on bottom of page 230.

CPR PRACTICE SESSIONS 8–17 THROUGH 8–21

8–17 12678547XX (UPIN/NPI)

8–18 95 0731067 (hospital provider number)

8–19 72 57130XX (employer federal tax identification number—EIN)

8–20 3664021CC (employer group tax identification number)

8–21 43050047XX (PIN/NPI)

CPR REVIEW SESSIONS 8–22 THROUGH 8–24

8–22 (1) Handwritten by physician
(2) Handwritten by physician's representative
(3) Signature stamp (facsimile)
(4) Electronic signature

8–23 (1) Physician's name preprinted on form
(2) Provider has a notarized authorization on file

8–24 (1) Electronic signature
(2) Digital signature

CPR REVIEW SESSIONS 8–25 THROUGH 8–27

8–25 (1) Manage appointment schedule
(2) Store diagnostic and procedural codes
(3) Store medical records
(4) Function as word processor
(5) Manage financial data

8–26 (1) Query patient eligibility
(2) Request prior authorization
(3) Submit electronic claims
(4) Send attachments
(5) Check claim status
(6) Receive RA statements using the same software

8–27 (1) Carrier-direct
(2) Clearinghouse

Answer for 8–12

SAFENET INSURANCE COMPANY
2277 CENTER STREET
TARZANA XY 12345-0001 (4)

1. MEDICARE MEDICAID CHAMPUS CHAMPVA (3) GROUP HEALTH PLAN FECA BLK LUNG OTHER ☐ (Medicare #) ☐ (Medicaid #) ☐ (Sponsor's SSN) ☐ (VA File #) ☒ (SSN or ID) ☐ (SSN) ☐ (ID)	1a. INSURED'S I.D. NUMBER (FOR PROGRAM IN ITEM 1) 7686960 (4) KED600
2. PATIENT'S NAME (Last Name, First Name, Middle Initial) DUNN KATHRYN E (1)	3. PATIENT'S BIRTHDATE MM DD YYYY 05 30 1970 (5) SEX M☐ F☐
4. INSURED'S NAME (Last Name, First Name, Middle Initial) SAME (3)	
5. PATIENT'S ADDRESS (No, Street) 587 CAMBRIA DRIVE (2)	6. PATIENT RELATIONSHIP TO INSURED Self ☒ Spouse ☐ (3) Child ☐ Other ☐
7. INSURED'S ADDRESS (No., Street)	
CITY SUMMERLAND STATE XY	8. PATIENT STATUS (5) Single ☒ Married ☐ Other ☐
CITY STATE	
ZIP CODE 12345 0001 TELEPHONE (include Area Code) (555) 658 2404	(3) Employed ☒ Full-Time Student ☐ Part-Time Student ☐
ZIP CODE TELEPHONE (Include Area Code) ( )	
9. OTHER INSURED'S NAME (Last Name, First Name, Middle Initial)	10. IS PATIENT'S CONDITION RELATED TO: (6)
11. INSURED'S POLICY GROUP OR FECA NUMBER	
a. OTHER INSURED'S POLICY OR GROUP NUMBER	a. EMPLOYMENT? (CURRENT OR PREVIOUS) ☐ YES ☒ NO
a. INSURED'S DATE OF BIRTH MM DD YYYY SEX M☐ F☐	
b. OTHER INSURED'S DATE OF BIRTH MM DD YYYY SEX M☐ F☐	b. AUTO ACCIDENT? ☐ YES ☒ NO PLACE (State)
b. EMPLOYER'S NAME OR SCHOOL NAME	
c. EMPLOYER'S NAME OR SCHOOL NAME	c. OTHER ACCIDENT? ☐ YES ☒ NO
c. INSURANCE PLAN NAME OR PROGRAM NAME	
d. INSURANCE PLAN NAME OR PROGRAM NAME	10d. RESERVED FOR LOCAL USE
d. IS THERE ANOTHER HEALTH BENEFIT PLAN? ☐ YES ☒ NO (3) *If yes, return to and complete item 9a-d*	
READ BACK OF FORM BEFORE COMPLETING & SIGNING THIS FIRM 12. PATIENT'S OR AUTHORIZED PERSON'S SIGNATURE. I authorize the release of any medical or other information necessary to process this claim. I also request payment of government benefits either to myself or to the party who accepts assignment below. SIGNED SOF DATE	13. INSURED'S OR AUTHORIZED PERSON'S SIGNATURE. I authorize payment of medical benefits to the undersigned physician or supplier for services described below. SIGNED SOF (6)

Answer for 8–13 to 8–16

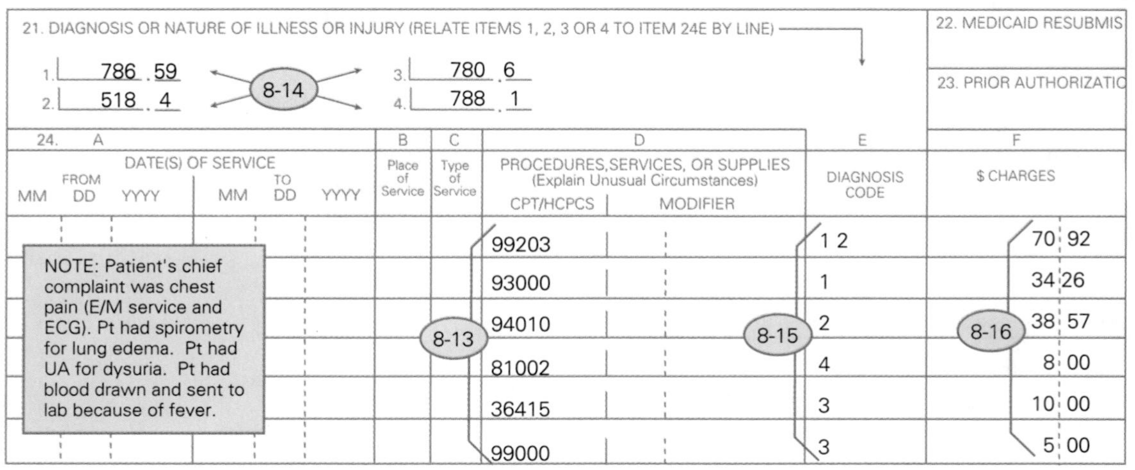

21. DIAGNOSIS OR NATURE OF ILLNESS OR INJURY (RELATE ITEMS 1, 2, 3 OR 4 TO ITEM 24E BY LINE)

1. 786 . 59
2. 518 . 4
3. 780 . 6
4. 788 . 1

(8-14)

22. MEDICAID RESUBMIS

23. PRIOR AUTHORIZATIC

24. A DATE(S) OF SERVICE FROM MM DD YYYY	TO MM DD YYYY	B Place of Service	C Type of Service	D PROCEDURES, SERVICES, OR SUPPLIES (Explain Unusual Circumstances) CPT/HCPCS	MODIFIER	E DIAGNOSIS CODE	F $ CHARGES
				99203		1 2	70 92
				93000		1	34 26
				94010		2	38 57
				81002		4	8 00
				36415		3	10 00
				99000		3	5 00

(8-13) (8-15) (8-16)

NOTE: Patient's chief complaint was chest pain (E/M service and ECG). Pt had spirometry for lung edema. Pt had UA for dysuria. Pt had blood drawn and sent to lab because of fever.

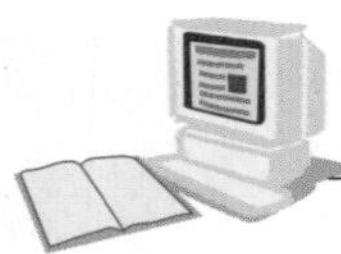

Resources

The HCFA-1500 form is in the process of being renamed and revised. Watch for the new name which will include the name Centers for Medicare and Medicaid Services (CMS). The revision may include a combination of the hospital insurance billing form (UB-92) and the outpatient billing form (HCFA-1500), and if so, you will need to take a class or seminar on rules for completing the new claim form. Access the Internet to locate up-to-date information on future changes.

For electronic transmission, you may wish to obtain details on the new Standard Code Set. The federal government has established compliance policies in the HIPAA where final regulations are published which may be helpful in answering questions you might have.

Following are web sites for quick access for all of this information.

Internet

- Health Insurance Claim Form (HCFA-1500), upcoming changes and ordering information. American Medical Association, 515 North State Street, Chicago, IL 60610
  Web site: http://www.ama-assn.org
- Health Insurance Portability and Accountability Act (HIPAA) regulations (free download)
- Standard Code Set (rules and information for electronic claim submission)
  Web site: http://aspe.hhs.gov

Objectives

After reading this chapter and completing the exercise sessions, you should be able to:

Learning Objectives:

- ✔ Compare private insurance with managed care plans.
- ✔ Describe fee-for-service and capitation reimbursement.
- ✔ State methods used to determine fees.
- ✔ Explain various types of discounted fees that occur in the physician's office.
- ✔ Define billed amount, allowed amount, and disallowed amount.
- ✔ List ways to communicate fees, collect fees, and respond to patient excuses not to pay.
- ✔ Identify types of managed care health plans.
- ✔ Give reasons for professional review organizations and explain how utilization review occurs.
- ✔ Define an independent practice association.
- ✔ Describe four types of referrals to obtain authorization for medical services, diagnostic tests, and procedures.

Performance Objectives:

- ✔ Complete the HCFA-1500 claim form for private insurance carriers and managed care plans.
- ✔ Complete a managed care authorization request for medical services.

Key Terms

actual charge
allowed amount
balance
Blue Cross
Blue Shield
capitation
carve-outs
competitive medical plan (CMP)
contractural adjustment
conversion factor (CF)
courtesy adjustment
direct referral
discount
disenrollment
exclusive provider organization (EPO)
fee-for-service
fee schedule
formal referral
foundations for medical care (FMC)
gatekeeper
health maintenance organization (HMO)
independent (or individual) practice association (IPA)
managed care organization (MCO)
network HMO
no charge (NC)
participating provider (par)
peer review
physician provider group (PPG)
physician's fee profile
point-of-service (POS) plan
preferred provider organization (PPO)
prepaid group practice model
prevailing charge
primary care physician (PCP)
professional courtesy
professional review organization (PRO)
relative value studies (RVS)
relative value unit (RVU)
resource-based relative value scale (RBRVS)
self-referral
staff model
tertiary care
usual, customary, and reasonable (UCR)
utilization review (UR)
verbal referral

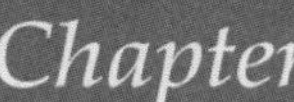
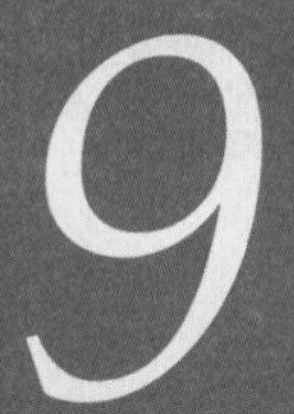

Chapter 9

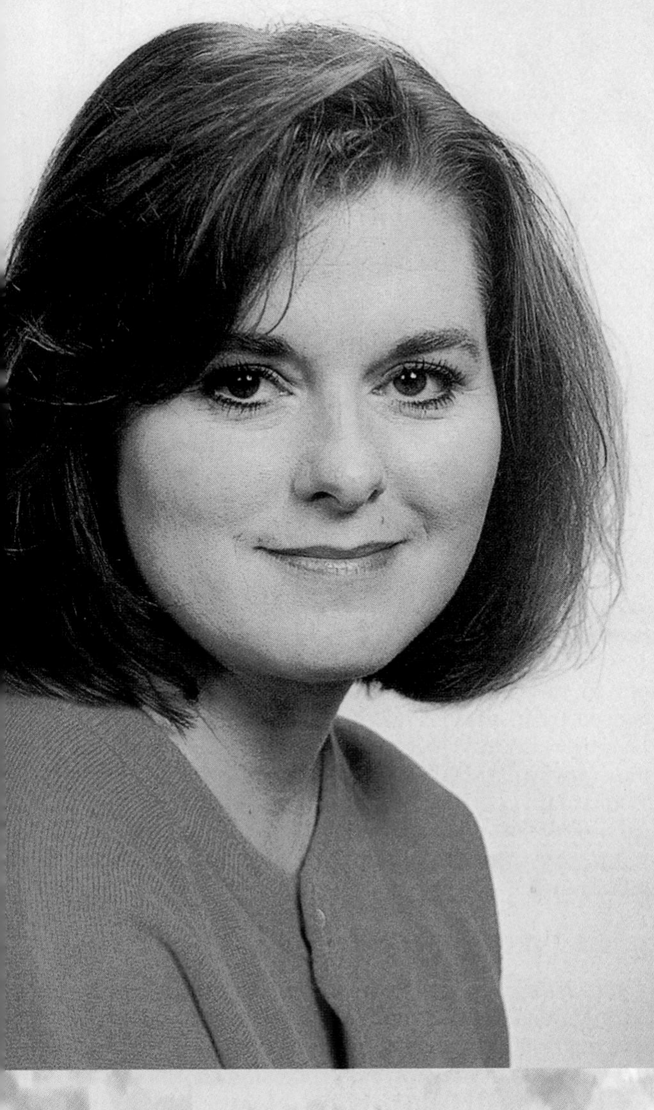

In 1989 I began my career in the medical field by taking a medical record and filing position with a private office. To expand my experience, I took a receptionist position in another practice and quickly took on responsibilities of billing and collections.

While working, I attained an accounting degree and did additional coursework in billing and medical terminology, as well as diagnostic and procedural coding.

In 1998 I began my tenure as operations manager with a family practice group. By combining education with practical experience, I have been able to enjoy a challenging career as operations manager overseeing a staff of twenty. I manage all aspects of day-to-day office operations, from patient reception to medical records and billing.

My current position constantly tests my working knowledge of PPOs, HMOs, and private pay health plans.

Holley Romero
Operations Manager
Family Practice Group

Fees: Private Insurance and Managed Care

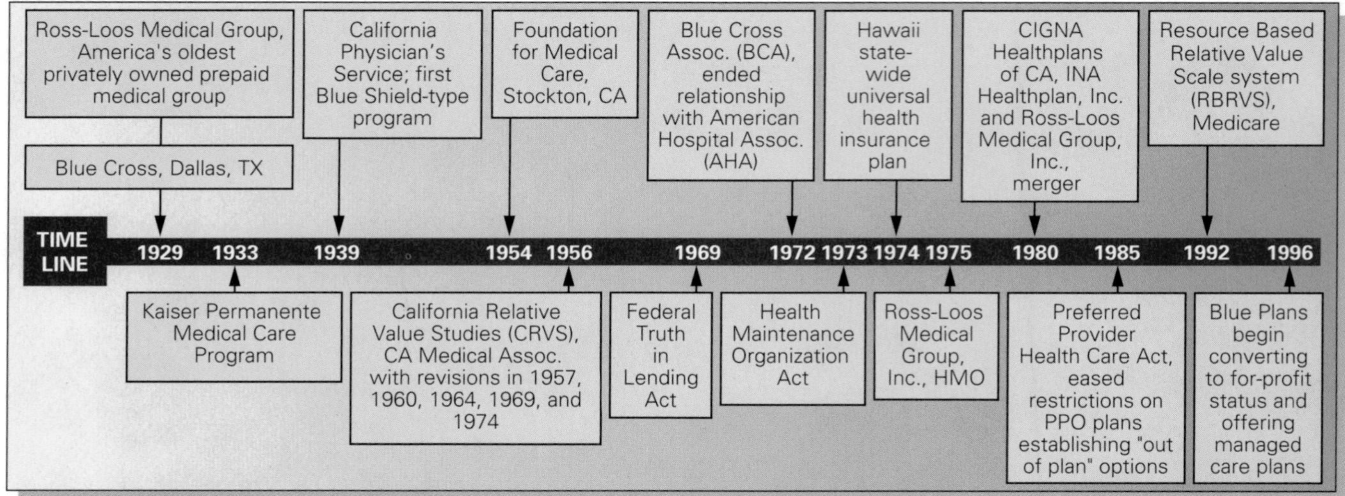

PRIVATE INSURANCE VERSUS MANAGED CARE PLANS

There are numerous private insurance companies and managed care plans with whom the physician may contract and send health insurance claims to. This chapter will explain the difference between private insurance and managed care, contract insurance and noncontract insurance, and fee-for-service reimbursement versus managed care capitation.

Participating Provider

A **participating provider (par),** has a contractual agreement with an insurance plan to render care to eligible beneficiaries and bill the insurance carrier directly. Each insurance carrier determines an **allowed amount** that it will pay for each procedure or service. The reimbursement is sent directly to the physician. The insurance carrier pays its portion of the allowed amount (e.g., 80%) and the provider bills the patient for the patient's portion of the allowed amount (e.g., 20%). The disallowed portion is the difference between the billed amount and the allowed amount (see Example 9–1) and is adjusted off (written off) of the account as a contract adjustment. Plans refer to participating providers as *member physicians, network physicians,* or *participating physicians.* With some insurance contracts the physician accepts the insurance reimbursement as payment in full and may not bill patients for amounts not covered by insurance.

It is important to refer to carrier provider manuals to obtain information on each contracted insurance, private or managed care. For easy reference, a summary of important information can be abstracted and included on an Insurance Plan Summary Sheet, as seen in Figure 9–1.

Nonparticipating Provider

A *nonparticipating provider* (nonpar) is a physician without a contractual agreement with an insurance plan. Nonparticipating providers are referred to as *out of network* providers and may or may not file an insurance claim as a courtesy to the patient. Nonpar physicians usually expect full payment at the time of service. The portion of the physician's bill that the insurance company pays to nonpar physicians will be less than that paid to par physicians. Patients seeing nonpar physicians will pay higher coinsurance payment amounts.

For most private insurance companies with whom the provider does not have a contractual agreement,

Example 9–1

Insurance Calculations To Determine Payment

Procedure or Service	Billed Amount	Allowed Amount	Insurance Carrier's Portion of Allowed Amount	Patient's Portion of Allowed Amount	Disallowed Amount or Contract Adjustment
CPT Code 20670	$125	$100	80% = $80	20% = $20	$25
Removal of implant	Amount charged according to fee schedule	Amount determined by insurance plan	Percent of allowed amount paid by insurance plan	Percent of allowed amount paid by patient	Difference between billed amount and allowed amount $125.00 − 100.00 $ 25.00

Insurance Plan Summary Sheet

Name of Carrier: West Coast Insurance Company

Address: 5500 Pacific Coast Highway, Santa Monica, XY

Telephone number: (555) 890-4600 Contact person: Frances

Eligibility Phone No. (555) 890-4610 Claim Status Phone No. (555) 890-4612

Mailing Address for Claims:	**Mailing Address for Appeals:**
P O Box 4960	P O Box 4970
Santa Monica	Santa Monica
XY 12345	XY 12345
Fax Claims To: (555) 896-1234	Fax Appeals To: (555) 896-1234

Managers of Claim Processing/Provider Relations

Jeff Bentley

Contracted Plan Type:

HMO	Co-Pay: ☑ Yes ☐ No amount $15.00
PPO	Discount Percentage
(POS) Select	see attached fee schedule
INDEMNITY	Referrals Required ☑ Yes ☐ No

Contracted Facilities

Hospital: College Hospital Laboratory: College Laboratory

Radiology: College Radiology Other: Western Physical Therapy

Preauthorization Requirements:
(List all services/procedures that apply to practice)

Surgical procedures

Diagnostic testing over $500.00

P.T.

Contract Payment Promised By: 30 days from billing date
(time from date of service or from billing date)

Figure 9–1. Example of a completed Insurance Plan Summary Sheet used to enter important information for each plan that the physician participates in for easy reference.

accepting assignment means that the insurance check will be sent to the provider's office rather than to the patient. The difference between the billed amount and the carrier's allowed amount is not written off but collected from the patient, as well as any copayment or deductible.

PRIVATE INSURANCE

There are numerous private insurance companies across the United States that offer health insurance to individuals and groups, most offering a variety of managed care plans. **Blue Cross** and **Blue Shield** plans are a pioneer in private insurance and had a nonprofit status that made them unique for many years among all private insurance carriers. Blue Cross plans were originally founded to cover hospital expenses. Blue Shield plans were primarily established to cover physician services.

Beginning with the 21st century, on the national level the Blue Cross and Blue Shield Association is a single corporation covering hospital expenses, outpatient care, other institutional services, home care, dental benefits, and vision care. Most have converted to for-profit status and operate in much the same way as other private insurance carriers. In some areas they are separate organizations, in some situations they may compete against each other, and Blue Cross/Blue Shield may act as a Medicare fiscal intermediary in certain regions. Because of their emergence to become like other private insurance companies, they no longer have nationally recognized rules and regulations or standardized claim form guidelines. Therefore, they have contracts like other types of private and managed care plans and will not be listed separately when describing types of fee structures, network physicians, managed care plans, and guidelines for completing the HCFA-1500 insurance claim form.

Fee-for-Service

Until the early 1970s, most health insurance was private and delivered through traditional fee-for-service plans. When billing **fee-for-service,** a fee is charged for each professional service or procedure the physician performs. The fee is obtained from a fee schedule. *While completing exercises for College Clinic, you will be using the mock fee schedule located in Appendix B.*

Fee Schedule

A **fee schedule** is a listing of accepted charges or established allowances for specific medical procedures. Medical practices generally set up a fee schedule for private insurance companies; however, they may operate with more then one fee schedule depending on the diversity of the patients seen unless specific state laws restrict this practice. Following are examples of situations where multiple fee schedules may be used:

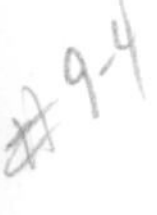

- Providers *participating* in the Medicare program would typically have a fee schedule listing "participating provider" fees for Medicare patients and a fee schedule for other private patients (see Medicare "Participating" mock fees in Appendix B).
- Providers seeing Medicare patients but *not participating* in the Medicare program would typically have two fee schedules, one based on limiting charges for each service set by the Medicare program, and one used for non-Medicare private patients (see Medicare "Nonparticipating" and "Limiting Charge" mock fees in Appendix B).
- Providers having a contractual arrangement with a managed care plan (e.g., HMO, PPO, IPA) would probably have additional fee schedules besides the one for private patients.
- Providers rendering services to patients who have sustained industrial accidents and illnesses would use a separate workers' compensation fee schedule (see Chapter 13).

Under federal regulations, a sign posted in the office along with a list, description, and fees for the most common services (including procedure code numbers) the physician offers must be available to all patients. It is important to determine which fee schedule applies to a patient before quoting fees and stating policies regarding the collection of fees. The physician may want to evaluate all fee schedules annually to determine if fees need to increase because of a rise in the cost of living. Whenever the fee schedule is changed, a notice should be placed in the reception room and a written communication sent to patients.

Determining Fees

There are a number of methods used to determine fees. Following is a brief description of two of the most common ways fees are determined.

Usual, Customary, and Reasonable

A complex system, in which three fees are considered in calculating payment is referred to as **usual, customary, and reasonable (UCR).** The *usual* fee (submitted fee) is the fee that a physician usually charges for a given service to a private patient. A fee is *customary* if it falls within the range of usual fees charged by providers of similar training and experience in a geographic area. Insurance companies often refer to this as the history of charges. The *reasonable* fee is the fee that meets the aforementioned criteria or is, in the opinion of the medical review committee, justifiable considering the special circumstances of the case. The lower of the two fees (usual and customary) determines the insurance company's approved or allowed amount on which reimbursement is based.

Many private health insurance plans that use this method of reimbursement will pay a physician's full charge if it does not exceed the UCR fee. If the physician's UCR fees are significantly lower than those of other practices in his or her area, document this and ask the insurance carrier for a review and possible adjustment to increase the physician's fee profile.

Two other factors that some insurance companies consider while assigning UCR fees are the actual and prevailing charge. The **actual charge** is the amount a physician actually bills a patient for a particular proce-

Example 9–2

Relative Value Scale

Procedure Code	Description Of Service	Unit Value
10060	Incision and drainage of cyst	0.8

Using a hypothetical figure of $153 per unit, this procedure would be valued at $122.40.

Math: $\$153.00 \times 0.8 = \$122.40$

Formula To Calculate Payment Using RBRVS

Code		Work		Overhead		Malpractice	
91000	RVUs	1.04		0.70		0.06	
	GAF*	× 1.028		× 1.258		× 1.370	
		1.07	+	0.88	+	0.08	= Total adjusted RVUs, 2.03

For 2002, the Conversion Factor for nonsurgical care is
$36.1992 × 2.03 = Allowed amount $73.48

** The medical practice location is Oakland, California*

Figure 9–2. Example of a formula used to calculate the fee for a specific procedure using the Resource-Based Relative Value Scale system.

dure or service. The **prevailing charge** is a charge that falls within the range of charges most frequently used in one local area for a particular medical service or procedure. Note that this is a general definition of UCR and various programs may define it in different ways.

Increasing numbers of plans are beginning to discontinue the UCR system and are adopting the Medicare Resource-Based Relative Value Scale (RBRVS) method for physician reimbursement. A description of this system follows the explanation of relative value studies.

Relative Value Studies

Relative value studies or scales (RVS), are a listing of coded procedures that are assigned *unit values* that indicate the relative value for each service performed. The time a service/procedure takes, as well as the skill involved to perform it, and the overhead costs that are required (e.g., business expenses and malpractice insurance) are three factors taken into account when determining the unit value (see Example 9–2).

A **conversion factor (CF)** is used, which is the dollar amount that is multiplied by each unit value in order to translate the actual units in the scale to dollar fees for each service. The units in this scale are based on median charges of all physicians during the time period in which the RVS was published. When used, insurance carriers pay a specific dollar amount for each unit listed. The dollar amounts may be different for each section of the CPT codebook (i.e., E/M, Anesthesia, Surgery, and so forth). These amounts are then computed for each procedure in the RVS codebook to determine fees.

It is legal to use an RVS guide for setting, realigning, or evaluating fees, as long as the physician does not enter into any price-fixing agreements.

Resource-Based Relative Value Scale

Resource-Based Relative Value Scale (RBRVS) is a type of RVS that was developed for the Centers for Medicare and Medicaid Services (CMS) to be used to devise a new type of Medicare fee schedule. The **relative value unit (RVU)** is based on (1) the amount of physician work RVU, (2) the practice expense RVU, and (3) the malpractice insurance RVU. Each local Medicare carrier adjusts the RVUs and determines a geographic adjustment factor (GAF) according to the cost of living in its region by using *geographic practice cost indices* (GPCIs), pronounced "gypsies." To convert a geographically adjusted relative value into a payment amount, a CF is used. This CF is updated to a new amount each year and published in Medicare bulletins and the *Federal Register* in November.

The formula for obtaining the Medicare fee involves three components: (1) a RVU for the service, (2) a GAF, and (3) a monetary CF. The formula looks like this:

RVU × GAF × CF = $ amount per Medicare service.

Figure 9–2 provides an example of calculating payment using the RBRVS system for one procedure (esophageal intubation).

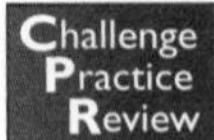

Pause and Practice CPR

PRACTICE SESSIONS 9–1 THROUGH 9–5

Directions: *Refer to listed examples and figures, as well as directions and explanation in the manuscript, to practice calculating fees for the physician's office.*

9–1 Refer to Example 9–1 and the section on "Participating Provider." The billed amount for a procedure is $220, the allowed amount is $180, and the insurance plan pays 80% of the allowed amount. The physician is a participating provider. Calculate the following:

(a) Insurance carrier's portion of allowed amount $ ____________

(b) Patient's portion of allowed amount $ ____________

(c) Difference between allowed amount and billed amount $ ____________

(d) Patient's responsibility $ ____________

(e) Total amount physician will receive $ ____________

(f) Disallowed portion (contract adjustment) $ ____________

9–2 The billed amount for a procedure is $160, the allowed amount is $135, and the insurance plan plays 70% of the allowed amount. The physician is a nonparticipating provider. Calculate the following:

(a) Insurance carrier's portion of allowed amount $ ____________

(b) Patient's portion of allowed amount $ ____________

(c) Difference between allowed amount and billed amount $ ____________

(d) Patient's responsibility $ ____________

(e) Total amount physician will receive $ ____________

(f) Disallowed portion (contract adjustment) $ ____________

9–3 If, for a specific procedure, the usual fee is $59 and the customary fee is $53, what is the reasonable fee that the insurance company would base its payment on? ____________

____

9–4 Refer to Example 9–2 and the explanation of the RVS system; then calculate the fee for a procedure having a unit value of 0.6 and a price of $125 per unit. ____________

9–5 Refer to the Formula to Calculate Payment Using RBRVS in Figure 9–2. Using the geographic adjustment factors (GAFs) shown in Figure 9–2, and the following relative value unit (RVU) figures, calculate the physician's fee.

(a) Work RVU 13.25 × GAF = ____________

(b) Overhead RVU 7.13 × GAF = ____________

(c) Malpractice RVU 1.42 × GAF = ____________

(d) Total adjusted RVU ____________

(e) Allowed amount (CF$36.1992) ____________

CHECK YOUR HEARTBEAT! Turn to the end of the chapter for answers to these practice sessions.

Copayments

As mentioned in Chapter 2, a *copayment* can be either a percentage of the fee (e.g., 20%) referred to as *coinsurance* payment, or a specific dollar amount (e.g., $5, $10, $15). Fixed copayments should be collected at the time of service, before the patient is seen. Percentage copayments are usually collected after the insurance company has paid its portion of the bill. If coinsurance payments are collected up front, it is wise to check the insurance contract to verify that this is legal.

Discounted Fees

A physician may choose to discount his or her fees for various reasons. A **discount** is a reduction of the normal fee and is based on a specific amount of money or a percentage of the charge. When a physician offers a discount, it must apply to the total amount of the bill, not just the portion that is paid by the patient, copayment or coinsurance amount. By following this rule, the physician is giving a discount both to the patient and to the insurance company. This practice could reduce the physician's fee profile with the insurance company and trigger a reduction in the physician's allowable reimbursement schedule; therefore, the physician should consider the outcome of discounting fees. All discounts must be noted on the patient's account/ledger (Example 9–3), and any financial reasons or special circumstances need to be documented in the patient's medical record. This will ensure complete

Example 9–3

Ledger

Date	Reference	Professional Service Description	Charge		Credits: Payments		Credits: Adjustments		Current Balance	
8/1/XX	99205	Level 5 NP	132	28					132	28
8/1/XX	Ck # 977	ROA Pt			92	60			39	68
8/1/XX	Discount 30%	Financial hardship					39	68	0	00

record keeping and safeguard any questions that may be brought up during a financial audit. Office policies regarding adjustments and discounts should be in writing, and all staff members informed.

Physician Profile

A **physician's fee profile** is a compilation of each physician's charges for specific professional services and the payments made to the physician over a given period of time. Each insurance company keeps a profile of compiled data (fees charged, procedure and diagnostic codes) on every provider for services that are processed for statistical purposes. As charges are increased or decreased, so are payments, and the profile is continually updated through the use of statistical computer data. To ensure accuracy of future profiles, it is important that the insurance billing specialist always use specific procedure and diagnostic codes, and not routinely discount fees.

Cash Discounts

Cash discounts may be offered (5%–20%) to patients who pay the entire fee, in cash, at the time of service. If a cash discount system is used, this policy should be posted in the office and every active patient sent notification.

Discount Clubs

An increase in both the number of uninsured patients and out-of-pocket expenses has incited several companies to form discount clubs that offer savings on doctor visits, prescription drugs, and other medical services. Patients can purchase annual memberships; fees range from $10 to $50. Members go to participating physicians and use their discount cards to pay on the spot, receiving discounts ranging from 10% to 70%.

Financial Hardship

The insurance billing specialist should never assume anything about a patient's financial status or judge the patient's ability to pay by his or her appearance. The physician needs to establish criteria to determine financial hardship that are the same for all patients requesting this type of discount. The Department of Health and Human Services annually publishes financial figures to be used as a guideline for poverty income in the Federal Register. This helps determine eligibility for uncompensated services for various federal programs. Physicians may access this information via the Federal Register on the Internet. These guidelines may be followed to direct patients to government-sponsored programs, to obtain public assistance, and to determine who is eligible for a hardship waiver which can vary from 25% to 100% of the bill. In order for the physician to make a reliable decision, patients seeking hardship waivers should sign a written explanation stating their financial hardship and be willing to bring in their wage and tax statement (W2 form), or tax return. The reason for a fee reduction must be noted in the patient's medical record. This will help in the collection process and allow the physician to accept the insurance as payment in full, in certain circumstances, without being suspected of insurance fraud.

Account Adjustments

A **courtesy adjustment** (write-off) is done for a debt that has been determined to be uncollectable and is therefore taken off (subtracted/credited) the accounting books. It is considered lost income but *may not* be claimed as a loss for tax purposes. The insurance specialist should obtain financial information on all patients who request a write-off. The physician must approve the portion of the charge to be credited to the financial record before the debt is forgiven.

A **contractual adjustment** is made when an insurance company has paid the *allowed* portion of a charge. The difference between the allowed amount and the billed amount is written off the accounting books as agreed upon in the insurance contract with the physician (refer to Example 9–1).

Professional Courtesy

Professional courtesy means making no charge to anyone, patient or insurance company, for medical care. The practice of professional courtesy is an old concept that was first established to build bonds between physicians and to reduce the incentive for physicians to treat their own families. It was often extended to others in the healthcare profession and to members of the clergy. Today, most physicians have insurance coverage for medical expenses and have since given up the practice of free care.

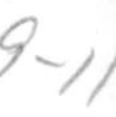

The law does not provide exceptions that allow professional courtesy to physicians in situations where the same courtesy could not be extended to *all* patients. Physicians must examine their policies on professional courtesy to ensure that they do not violate either the contractual terms in private or managed care insurance policies or Medicare/Medicaid laws and regulations.

No Charge

No charge (NC) means waiving the entire fee for professional care. However, it is considered different from professional courtesy and is permitted as long as it is *offered to all patients* and is not part of a fraudulent scheme. All NC visits must be fully documented in the clinical portion of the patient's medical record and in the financial record. An example of this would be free blood pressure checks for all patients.

Another instance when NC would occur on a patient's account is when follow-up visits are posted after a patient undergoes surgery that is considered under a surgical package or Medicare global fee structure. When posting such transactions in a computer system, CPT code 99024 (postoperative follow-up visits included in global fee) may be used.

Deductible and Copayment Waivers

Waiving deductible and copayment amounts is another way physicians have reduced the cost of medical care for patients in the past. By doing this, the physician accepts the insurance payment only and may be accused of not treating others with the same insurance coverage in an equal manner. A physician or insurance specialist cannot assess a fee for services for which the insurance company does not approve as a way of trying to satisfy a patient's deductible.

In most situations, both private insurers and the federal government ban waiving deductibles and copayments. It is, therefore, not recommended. There is one exception to this rule: Medicare recognizes a credit adjustment for this purpose on a doctor-to-doctor basis.

Reduced Fee

Fee adjustments have already been discussed; however, reduction of fees for other reasons needs to be addressed. Precautions need to be taken before reducing the fee of a patient who dies. The doctor's sympathy in this case could be misinterpreted and result in a malpractice suit. A fee reduction should never be based on a poor result in the treatment of a patient.

If a patient is disputing a fee and the physician agrees to settle for a reduced fee, the agreement should be in writing with a definite time limit for payment and the words "without prejudice" inserted. By doing this, the physician protects the right to collect the original sum if the patient fails to pay the reduced fee. The physician and the patient should sign the agreement and each receive a copy.

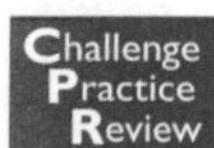

Pause and Practice CPR

REVIEW SESSIONS 9–6 THROUGH 9–9

Directions: *Complete the following questions as a review of information you have just read.*

9–6 Name two types of copayments.

(a) ______________________

(b) ______________________

9–7 State two criteria the patient must meet to receive a cash discount, and two criteria the office policy should incorporate before offering a cash discount.

(a) ______________________

(b) ______________________

(c) ______________________

(d) ______________________

9–8 A write-off that is made according to the insurance contract when the insurance company has paid its portion of the allowed amount is called a ______________________.

9–9 In most situations, how do private insurance carriers and the federal government view waiving of deductibles and copayment amounts? ______________________

CHALLENGE SESSION 9–10

Directions: *Study the information presented about the physician's fee profile and use critical thinking skills to answer the following question.*

9–10 If a physician routinely discounts fees to patients, how would this affect his or her fee profile, the physician's reimbursement, and why? ______________________________

____

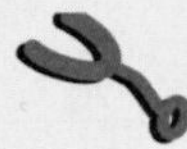

CHECK YOUR HEARTBEAT! Turn to the end of the chapter for answers to these review and challenge sessions.

Communicating Fees

People have a difficult time talking about financial obligations and asking each other for money. Financial arrangements should be discussed up front and in great detail before any services are provided. Many medical practices create their own collection problems by not being clear about *how* and *when* they expect to be paid. If you do not tell patients that payment is due at the time of service, most will assume they can pay at a later time. Following are some guidelines to help communicate effectively about money.

1. Request money using a firm, business-like approach.
2. State the payment policy, informing each patient of the fee and any deductible and balance due in a clear manner.
3. Verify the patient's copayment listed on his or her insurance card and collect this amount before the patient is seen.
4. Be courteous at all times regardless of how the patient responds; never offend, badger, or intimidate a patient into paying.
5. Make it more likely for the patient to pay, rather than leave without making payment, by *not* asking if they would like to pay now or have a bill sent.
6. Motivate the patient to pay by appealing to his or her honesty, integrity, and pride.

Following are examples of communicating in a positive manner and letting the patient know exactly what is expected.

- "The office visit is $62, Mrs. Smith. Would you like to pay by cash, check, or credit card?"
- "Your copayment will be $10, Mr. Jones. I will be collecting it prior to your office visit."
- "Miss Rodriguez, your insurance policy shows a deductible of $100 that has not been met. This is your responsibility so you will need to pay the full fee today, which is $75. An insurance claim will be submitted so that the amount paid can be applied toward your deductible."

Collecting Fees

Payment at Time of Service

Patients do not make healthcare bills a priority, so the importance of collecting outstanding bills, copayments, coinsurance amounts, and money from cash-paying patients up front should be communicated to office staff. Collect all fixed copayments before the patient is seen to alleviate billing for small amounts.

One-on-one communication is the best way to motivate a debtor. Be prepared by reviewing each patient's account **balance** (amount due) before his or her appointment. If the appointment schedule is on a computer system, print the account balance by each patient's name. If an appointment book is used, make a copy of the page showing the day's schedule and write overdue balances obtained from the ledger card by each patient's name. This information should also be recorded on the transaction slip for that day's visit and may be "flagged" when the transaction slips are printed or written. Treat this information confidentially by keeping it out of view of other patients. When a patient arrives whose name is flagged, alert the Patient Accounts Manager.

To maintain confidentiality and assure effective preappointment collection counseling, the patient should be led to a quiet area away from the general activity of the office. Sit down with the patient and discuss the situation. Use an understanding attitude and project a helpful nature while verbalizing phrases such as "I understand" and "I can help." Ask direct questions to learn exactly what problems the patient is facing. Answers to questions such as "What resources do you have available to pay your bill?" and "How much are you able to pay and how soon?" will help determine your strategy. Your goal should be to try and collect the full amount. If that is not possible, try to collect a portion of the balance. Get a promise to pay for the remaining balance by a specific date. If the patient is unable to comply, then set up a payment plan. The chances of reaching a mutually satisfactory resolution are greatly improved when the two parties are face to face. Document whatever agreement is reached in writing. Payment plans are discussed in Chapter 14.

Patient Excuses

Do not miss the opportunity to ask for payment at the time of service. Nonpayers show a tendency to dismiss financial arrangements with curt remarks. Look directly at the patient, and be confident in your expectation to collect payment. Demonstrate to the patient that you feel secure in knowing you have the right to request payment. If excuses are offered, be prepared to respond to them. Table 9–1 shows some examples of patients' excuses and possible responses.

When a patient chatters nervously it may be a way of setting up reasons to rationalize not paying. Do not

Table 9–1 Responses to Patients Avoiding Payment

Excuse	Response
"Just bill me."	"As we explained when we made your appointment, Mr. Barkley, our practice bills for charges over $50. Amounts under $50 are to be paid at the time of the visit. That will be $25 for today's visit please."
"I have insurance to cover this."	"We will be billing your insurance for you, Miss Butler, but your policy shows a deductible in the amount of $300 that still needs to be met. We need to collect the full fee for today's visit, which is $150, to meet that deductible responsibility."
"I get paid on Friday; you know how it is."	"I understand. Why don't you write the check today and postdate it for Saturday. We will hold the check and deposit it on the next business day" (depending on office policy).
"If I pay for this I won't be able to pay for the prescription."	"Our payment policy is very much like the pharmacy; we expect payment at the time of service. Let me check and see if the doctor can dispense some medication samples to last you until you can get your prescription filled."
"I don't have that much with me."	"How much can you pay, Mrs. Fish? I can accept $10 now and give you an envelope to send us the balance within the week, or I can put it on your credit card."
"I'll take care of it."	"I know you will, Mr. Stone; I just need to know when that will be so I can document your intentions for our bookkeeper." (Get a commitment and write down the date on a tickler calendar or on the patient's ledger card while in view of the patient. Hand him or her an envelope with the amount due written under the sealing flap.)
"I forgot my checkbook."	"We take Visa, MasterCard, and American Express, Mr. Storz." (If the patient still does not pay, provide him with a self-addressed envelope and write the patient's name, account number, date of service, amount due, and expected payment date under the sealing flap. Restate the expected payment date as you hand the patient the envelope. Note the date on a tickler calendar or on the patient's ledger card while the patient is watching.)

let this distract you. Pause after asking for payment and do not say another word until the patient responds. Many people feel uncomfortable with silence, but pauses may work to your advantage and help you complete a transaction. By taking this approach you will help increase the cash flow and collection ratio, while decreasing billing chores and collection costs. You will also be able to quickly identify nonpayers and notify the person responsible for collections.

Payment by Check

Check Verification

A personal check is the most common method of payment in most medical offices, but it is not a personal guarantee of payment. Check verification requires the insurance specialist to become familiar with the appearance of a good check. A driver's license and one other form of identification should always be required. Check these against existing records. Call the bank to verify all out-of-state and suspicious checks. A verification service, which is a private company with resources to quickly identify patient information over the telephone, or a check authorization system, may be worthy of consideration for clinics and larger group practices.

Check Forgery

Forgery is false writing or alteration of a document to injure another person or with intent to deceive (e.g., signing, without permission, another person's name on a check to obtain money or to pay off a debt). To guard against forgery, always check to be sure the endorsement on the back of the check matches the name on the front. It may also be checked against the patient's signature on the patient registration form. Be suspicious if the beneficiary or provider states that he or she did not receive the check but the insurance company shows it as being cashed, or if the payee of the check claims that the signature is not his or hers.

Unsigned Checks

If you discover that a check has not been signed, you can ask the patient to come to the office and sign the check or send a new one. If you are unable to reach the patient or if there is a transportation or time limitation problem, you can write the word "over" or "see reverse" on the signature line on the front of the check. On the back of the check, where the endorsement would appear, write "lack of signature guaranteed," your practice's name, and your name and title. Your endorsement is, in effect, a guarantee that you

Expressions from Experience

As operations manager, I am charged with maintaining the often-complex relationships among the patient, the patient's health insurance carrier, and our family practice group. I use interpersonal and supervisory skills to encourage my staff to focus on teamwork, customer service, and exemplary patient care. I try to set an example of integrity and professionalism in conducting business with the variety of health care providers.

Holley Romero
Operations Manager
Family Practice Group

will absorb the loss if the patient or the patient's bank does not honor the check.

Returned Checks

When the physician's office receives notice that a check was not honored, the reason should be stated on the back of the check. The most common reason is nonsufficient funds (NSF). Call the bank or patient to see if redepositing it is suggested. It may be an oversight or miscalculation by the patient. If it is not worth redepositing, or you receive a second NSF notice, call the patient immediately. Be courteous but straight to the point. Inform the patient that payment is due by cash, money order, or certified check within 3 days. If you do not receive restitution within 3 days, you need to start the legal process of notifying the patient in writing. Send an NSF demand letter (Fig. 9–3) by certified mail with return receipt requested, and include the following:

1. Check date
2. Check number
3. Bank the check is drawn on
4. The payee
5. Check amount
6. Any allowable service charge
7. Total amount due
8. Number of days the check writer has to take action

Once a patient has been informed of the returned check, explain that your facility will no longer be able to accept checks as payment. Future payments need to be in the form of cash, money order, or a cashier's check. It the patient wishes the check returned, photocopy it and keep it in the financial record because it serves as an acknowledgment of the debt. The bad check may be returned to the patient after it has been replaced with a valid payment. Place a notation on the patient's record to this effect.

To guard against bad checks, it is wise to consider a check authorization system. To help discourage bad checks, charge a penalty for returned checks. This information should be included in the new patient brochure and posted in the office for all patients to

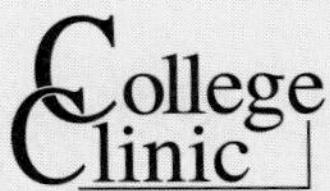

4567 Broad Avenue
Woodland Hills, XY 12345-0001
Tel. (555) 486-9002
FAX (555) 487-8976

August 15, 20XX

Mrs. Maxine Holt
444 Labina Lane
Woodland Hills, XY 12345-0001

Dear Mrs. Holt:

The following check has been dishonored by the bank and returned without payment:

Date:	08/04/20XX
Check No.:	755
Amount:	$106.11
Payable to:	Perry Cardi, MD
Bank:	Woodland Hills National Bank
Reason:	Nonsufficient funds

This is a formal notice demanding payment in the amount of $106.11 within 15 days from today's date or your account will be considered for legal action.

Please make payment immediately by cash, cashier's check, or money order at the above address. Your immediate attention will be appreciated.

Sincerely,

Delores Yee, CMA-A

Patient Accounts Manager
for Perry Cardi, MD

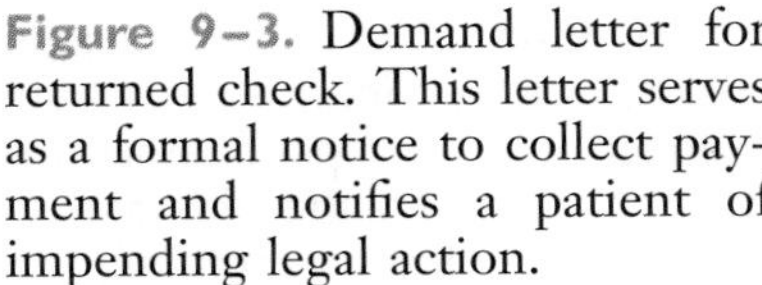

Figure 9–3. Demand letter for returned check. This letter serves as a formal notice to collect payment and notifies a patient of impending legal action.

view. You may need to make reference to the particular section of your state's civil codes provisions regarding checks for nonsufficient funds if you want to collect more than the face value of the check.

If you are notified that the checking account is closed, do not waste time trying to contact the patient. Send a demand letter immediately. In most states, if the patient has not responded in 30 days, legal action can be taken. Consider filing a claim in small claims court. Most states have written codes or statutes pertaining to bad checks. Often legislation allows the creditor to add punitive damages to the amount of the debt being collected, sometimes up to three times the amount of the check.

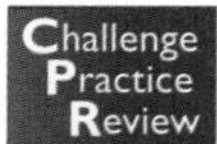

Pause and Practice CPR

REVIEW SESSIONS 9–11 THROUGH 9–14

Directions: *Complete the following questions as a review of information you have just read.*

9–11 Patients can be motivated to pay by appealing to their ________________, ________________, and ________________.

9–12 How can you prepare to collect money from a patient prior to his or her arrival at the office for an appointment? ________________

9–13 What is the best time to ask for payment? ________________

9–14 What is the most common method of payment in the physician's office? ________________

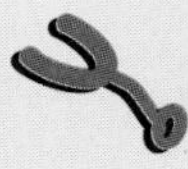

CHECK YOUR HEARTBEAT! Turn to the end of the chapter for answers to these review sessions.

MANAGED CARE

Over the past 60 years there have been many reforms of the healthcare system. Medical practices have made transitions from rural to urban, from generalist to specialist, from solo to group practice, and from fee-for-service to capitated reimbursement. The expansion of healthcare plans to a number of different types of delivery systems that try to manage the cost of healthcare resulted in managed care.

Health maintenance organizations (HMOs) were the first type of **managed care organization (MCO)** developed to control the expenditure of healthcare dollars and manage patient care. At the inception of managed care, one would use the term HMO when referring to all managed care; therefore, early managed care laws and regulations have been structured to also use this term.

In prepaid group plans, patients join the plan and pay monthly medical insurance premiums, either individually or through their employer. Physicians join the managed care plan and patients choose a physician from the list of contracted network physicians to manage all of their healthcare needs. The physician renders service to the patient, and the patient usually pays a small copayment and occasionally a deductible as required by the plan. Providers that join the plan are referred to as *preferred providers* and are paid using the capitation method. For individuals who have signed with a managed care plan, the assignment of benefits is automatic and all reimbursement is sent directly to the physician.

Eligibility

Those who have voluntarily enrolled in an HMO plan from a specific geographic area (service area) or who are covered by an employer who has paid an established sum per person to be covered by the plan are eligible. The law states that an employer employing 25 or more persons may offer the services of an HMO as an alternative health plan for employees. Medicare and Medicaid beneficiaries may also become members of managed care plans whether retired or employed.

Primary Care Physician

Most managed care plans use a **primary care physician (PCP)** as a gatekeeper. A **gatekeeper** is a physician who controls patient access to specialists and diagnostic testing services. PCPs are physicians who try to take care of most of the patient's needs. They usually practice in the fields of internal medicine, family practice, general practice, or pediatrics. Although obstetrics and gynecology (OB-GYN) is considered specialty care, the OB-GYN physician may be contracted as a PCP by some plans.

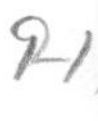

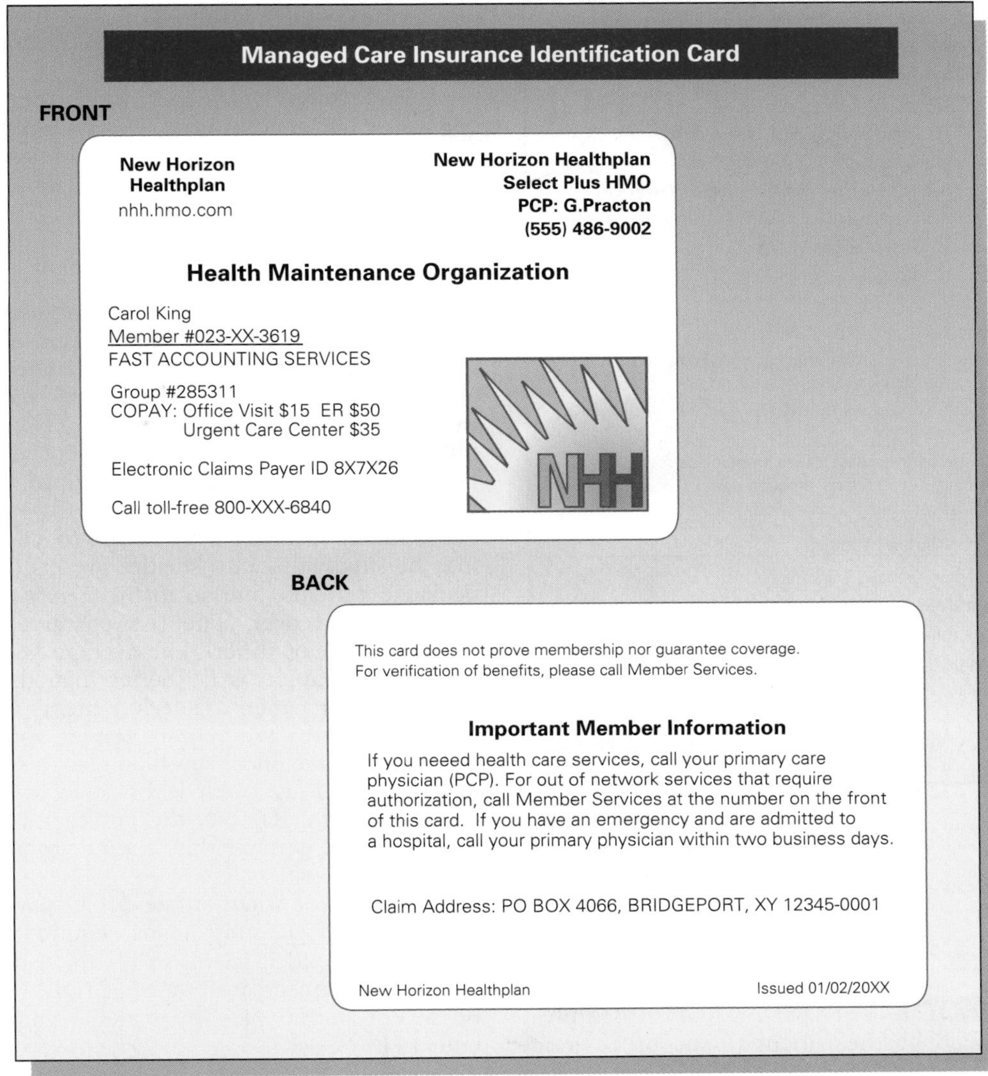

Figure 9–4. Front (top) and back (bottom) sides of a managed care insurance card.

Identification Card

Each enrollee of a managed care plan is given an identification card, as shown in Figure 9–4. The card usually lists the group number, member number, and primary care physician. The name of the MCO and the abbreviation for the type of plan with the amount of copayment for various outpatient services (e.g., hospital, emergency room, office visit, urgent care center, and pharmacy) are also included.

Photocopy both sides of the patient's card because the insurance address, telephone numbers used for inquiries and authorizations, or other important information may be listed on the front and/or back of the card.

Benefits

Benefits under the HMO act fall under two categories: basic and supplemental health services. These are listed in Table 9–2.

Future of Managed Care

Much has been printed in the last few years regarding the viability of managed care. Prices have been undercut to compete with the market share of patients seeking affordable healthcare and this has had a negative effect on the profitability of many managed care firms. The increased competition, along with the rising costs of healthcare, has forced many MCOs to offer "open access." Plans with more options and less reliance on the primary care physician are beginning to take over and premiums, no doubt, will increase.

Financial Management

Payment of Deductibles

Usually, there is no deductible for patients who belong to a managed care plan. However, if there is one (e.g., POS and PPO plans), be sure to collect it in the early

Table 9–2 Health Maintenance Organization Act Benefits of 1973

Basic Health Services
Alcohol, drug abuse, and addiction medical treatment
Dental services (preventive) for children younger than age 12 years
Diagnostic laboratory, x-ray, and therapeutic radiology services
Emergency health services in or out of the HMO service area
Family planning and infertility services
Health education and medical social services
Home health services
Hospital services (inpatient and outpatient)
Mental health services on an outpatient basis, short-term (not to exceed 20 visits) ambulatory, evaluative, and crisis intervention
Physicians' services and consultant or referral services without time or cost limits
Preventive health services (e.g., physical examinations for adults, vision and hearing tests for children through age 17 years, well-baby care, immunizations, health education).
Supplemental Health Services
Dental care not included in basic benefits
Extended mental health services not included in basic benefits
Eye examinations for adults
Intermediate and long-term care (nursing facilities and nursing homes)
Prescription drugs
Rehabilitative services and long-term physical medicine (e.g., physical therapy)

months of the year (January through April) by asking patients if they have met their deductible.

Copayment

In a managed care plan, a copayment (copay) is a predetermined fee paid by the patient to the provider at the time service is rendered. It is a form of cost sharing because the managed care plan or insurance company pays the remaining cost.

Always collect the copay when the patient arrives for his or her appointment. Copays are commonly collected for office visits, urgent care visits, emergency department visits, prescription drugs, and inpatient mental health services.

Capitation

Capitation is a system of payment used by managed care plans in which physicians and hospitals are paid a fixed per capita amount for each patient enrolled over a stated period of time, regardless of the type and number of services provided. The HMOs are also reimbursed by the federal government on a per capita basis. Patients are usually divided into two basic categories, commercial and senior. *Commercial* patients range in age from birth up to age 65 years. This group may be subdivided into smaller groups (e.g., newborns, pediatric patients, and so forth). *Senior* patients are 65 years old and over. The risk characteristics of these two basic groups differ. The average health status of a commercial patient is far better than the typically less healthy senior patient. Elderly patients are hospitalized more frequently and require longer appointments because they have more problems to discuss, ask more questions, and are often less rushed for time. Because of these varying factors, the per capita payment for a senior patient is more than the per capita payment for a commercial patient.

Regardless of whether the MCO pays by capitation or fee-for-service, most plans require that the physician's office send in claim forms for each patient seen. The claim form creates an audit trail which is used to verify use of the plan by patients and track services rendered.

Challenge Practice Review

Pause and Practice CPR

REVIEW SESSIONS 9–15 THROUGH 9–17

Directions: *Complete the following questions as a review of information you have just read.*

9–15 Name five situations where copayments are commonly collected.

(a) ______________________

(b) ______________________

(c) ______________________

(d) ______________________

(e) ______________________

9–16 Define capitation. ______________________

____

____

9–17 How many employees must an employer have to be able to offer an HMO plan to employees? __________

PRACTICE SESSIONS 9–18 THROUGH 9–22

Directions: *View Figure 9–4 and abstract information to answer the following questions.*

9–18 What type of managed care plan does the patient have? ____________________

9–19 What is the member and group number? ____________________

9–20 List the copayment amounts for: office visit ________, emergency room ________, urgent care center ________.

9–21 What telephone number should you call to receive authorization for out-of-network services? ____________________

9–22 What address should the claim be sent to? ____________________

____

CHALLENGE SESSION 9–23

Directions: *Refer to the section on capitation and use critical thinking skills to answer the questions presented in the following scenario.*

9–23 Nancy Darwin is a commercial patient enrolled in ABC Managed Care plan. Dr. Practon receives $36 per month capitation for commercial patients. In November, Nancy was completely healthy and did not have to go to the doctor. In December, Nancy got sick and saw Dr. Practon three times totaling $357. How much did her managed care plan pay Dr. Practon for (1) the month of November ____________, and (2) the month of December? ____________.

CHECK YOUR HEARTBEAT! Turn to the end of the chapter for answers to these review, practice, and challenge sessions.

Types of Managed Care Organizations

When referring to managed care and prepaid health plans (PHPs), not only is the health care delivery system different from traditional care but the financial structure also differs. Following are different types of managed care plans and discussion on how plans are administered and managed.

Health Maintenance Organizations

The oldest of all the prepaid health plans is the **health maintenance organization (HMO)** whose definition has evolved along with the changes in managed care. An HMO is a comprehensive healthcare financing and delivery organization that provides a wide range of healthcare services, with an emphasis on preventive medicine, to enrollees within a geographic area through a panel of providers. Physicians are usually reimbursed by a fixed periodic payment, called capitation, regardless of the amount of actual services used. If a health insurance carrier administers and manages the HMO, it contracts to pay in advance for the full range of health services to which the insured is entitled under the terms of the health insurance contract. Numerous HMOs are loosening up their requirements, so many different arrangements are now in place.

HMO Models

There are important differences in the structure of various HMOs that influence the way physicians practice and, perhaps, the quality of medical care delivered. Following are several types of HMO models.

PREPAID GROUP PRACTICE MODEL. The **prepaid group practice model** delivers services at one or more locations through a group of physicians who either (1) contract with the HMO to provide care, or (2) are employed by the HMO. For example, Kaiser Permanente is a prepaid group practice model where physicians form an independent group contract (Permanente) with a health plan (Kaiser) to provide medical treatment to members enrolled by the plans. Although the physicians work for a salary, it is paid by their own independent group, not by the administrators of the health plan. This is designed to permit the physicians to concentrate on medicine.

STAFF MODEL. The **staff model** is a type of HMO in which the health plan hires physicians directly and pays them a salary instead of contracting with a medical group.

NETWORK HMO. A **network HMO** contracts with two or more group practices to provide health services.

Competitive Medical Plan

A **competitive medical plan (CMP)** is a state-licensed health plan, similar to an HMO, that delivers comprehensive, coordinated services to voluntarily enrolled members on a prepaid, capitated basis. CMP status may be granted by the federal government for the enrollment of Medicare beneficiaries into managed care plans, without having to qualify as an HMO.

Exclusive Provider Organization

An **exclusive provider organization (EPO)** is a type of managed care plan that combines features of HMOs (e.g., enrolled population, limited provider network, gatekeepers, utilization management, capitation reimbursement, authorization system) and PPOs (e.g., flexible benefit design, negotiated fees, and fee-for-service payments). It is referred to as exclusive because it is offered to large employers who agree not to contract with any other plan. The member must choose medical care from network providers with certain exceptions for emergency or out-of-area services. If a patient decides to seek care outside the network, generally he or she will not be reimbursed for the cost of treatment. Technically, many HMOs can be considered EPOs. However, EPOs are regulated under insurance statutes rather than federal and state HMO regulations.

Foundations for Medical Care

Foundations for medical care (FMC) are organizations of physicians sponsored by a state or local medical association concerned with the development and delivery of medical services and the cost of healthcare.

Expressions from Experience

As the primary contact for a multitude of health insurance carriers, I recognize that I'm not just representing a family practice group, I'm also representing the patient. Anyone interested in the medical authorization process, insurance billing, and office management needs to demonstrate confidentiality, compassion, empathy, loyalty, and patience.

Holley Romero
Operations Manager
Family Practice Group

Foundations usually deal with employer groups, government groups, and county and city employees. However, a small percentage of plans are open to individual subscribers.

There are basically two types of foundations for medical care and each functions differently: (1) a *comprehensive type of foundation,* which designs and sponsors prepaid health programs or sets minimum benefits of coverage, and (2) a *claims-review type of foundation,* which provides evaluation of the quality and efficiency of services by a panel of physicians to the numerous fiscal agents or carriers involved in its area. These reviews are done for services and/or fees that exceed local community guidelines.

A key feature of the foundation is its dedication to an incentive reimbursement system. For a participating physician, income is received in direct proportion to the number of medical services delivered (i.e., fee-for-service) rather than payment through capitation. The FMC offers a managed care plan fee schedule to be used by member physicians. The patient is responsible for paying a deductible, coinsurance, and all nonbenefit items. The patient may or may not be billed for the difference between the charged amount and the allowed amount, depending on the plan.

The patient may select a member or nonmember physician. The member physician agrees to submit insurance claims directly to the foundation, and nonmember physicians may wish to collect directly from the patient. Claims are transmitted electronically, or submitted on the HCFA-1500 form.

Independent Practice Association

Another type of MCO is the **independent (or individual) practice association (IPA)** in which the physicians are not employees and are not paid salaries. Instead, they are paid for their services on a capitation or fee-for-service basis out of a fund drawn from the premiums collected from the subscriber, union, or corporation by an organization that markets the health plan. A discount of up to 30% is withheld to cover costs of operating the IPA. IPA physicians make contractual arrangements to treat HMO members out of their own offices. A participating physician may also treat non-HMO patients.

Physician Provider Group

A **physician provider group (PPG)** is a physician-owned business entity that has the flexibility to deal with all forms of contract medicine and still offer its own packages to business groups, unions, and the general public. One division may function as an IPA under contract to an HMO. Another section may act as the broker in a PPO that contracts with hospitals as well as other physicians to market services or medical supplies to employers and other third parties. And still another segment might participate in joint ventures with hospitals, laboratories, and so on.

The difference between an IPA and a PPG is that an IPA may not be owned by its member physicians whereas a PPG is physician-owned. The ability of the PPGs to combine services (joint purchasing, marketing, billing, collections, attorneys, and accountant fees) is an advantage because it cuts the cost of running a business and allows each physician to retain his or her own practice in addition to these joint ventures. The physicians turn over a small percentage of their income to the PPG for expenses. Patients call one telephone number to make appointments and the billing is done in one location.

Point-of-Service Plan

A **point-of-service plan (POS)** is a type of managed care plan in which members are given a choice as to how to receive services, whether through an HMO, PPO, or fee-for-service plan. The decision is made at the time the service is needed (i.e., "at the point of service"). A patient can refer himself or herself to a specialist or see a nonprogram provider for a higher coinsurance payment, thus being given an incentive to stay within the network. The key advantage of POS programs is the combination of HMO-style cost management and PPO-style freedom of choice. POS plans are also referred to as open-ended HMOs, swing-out HMOs, self-referral options, or multiple option plans.

Preferred Provider Organization

A **preferred provider organization (PPO)** is a form of contract medicine in which a large employer or organization, which can produce a large number of patients, contracts with a hospital or a group of physicians (designated as "preferred") to offer medical care at reduced rates. A PPO is not a prepaid plan, but uses utilization management techniques for long-term cost savings. PPO contracts offer a variety of health plans from which patients have free choice of providers, but are given financial incentives to use a preferred provider network. There are usually coinsurance requirements and deductibles. As with major medical policies, the coinsurance stipulation requires the patient to pay 20% to 25% of the allowed amount up to a certain dollar amount (e.g., $1,500). When the patient's out-of-pocket expenses reach that amount, then the PPO pays 100% of all charges after that.

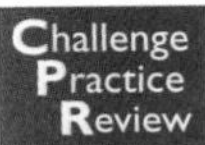

Pause and Practice CPR

REVIEW SESSIONS 9–24 THROUGH 9–27

Directions: *Complete the following questions as a review of information you have just read.*

9–24 What is the oldest type of prepaid health plan? ______________________

9–25 When a large employer contracts directly with an MCO to provide care and agrees not to contract with any other plan, this type of prepaid health plan is called a/an

______________________.

9–26 When a physician has a contractual arrangement to treat HMO members out of his or her own office and receive fee-for-service or capitated reimbursement, this type of arrangement is called a/an ______________________.

9–27 Which managed care plan offers flexibility, giving members a choice as to how they receive services (through an HMO, PPO, or fee-for-service plan)?

____

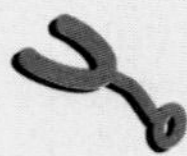

CHECK YOUR HEARTBEAT! Turn to the end of the chapter for answers to these review sessions.

Medical Review

Professional Review Organizations

A **professional review organization (PRO)** determines and assures the quality and operation of healthcare through a process called peer review. **Peer review** is an evaluation of the quality and efficiency of services rendered by a practicing physician. Practitioners in a managed care program may come under peer review by a PRO. In this type of review, one or more physicians working with the federal government use federal guidelines to evaluate another physician in regard to the quality and efficiency of professional care. The review may be used to examine evidence for admission and discharge of a hospital patient and to settle disputes on fees. PROs are not restricted to MCO programs; they also play a role in Medicare inpatient cases.

Utilization Review

In a managed care setting, a management system called **utilization review (UR),** or *utilization management,* is necessary to control costs. UR is a formal assessment of the cost and use of components of the healthcare system. The utilization review committee examines individual cases to determine the necessity for medical tests and procedures. It also watches over how providers use medical resources. If medical care, tests, or procedures are denied, then the patient's physician must inform the patient of the need for the denied service, the risks of not having it, and the cost and obligation to pay for the service.

Management of Plans

To make a knowledgeable financial decision on how a managed care plan will impact an existing medical practice, it is important to evaluate existing fees and contracts, know how to negotiate with managed care firms, weigh practice expansions (i.e., adding partners or other office locations), and understand managed care contracts.

Contracts

Before signing a contract with a managed care plan, a physician should have the contract reviewed by an attorney. Many clinics and large group practices hire administrators who have a legal background, which is helpful when deciphering the language in managed care contracts. When an MCO contracts with a physician group, several important considerations are:

1. How many patients will the MCO provide?
2. What is the per capita rate (capitation dollar amount per patient)?
3. What services are included in the capitated amount?

Carve-Outs

Medical services not included in the contract benefits are called **carve-outs.** Such services may be contracted for separately. For example, if an internist contracts with an MCO, all Evaluation and Management services as well as routine testing done by the internist (i.e., ECGs, spirometries, hematocrits, fasting blood sugar tests, and urinalyses) might be included in the capitation amount. Regardless of whether any MCO patients were seen, or whether any of these services were rendered, the physician would be paid a monthly capitated amount (e.g., $11 per capita) for each person who has signed up for the MCO plan. However, nonroutine or expensive tests (e.g., sigmoidoscopies) and hospital visits might be "carved out" of the contract and paid on a fee-for-service basis.

Preauthorization or Prior Approval

Most managed care plans require some type of prior approval for diagnostic services, hospitalization, and specialist care. In Chapter 2, preauthorization was defined. Following, are several types of referrals that a plan may use for different levels of prior approval.

1. **Formal referral**—Authorization request required by the MCO contract to determine medical necessity. This preauthorization may be obtained via telephone or a completed authorization form mailed or transmitted via fax (Fig. 9–5).
2. **Direct referral**—A simplified authorization request form is completed and signed by the physician and handed to the patient at the time of referral. Certain services may not require a formal referral (e.g., obstetric care, dermatology).
3. **Verbal referral**—The primary care physician informs the patient that he or she would like to refer them to a specialist. The physician telephones the specialist and indicates the patient is being referred for an appointment.
4. **Self-referral**—Patient refers himself or herself to a specialist. The patient may be required to inform the primary care physician. POS plans and some PPO plans use self-referral.

Patients may be unaware of preapproval requirements, and such requirements may change, so, as a precaution, ask the patient about insurance coverage at the time the appointment is made. If the patient is a member of a managed care plan, carefully review the patient's preauthorization requirements and if approval is needed for certain situations, inform the patient of this before he or she sees the physician.

If the patient has obtained written authorization for the appointment or procedure, then remind him or her to bring that document at the time of the scheduled visit. If the authorization is delayed and the patient comes in for the appointment, try to call the plan and obtain a verbal authorization. Document the date, time, authorization number, and name of the authorizing person. If the managed care plan refuses to authorize the service over the telephone, the patient either needs to sign a waiver indicating that if not approved he or she will pay for the service, or reschedule the appointment. More and more managed care companies are not issuing retroactive (after the fact) authorizations. All referral recommendations must be documented in the patient's record and, if applicable, sent to the referring physician. Approved authorization numbers need to be entered in Block 23 of the HCFA-1500 insurance claim form and a hard copy attached, if necessary.

A tracking system, such as a referral tracking log, needs to be in place for pending referrals so that care may be rendered in a timely manner and patients do not get lost in the system (Fig. 9–6). This log should include the date the authorization was requested, the patient's name, the procedure or consultant requested, and the insurance plan, as well as dates of follow-up, the name of the person who approved or denied request, and the appointment date for the consult or procedure. Sometimes authorization approvals are sent to the primary care physician and not to the refer-

Managed Care Plan
Treatment Authorization Request

TO BE COMPLETED BY PRIMARY CARE PHYSICIAN OR OUTSIDE PROVIDER

Health Net	☐	Met Life	☐
Pacificare	☐	Travelers	☒
Secure Horizons	☐	Pru Care	☐

Member No. 1357906

Patient Name: Louann Campbell Date: 7-14-20XX

M____ F X Birthdate 4-7-1952 Home telephone number 555-450-1666

Address 2516 Encina Avenue, Woodland Hills, XY 12345-0439

Primary Care Physician Gerald Practon, MD Provider ID# TC 14021

Referring Physician Gerald Practon, MD Provider ID# TC 14021

Referred to Raymond Skeleton, MD Address 4567 Broad Avenue

Woodland Hills, XY 12345-0001 Office telephone no. 555-486-9002

Diagnosis Code 724.2 Diagnosis Low back pain

Diagnosis Code 722.10 Diagnosis Sciatica

Treatment Plan: Orthopedic evaluation of lumbar spine R/O herniated disc L4, 5

Authorization requested for procedures/tests/visits:

Procedure Code 99244 Description New patient consultation

Procedure Code ________ Description ________

Facility to be used: ________ Estimated length of stay ________

Office ☒ Outpatient ☐ Inpatient ☐ Other ☐

List of potential consultants (i.e., anesthetists, assistants, or medical/surgical):

Raymond Skeleton, MD - Orthopedic

Physician's signature [signature]

TO BE COMPLETED BY PRIMARY CARE PHYSICIAN

PCP Recommendations: See above PCP Initials [initials]

Date eligibility checked 7-14-20XX Effective date 1-15-20XX

TO BE COMPLETED BY UTILIZATION MANAGEMENT

Authorized ________ Not authorized ________

Deferred ________ Modified ________

Authorization Request# ________

Comments: ________

Figure 9–5. Example of a managed care plan treatment authorization request form completed by a primary care physician for preauthorization of a professional service.

Authorization Request Log

Date requested	Patient name	Procedure/ consult	Insurance plan	1st F/U	2nd F/U	3rd F/U	Approved	Scheduled date
2/8/XX	Juan Percy	Bone scan- full body	Health Net	2/20			J. Smith	2/23/XX
2/8/XX	Nathan Takai	MRI-L-knee	Pru-Care	2/20	3/3			
2/9/XX	Lori Smythe	Consult-Neuro G. Frankel MD	FHP	2/22			T. Hope	2/26/XX
2/10/XX	Bob Mason	Cervical collar	Secure Horizons	2/22	3/5	3/19		

Figure 9–6. Example of an authorization request log to be used as a system for tracing referral of patients for diagnostic testing, consultations, and procedures.

ring/ordering physician. In these cases, follow-up must be made with the PCP. Allow a maximum 2-week turnaround time for routine authorizations, track all authorization requests, and expedite emergent requests via telephone or fax.

In some managed care plans, when a PCP sends a patient to a specialist for consultation who is not in the managed care plan, the specialist bills the PCP. This is done because the PCP receives a monthly capitation check from the plan and any care for the patient must come from the capitation pool. This type of plan encourages PCPs not to refer patients in order to retain profits.

If a specialist recommends a referral to another specialist, this is referred to as **tertiary care.** Be sure the referral is tracked as mentioned before. The approval or denial may be sent directly to the PCP and/or the second specialist, leaving the requesting physician uninformed. If the patient refuses to be referred, be sure this is documented in the medical record.

If a referral *form* is required by the managed care plan, do NOT telephone or write a letter. Complete the proper form and channel it as directed; otherwise the managed care plan may refuse payment.

When receiving a referral authorization form, make a copy of the form for each approved office visit, laboratory test, or series of treatments. Then use the copy as a reference to bill for the service. When all copies are used, this indicates all the services that the patient's plan had approved are completed. Request a new authorization, if necessary to continue treatment of the patient. The request should be generated in a timely manner so that treatment is not delayed.

Network Facilities

Managed care plans require that patients go to *network facilities* for surgery and diagnostic testing, such as laboratory and radiology services. Obtain authorization, when necessary, for such services and educate patients regarding this requirement.

Call to obtain precertification when there is doubt about covered services. If the recommended service is uncovered, disclose the cost and have the patient sign a waiver agreement stating that the patient has been informed the insurance plan will not pay for the specified service. This will allow the physician to bill the patient and receive payment. If authorization is denied stating the service is not "medically necessary," advise the physician, and, if the physician wishes to appeal, the physician can dictate a letter presenting clinical reasons to the MCO's review board to request reconsideration.

Managed Care Guide

One of the most confusing aspects of handling various managed care plans in the physician's office is keeping track of all the plans the physician belongs to as well as the specifics about each plan. To assist with this difficult task, create a grid of all MCOs that the practice has contracts with. Figure 9–7 shows a Managed Care Plan Reference Guide with suggested titles for column categories. Reference to such a guide will save time by giving office staff information at a glance to help with patient inquiries, collection of copayments, use of network facilities, and so forth.

Plan Administration

In order to administer a managed care plan successfully, all patients need to be informed of what you expect from them and what they can expect from you. Post a sign in the waiting room advising managed care patients to check with the receptionist regarding participating plans.

A patient information letter should outline expectations for copayment, possible requirements for preauthorization, possible noncovered items, and names of the managed care plans in which your physician participates. Note that if the patient neglects to obtain necessary authorization or to notify the office of any change regarding eligibility status in the plan, such as

Managed Care Plan Reference Guide

PLAN NAME/ADDRESS	TELEPHONE ELIGIBILITY	COPAY	PREAUTHORIZATION REQUIREMENTS	TEST RESTRICTIONS	CONTRACTED LAB(S) RADIOLOGY	CONTRACTED HOSPITAL(S)
Aetna PPO P O Box 43 WH XY 12345	555-239-0067	$5	hosp/surg/all dx tests	PE 1/yr	ABC Labs	College Hosp
Blue PPO P O Box 24335 WH XY 12345	555-245-0899	$8	referral specialist	PE 1/yr	Main St. Lab	St. John MC
Health Net P O Box 54000 WH XY 12345	555-408-5466	$5	hosp/surg see check list referrals	Mammogram 1/yr	Valley Lab	St. Joseph MC
Travelers MCO P O Box 1200 WH XY 12345	555-435-9877	$10	surg/hosp admit referrals	Pap >50 q3yr <50 q1yr	College Hosp. Metro Lab	College Hosp

Figure 9–7. Managed Care Plan Reference Guide used to list all MCOs the physician participates in and categorize specific information for each managed care plan for efficient retrieval.

disenrollment, the patient is held personally responsible for the bill.

Medical Records

Medical record management may differ when handling multiple managed care contracts. To save time in identifying managed care plans so that individual plan requirements can be met, file folders for different types of plans (e.g., HMO, EPO, IPA) can be flagged by using differently colored charts, or by placing colored markers (adhesive dots or labels) on the files.

Scheduling Appointments

Screen patients when they call for appointments to determine whether they belong to the same prepaid health plan as the physician. You may ask the patient to read directly from the insurance card to determine whether the physician's name is listed as the patient's PCP. Check the Managed Care Plan Reference Guide to determine plan requirements. If the patient is not in a participating plan and still wishes to schedule a visit, inform him or her that payment at the time of the service is required and the amount is determined by the private fee schedule.

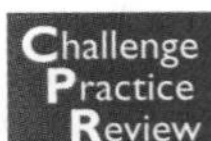

Pause and Practice CPR

REVIEW SESSIONS 9–28 THROUGH 9–32

Directions: *Complete the following questions as a review of information you have just read.*

9–28 When a physician evaluates another physician (using federal guidelines) in regard to the quality and efficiency of professional care, this is referred to as ______________________.

9–29 To help control costs in a managed care setting, a system called ______________________ is used to examine individual cases to determine medical necessity.

9–30 State three important considerations when contracting with a managed care plan.

(a) ____

(b) ____

(c) ____

9–31 Medical services that are not included in the contract benefits and are not paid under capitation are called ______________________________.

9–32 Where must managed care patients be directed when receiving surgery, laboratory testing, and radiology services? ______________________________

CHALLENGE SESSIONS 9–33 THROUGH 9–35

Directions: *Study the various types of referrals, then read the following scenarios. Use critical thinking skills to determine and list what type of referral is needed.*

9–33 Yvonne Graham has numerous skin lesions on various parts of her body that she is concerned about. Dr. Practon, her PCP, examines her and then completes and signs a form for her to see Dr. Cutis. ______________________________

9–34 Dr. Cardi sees Lawrence Parker for back pain. Upon examination, Dr. Cardi discovers that the patient's kidneys are very tender and he notices crystals in the patient's urine. He telephones Dr. Ulibarri and asks how soon he can see Mr. Parker and an appointment is made. ________ ______________________________

9–35 Elliott Baxter, a 4-year-old patient, sees Dr. Atrics for a severe earache. Upon Dr. Atrics' request, his medical insurance billing specialist completes a form requesting that the patient see Dr. Antrum as soon as possible for a chronic ear infection. ______________________________

CHECK YOUR HEARTBEAT! Turn to the end of the chapter for answers to these review and challenge sessions.

SUMMATION AND PREVIEW

You have now been introduced to private insurance and managed care plans and are able to describe some of their similarities and differences. You will be practicing completion of the HCFA-1500 insurance claim form for private carriers and managed care plans in Billing Break exercises at the end of this chapter. You will abstract patient and insurance information from the Patient Registration form, use Encounter forms to abstract physician information, and post entries on the patient's ledger.

In the final Billing Break exercise and in all remaining chapters, you will use chart notes to abstract information and practice your coding skills as you fill out the HCFA-1500 claim form. Different types of insurance plans and programs are presented in Chapters 10, 11, 12, and 13. Medicaid, presented in Chapter 10, is jointly funded by the state and federal governments and operated by regional state agencies. It has its own rules and regulations, including specific rules for filing a HCFA-1500 claim form. You will have an opportunity to learn the rules and practice Medicaid guidelines as you complete Medicaid cases.

GOLDEN RULE

Play it safe. Check authorization requirements on all patients.

Chapter 9 Review and Practice

Study Session

Directions: *Review the objectives, key terms, and chapter information before completing the following study questions.*

9–1 Participating providers are also referred to as:

(a) member physicians

(b) network physicians

(c) participating physicians

9–2 Nonparticipating providers are also referred to as out of network providers.

9–3 Where will private insurance plans send most insurance payments for a nonparticipating provider who accepts assignment? Provider's office rather than to the patient

9–4 Name some situations where multiple fee schedules may be used.

(a) pg 236 a (bottom left)

(b) pg 236 b

(c) pg 236 c

(d) pg 236 d (top Right)

9–5 When there is a change in the fee schedule in a physician's office, what is the standard protocol to notify patients? A notice should be placed in the reception room and a written communication sent to patients.

9–6 In the usual, customary, and reasonable (UCR) system for determining fees, give the description of these key terms:

(a) usual is the fee that a physician usually charges for a given service to a private patient

(b) customary if it falls within the range of usual fees charged by providers of similar training + experience in a geographic area.

(c) reasonable fee that meets the aforementioned criteria

9–7 What three factors are taken into account to determine the unit value of a procedure?

(a) The time a service/procedure takes

(b) the skill involved to perform it.

(c) overhead costs that are required.

9–8 Who was the Resource-Based Relative Value Scale (RBRVS) developed for?

Centers for Medicare and Medicaid Services.

238 9–9 State when the two types of copayment amounts are typically collected:

(a) Percentage of fee: after insurance company has paid.

(b) Fixed amount: at time of service – before the patient is seen

238 9–10 The rule to follow when a physician discounts a fee is, it must apply to the total amount of the bill

Pg 239+240 9–11 State three reasons why a "professional courtesy" is not usually given to physicians and other healthcare professionals today?

(a) Most physicians have insurance coverage for medical expenses.

(b) law does not provide exceptions that allow professional courtesy to physicians in situations where same courtesy not extended to all patients

(c) Must examine policies on professional courtesy to ensure do not violate either contractual terms in private OR managed care insurance policies OR medicare/medicaid laws & regulations.

240 9–12 Why is it not advisable for a physician to reduce the fee of a patient who has had a poor result from treatment or died? The doctor's sympathy could be misinterpreted and result in a malpractice suit.

241 9–13 Where should preappointment collection counseling take place? patient should be led to a quiet area away from general activity of office.

242 9–14 What should you ask for to verify a personal check when one is presented in the physician's office? Driver's License + one other form of ID.

243 9–15 If a check is returned stating "nonsufficient funds," what is the first step that should be taken? call Bank or patient to see if redepositing it is suggested.

244 9–16 What are the primary duties of a primary care physician? Control patient access to Specialists & diagnostic testing services.

248 9–17 Which HMO model hires physicians directly and pays them a salary? Staff model

249 9–18 What type of MCO is not a prepaid plan, but utilizes management techniques for long-term cost savings and contracts with large employers to offer medical care at reduced rates? Preferred Provider Organization (PPO)

249 9–19 What is the name of an organization that determines and assures the quality and operation of healthcare? Professional Review Organization (PRO)

252 9–20 A specialist referring a patient to another specialist is referred to as Tertiary Care.

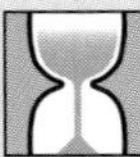

Billing Break

Case 9–1 April P. Tennyson

Time Started
Time Finished
Total Time

Directions: *Follow these steps to complete the HCFA-1500 insurance claim form for a private insurance case using OCR guidelines.*

1. Copy the HCFA-1500 insurance claim form found in Appendix F (Form 09).
2. Refer to the Patient Registration form for Case 9–1 and abstract information to complete the top portion of the HCFA-1500 claim form.
3. Refer to the Encounter form for Case 9–1 to abstract information for the bottom portion of the HCFA-1500 claim form.
4. Use the "HCFA-1500 Claim Form Block by Block Instructions" for All Private Patients found in Appendix D and the Private Insurance template (Figure D–3) for guidance and block help.
5. Date the claim 7/7/20XX.
6. Copy and prepare the ledger card found in Appendix F (Form 07) for the patient. Complete the ledger by posting each transaction in this case and indicating when you have billed the insurance carrier. Note: Since the patient is a minor, the ledger card is made out in the patient's name and on the second line the name of the responsible party should be included (e.g., April Tennyson, c/o Ann Michele Tennyson).

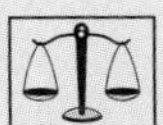

Weigh your progress. Turn to the Assignment Score Sheet in Appendix F (Form 10) and enter the information to track your success. Your instructor may ask that you include a Performance Evaluation Checklist, and if so, copy Form 11 found in Appendix F and attach it to your insurance claim.

4567 Broad Avenue
Woodland Hills, XY
12345-0001
Tel (555) 486-9002
Fax (555) 487-8976

REGISTRATION
(PLEASE PRINT)

Account # 3974 Today's Date: 04/21/02

PATIENT INFORMATION

Name Tennyson (Last Name) April (First Name) P (Initial) Soc. Sec. # 884-XX-1044

Address 912 Eagle Court Home Phone (555) 486-8892

City Woodland Hills State XY Zip 12345

Single ✓ Married ___ Separated ___ Divorced ___ Sex M ___ F ✓ Birthdate 04/07/02

Patient Employed by N/A Occupation

Business Address Business Phone

Spouse's Name Ann-Michele (Mother) Employed by: Halsey, Jenner and ~~Owens Family Law~~ Occupation Legal Secretary

Business Address 500 Pismo Street Woodland Hills Business Phone (555) 486-7200

Reason for Visit check up and DPT injection If accident: ___ Auto ___ Employment ___ Other ___

By whom were you referred? Ann-Michele Tennyson (mother)

In case of emergency, who should be notified? Mr/Mrs Richard Tennyson (Name) (parents) (Relation to Patient) Phone (555)486-7200

PRIMARY INSURANCE

Insured/Subscriber Tennyson (Last Name) Ann-Michele (First Name) (Initial)

Relation to Patient mother Birthdate 05/02/74 Soc. Sec.# 406-XX-2971

Address (if different from patient's) same

City State Zip

Insurance Company AmeriPlan Insurance Company

Insurance Address 1200 Broadway Avenue, Maddison, XY 12345

Insurance Identification Number 24069-72 Group # 0684

ADDITIONAL INSURANCE

Is patient covered by additional insurance? Yes ___ No ✓

Subscriber Name Relation to Patient Birthdate

Address (if different from patient's) Phone

City State Zip

Subscriber Employed by Buisness Phone

Insurance Company Soc. Sec. #

Insurance Address

Insurance Identification Number Group #

ASSIGNMENT AND RELEASE

I, the undersigned, certify that I (or my dependent) have insurance coverage with AmeriPlan Insurance Company (Name of Insurance Company(ies)) and assign directly to Dr. Pedro Atics insurance benefits, if any, otherwise payable to me for services rendered. I understand that I am financially responsible for all charges whether or not paid by insurance. I hereby consent for the doctor to release all information necessary to secure the payment of benefits. I authorize the use of this signature on all insurance submissions.

Responsible Party Signature April P Tennyson Relationship self Date 04/21/02

ORDER # 58-8426 @BIBBERO SYSTEMS, INC. •PETALUMA, CALIFORNIA• TO REORDER CALL TOLL FREE (800)242-9330

TAX ID #3664021CC
Medicaid #HSC12345F

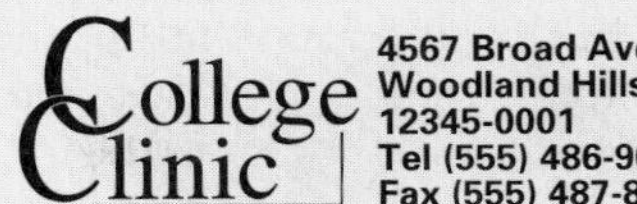

4567 Broad Avenue
Woodland Hills, XY
12345-0001
Tel (555) 486-9002
Fax (555) 487-8976

Doctor No. 2

☒ PRIVATE ☐ MANAGED CARE ☐ MEDICAID ☐ MEDICARE ☐ TRICARE ☐ W/C

ACCOUNT #	PATIENT'S LAST NAME	FIRST	INITIAL	TODAY'S DATE
3974	Tennyson	April	P	07/ 07 / 02

ASSIGNMENT: I hereby assign payment directly to College Clinic of the surgical and/or medical benefits, if any, otherwise payable to me for his/her services as described below.
SIGNED (Patient, or Parent, if Minor) Ann Michele Tennyson DATE: 07/07/02

✓	DESCRIPTION	CPT-4/MD	FEE	✓	DESCRIPTION	CPT-4/MD	FEE	✓	DESCRIPTION	CPT-4/MD	FEE
	OFFICE VISIT–NEW PATIENT				**WELL BABY EXAM**				**LABORATORY**		
	Level 1	99201			Initial	99381			Glucose Blood	82962	
	Level 2	99202		✓	Periodic	99391	35.00		Hematocrit	85013	
	Level 3	99203			**OFFICE PROCEDURES**				Occult Blood	82270	
	Level 4	99204			Anoscopy	46600			Urine Dip	81000	
	Level 5	99205			ECG 24-hr	93224			**X-RAY**		
	OFFICE VISIT–ESTAB. PATIENT				Fracture Rpr Foot	28470			Foot – 2 view	73620	
	Level 1	99211			I & D	10060			Forearm - 2 view	73090	
	Level 2	99212			Suture Repair				Nasal Bone - 3	70160	
	Level 3	99213							Spine LS - 2 view	72100	
	Level 4	99214			**INJECTIONS/VACCINATIONS**						
	Level 5	99215		✓	DPT	90701	34.00		**MISCELLANEOUS**		
	OFFICE CONSULT-NP/EST				IM-Antibiotic	90788			Handling of Spec	99000	
	Level 3	99243			OPU-Poliovirus	90712			Supply	99070	
	Level 4	99244			Tetanus	90703			Venipuncture	36415	
	Level 5	99245									

COMMENTS:

Physician: [signature] MD

RETURN APPOINTMENT
____ Week(s) 1 Month(s)

DIAGNOSIS:	DESCRIPTION	CODE
Primary:	routine infant health check	V20.2
Secondary:		

REC'D BY:
☐ BANK CARD
☐ CASH
☐ CHECK
____

PREVIOUS BALANCE	-0-
TODAY'S FEE	69.00
AMOUNT REC'D/CO-PAY	-0-
BALANCE	69.00

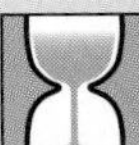

Billing Break

Case 9–2 Darrell T. Livingston

Time Started
Time Finished
Total Time

Directions: *Follow these steps to complete the HCFA-1500 insurance claim form for a private insurance case using OCR guidelines.*

1. Copy the HCFA-1500 insurance claim form found in Appendix F (Form 09).
2. Refer to the Patient Registration form for Case 9–2 and abstract information to complete the top portion of the HCFA-1500 claim form.
3. Refer to the Encounter form for Case 9–2 to abstract information for the bottom portion of the HCFA-1500 claim form.
4. Use the "HCFA-1500 Claim Form Block by Block Instructions" for All Private Patients found in Appendix D and the Private Insurance template (Figure D–3) for guidance and block help.

5. Date the claim 8/31/XX.

6. Copy and prepare the ledger card found in Appendix F (Form 07) for the patient. Complete the ledger by posting each transaction in this case and indicating when you have billed the insurance carrier.

7. Note: If the private insurance carrier accepts HCPCS Level II modifiers, how would you apply them to this case? ____

____

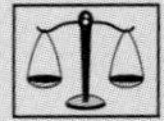

Weigh your progress. Turn to the Assignment Score Sheet in Appendix F (Form 10) and enter the information to track your success. Your instructor may ask that you include a Performance Evaluation Checklist, and if so, copy Form 11 found in Appendix F and attach it to your insurance claim.

4567 Broad Avenue
Woodland Hills, XY
12345-0001
Tel (555) 486-9002
Fax (555) 487-8976

REGISTRATION
(PLEASE PRINT)

Account # 2368 Today's Date: 08/31/XX

PATIENT INFORMATION

Name Livingston (Last Name) Darrell (First Name) T (Initial) Soc. Sec. # 481-XX-2600

Address 394 Chapel Street Home Phone (555) 967-1101

City Orange Grove State XY Zip 12345

Single___ Married ✓ Separated___ Divorced___ Sex M ✓ F___ Birthdate 03/20/69

Patient Employed by Bridgeport Honda Occupation Mechanic

Business Address 8569 Bridgeport Blvd Orange Grove XY Business Phone (555) 967-4001

Spouse's Name Julie Employed by: Anchorage Appliance Occupation Bookkeeper

Business Address 71631 Crestview Street Orange Grove Business Phone (555) 967-5969

Reason for Visit foot pain If accident:___ Auto___ Employment___ Other ✓

By whom were you referred? Gerald Practon MD

In case of emergency, who should be notified? Troy Livingston (Name) brother (Relation to Patient) Phone (555) 369-7126

PRIMARY INSURANCE

Insured/Subscriber Livingston (Last Name) Darrell (First Name) T (Initial)

Relation to Patient self Birthdate 03/20/69 Soc. Sec.# 481-XX-2600

Address (if different from patient's) same

City___ State___ Zip___

Insurance Company Northern Insurance Company

Insurance Address 4200 El Capitan Blvd, Rochester, XY 12345

Insurance Identification Number 481-XX-2600 Group # BH12

ADDITIONAL INSURANCE

Is patient covered by additional insurance? Yes___ No ✓

Subscriber Name___ Relation to Patient___ Birthdate___

Address (if different from patient's)___ Phone___

City___ State___ Zip___

Subscriber Employed by___ Buisness Phone___

Insurance Company___ Soc. Sec. #___

Insurance Address___

Insurance Identification Number___ Group #___

ASSIGNMENT AND RELEASE

I, the undersigned, certify that I (or my dependent) have insurance coverage with Northern Insurance Company (Name of Insurance Company(ies)) and assign directly to Dr. Raymond Skeleton insurance benefits, if any, otherwise payable to me for services rendered. I understand that I am financially responsible for all charges whether or not paid by insurance. I hereby consent for the doctor to release all information necessary to secure the payment of benefits. I authorize the use of this signature on all insurance submissions.

Darrell T Livingston (Responsible Party Signature) Self (Relationship) Date 08-31-XX

ORDER # 58-8426 @BIBBERO SYSTEMS, INC •PETALUMA, CALIFORNIA• TO REORDER CALL TOLL FREE (800)242-9330

TAX ID #3664021CC
Medicaid #HSC12345F

4567 Broad Avenue
Woodland Hills, XY
12345-0001
Tel (555) 486-9002
Fax (555) 487-8976

Doctor No. 9

☒ PRIVATE ☐ MANAGED CARE ☐ MEDICAID ☐ MEDICARE ☐ TRICARE ☐ W/C

ACCOUNT #	PATIENT'S LAST NAME	FIRST	INITIAL	TODAY'S DATE
2368	Livingston	Darrell	T	08/ 31 / XX

ASSIGNMENT: I hereby assign payment directly to College Clinic of the surgical and/or medical benefits, if any, otherwise payable to me for his/her services as described below.
SIGNED (Patient, or Parent, if Minor) *Darrell T Livingston* DATE: *08-31-XX*

✓	DESCRIPTION	CPT-4/MD	FEE	✓	DESCRIPTION	CPT-4/MD	FEE	✓	DESCRIPTION	CPT-4/MD	FEE
	OFFICE VISIT–NEW PATIENT				**WELL BABY EXAM**				**LABORATORY**		
	Level 1	99201			Initial	99381			Glucose Blood	82962	
✓	Level 2	99202	51.91		Periodic	99391			Hematocrit	85013	
	Level 3	99203			**OFFICE PROCEDURES**				Occult Blood	82270	
	Level 4	99204			Anoscopy	46600			Urine Dip	81000	
	Level 5	99205			ECG 24-hr	93224			**X-RAY**		
	OFFICE VISIT–ESTAB. PATIENT			✓	Fracture Rpr Foot	28470	167.79	✓	Foot – 2 view	73620	31.61
	Level 1	99211			I & D	10060			Forearm - 2 view	73090	
	Level 2	99212			Suture Repair				Nasal Bone - 3	70160	
	Level 3	99213							Spine LS - 2 view	72100	
	Level 4	99214			**INJECTIONS/VACCINATIONS**						
	Level 5	99215			DPT	90701			**MISCELLANEOUS**		
	OFFICE CONSULT-NP/EST				IM-Antibiotic	90788			Handling of Spec	99000	
	Level 3	99243			OPU-Poliovirus	90712		✓	Supply	99070	25.00
	Level 4	99244			Tetanus	90703			Venipuncture	36415	
	Level 5	99245									

COMMENTS: *Dropped sack of cement on L foot today at home*
**Supply: Cast materials*
Physician: *Raymond Skeleton MD*

RETURN APPOINTMENT: *3* Week(s) ____ Month(s)

DIAGNOSIS:	DESCRIPTION	CODE
Primary:	*Fracture, metatarsal*	*825.25*
Secondary:		

REC'D BY: ☐ BANK CARD ☐ CASH ☐ CHECK #______

PREVIOUS BALANCE	-0-
TODAY'S FEE	276.31
AMOUNT REC'D/CO-PAY	0.00
BALANCE	276.31

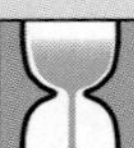

Billing Break

Case 9–3 Marina L. Nonn

Time Started
Time Finished
Total Time

Directions: *Follow these steps to complete the HCFA-1500 insurance claim form for a managed care insurance case using OCR guidelines.*

1. Copy the HCFA-1500 insurance claim form found in Appendix F (Form 09).

2. Refer to the Patient Registration form for Case 9–3 and abstract information to complete the top portion of the HCFA-1500 claim form.

3. Refer to the Encounter form for Case 9–3 to abstract information for the bottom portion of the HCFA-1500 claim form.

4. Use the "HCFA-1500 Claim Form Block by Block Instructions" for All Private Patients found in Appendix D and the Private Insurance template (Figure D-3) for guidance and block help.

5. Date the claim 6/27/XX.

6. Copy and prepare the ledger card found in Appendix F (Form 07) for the patient. Complete the ledger by posting each transaction in this case. Indicate payment received and when you have billed the insurance carrier.

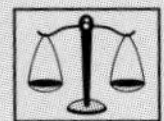

Weigh your progress. Turn to the Assignment Score Sheet in Appendix F (Form 10) and enter the information to track your success. Your instructor may ask that you include a Performance Evaluation Checklist, and if so, copy Form 11 found in Appendix F and attach it to your insurance claim.

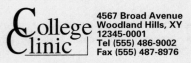

4567 Broad Avenue
Woodland Hills, XY
12345-0001
Tel (555) 486-9002
Fax (555) 487-8976

REGISTRATION
(PLEASE PRINT)

Account # 1502 Today's Date: 02/12/XX

PATIENT INFORMATION

Name Nonn (Last Name) Marina (First Name) L. (Initial) Soc. Sec. # 291-XX-8869

Address 1115 Gaviota Road Home Phone (555) 487-3988

City Woodland Hills State XY Zip 12345

Single___ Married ✓ Separated___ Divorced___ Sex M___ F ✓ Birthdate 01/10/53

Patient Employed by Cottage Nursery School Occupation Nursery School Administrator

Business Address 300 Cathedral Oaks Rd Woodland Hills Business Phone (555) 487-1023

Spouse's Name James Employed by: Peach Tree Vineyard Occupation Wine Maker

Business Address 2 Peachy Canyon Rd Temple XY Business Phone (555) 523-WINE

Reason for Visit physical exam If accident:___ Auto___ Employment___ Other___

By whom were you referred? mother – Peggy Becchio

In case of emergency, who should be notified? Jim Nonn (Name) husband (Relation to Patient) Phone (555) 523-WINE

PRIMARY INSURANCE

Insured/Subscriber Nonn (Last Name) James (First Name) A (Initial)

Relation to Patient husband Birthdate 09/03/52 Soc. Sec.# 802-XX-2463

Address (if different from patient's) same

City___ State___ Zip___

Insurance Company Western Insurance Company

Insurance Address P O Box 4500, Encina XY 12345

Insurance Identification Number 596820 Group # 42

ADDITIONAL INSURANCE

Is patient covered by additional insurance? Yes___ No ✓

Subscriber Name___ Relation to Patient___ Birthdate___

Address (if different from patient's)___ Phone___

City___ State___ Zip___

Subscriber Employed by___ Buisness Phone___

Insurance Company___ Soc. Sec. #___

Insurance Address___

Insurance Identification Number___ Group #___

ASSIGNMENT AND RELEASE

I, the undersigned, certify that I (or my dependent) have insurance coverage with Western Insurance Company (Name of Insurance Company(ies)) and assign directly to Dr. Gerald Practon insurance benefits, if any, otherwise payable to me for services rendered. I understand that I am financially responsible for all charges whether or not paid by insurance. I hereby consent for the doctor to release all information necessary to secure the payment of benefits. I authorize the use of this signature on all insurance submissions.

Marina L Nonn (Responsible Party Signature) self (Relationship) 2-12-XX (Date)

ORDER # 58-8426 @BIBBERO SYSTEMS, INC. •PETALUMA, CALIFORNIA• TO REORDER CALL TOLL FREE (800)242-9330

TAX ID #3664021CC
Medicaid #HSC12345F

4567 Broad Avenue
Woodland Hills, XY
12345-0001
Tel (555) 486-9002
Fax (555) 487-8976

Doctor No. 8

☐ PRIVATE ☒ MANAGED CARE ☐ MEDICAID ☐ MEDICARE ☐ TRICARE ☐ W/C

ACCOUNT #	PATIENT'S LAST NAME	FIRST	INITIAL	TODAY'S DATE
1502	Nonn	Marina	L	06/27/XX

ASSIGNMENT: I hereby assign payment directly to College Clinic of the surgical and/or medical benefits, if any, otherwise payable to me for his/her services as described below.
SIGNED (Patient, or Parent, if Minor) *Marina L Nonn* DATE *6-27-XX*

✓	DESCRIPTION	CPT-4/MD	FEE	✓	DESCRIPTION	CPT-4/MD	FEE	✓	DESCRIPTION	CPT-4/MD	FEE
	OFFICE VISIT–NEW PATIENT				**WELL BABY EXAM**				**LABORATORY**		
	Level 1	99201			Initial	99381			Glucose Blood	82962	
	Level 2	99202			Periodic	99391			Hematocrit	85013	
	Level 3	99203			**OFFICE PROCEDURES**			✓	Occult Blood	82270	4.05
	Level 4	99204		✓	Anoscopy	46600	32.86		Urine Dip	81000	
	Level 5	99205			ECG 24-hr	93224			**X-RAY**		
	OFFICE VISIT–ESTAB. PATIENT				Fracture Rpr Foot	28470			Foot – 2 view	73620	
	Level 1	99211			I & D	10060			Forearm - 2 view	73090	
	Level 2	99212			Suture Repair				Nasal Bone - 3	70160	
✓	Level 3	99213	40.20						Spine LS - 2 view	72100	
	Level 4	99214			**INJECTIONS/VACCINATIONS**						
	Level 5	99215			DPT	90701			**MISCELLANEOUS**		
	OFFICE CONSULT-NP/EST				IM-Antibiotic	90788			Handling of Spec	99000	
	Level 3	99243			OPU-Poliovirus	90712			Supply	99070	
	Level 4	99244			Tetanus	90703			Venipuncture	36415	
	Level 5	99245									

COMMENTS: *Schedule Lower GI-Need Autho*

RETURN APPOINTMENT *After test*
____ Week(s) ____ Month(s)

Physician: *[signature] MD*

DIAGNOSIS:	DESCRIPTION	CODE
Primary:	*Rectal bleeding*	*569.3*
Secondary:	*Rectal pain*	*569.42*

REC'D BY:
☐ BANK CARD
☐ CASH
☒ CHECK
\# *401*

PREVIOUS BALANCE	*-0-*
TODAY'S FEE	*77.11*
AMOUNT REC'D/CO-PAY	*15.00*
BALANCE	*62.11*

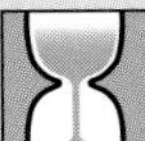

Billing Break

Case 9–4 Grace L. Ventura

Time Started
Time Finished
Total Time

Directions: *Follow these steps to complete the HCFA-1500 insurance claim form for a managed care case using OCR guidelines.*

1. Copy the HCFA-1500 insurance claim form found in Appendix F (Form 09).
2. Refer to the Patient Information form for Case 9–4 and abstract information to complete the top portion of the HCFA-1500 claim form.
3. Refer to the Medical Record for Case 9–4 to abstract information for the bottom portion of the HCFA-1500 claim form. See page 266 for directions.
4. Copy the Medical Record Coding Worksheet found in Appendix F (Form 12) to use when abstracting information from the chart note.

5. Use the "HCFA-1500 Claim Form Block by Block Instructions" for All Private Patients found in Appendix D and the Private Insurance template (Figure D–3) for guidance and block help.

6. Use your procedure codebook to determine the correct code number(s) and modifier(s) for each professional service/procedure rendered.

7. Refer to the fee schedule in Appendix B for mock fees.

8. Use your diagnostic codebook to determine the correct diagnosis.

9. Date the claim 01/19/20XX.

10. Copy and prepare the ledger card found in Appendix F (Form 07) for the patient. Complete the ledger by posting each transaction in this case and indicating when you have billed the insurance carrier.

Abstract Data from a Medical Record and Code Procedures and Diagnoses

Directions: This is the first assignment in which you will abstract data from the patient's medical record and apply procedure and diagnostic codes to insert on the HCFA-1500 insurance claim form. For each case that includes a chart note, copy the Medical Record Coding Worksheet found in Appendix F (Form 12) and follow these guidelines.

1. Read the patient's medical record and locate all symptoms, diagnoses, and services/procedures.

2. Highlight each of these three components with colors as indicated in the example.

3. List each symptom, diagnosis, and service/procedure according to the date of service (DOS). Six lines are provided to correspond with the six lines on the HCFA-1500 claim form; however, each case may not use all six lines.

4. Determine if a formal diagnosis has been made for each symptom and if so, code the diagnosis. If not, code the symptom. Note: Additional symptoms may be coded for practice; however, if the diagnosis includes the symptom, it should not appear on the HCFA-1500 claim form.

5. Code all services and procedures.

6. Transfer service/procedure codes and diagnostic codes to the claim form.

Chart Note Example

02/12/XX An established patient, Mary Beth Williams presents complaining of a severe headache and fatigue. I performed an EPF HX/PX with L/MDM. History and symptoms are consistant with a classic migraine headache. Blood is drawn for a red blood cell count (spun microhematocrit) which determines iron deficient anemia (34%). A sample is sent to an outside laboratory for a general health panel. Patient is prescibed iron and pain medication and advised to stay at complete bed rest for 3 days. RTO in 3 days for follow up and test results.

Gerald Practon, MD

DOS	Symptom/code		Diagnosis/code		Services and Procedures /code	
2/12/XX	1. headache	784.0	1. classic migraine	346.00	1. EST. PT E/M EPF HX/PX L/MDM	99213
	2. fatigue	780.79	2. iron deficient anemia	280.9	2. Venipuncture	36415
	3.		3.		3. Microhematocrit	85013
	4.		4.		4. Specimen handling	99000
	5.		5.		5.	
	6.		6.		6.	

Rationale: Because "severe headache" is a symptom of the diagnosis "classic migraine headache," it will not appear on the claim form. Because "fatigue" is a symptom of the diagnosis "iron deficiency anemia," it will not appear on the claim form. There will be a total of two diagnoses on the HCFA-1500 form. The symptoms (headache and fatigue) may be coded for practice. Each diagnosis should be properly linked with each procedure/service (i.e., both would apply to the E/M service and iron deficiency anemia would be linked to the blood draw and hematocrit).

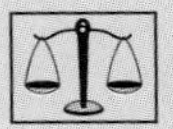

Weigh your progress. Turn to the Assignment Score Sheet in Appendix F (Form 10) and enter the information to track your success. Your instructor may ask that you include a Performance Evaluation Checklist, and if so, copy Form 11 found in Appendix F and attach it to your insurance claim.

4567 Broad Avenue
Woodland Hills, XY
12345-0001
Tel (555) 486-9002
Fax (555) 487-8976

REGISTRATION
(PLEASE PRINT)

Account # 2415 Today's Date: 01/08/01

PATIENT INFORMATION

Name Ventura (Last Name) Grace (First Name) L. (Initial) Soc. Sec. # 196-XX-8941

Address 459 Devanshire Way Home Phone (555) 985-4502

City Meadowridge State XY Zip 12345

Single ✓ Married ___ Separated ___ Divorced ___ Sex M ___ F ✓ Birthdate 08/05/87

Patient Employed by Full time student Occupation ___

Business Address N/A Business Phone (555) 967-4001

Spouse's Name Beatrice (mother) Employed by: Hamilton Hardware Occupation sales clerk

Business Address 444 Seabreeze Way Meadowridge Business Phone (555) 986-2540

Reason for Visit runny nose, constant cold If accident: ___ Auto ___ Employment ___ Other ___

By whom were you referred? Pedro Atrics MD

In case of emergency, who should be notified? Beatrice Ventura (Name) mother (Relation to Patient) Phone (555) 986-2540

PRIMARY INSURANCE

Insured/Subscriber Ventura (Last Name) Beatrice (First Name) J (Initial)

Relation to Patient mother Birthdate 08/20/67 Soc. Sec.# 501-XX-5103

Address (if different from patient's) same

City ___ State ___ Zip ___

Insurance Company Pru Care Health Maintenance Organization

Insurance Address 20163 San Mateo Avenue, San Mateo, XY 12345

Insurance Identification Number 9876500 Group # PC 005

ADDITIONAL INSURANCE

Is patient covered by additional insurance? Yes ___ No ✓

Subscriber Name ___ Relation to Patient ___ Birthdate ___

Address (if different from patient's) ___ Phone ___

City ___ State ___ Zip ___

Subscriber Employed by ___ Buisness Phone ___

Insurance Company ___ Soc. Sec. # ___

Insurance Address ___

Insurance Identification Number ___ Group # ___

ASSIGNMENT AND RELEASE

I, the undersigned, certify that I (or my dependent) have insurance coverage with Pru Care HMO (Name of Insurance Company(ies)) and assign directly to Dr. Cocha Antrum insurance benefits, if any, otherwise payable to me for services rendered. I understand that I am financially responsible for all charges whether or not paid by insurance. I hereby consent for the doctor to release all information necessary to secure the payment of benefits. I authorize the use of this signature on all insurance submissions.

Responsible Party Signature Beatrice Ventura Relationship mother Date 1/8/01

Medical Record

Account number: 2415
Patient's name: Ventura, Grace L
Date of birth: 08/05/87

Date	Progress Notes

01/08/XX Patient referred by Dr. Pedro Atrics (PCP) for consultation and evaluation of possible allergies. Dr. Atrics is treating this patient for chronic rhinitis and acute sinusitis with a broad-spectrum antibiotic. Patient is also experiencing a cough and acute pharyngitis.

An EPF HX is taken which reveals typical onset of allergic reaction manifesting in secondary infection. An EPF PX is performed. I discussed various disease and allergy testing with the patient and patient's mother to determine the cause of the allergic rhinitis and possible treatment options. patient to return after symptoms have decreased or resolved to undergo testing. SF MDM.

Concha Antrum, MD

01/19/XX Patient returns for disease and allergy testing. Coccidioidomycosis skin test and tuberculosis intradermal test applied to the patient's left anterior forearm per Dr. Antrums' order. Patient to return in 3 days for reading and appointment with Dr. Antrum. She will then start a series of scratch and patch tests to determine the source of the allergic rhinitis.

Jill Quintin, CMA

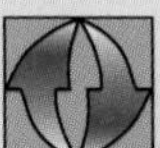

Exercise Exchange

9–1 Complete Managed Care Plan Authorization Request

Directions:

1. Complete the authorization Form 12 found in Appendix F.
2. Refer to the section on Preauthorization or Prior Approval and Figure 9–5 for guidance.
3. Abstract data from the Patient Registration form and Patient Record for Grace Ventura listed in Billing Break Exercise 9–4.
4. The authorization request is from the primary care physician requesting approval for the patient to see an otolaryngology specialist. The request is made on 1/2/XX.
5. Use the physician's state license number as the provider identification for the managed care plan.
6. Use the primary diagnosis as the reason for the consultation.
7. Date the request January 2, 20XX.

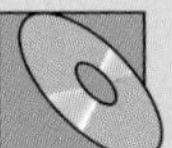

Computer Session—Cases 1 through 6

Directions: *Insert the CD-ROM into the computer. Print directions when they are offered from each screen and read before attempting the first case. Locate Case 1 from the file folder and follow the instructions on the screen. Continue completing Cases 2, 3, 4, 5, and 6 for private insurance plans.*

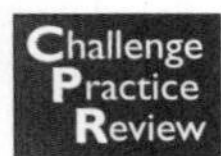

CPR Session: Answers

CPR PRACTICE SESSIONS 9–1 THROUGH 9–5

9–1 (a) $144 (80% of $180 or 180 × .80)
(b) $36 (20% of $180 or 180 × .20)
(c) $40 ($220-$180)
(d) $36 (20% of allowed amount)
(e) $180 (insurance portion—80%, and patient portion—20%, of allowed amount)
(f) $40 ($220-$180)

9–2 (a) $94.50 (70% of $135 or 135 × .70)
(b) $40.50 (30% of $135 or 135 × .30)
(c) $25 ($160-$135)
(d) $65.50 ($40.50 − 30% plus $25 difference between billed amount and allowed amount)
(e) $160 (total allowed amount, or $94.50 + $40.50 + $25)
(f) None

9–3 $53, because it is the lower of the two (usual and customary)

9–4 $75 ($125 × .60)

9–5 (a) 13.621 (13.25 × 1.028)
(b) 8.96954 (7.13 × 1.258)
(c) 1.9454 (1.42 × 1.370)
(d) 24.53594 (13.621 + 8.96954 + 1.9454)
(e) $888.31171 = rounded to $888.31 (24.53954 × 36.1992)

CPR REVIEW SESSIONS 9–6 THROUGH 9–9

9–6 (a) percentage of fee (e.g., 20%)
(b) fixed amount (e.g., $15)

9–7 (a) pay in cash at the time of service
(b) pay the entire amount
(c) post cash discount policy in office
(d) send every active patient a notice of the cash discount policy

9–8 contractural adjustment

9–9 they ban waiving deductibles and copayment amounts

CPR CHALLENGE SESSION 9–10

9–10 It would lower his or her fee schedule and decrease payments because as charges are decreased, so is the physician's fee profile—that is, the record of all charges that the insurance company has on file from that physician.

CPR REVIEW SESSIONS 9–11 THROUGH 9–14

9–11 honesty, integrity, and pride

9–12 review each patient's account and flag accounts that have an outstanding balance

9–13 at the time of service

9–14 personal check

CPR REVIEW SESSIONS 9–15 THROUGH 9–17

9–15 (a) office visits
(b) urgent care visits
(c) emergency department visits
(d) prescription drugs
(e) inpatient mental health services

9–16 Payment system used by managed care plans in which physicians and hospitals are paid a fixed per capita amount for each patient enrolled over a stated period of time, regardless of the type and number of services provided.

9–17 25 or more

CPR PRACTICE SESSIONS 9–18 THROUGH 9–22

9–18 Select Plus HMO

9–19 member number 023-XX-3619, group 285311

9–20 $15, $50, $35

9–21 800-XXX-6840

9–22 P.O. Box 4066, Bridgeport, XY 12345-0001

CPR CHALLENGE SESSION 9–23

9–23 (1) $36. (2) $36. Rationale: The physician receives the capitated amount regardless of how many times the patient sees the physician.

CPR REVIEW SESSIONS 9–24 THROUGH 9–27

9–24 health maintenance organization (HMO)

9–25 exclusive provider organization (EPO)

9–26 independent (or individual) practice association (IPA)

9–27 point-of-service-plan (POS)

CPR REVIEW SESSIONS 9–28 THROUGH 9–32

9–28 peer review

9–29 utilization review

9–30 (a) number of patients the MCO will provide
(b) capitation rate
(c) services included in the capitated amount

9–31 carve-outs

9–32 network providers/facilities

CPR CHALLENGE SESSIONS 9–33 THROUGH 9–35

9–33 direct referral

9–34 verbal referral

9–35 formal referral

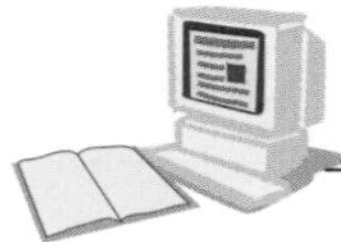

Resources

As you practice claim form completion, organize samples of completed claim forms into a binder for future reference. Changes occur daily so keep well informed by reading carrier and local medical society bulletins. Maintain a binder with a chronological file on each of these bulletins for quick reference, always keeping the latest bulletin on top. Attend training workshops and educational seminars in your locale to keep current on insurance practices for private and managed care plans. Converse with other insurance specialists to compare policies and discuss common problems. Network with individuals in your region who are working in the same specialty that you are to compare notes on billing and reimbursement from various plans.

You may be accessing the Internet and using a *web browser* (search engine) to go to a specific address to obtain current legal and regulatory information from insurance programs and federal agencies and downloading data or attachments from the web. Following are associations, reference books and Web site addresses for obtaining additional information.

Organizations

Managed Care Plans and Foundations

- American Association of Health Plans (AAHP) [formerly known as American Managed Care and Review Association and American Association of Foundations for Medical Care], 1129 20th Street NW, Suite 600, Washington, DC 20036, (202) 778-3200.
  Web site: www.aahp.org
- Office of Health Maintenance Organizations, Centers for Medicare and Medicaid Services, Room 4350—Cohen Building, 330 Independence Avenue SW, Washington, DC 20201.
  Web site: www.hefa.gov

Internet

- *Federal Register*
  Web site: www.gpo.gov

Reference Books

- *Managed Care Handbook,* Kongsvedt, Peter R., Aspen Publishers, Inc., 7201 McKinney Circle (21704), P.O. Box 990, Frederick, MD 21705-9727, (800) 638-8437.
- *St Anthony's Relative Values for Physicians (RVP),* St. Anthony/Ingenix Publishing Group, 11410 Isaac Newton Square, Reston, VA 22090 or P.O. Box 96561, Washington, DC 20044-4212, (800) 632-0123 or (703) 904-3900, fax (703) 706-5830.

NOTES

Objectives

After reading this chapter and completing the exercise sessions, you should be able to:

Learning Objectives:

- ✔ Understand the benefits and nonbenefits of Medicaid.
- ✔ Define terminology inherent to the Medicaid program.
- ✔ Interpret Medicaid abbreviations.
- ✔ Name the two classifications in which all Medicaid-eligible individuals are grouped.
- ✔ List important information to abstract from the patient's Medicaid card.
- ✔ State eligibility requirements and benefits for the Maternal and Child Health Program.
- ✔ Identify those eligible for the Medicaid Qualified Medicare Beneficiaries program.
- ✔ Explain basic operations of a Medicaid managed care system.

Performance Objectives:

- ✔ Demonstrate basic Medicaid claim procedure guidelines while completing the HCFA-1500 claim form for a Medicaid case.
- ✔ File claims for patients who have Medicaid and other coverage.

Key Terms

categorically needy

covered services

Early and Periodic Screening, Diagnosis, and Treatment (EPSDT)

Maternal and Child Health Program (MCHP)

Medicaid (MCD)

Medi-Cal

medically indigent

medically needy (MN)

prior approval

recipients

reciprocity

share of cost (SOC)

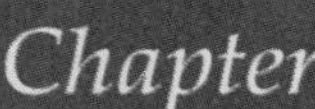
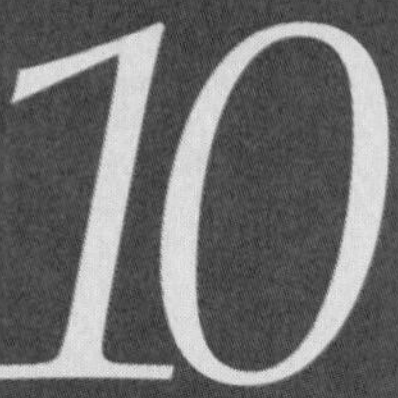

Chapter 10

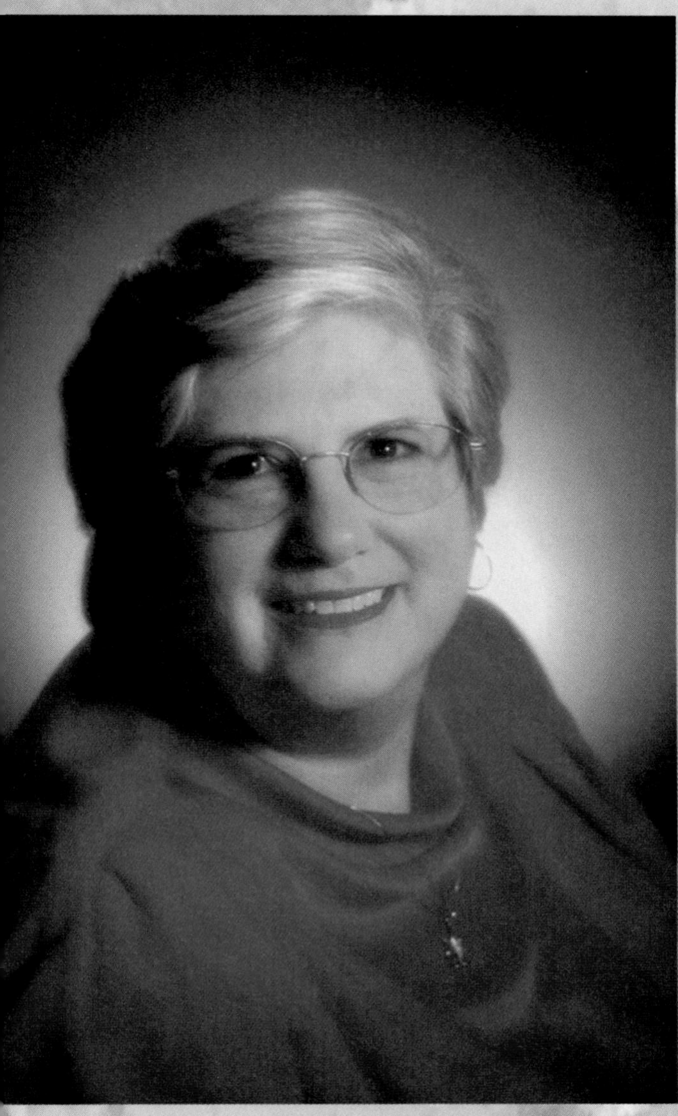

I am a CMA-A, specializing in medical billing. I began my career in medicine as a secretary in the neurology department at a major university. Then, I managed a neurology practice, did consulting work, and billed for pathology and anesthesiology. Currently I am employed as the billing and collection specialist for a federally qualified health center (FQHC) with 6 clinics. Most of our clients are uninsured or underinsured individuals. The most challenging aspect of FQHC billing is interpreting insurance regulations and applying them to FQHC guidelines. Reimbursement by Medicare and Medicaid is based upon the costs of providing our services. This is similar to the way a hospital is reimbursed. Only certain "core" provider services are billable and services without an office visit by one of these providers may not be billed.

Jane Seelig, CMA-A
Billing and Collection Specialist
Federally Qualified Health Center

The Medicaid Program

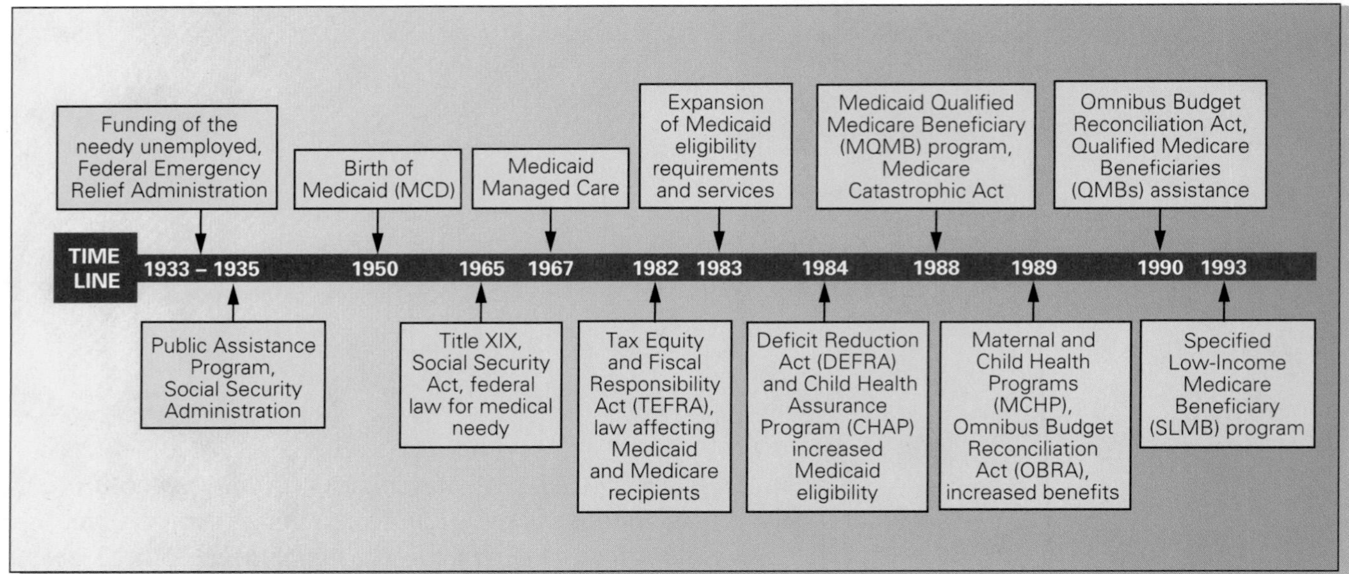

THE BIRTH OF MEDICAID

When public assistance was first established, no provisions were made for medical aid. However, the federal government paid a share of the monthly assistance payments, which were made directly to the recipient and could be used to meet the cost of medical care. A healthcare assistance program mandating states to meet minimum requirements followed approximately 15 years later. As a result of this mandate, states set up **Medicaid (MCD)** programs. *Vendor payments* for medical care were authorized by Congress, which went directly from the welfare agency to physicians, healthcare institutions, and other providers of medical services.

After another 15 years, Medicaid legally came into being as part of a federal law. The program has always had somewhat of a split personality. On one hand, it is viewed as an attempt on the part of the government to provide comprehensive quality healthcare to those unable to afford it. On the other hand, Medicaid has been seen as merely a bill-paying mechanism whose purpose is to administer the provision of healthcare using the most efficient and economic system possible.

Medicaid Administration

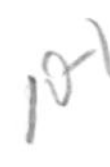

The program that provides medical assistance for certain low-income individuals and families is known as Medicaid in 48 states and **Medi-Cal** in California. Arizona is the only state without a Medicaid program like those existing in other states. It has received federal funds under a demonstration waiver and set up an alternative medical assistance program (prepaid care) for low-income persons called the Arizona Health Care Cost Containment System (AHCCCS).

Medicaid is administered by state governments with partial federal funding. Coverage and benefits vary widely from state to state because the federal government sets minimum requirements and states are free to enact more benefits. Thus, each state designs its own Medicaid program within federal guidelines. Since the restructuring of the Health Care Financing Administration (HCFA), the Center for Medicaid and State Operations, a division of the Centers for Medicare and Medicaid Services (CMS), is responsible for the federal aspects of Medicaid. The center focuses not only on Medicaid but also on insurance regulations as well as other joint federal-state programs such as the State Children's Health Insurance Program. The goal is to improve communication between beneficiaries, physicians, and the governmental agencies that are responsible for these programs. Medicaid is not so much an insurance program as an assistance program.

Accepting Medicaid Patients

The physician may accept or refuse to treat Medicaid patients but must make the decision on the basis of the *entire* Medicaid program, not an individual patient's personality, medical situation, or other discriminating factor. It is important that the patient receive quality care and be treated the same as the paying patient. Each medical practice, or individual physicians within a medical practice, may have their own office procedures for handling Medicaid patients.

If the physician decides to take Medicaid patients, he or she must accept the Medicaid allowance as payment in full. A patient can be on Medicaid 1 month and off the following month, or on the program for several months or years; therefore, each case is different. When obtaining personal information from the patient at the time of the first visit, or a follow-up visit in the case where the physician treats the patient initially in the hospital, make sure all information is accurate and complete. Some Medicaid individuals are homeless and may list fake addresses, which makes locating them difficult.

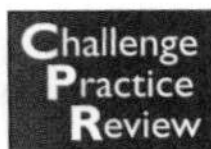

Pause and Practice CPR

REVIEW SESSIONS 10–1 AND 10–2

Directions: *Complete the following questions as a review of information you have just read.*

10–1 Medicaid is administered by ______________________.

10–2 What reimbursement must the physician accept when agreeing to treat Medicaid patients?

____

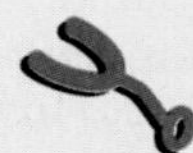

CHECK YOUR HEARTBEAT! Turn to the end of the chapter for answers to these review sessions.

MEDICAID ELIGIBILITY

Changes have been made along the way to allow more people into the program. Medicaid is available to certain needy and low-income people, such as the aged (65 years or older), the blind, the disabled, and members of families with dependent children deprived of the support of at least one parent and financially eligible on the basis of income and resources. If a person is eligible for Medicaid, he or she goes to the local welfare office and applies for benefits. Each state decides what services are covered and what the reimbursement will be for each service. Following, two classifications (categorically needy and medically needy) that contain several basic groups of needy and low-income individuals are described. For a clear, simple understanding of the classes and basic groups that qualify for Medicaid, see Figure 10–1.

Categorically Needy

The first classification, the **categorically needy** group, categorizes three groups of people who qualify for benefits: (1) families, pregnant women, and children, (2) the aged and disabled, and (3) persons receiving institutional or other long-term care. Figure 10–1 further defines subgroup titles which incorporate people from within each group.

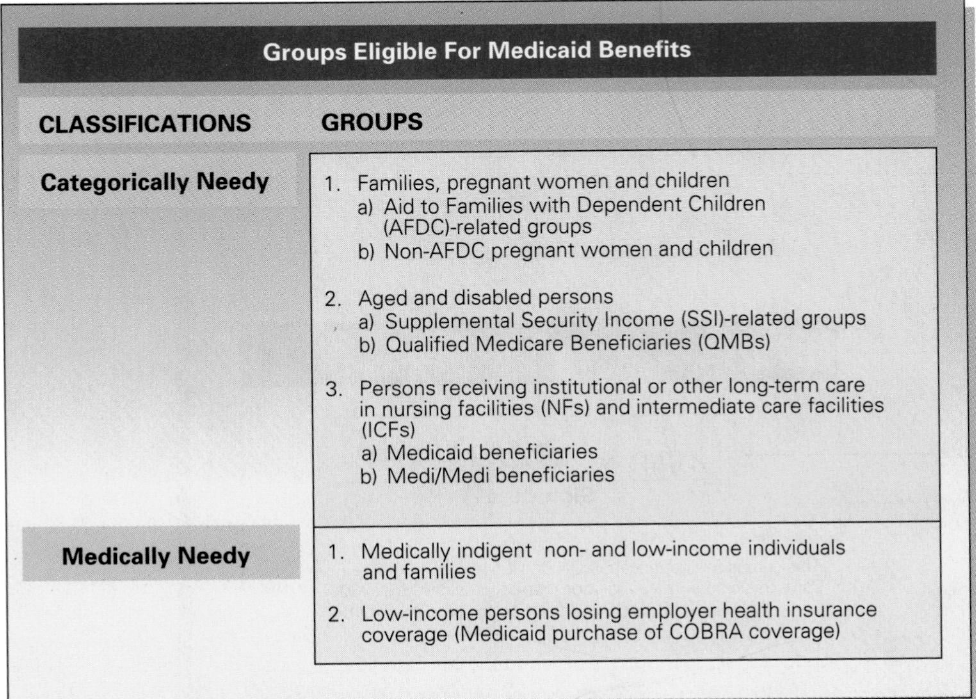

Figure 10–1. Classifications and basic groups eligible for Medicaid benefits.

Medically Needy

The second classification, the **medically needy (MN)** group, involves state general assistance programs for the following groups: (1) medically indigent, non- and low-income individuals and families, and (2) low-income persons losing employer health insurance coverage.

For those individuals who may become **medically indigent** as a result of high medical expenses and inadequate health insurance coverage, a number of states have adopted a State Program of Assistance for the Medically Indigent. The costs of medical care are financially supported by the federal government according to the minimum assistance level, and states must wholly support any part of the program that goes beyond the federal minimum. This is referred to as *state share.*

Some Medicaid **recipients** in this category must pay coinsurance and/or deductible amounts, which must be met within the eligible month or other specified time frame before they can receive state benefits. The amount to be paid is determined according to the income earned for each eligible time frame or month, and is known as a share of cost (SOC). Types of copayment and SOC requirements will be discussed later in this section.

Identification Card

After acceptance into the program, a plastic or paper Medicaid identification card is issued to the recipient indicating that he or she has qualified for Medicaid. The card may be referred to as a *benefits identification card (BIC)* in some states (Fig. 10–2). Instead of a card, some states issue coupons to be placed on the billing form when Medicaid services are provided. These "proof of eligibility" (POE) coupons have adhesive labels listing the months of eligibility. Depending on state policy and classifications of eligibility, the

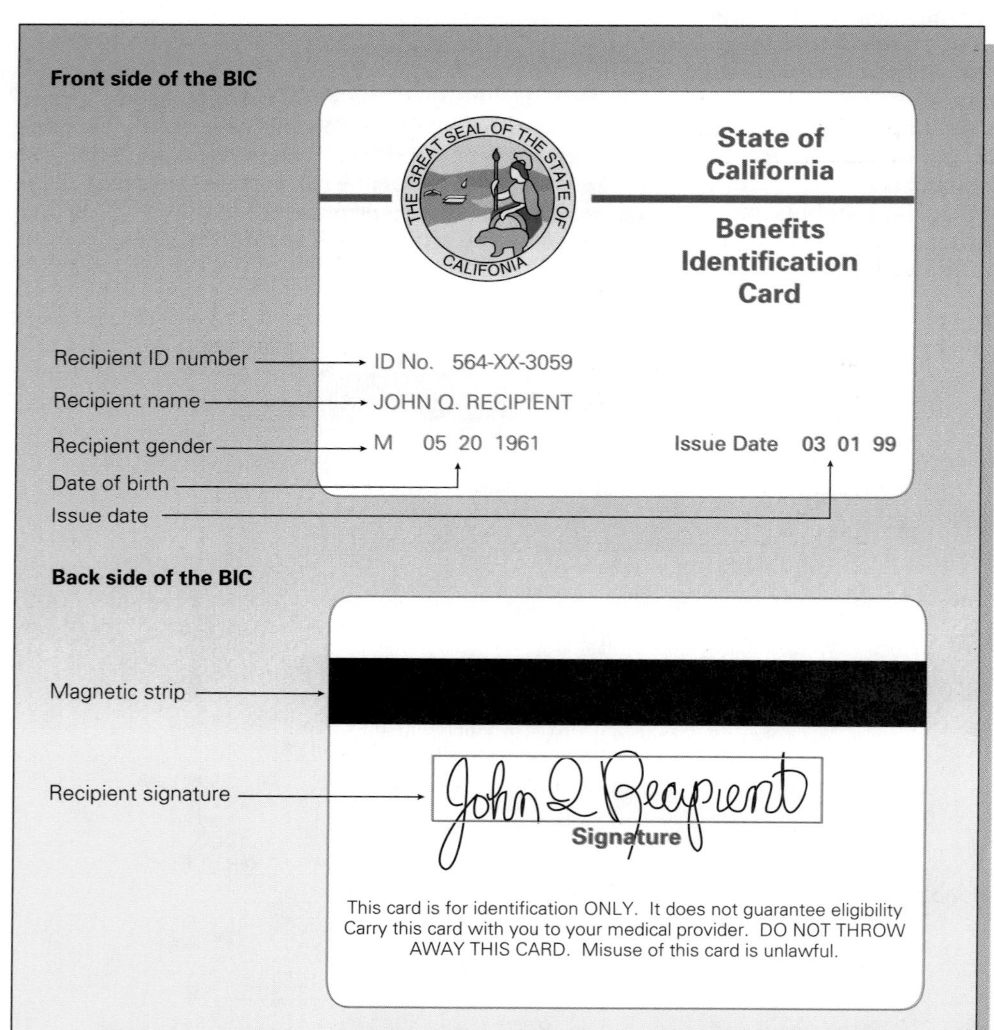

Figure 10–2. Sample plastic Medi-Cal benefits identification card (BIC).

card/coupons may be issued on the 1st and/or 15th of the month, or every 2, 3, or 6 months. Typically, eligibility is determined on a monthly basis. Paperwork is sometimes presented by the patient stating that he or she has Medicaid but the card has not been issued. Care must be taken to confirm that the patient is actually eligible for the date of service and that the paperwork is not just proof of application. Sometimes a mother is issued an identification card for an unborn child to be used for services promoting the life and health of the fetus. Often, infants use the mother's identification card until application has been made on their behalf and a card has been issued. This occurs at approximately 2 months of age.

Verifying Eligibility

A person may have a Medicaid card, but this does not indicate proof of eligibility. It is the provider's responsibility to verify that the person to receive care is eligible for the date the service is rendered and is, indeed, the individual to whom the card was issued. Obtain a photocopy of the front and back of the card, or of the coupon. Match the name and signature on the card against the signature on a valid driver's license, picture identification card, or other credible identification document.

Eligibility, which is verified at the first of the month, is valid for the entire month of service. The insurance billing specialist should keep the verification number in the recipient's file and use it as proof of eligibility for the entire month. Note whether the patient has other insurance, copayment requirements, or restrictions, such as being eligible for only certain types of medical services (e.g., pregnancy).

Eligibility for the month of service may be verified in a number of ways. The Potomac Group, Inc., in Nashville, Tennessee, has developed MediFAX to be used by several states. This is a machine that allows the user to verify coverage in seconds. In other states, the state provides electronic systems for Medicaid verification via touch-tone telephone, software with modem, or specialized Medicaid terminal equipment (Fig. 10–3). For states that issue coupons containing adhesive labels, the patient's name, date of birth, Medicaid number, and month of eligibility listed on the label suffice as eligibility verification requirements.

Copayment Requirements

Fixed Copayment

There are two types of copayment requirements that may apply to the Medicaid patient. Some states require a small fixed copayment paid to the provider at the time of service (e.g., $1 or $2). This policy was instituted to help pay some of the administrative costs of physicians participating in the Medicaid program. There may be certain groups of patients that are exempt from this copayment requirement (e.g., persons under 18 years of age, women receiving perinatal care, persons receiving emergency service, and so forth), so check carefully when collecting this amount.

Share of Cost

Another requirement is the **share of cost (SOC)** copayment. A Medicaid recipient may have a share of cost one month and not the next, or the amount may change from month to month. First, identify if an SOC is required, and second, verify the amount each time it is collected. It is important to obtain this copay amount when the patient comes in for medical care and report the amount collected on the claim form. Often, the equipment used to verify eligibility will also supply information about the patient's SOC, if applicable (Fig. 10–3C). When the patient pays, the amount can be entered into the system and Medicaid will clear the patient's SOC. This transaction records the patient's eligibility for that month and enables the patient to receive Medicaid benefits.

Prior Approval

Usually, prior authorization forms are completed to obtain permission for a specific service or hospitalization (Fig. 10–4). The form is mailed or faxed to the department of health or a designated office in the region for approval. Response may take 10 to 15 days. In emergent cases, time does not allow for a written request to be sent for **prior approval.** In such cases, an immediate authorization can be obtained via a telephone call to the proper department in your locale. Note the date and time the authorization was given, the name of the person who gave authorization, and any verbal number given to you by the field office. Usually a treatment authorization form indicating that the service was already authorized must be sent to the field office as follow-up to the telephone call. If the authorization request is for hospital services, send a copy of the approved authorization form to the hospital.

The Medicaid field office or provider manual for your area usually contains a benefit and nonbenefit list. These lists indicate which services are covered, which require prior approval, and which are not a benefit. Some of the services requiring prior approval might be:

- Durable medical equipment (DME)
- Hearing aids
- Hemodialysis
- Home healthcare
- Inpatient hospital care
- Long-term facility services
- Medical supplies
- Medications
- Prosthetic/orthotic appliances
- Surgical procedures
- Transportation
- Vision care, depending on diagnosis

The treatment authorization request (TAR) form has been redesigned as an e-TAR (electronic treatment

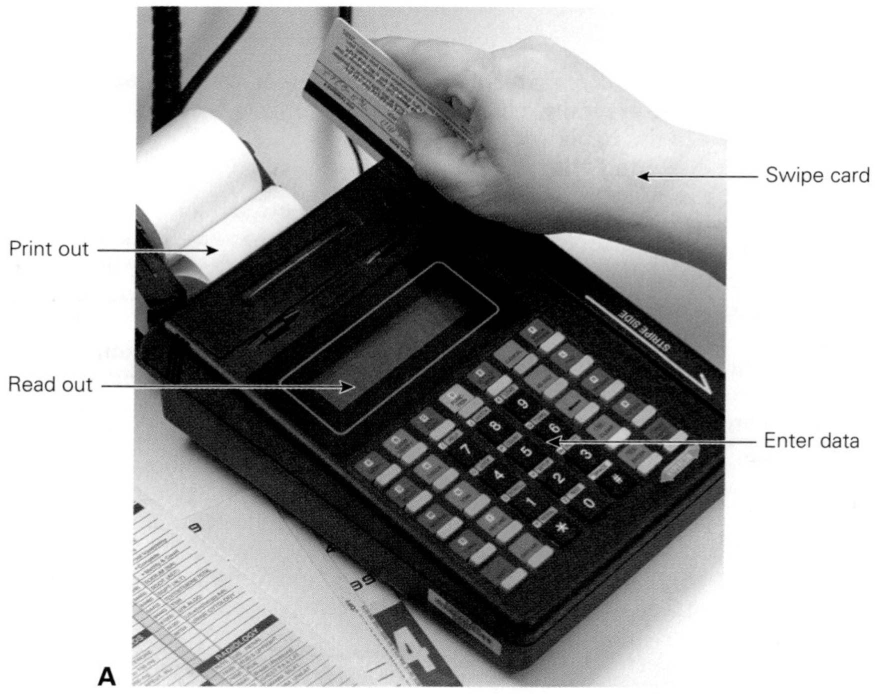

POS Device: Medi-Service Printout

EDS BROAD AVENUE TERMINAL T309006
XX-02-15
17:16:36

PROVIDER NUMBER:
12345F

TRANSACTION TYPE: MEDI-SERVICES

RECIPIENT ID:
5077534XX

YEAR & MONTH OF BIRTH:
1975-12

DATE OF ISSUE:
XX-02-15

DATE OF SERVICE:
XX-02-15

PROCEDURE CODE:
45339

LAST NAME: MORRISON MEDI SVC
RESERVATION APPLIED

B

POS Device: Share of Cost Printout

EDS BROAD AVENUE TERMINAL T309006
XX-02-15
17:16:36

PROVIDER NUMBER:
12345F

TRANSACTION TYPE: SHARE OF COST

RECIPIENT ID:
5077534XX

YEAR & MONTH OF BIRTH:
1984-10

DATE OF ISSUE:
XX-02-15

DATE OF SERVICE:
XX-02-15

CASE NUMBER:

PROCEDURE CODE:
90945

PATIENT APPLIED AMOUNT:
$50.00

TOTAL BILLED AMOUNT:
$100.00

LAST NAME: ADAMS
AMOUNT DEDUCTED: $50.00
SHARE OF COST HAS BEEN MET

C

Figure 10–3. *A*, An insurance biller using a point-of-service (POS) device machine. *B*, Sample printout from a POS device for Medi-Service. *C*, Sample printout from a POS device for share of cost (SOC).

STATE USE ONLY

SERVICE CATEGORY

3

TYPEWRITER ALIGNMENT Elite Pica

CONFIDENTIAL PATIENT INFORMATION

FOR F.I. USE ONLY

CCN

TREATMENT AUTHORIZATION REQUEST

STATE DEPARTMENT OF HEALTH SERVICES

F.I. USE ONLY 40 41 42 43

TYPEWRITER ALIGNMENT Elite Pica

(PLEASE TYPE) FOR PROVIDER USE (PLEASE TYPE)

VERBAL CONTROL NO.

TYPE OF SERVICE REQUESTED: DRUG [ ] OTHER [X]

REQUEST IS RETROACTIVATE? YES [ ] NO [X]

IS PATIENT MEDICARE ELIGIBLE? YES [ ] NO [X]

PROVIDER PHONE NO. (555) 486-9002 AREA

PATIENT'S AUTHORIZED REPRESENTATIVE (IF ANY) ENTER NAME AND ADDRESS

PROVIDER NO. HSC12345F

PROVIDER NAME AND ADDRESS

PLEASE TYPE YOUR NAME AND ADDRESS HERE

BERTHA CAESAR MD
4567 BROAD AVENUE
WOODLAND HILLS, XY
12345

COUNTY CODE 30 AID CODE 83

FOR STATE USE

33 PROVIDER; YOUR REQUEST IS:

1 [X] APPROVED AS REQUESTED [ ] [ ] DEFERRED

2 [ ] APPROVED AS MODIFIED (ITEMS MARKED BELOW AS AUTHORIZED MAY BE CLAIMED) [ ] JACKSON VS RANK PARAGRAPH CODE

BY John Doe MD MEDICAL CONSULTANT

I.D. # 34 01 DATE 35 08 20 XX REVIEW COMMENTS INDICATOR 44

NAME AND ADDRESS OF PATIENT

PATIENT NAME (LAST, FIRST, M. I.) APPLEGATE, NANCY

MEDICAL IDENTIFICATION NO. 253971060 CHECK DIGIT

STREET ADDRESS 1515 RIVER ROAD

SEX F AGE 32 DATE OF BIRTH 06 18 70

CITY, STATE, ZIP CODE WOODLAND HILLS, XY 12345

PATIENT STATUS: [X] HOME [ ] BOARD AND CARE [ ] SNF/ICF [ ] ACUTE HOSPITAL

PHONE NUMBER (555) 545-1123

COMMENTS/ EXPLANATION

DIAGNOSIS DESCRIPTION: ENDOMETRIOSIS

ICD-9-CM DIAGNOSIS CODE 617.9

MEDICAL JUSTIFICATION:
COLLEGE HOSPITAL - 4500 BROAD AVE, WOODLAND HILLS, XY

UNCONTROLLABLE ENDOMETRIOSIS

RETROACTIVE AUTHORIZATION GRANTED IN ACCORDANCE WITH SECTION 51003 (B)

36 1 2 3 4 5 6

	AUTHORIZED YES	NO	APPROVED UNITS	SPECIFIC SERVICES REQUESTED	UNITS OF SERVICE	PROCEDURE OR DRUG CODE	QUANTITY	CHARGES
1	9 X		10 3	DAYS: 3 HOSPITAL DAYS REQUESTED		11	12	$
2	13 X		14 1	HYSTERECTOMY	1	15 5815070	16 1	$ $1300.00
3	17		18			19	20	$
4	21		22			23	24	$
5	25		26			27	28	$
6	29		30			31	32	$

TO THE BEST OF MY KNOWLEDGE, THE ABOVE INFORMATION IS TRUE, ACCURATE AND COMPLETE AND THE REQUESTED SERVICES ARE MEDICALLY INDICATED AND NECESSARY TO THE HEALTH OF THE PATIENT.

Bertha Caesar — SIGNATURE OF PHYSICIAN OR PROVIDER

MD — TITLE

8-10-XX — DATE

AUTHORIZATION IS VALID FOR SERVICES PROVIDED

37 FROM DATE 09 01XX 38 TO DATE 093 0XX

TAR CONTROL NUMBER

36 OFFICE 12 SEQUENCE NUMBER 61240229 PI 0

NOTE: AUTHORIZATION DOES NOT GUARANTEE PAYMENT. PAYMENT IS SUBJECT TO PATIENT'S ELIGIBILITY. BE SURE THE IDENTIFICATION CARD IS CURRENT BEFORE RENDERING SERVICE. SEND TO FIELD SERVICES (F.I. COPY)

SEE YOUR PROVIDER MANUAL FOR ASSISTANCE REGARDING THE COMPLETION OF THIS FORM. 50-1 12/87

Figure 10–4. Example of a completed treatment authorization request form for the Medicaid program.

authorization request) and is being made available via a Medi-Cal web site for the state of California. Other states may soon follow this easy method of form completion and submission.

Retroactive Eligibility

There are a number of situations where retroactive eligibility may be granted to a patient. When patients who are seeking medical care are in hope of qualifying for Medicaid but have not done so at the time of service (e.g., emergency, pregnancy), the account must be set up as a cash account until retroactive eligibility has been established. As described and shown in the previous chapter, a waiver of liability agreement (Advance Beneficiary Notice) rewritten to specify the Medicaid program and signed by the patient might be used in such cases. If the patient qualifies and provides documentation or a retroactive card confirming prior services during the covered retroactive period, and the patient paid for such services, then a refund must be immediately made to the patient and Medicaid billed.

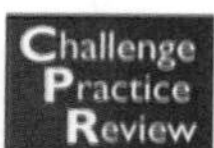

Pause and Practice CPR

REVIEW SESSIONS 10–3 THROUGH 10–5

Directions: *Complete the following questions as a review of information you have just read.*

10–3 Name the two classifications under which all Medicaid recipients can be categorized.

(a) ______________________________

(b) ______________________________

10–4 Typically, Medicaid eligibility is determined on a ______________ basis.

10–5 Two types of copayment requirements are:

(a) ______________________________

(b) ______________________________

CHECK YOUR HEARTBEAT! Turn to the end of the chapter for answers to these review sessions.

MEDICAID ASSISTANCE PROGRAMS AND BENEFITS

Under federal guidelines, state Medicaid programs establish basic Medicaid benefits that are offered to eligible recipients. Basic benefits include **covered services** as shown in Table 10–1. Other Medicaid-sponsored programs and benefits are described and listed in the following section.

Early and Periodic Screening, Diagnosis, and Treatment

Early and Periodic Screening, Diagnosis, and Treatment (EPSDT) is a program of prevention, early detection, and treatment of welfare children who are younger than age 21 years. In California, it is known as the Child Health and Disability Prevention (CHDP) program and in New York as the Child Health Assurance Program (CHAP).

Benefits

The EPSDT benefit guidelines include a medical history and physical examination; immunization status assessment; dental, hearing, and vision screening; developmental assessment; and screening for anemia and lead absorption, tuberculosis, bacteriuria, and sickle cell trait or disease. States are required to provide necessary health care, diagnostic services, treatment, and other services to correct physical or mental defects found.

Maternal and Child Health Programs

All states and certain other jurisdictions, including territories and the District of Columbia, operate a total of 56 **Maternal and Child Health Programs (MCHPs)** with federal grant support under Title V of the Social Security Act. MCHP is a state and federal program for

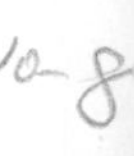

Table 10–1 MEDICAID BASIC BENEFITS

Family planning
Home healthcare
Immunizations
Inpatient hospital care
Laboratory and x-ray
Outpatient hospital care
Physicians' care
Screening, diagnosis, and treatment of children younger than 21 years of age
Skilled nursing care
Transportation to and from healthcare providers

Additional services in some states might include the following:

Allergy care
Ambulance services
Cosmetic procedures (limited)
Chiropractic services
Clinic care
Dental care
Dermatologic care
Diagnostic, screening, preventive, and rehabilitative services (e.g., physical therapy)
Emergency department care
Eyeglasses and eye refraction
Hospice care
Intermediate care
Occupational therapy
Optometric services
Podiatric care
Prescription drugs
Private duty nursing
Prosthetic devices
Psychiatric care
Respiratory care
Speech therapy

children who are under 21 years of age and have special healthcare needs. It assists parents with financial planning and may assume part or all of the costs of treatment, depending on the child's condition and the family's resources. The state agency tries to locate mothers, infants, and children younger than 21 years of age who may have conditions eligible for treatment under the MCHP.

Specific conditions qualify a child for benefits. Qualifying conditions may change from state to state; however, all state laws include children who have some kind of handicap that needs orthopedic treatment or plastic surgery. Following is a list of the types of conditions that qualify children for MCHP:

- Cerebral palsy
- Chronic conditions affecting bones and joints
- Cleft lip and palate
- Clubfoot
- Cystic fibrosis*
- Epilepsy*
- Hearing problems*
- Mental retardation*
- Multiple handicaps*
- Paralyzed muscles
- Rheumatic and congenital heart disease*
- Vision problems requiring surgery*

Benefits

After a child is examined at an MCHP clinic and a diagnosis is made, the parents are advised about the treatment that will benefit the child. The state agency then helps them locate this care. If the parents cannot afford the necessary care, the agency assists them with financial planning and may assume part or all of the cost of treatment (including hospitalization), depending on the child's condition and the family's resources.

Federal funds are granted to states for the MCHP enabling them to:

- Provide low-income mothers and children access to quality maternal and child health services.
- Reduce infant mortality and the incidence of preventable diseases and handicapping conditions among children.
- Increase the number of children immunized against disease.
- Increase the number of low-income children receiving health assessments and follow-up diagnostic services and treatment.
- Promote the health of mothers and infants by providing prenatal, delivery, and postpartum care for low-income, at-risk pregnant women.
- Provide preventive and primary care services for low-income children.
- Provide rehabilitation services for the blind and disabled younger than 16 years of age.
- Provide, promote, and develop family-centered, community-based, coordinated care for children with special healthcare needs.

Low-Income Medicare Recipients

There are three programs that aid Medicare patients over 65 years of age who have low incomes and have difficulty paying Medicare premiums, copayments, and deductibles. Each program addresses a different financial category, and the monthly income figures are adjusted each year. The programs are usually administered through county social service departments, the same ones that administer Medicaid. One application is completed that pertains to all three programs, and an individual is placed in one of the programs, depending on how he or she qualifies financially. Next is a description of the three programs that list qualified individuals and benefits.

*Only some states include this item in their Maternal and Child Health Program.

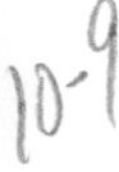

Medicaid Qualified Medicare Beneficiary Program

The *Medicaid Qualified Medicare Beneficiary (MQMB)* program allows the qualified Medicare beneficiaries (QMBs—pronounced "kwim-bees") limited Medicaid coverage. They must be aged and disabled, qualify for Medicare benefits, have annual incomes below the federal poverty level, and have limited other financial resources.

Benefits

The state must pay QMBs Medicare Part B premiums (and if applicable, premiums for Part A), along with required Medicare deductibles and coinsurance amounts. Benefits are limited to Medicare cost sharing as described above unless the beneficiary qualifies for Medicaid in some other way. Medicaid will not pay for the service if Medicare considers it a noncovered service.

States are also required to pay Part A premiums, but not other expenses, for qualified disabled and working individuals. It is optional for states to provide full Medicaid benefits to QMBs who meet a state-established income standard.

Specified Low-Income Medicare Beneficiary Program

The Specified Low-Income Medicare Beneficiary (SLMB—pronounced "slim-bee") program was established for elderly individuals whose incomes are 20% above the federal poverty level.

Benefits

Benefits for SLMBs include payment of the entire Medicare Part B premium. The patient must pay the deductible, copay, and all noncovered service fees.

Qualifying Individuals Program

The *Qualifying Individuals (QIs)* program for old age security (OAS) assistance was created for individuals who are 135% above the poverty standard.

Benefits

Benefits for QIs also include payment of the Medicare Part B premium.

Disallowed Services

If a claim is denied stating a service is totally disallowed by Medicaid, a physician is within legal rights to bill the patient. However, if the service to be provided has been a denied service from known past claim submission experience, it is wise to have the patient sign a waiver of liability agreement and collect the payment at the time of service. An example of a waiver of liability agreement is shown in Chapter 11, Figure 11–9. To obtain up-to-date information and details on the Medicaid program in your state, write or telephone your state agency.

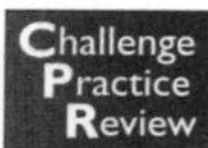

Pause and Practice CPR

REVIEW SESSIONS 10–6 AND 10–7

Directions: *Complete the following questions as a review of information you have just read.*

10–6 Refer to Table 10–1 and indicate by checking (✓) whether the following services are *basic*, *additional services* sometimes offered, or *not covered* services in the Medicaid program.

Service	Basic	Additional	Not covered
(a) Allergy care	______	______	______
(b) Hospice care	______	______	______
(c) Massage therapy	______	______	______
(d) Prescription drugs	______	______	______
(e) Over-the-counter drugs	______	______	______
(f) Immunizations	______	______	______
(g) Home healthcare	______	______	______

10–7 List the acronym for the program that provides prevention, early detection, and treatment of welfare children who are younger than age 21. ______________________

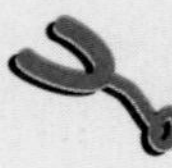

CHECK YOUR HEARTBEAT! Turn to the end of the chapter for answers to these review sessions.

MEDICAID MANAGED CARE

As early as 1967, some states began incorporating managed care in their Medicaid program. In the past decade, many states have adopted pilot projects to evaluate benefits and see whether a managed care system will work. Mainly, this has been done as an effort to control escalating healthcare costs by emphasizing preventive care and curbing unnecessary emergency department and other healthcare visits.

When the last state, Arizona, joined Medicaid, most states had been struggling with Medicaid for nearly 20 years. Arizona chose to structure a prepaid healthcare Medicaid system, rather than adopt a system similar to what most states were using.

In Medicaid managed care systems, the recipient enrolls in a plan similar to a health maintenance organization (HMO). The enrollment may be automatic once the recipient qualifies for Medicaid and lives in an area where a managed care plan is in place. The patient usually has a primary care physician (PCP) and can choose or be assigned this gatekeeper, who must approve all specialty care and hospital treatment. Patients must use physicians, clinics, and hospitals participating in their assigned plan. Patients can be cared for side by side with private-paying patients. Persons with complicated medical problems may receive help through a case management department.

Some states have adopted capitated (flat fee per patient) rather than fee-for-service reimbursement. There may be a small copayment for services. In programs that have been in existence for a number of years, it has been found that if they are well managed, there is better access to primary healthcare and lower costs for the delivery of care.

CLAIM PROCEDURES

Medicaid policies and claim procedures regarding placement of share of cost and prior authorization information on the claim form, claim submission time limits, and claim form completion vary from state to state. Following are general guidelines for submitting claims. Although some states may use their own claim form, many states use the universal claim form (HCFA-1500); therefore, the HCFA-1500 claim form template (see Fig. D–5 in Appendix D) is used to illustrate block-by-block requirements. For specific state guidelines, consult your current Medicaid Handbook and/or state fiscal agent.

Reporting the Share of Cost

When the patient pays his or her share of cost it must be reported on the claim form. The block used to report the SOC varies from state to state. In the state of California, the SOC is entered in Block 10d without any dollar sign or decimal point to indicate the dollar amount (e.g., $50 would be entered as SOC 5000, as seen in Fig. 10–5).

10d. RESERVED FOR LOCAL USE
SOC 5000

Figure 10–5. Block 10d of the HCFA-1500 claim form illustrating a share of cost (SOC) entry.

Reporting Prior Approval

When submitting the insurance claim for authorized services, indicate the authorization approval number in Block 23 of the claim form and enclose a copy with the form.

Time Limit

Each state has its own time limit for the submission of a claim. The time limit can vary from 2 months to 1 year from the date or month of service. If a bill is submitted after the time limit, it most likely will be rejected unless a valid justification that the state recognizes accompanies the claim. Justification may include retroactive eligibility, county error, reversal of decision on appealed authorization request, and so forth.

Some states have separate procedures for billing *over-one-year* (OOY) claims. A percentage of the claim may be reduced according to the date of a delinquent submission unless an approved billing limit exception code is noted. Example 10–1 illustrates a state (California) where such as system is in place.

Reciprocity

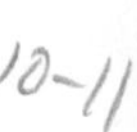

Reciprocity is the mutual exchange of privileges or services. In the case of a Medicaid patient, reciprocity applies to the patient who obtains services while out of the state in which he or she receives benefits. Most states have reciprocity agreements for a Medicaid patient who requires medical care while out of state. To process a claim, contact the Medicaid intermediary in the patient's home state and ask for the appropriate

> **Example 10–1**
>
> **Percentage of Claim Amounts Paid According to Submission Dates**
>
> **BILLING TIME LIMIT**
> **SIX MONTHS FROM MONTH OF SERVICE**
>
> - Claim submitted within 6 months of billing limit—paid at 100%
> - Claim submitted 7–9 months after the month of service—paid at 75%
> - Claims submitted 10–12 months after the month of service—paid at 50%
> - Claims submitted over 1 year from the month of service—not paid
>
> *Note: When a qualified exception code accompanies a late claim, it will be paid at a higher amount.*

Expressions from Experience

Use the telephone whenever possible to get a pending claim processed. Through years of experience I have learned to work the mail daily and process denied claims according to the policy of the employer. It is very important to keep your work current in the billing arena because time is unkind to unpaid claims.

Jane Seelig, CMA-A
Billing and Collection Specialist
Federally Qualified Health Center

form. If the case was an emergency, state this on the form and file the papers with the Medicaid intermediary in the patient's home state. Reimbursement will be at that state's rate.

Claim Form

Federal law mandates that the universal claim form be adopted for the processing of Medicaid claims in all states that do not optically scan their claims. States that use optical scanners must adopt a form that is as close as possible to the format of the universal claim form. Be sure to use the required form, and if documentation or additional information is necessary to accompany the claim, state your case briefly.

General block-by-block instructions for the completion of the HCFA-1500 claim form for a Medicaid patient are found in Appendix D. Because guidelines vary among Medicaid intermediaries, refer to your local Medicaid intermediary for specific directions. Figure D–5 is a template emphasizing placement of basic elements on the claim form.

Unique Claim Form Requirements

Medicaid has the least number of mandatory blocks to be completed on the HCFA-1500 claim form. Refer to the shaded areas in Figure D–5 for a visual illustration of blocks that are not required. Following are a few of the unique requirements encountered when completing the claim form.

Assignment of Benefits/Claim Submission

For Medicaid cases, there is no assignment of benefits unless the patient has other insurance in addition to Medicaid. Claims are submitted to a fiscal agent, which might be an insurance company, or directly to the local department of social services. Prescription drugs and dental services are often billed to a different intermediary than services performed by a physician, depending on state guidelines.

Block 24

There are a few special rules that should be noted when completing some subsections of Block 24. Refer to Figure 10–6 for a visual illustration of the following subsections.

- Block 24A (To)—There is no date ranging on Medicaid claims; therefore this block is not used.
- Block 24C (Type of Service)—This block has not been completed for the programs previously described. However, Medicaid requires this block, and a brief list of codes with their descriptions used in this block is found in Figure D–2 in Appendix D.
- Block 24H (EPSDT)—As described earlier, Early and Periodic Screening, Diagnosis, and Treatment is a preventive program. When EPSDT services are provided, enter an "E" in this block. When family planning services are provided, enter an "F" in this block.
- Block 24I (EMG)—This block is used to indicate when an emergency (EMG) service has been provided in a hospital emergency department. Enter an "X" in this block when applicable and describe the emergency in Block 19.
- Block 24J (COB)—Is used to indicate when a patient has other insurance in addition to Medicaid to which the coordination of benefits rule would apply.
- Block 24K (Reserved for Local Use)—Is not recognized by Medicaid; leave blank.

	24. A DATE(S) OF SERVICE FROM MM DD YY	TO MM DD YY	B Place of Service	C Type of Service	D PROCEDURES, SERVICES, OR SUPPLIES (Explain Unusual Circumstances) CPT/HCPCS	MODIFIER	E DIAGNOSIS CODE	F $ CHARGES	G DAYS OR UNITS	H EPSDT Family Plan	I EMG	J COB	K RESERVED FOR LOCAL USE
1	051220XX		11	5	86580		1	11 34	1	E			
2	051320XX		11	1	99213		2	40 20	1	F			
3	051420XX		23	1	99281		3	24 32	1		X		
4	051520XX		11	1	99212		4	24 32	1			X	

Figure 10–6. Block 24 of the HCFA-1500 claim form illustrating Block 24A—"To" and 24K shaded (nonused) areas, and entries for Block 24C—type of service, 24H—Early and Periodic Screening, and Diagnostic Testing and Family Planning, 24I—emergency service provided in Emergency Department, and 24J—coordination of benefits.

Name and Address of Facility Where Services Were Rendered

Although Medicaid guidelines for Block 32 state to use Medicare guidelines, in many states it is sufficient to list the facility provider number alone and not list the name and address of the facility (Fig. 10–7).

32. NAME AND ADDRESS OF FACILITY WHERE SERVICES WERE RENDERED (if other than home or office)

HSC 43700F

Figure 10–7. Block 32 of the HCFA-1500 claim form illustrating entry of College Hospital facility provider number.

Provider Support Center

Most Medicaid programs have a provider support center (PSC) or similar place where providers and representatives may call to ask questions and obtain information. Specific information may be available via a voice response system (e.g., authorization status, claim status, mailing information), while help desks, hotlines, and specific units serve other needs and concerns.

Medicaid Managed Care

When filing a claim for a Medicaid managed care patient, send the bill to the managed care organization (MCO), not to the Medicaid fiscal agent. The MCO receives payment for services rendered to eligible members via the capitation method.

Maternal and Child Health Program

Each jurisdiction operates its own Maternal and Child Health Program (MCHP) that has unique administrative characteristics. Thus, each has its own system and forms used for billing. The official plans and documents are retained in the individual state offices and are not available on either a regional or national office basis. For specific information about your state's policies, write to the MCHP state agency.

Medicaid and Private Insurance

When Medicaid and a third party payer cover the patient, Medicaid is always considered the payer of last resort. The third party payer is billed first, using its guidelines. Have the patient sign an assignment of benefits for the private payer. When the primary carrier pays, attach the explanation of benefits (EOB) to the Medicaid claim and submit for payment. In most cases, the Medicaid carrier will not pay because the primary carrier's payment exceeds the Medicaid fee schedule; however, sometimes Medicaid will pick up services not covered by the primary carrier.

Medicaid and Government Programs

When a Medicaid patient has Medicare (referred to as a Medi-Medi case), TRICARE, or CHAMPVA, obtain an assignment of benefits for the government program and send the insurance claim first to the federal program fiscal agent servicing your region. If the federal program does not automatically cross over the claim to Medicaid, bill Medicaid second and enclose the remittance advice/explanation of benefits (RA/EOB) that has been received from the federal program. Send in a claim only if the other coverage denies payment or pays less than the Medicaid fee schedule, or if Medicaid covers services not covered by the other policy. Chapter 11 gives additional information on Medi-Medi claim submission. Refer to Chapter 12 for further information on patients who receive benefits from TRICARE and CHAMPVA.

Medicaid and Aliens

Process claims for aliens as you would any other Medicaid claim. However, if an alien is older than 65 years and on Medicaid (Medi-Cal in California) and not eligible for Medicare benefits, send the claim to Medicaid and indicate in Block 19 of the HCFA-1500 claim form, "Alien is older than 65 years and not eligible for Medicare benefits."

MEDICAID FRAUD CONTROL

Each state has a Medicaid Fraud Control Unit (MFCU), which is a federally funded state law enforcement entity usually located in the state attorney general's office. The MFCU investigates and prosecutes cases of fraud and other violations, including complaints of mistreatment in long-term care facilities. The state Medicaid agency must cooperate and ensure access to records by the MFCU and agree to refer suspected cases of provider fraud to this division of the attorney general's office for investigation.

Expressions from Experience

Over the years I have had experiences with billing situations that have been both gratifying and educational. The collection call was always the most difficult but the most rewarding as well. My primary objective was to maintain a friendly soft-spoken voice and offer manageable recommendations to resolution of the outstanding debt. If the verbal response to my call was irate and irrational, I would speak more softly and slowly until the patient calmed down.

Jane Seelig, CMA-A
Billing and Collection Specialist
Federally Qualified Health Center

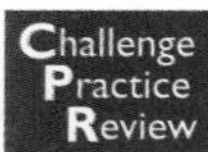

Pause and Practice CPR

PRACTICE SESSIONS 10–8 AND 10–9

Directions: *Complete the following questions by applying the information you have just read.*

10–8 Indicate how a share of cost in the amount of $75.25 would be entered on the claim form.

____

10–9 Dr. Gerald Practon goes to a patient's home to deliver hospice care on 10/13/20XX (99342). The primary diagnosis is breast cancer. Refer to Medicaid instructions for Block 24 in Appendix D and the mock fee schedule in Appendix B to complete this section of the claim form.

24. A DATE(S) OF SERVICE FROM			TO			B	C	D PROCEDURES, SERVICES, OR SUPPLIES (Explain Unusual Circumstances)		E	F	G	H	I	J	K
MM	DD	YYYY	MM	DD	YYYY	Place of Service	Type of Service	CPT/HCPCS	MODIFIER	DIAGNOSIS CODE	$ CHARGES	DAYS OR UNITS	EPSDT Family Plan	EMG	COB	RESERVED FOR LOCAL USE

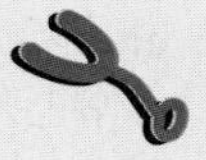

CHECK YOUR HEARTBEAT! Turn to the end of the chapter for answers to these practice sessions.

SUMMATION AND PREVIEW

Although individual states have specific forms and requirements for billing Medicaid patients, once the state's protocol is known and adhered to, processing claims for Medicaid can be done with expertise. A medical biller specializing in Medicaid claims will always be sought after, and employment opportunities are numerous. Knowing the ins and outs of federal and state regulations is sometimes a daunting task; however, once they are known, it is easier to keep up with changes and bill clean claims according to regulations.

Next, you will continue to deal with federal laws and ordinances as you learn about another federal program, Medicare. It, too, is a major building block because it is available throughout all states, in every town and city, no matter how big or small.

GOLDEN RULE

Use all required forms and STATE your case briefly.

Chapter 10 Review and Practice

Study Session

Directions: *Review the objectives, key terms, and chapter information before completing the following study questions.*

10–1 Medicaid exists in 48 states. It is called Medi-Cal in California, and the state of Arizona has a prepaid alternative assistant program.

10–2 Medicaid is referred to as a/an assistance program instead of an insurance program.

10–3 The physician's decision to accept or not accept Medicaid patients must be based on the entire Medicaid program, not an individual patient's personality, medical situation, or other discriminating factor.

10–4 Where does a patient go to apply for Medicaid benefits? local welfare office

10–5 An infant is issued a Medicaid identification card at approximately 2 months of age.

10–6 Name ways in which Medicaid eligibility can be verified.

(a) mediFAX

(b) touch tone telephone

(c) Software with modem

(d) Specialized Medicaid terminal equipment

(e) Coupons containing adhesive labels

10–7 If a Medicaid patient needs surgery, you must first obtain prior approval.

10–8 What is the Medicaid program that is available in all states to provide special-needs children (e.g., handicapped), under age 21, with medical care? (MCHP) Maternal & Child Health Programs

10–9 List the three Medicaid programs that aid Medicare patients over 65 years of age who have low incomes and have difficulty paying Medicare premiums, copayments, and deductibles.

(a) Medicaid Qualified Medicare Beneficiary Program

(b) Specified Low-Income Medicare Beneficiary Program

(c) Qualifying Individuals Program

10–10 Medicaid managed care systems exist that are similar to a/an HMO.

10–11 When a Medicaid patient is out of state and needs medical treatment, reciprocity applies and the medical insurance billing specialist should contact the Medicaid intermediary in which state? The patient's home state

10–12 An assignment of benefits [is, is not] required for a Medicaid patient with no other insurance.

10–13 If you have questions about the Medicaid program, where do you call? ____________

10–14 When Medicaid and a third party payer cover the patient, Medicaid is billed [first, second] because it is always considered ____________

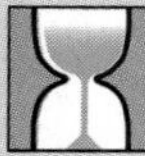

Billing Break—

Case 10–1 Salvador A. Winton

Time Started
Time Finished
Total Time

Directions: *Follow these steps to complete the HCFA-1500 insurance claim form for a Medicaid case using OCR guidelines.*

1. Copy the HCFA-1500 insurance claim form found in Appendix F (Form 09).
2. Refer to the Patient Information form for Case 10–1 and abstract information to complete the top portion of the HCFA-1500 claim form.
3. Refer to the Medical Record for Case 10–1 to abstract information for the bottom portion of the HCFA-1500 claim form.
4. Copy the Medical Coding Worksheet found in Appendix F (Form 12) to use when abstracting information from the chart note.
5. Use the "HCFA-1500 Claim Form Block-by-Block Instructions" for Medicaid patients found in Appendix D and the Medicaid template (Fig. 10–5) for guidance and block help.
6. Use your procedure codebook to determine the correct code number(s) and modifier(s) for each professional service/procedure rendered.
7. Use your HCPCS Level II codebook or Appendix C to apply HCPCS codes and modifiers when applicable.
8. Refer to the fee schedule in Appendix B for mock fees.
9. Use your diagnostic codebook to determine the correct diagnoses.
10. Address the claim to Medicaid and date the claim 09/25/20XX.
11. Copy and prepare the ledger card found in Appendix F (Form 7) for the patient. Complete the ledger by posting each transaction in this case and indicating when you have billed the insurance carrier.

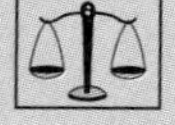

Weigh your progress. Turn to the Assignment Score Sheet in Appendix F (Form 10) and record information to track your success. Your instructor may ask that you include a Performance Evaluation Checklist, and if so, copy Form 11 found in Appendix F and attach it to your insurance claim.

4567 Broad Avenue
Woodland Hills, XY
12345-0001
Tel (555) 486-9002
Fax (555) 487-8976

REGISTRATION
(PLEASE PRINT)

Account # 1727 Today's Date: 03/16/XX

PATIENT INFORMATION

Name: Winton (Last Name) Salvador (First Name) A. (Initial) Soc. Sec. # 301-XX-2987

Address 726 Bouquet Canyon Home Phone (555) 486-1523

City Woodland Hills State XY Zip 12345

Single___ Married ✓ Separated___ Divorced___ Sex M ✓ F___ Birthdate 09/07/1996

Patient Employed by Saturn Strawberry Company Occupation Picker

Business Address PO Box 389A Crest City, XY Business Phone (555) 840-9696

Spouse's Name Sally (Mother) Employed by: N/A Occupation ___

Business Address ___ Business Phone ___

Reason for Visit Sore throat If accident:___ Auto___ Employment___ Other___

By whom were you referred? Mother

In case of emergency, who should be notified? Sally Winton (Name) Wife (Relation to Patient) Phone (555) 486-1523

PRIMARY INSURANCE

Insured/Subscriber Winton (Last Name) Salvador (First Name) A. (Initial)

Relation to Patient Self Birthdate 09/07/1996 Soc. Sec.# 301-XX-2987

Address (if different from patient's) ___

City ___ State ___ Zip ___

Insurance Company Medicaid

Insurance Address 1515 Center Court El Capitan, XY 12345

Insurance Identification Number 7249-900-61104 Group # ___

ADDITIONAL INSURANCE

Is patient covered by additional insurance? Yes___ No ✓

Subscriber Name ___ Relation to Patient ___ Birthdate ___

Address (if different from patient's) ___ Phone ___

City ___ State ___ Zip ___

Subscriber Employed by ___ Buisness Phone ___

Insurance Company ___ Soc. Sec. # ___

Insurance Address ___

Insurance Identification Number ___ Group # ___

ASSIGNMENT AND RELEASE

I, the undersigned, certify that I (or my dependent) have insurance coverage with Medicaid (Name of Insurance Company(ies)) and assign directly to Dr. Pedro Atrics insurance benefits, if any, otherwise payable to me for services rendered. I understand that I am financially responsible for all charges whether or not paid by insurance. I hereby consent for the doctor to release all information necessary to secure the payment of benefits. I authorize the use of this signature on all insurance submissions.

Salvador A Winton (Responsible Party Signature) Self (Relationship) 03/16/XX (Date)

ORDER # 58-8426 @BIBBERO SYSTEMS, INC. •PETALUMA, CALIFORNIA• TO REORDER CALL TOLL FREE (800)242-9330

Medical Record

Account number: 1727
Patient's name: Winton, Salvador A.
Date of birth: 09/07/96

Date	Progress Notes

09/25/XX While doing rounds at College Hospital I saw patient Salvador Winton in the waiting area of the Emergency Room. He was crying and I asked him what had happened. Mrs. Winton explained that a barbell fell off of a shelf in the garage smashing 3 of his left fingers. I asked Salvador if he would like for me to take care of him and he shook his head up and down while sobbing. I advised the emergency room staff that I was going to examine one of my patients and took a PF HX.

I performed a PF PX and normal active and passive range of motion (ROM) occurs in both the flexion and extension positions of the left index finger and left ring finger. The left long finger has decreased ROM in the extended position. I sent the patient to the radiology department for x-rays which shows a mid-phalanx fracture of the left long finger. SF MDM.

There is a 3 mm laceration (superficial injury) on the flexor part of the mid-phalanx of the left long finger and a 4 mm abrasion at the base of the nail bed. Local anesthesia is applied and the wound is cleansed and examined closely. I decided not to suture the laceration. Closed treatment of the phalangeal shaft fracture is performed and the fracture is stabilized with a static splint.

The patient and the patient's mother are advised to soak the wound 3 times a day in tepid soapy water beginning tomorrow, replace the splint and keep the hand elevated. Follow-up in the office in 1 week.

Pedro Atrics, MD

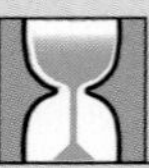

Billing Break—

Time Started
Time Finished
Total Time

Case 10–2A and B: Leslee K. Knight

Directions: *Follow these steps to complete two HCFA-1500 insurance claim forms for this Medicaid case using OCR guidelines.*

1. Make two copies of the HCFA-1500 insurance claim form found in Appendix F (Form 9).
2. Refer to the Patient Information form for Case 10–2 and abstract information to complete the top portion of two HCFA-1500 claim forms.
3. Refer to the Medical Record for Case 10–2 to abstract information for the bottom portion of the HCFA-1500 claim forms. Although two claims are being filed for separate dates of service, the patient's medical record and worksheet can be used to record all symptoms, diagnoses, and services/procedures.
4. Copy the Medical Record Coding Worksheet found in Appendix F (Form 12) to use when abstracting information from the chart note.
5. Complete the first claim (A) for DOS 5/6/20XX and use this date to file the claim to Medicaid.

(Continued on page 294)

4567 Broad Avenue
Woodland Hills, XY
12345-0001
Tel (555) 486-9002
Fax (555) 487-8976

REGISTRATION
(PLEASE PRINT)

Account # 3452 Today's Date: 09/21/XX

PATIENT INFORMATION

Name Knight (Last Name) Leslee (First Name) K. (Initial) Soc. Sec. # 660-XX-8573

Address 1162 Los Osos Street Home Phone (555) 967-3619

City Orange Grove State XY Zip 12345

Single___ Married___ Separated ✓ Divorced___ Sex M___ F ✓ Birthdate 07/04/1967

Patient Employed by Unemployed Occupation ___

Business Address ___ Business Phone ___

Spouse's Name Jim Knight Employed by: Foodaholic Rest Occupation Owner

Business Address 131 Kelp Street Oceanland, XY Business Phone (555) 676-3152

Reason for Visit Breast Pain If accident:___ Auto___ Employment___ Other___

By whom were you referred? Phone Book

In case of emergency, who should be notified? Leann Hollister (Name) Sister (Relation to Patient) Phone (555) 967-6767

PRIMARY INSURANCE

Insured/Subscriber Knight (Last Name) Leslee (First Name) K. (Initial)

Relation to Patient Self Birthdate 07/04/1967 Soc. Sec.# 660-XX-8573

Address (if different from patient's) Same

City ___ State ___ Zip ___

Insurance Company Medicaid

Insurance Address 1515 Center Court El Capitan, XY 12345

Insurance Identification Number 6295-800-62323 Group # ___

ADDITIONAL INSURANCE

Is patient covered by additional insurance? Yes___ No ✓

Subscriber Name ___ Relation to Patient ___ Birthdate ___

Address (if different from patient's) ___ Phone ___

City ___ State ___ Zip ___

Subscriber Employed by ___ Buisness Phone ___

Insurance Company ___ Soc. Sec. # ___

Insurance Address ___

Insurance Identification Number ___ Group # ___

ASSIGNMENT AND RELEASE

I, the undersigned, certify that I (or my dependent) have insurance coverage with Medicaid (Name of Insurance Company(ies)) and assign directly to Dr. Berta Caesar insurance benefits, if any, otherwise payable to me for services rendered. I understand that I am financially responsible for all charges whether or not paid by insurance. I hereby consent for the doctor to release all information necessary to secure the payment of benefits. I authorize the use of this signature on all insurance submissions.

Leslee K. Knight (Responsible Party Signature) self (Relationship) 09/21/XX (Date)

ORDER # 58-8426 @BIBBERO SYSTEMS, INC. •PETALUMA, CALIFORNIA• TO REORDER CALL TOLL FREE (800)242-9330

Medical Record

Account number: 3452
Patient's name: Knight, Leslee K.
Date of birth: 07/04/67

Date	Progress Notes
	05/06/XX A 26-year-old established female patient presents in office complaining of heavy menstruation. She has an abnormal weight gain of 48 pounds since visit on 4/12 of last year. Height 70", weight 297 pounds, BP 186/88, Temp. 98.8, last menstrual period 04/21/XX. She states she has had to use 2 super tampons and 1 super pad at a time changing approximately every 1 to 2 hours during heaviest menses. Spotting (dark blood), day 1 through 3, heavy bleeding day 4 through 7, spotting light red blood last 5 days; total 15 day menstrual period. Patient also complains of vaginal discharge. Performed a D HX/PX. Collected cell samples from cervix and endocervical canal for Pap smear which was sent to an outside laboratory. Cervicitis is present along with leukorrhea (watery discharge). Breast examination reveals no lumps–consistent with previous exam. Collected blood sample and sent to outside laboratory for general health panel. Prescribed vaginal cream for cervicitis. Patient to return in 1 week for BP check, test results, and treatment options for excess weight and menorrhagia. M/MDM Bertha Caesar, MD
	05/14/XX Patient returns for Pap smear and blood test results (EPF HX/PX). Blood panel shows reduced T_4 level. Blood drawn and sent to outside laboratory for additional thyroid tests. Impression: severe hypothyroidism disease (myxedema) (M/MDM). Discussed treatment options and prescribed therapeutic thyroid hormone treatment. Abnormal Pap smear indicates cervical dysplasia. Patient to continue vaginal cream for next 3 weeks then return for colposcopy and laser treatment of cervical dysplasia. Return to office in 3 weeks. Bertha Caesar, MD

6. Complete the second claim (B) for DOS 5/14/20XX and use this date to file the claim to Medicaid.
7. Use the "HCFA-1500 Claim Form Block-by-Block Instructions" for Medicaid patients found in Appendix D and the Medicaid template (Fig. D–5) for guidance and block help.
8. Use your procedure codebook to determine the correct code number(s) and modifier(s) for each professional service/procedure rendered.
9. Use your HCPCS Level II codebook or Appendix C to apply HCPCS codes when applicable.
10. Refer to the fee schedule in Appendix B for mock fees.
11. Use your diagnostic codebook to determine the correct diagnoses.
12. Address each claim to Medicaid.
13. Copy and prepare the ledger card found in Appendix F (Form 07) for the patient. Complete the ledger by posting each transaction in this case and indicating each time you have billed the insurance carrier.

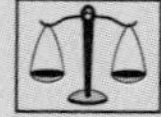

Weigh your progress. Turn to the Assignment Score Sheet in Appendix F (Form 10) and record and enter the information to track your success. Your instructor may ask that you include a Performance Evaluation Checklist, and if so, copy Form 11 found in Appendix F and attach it to your insurance claim.

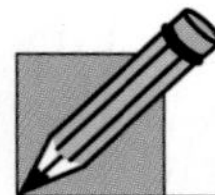

CPR Session: Answers

CPR REVIEW SESSIONS 10–1 AND 10–2

10–1 state governments with partial federal funding.
10–2 the Medicaid allowable amount as payment in full.

CPR REVIEW SESSIONS 10–3 THROUGH 10–5

10–3 (a) categorically needy
(b) medically needy
10–4 monthly
10–5 (a) fixed copayment (e.g., $1 or $2)
(b) share of cost (SOC)

CPR REVIEW SESSIONS 10–6 AND 10–7

10–6 (a) additional
(b) additional
(c) not covered
(d) additional
(e) not covered
(f) basic
(g) basic
10–7 EPSDT

CPR PRACTICE SESSIONS 10–8 AND 10–9

10–8 SOC 7525
10–9

A					B	C	D		E	F		G	H	I	J	K
DATE(S) OF SERVICE FROM DD YYYY		TO MM	DD	YYYY	Place of Service	Type of Service	PROCEDURES,SERVICES, OR SUPPLIES (Explain Unusual Circumstances) CPT/HCPCS	MODIFIER	DIAGNOSIS CODE	$ CHARGES		DAYS OR UNITS	EPSDT Family Plan	EMG	COB	RESERVED FOR LOCAL USE
)1320XX					12	D	99342		1	91	85	1				

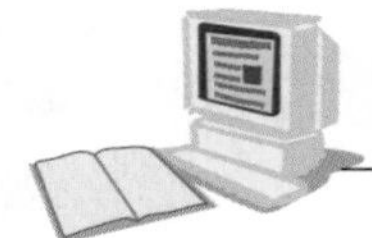

Resources

Obtain your state-published handbook with updates of Medicaid rules. Read and implement the rule changes to avoid rejected claims. Study the current bulletins or newsletters on the Medicaid or Medi-Cal program published by the fiscal agent in your state. Newsletters contain new information, changes in procedures and policies, and guidelines for frequent errors that occur in the Medicaid program.

Internet

- *Federal Register* (see Resources for Chapter 11, The Medicare Program).

Many states have Medicaid web sites. Get the Internet address for your state by contacting your local Medicaid office. To obtain general data or compare state Medicaid programs, contact the Center for Medicare and Medicaid Services' web site. This agency's web site and links continue to use "hcfa" within the web addresses.

Web site: http://www.hcfa.gov/Medicaid

- Medi-Cal—the state of California has a web site to obtain eligibility verification, perform share of cost transactions, initiate treatment authorization requests, and view updated bulletins, technical publications, and their provider manual. Program information, billing policy, and code descriptions may be found via a variety of search capabilities, and sections may be downloaded for hardcopy.

Web site: http://www.medi-col.ca.gov

Reference Books

- *Medicare/Medicaid Select,* IHS Health Group. (Specific topics may be chosen that include many reference materials.)

Web site: http://www.ihshealthgroup.com

Objectives

After reading this chapter and completing the exercise sessions, you should be able to:

Learning Objectives:

- ✔ Explain eligibility criteria for Medicare.
- ✔ Name important information to abstract from a patient's Medicare card.
- ✔ Identify the benefits and nonbenefits of Medicare.
- ✔ Differentiate between standard Medicare and managed care Medicare.
- ✔ State basic coverage for Medicare Part A, Part B, and Part C.
- ✔ Explain when to obtain a patient's signature on an advance beneficiary notice.
- ✔ State the fee schedule used and reimbursement criteria for participating versus nonparticipating physicians.
- ✔ List situations for using a release of information document and a lifetime beneficiary authorization to assign benefits.
- ✔ Determine the time limit for submitting Medicare claims and claims with Medicare and other insurance plans.

Performing Objectives:

- ✔ Demonstrate claims submission for individuals who have Medicare insurance.
- ✔ Fill in HCFA-1500 blocks that require Medigap information, Medicaid information, and information for primary insurance plans when submitting crossover or combination claims.

Key Terms

accepting assignment
benefit period
Centers for Medicare and Medicaid Services (CMS)
correct coding initiative (CCI)
crossover claim
end-stage renal disease (ESRD)
fiscal intermediary (FI)
hospice
insurance claim number
intermediate care facilities (ICFs)
medical necessity
Medicare Part A
Medicare Part B
Medicare Part C
Medicare/Medicaid (Medi-Medi)
Medicare Secondary Payer (MSP)
Medigap (MG)
nursing facility (NF)
peer review organization (PRO)
prospective payment system (PPS)
reasonable fee
respite care
Supplemental Security Income (SSI)

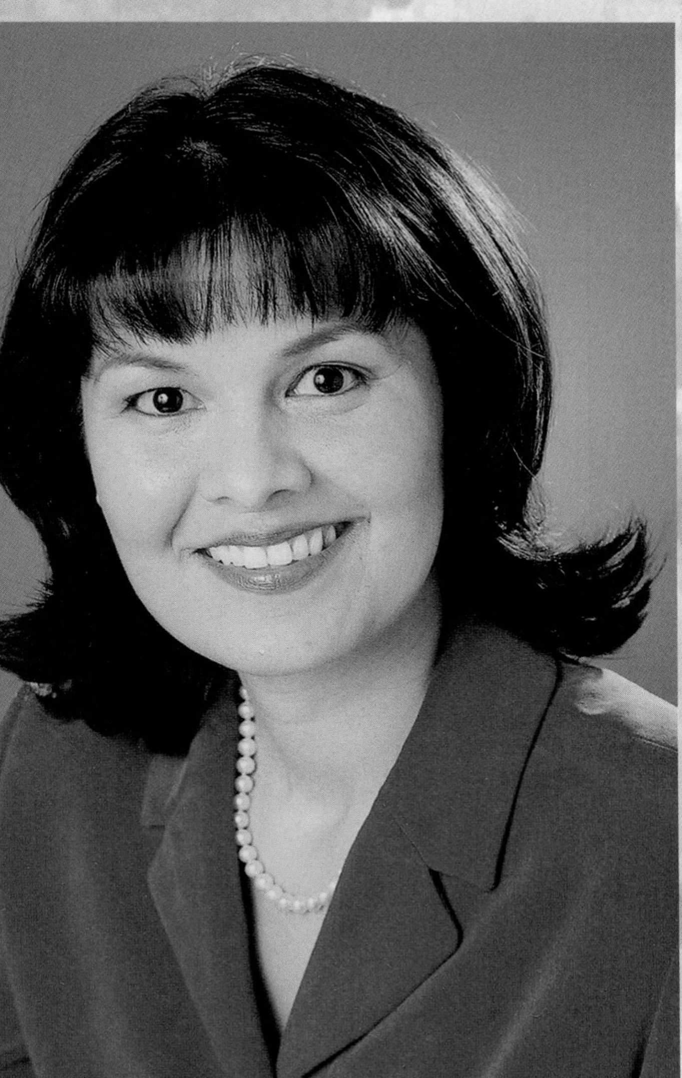

Chapter

11

Before my present position I was a manager for an executive search firm. Although I loved my job, my goal was to run my own business.

After receiving a medical insurance billing certificate from an adult school program, I created a marketing package and hit the pavement. I enclosed professional reference letters, a brochure detailing the services my company offers and explaining how I can save the physician money, and a calendar and pen. I needed a "hook" to open the door, so I included candy wrapped with a beautiful ribbon. This package broke the ice and my information got forwarded to the physician.

I soon met with a physical therapist and got the job. I was excited, I was scared, I was challenged, but I was having so much fun! Then, an endocrinologist called and we worked together to create a superbill. She is my most challenging, but also the most profitable, client.

Laura M. Garcia
President
LMG Medical Management

The Medicare Program

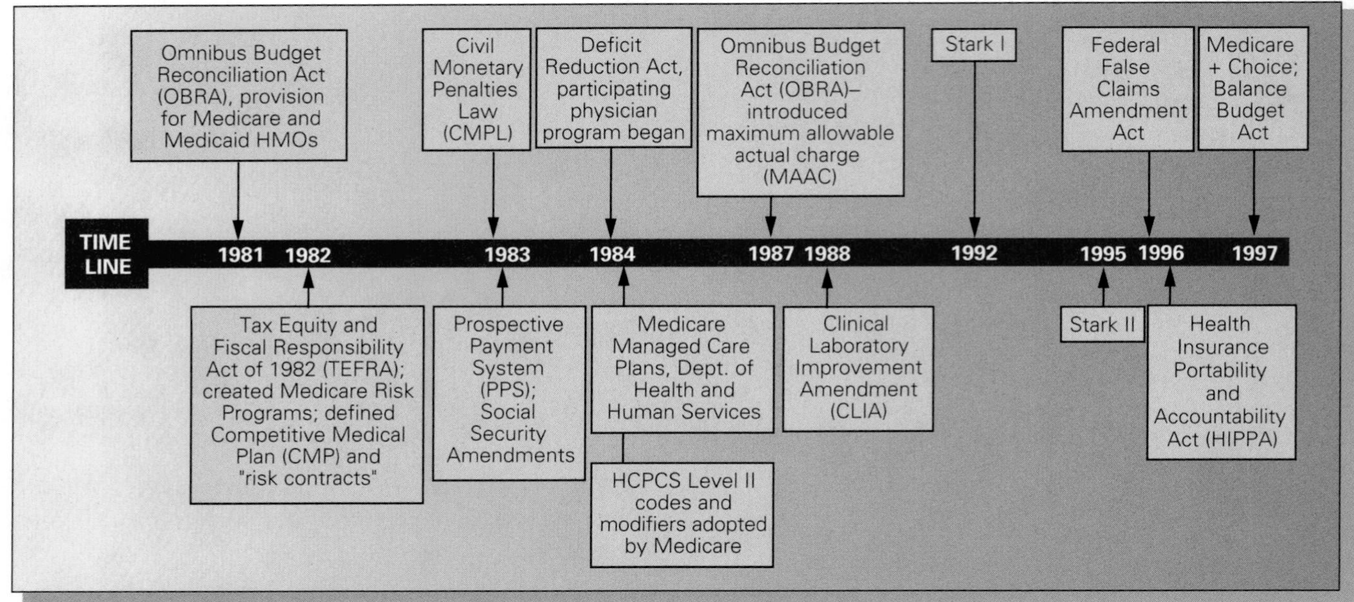

MEDICARE POLICIES AND REGULATIONS

Medicare is a federally funded program administered by the **Centers for Medicare and Medicaid Services (CMS),** formerly known as the *Health Care Financing Administration (HCFA).* CMS is subdivided into three divisions with the following responsibilities:

1. *The Center for Medicare Management* oversees traditional fee-for-service Medicare, including development of payment policy and management of fee-for-service contractors.
2. *The Center for Beneficiary Choices* provides beneficiaries with information on Medicare, Medicare Select, and Medicare Plus (+) Choice programs and Medigap options. It also manages the Medicare + Choice plans, consumer research, and grievance and appeals functions.
3. *The Center for Medicaid and State Operations* focuses on federal-state programs, such as Medicaid, the State Children's Health Insurance Program, insurance regulations, and the Clinical Laboratory Improvements Act (CLIA).

Medicare policies are intricate and their regulations are numerous, ever-changing, sometimes contradictory, and often difficult to understand. Dealing with the Medicare patient can be a challenge because sometimes they may be hard of hearing, visually impaired, have poor memory retention, or have difficulty in getting around. Contacting the Medicare fiscal intermediary can also be a formidable task. You may spend hours on the telephone, on hold, or transferring around their voice-mail system trying to find out information only to eventually become disconnected.

Keeping a positive attitude and a humorous outlook will help when dealing with the myriad of situations that can cause stress and frustration. A sampling of quotes shown in Figure 11–1 perhaps says it best. A sense of humor serves to lighten several situations when dealing with Medicare and may help in the development of patience, patience, and more patience!

Eligibility Requirements

Local Social Security Administration (SSA) offices take applications in person or via telephone and provide information about the Medicare program. The Medicare program was devised to provide health insurance for the following categories of people:

1. People age 65 years or older who are retired or eligible for Social Security.
2. People age 65 or older who are retired from the railroad or civil service.
3. Blind individuals.
4. Disabled individuals who are eligible for Social Security disability benefits* and are in the following categories:
   a. Disabled workers of any age.
   b. Adults disabled before age 18 whose parents are eligible for or retired on Social Security.
   c. Disabled widows of workers who are insured through the federal government, civil service, SSA, **Supplemental Security Income (SSI),** or the Railroad Retirement Act, and whose husbands qualified for benefits under one of these programs.
5. Children and adults who have chronic kidney disease requiring dialysis or **end-stage renal disease (ESRD)** requiring kidney transplant.

*In the disabled categories, a person must be disabled for at least 12 months to apply for disability benefits. A disabled beneficiary must receive disability benefits for 24 months before Medicare benefits begin.

MEDICARE MANIA

- Coding is an art, not an exact science and Medicare uses a wide brush and a bottle of turpentine when it comes to creating and changing coding rules.
- When calling Medicare customer service, I realized I was not dealing with the brightest crayon in the box.
- The hours spent taking care of the hard of hearing, the blind, the crippled, and the senile will be reimbursed according to a fee schedule made in Medicare heaven.
- If you don't like the answer to a question that Medicare gives you, call back and get another representative—you are bound to get another answer.
- Just as you pat yourself on the back thinking you have finally figured out the Medicare system, a pile of mail arrives with a one pound document informing you of Medicare changes.
- Medicare produces acronym-phobia when it says things like: CMS mandates use of NDCs along with CPT, HCPCS Level II, HCPCS Level III, and ICD-9-CM on the HCFA-1500.
- The "clean claim" is just a myth!!!

Figure 11–1. Amusing quotes which refer to different situations encountered when dealing with the Medicare system and its rules and regulations. (Permission granted by Sharon LaScala, NCICS and Linda L. French, CMA-C, NCICS.)

6. Kidney donors; all expenses related to the kidney transplantation.

Medicare Enrollment

All persons who meet one of the previously stated eligibility requirements are eligible for Medicare Part A (hospital coverage). An individual is eligible to enroll in Medicare 3 months before his or her 65th birthday, and the enrollment period ends 3 months after the month in which the person turns 65. If the enrollment period is missed, the individual must wait until the next general enrollment period—January 1 through March 31. Persons who fail to enroll prior to age 65 or who drop out and reenroll, will be assessed a 10% Part B premium penalty for each 12 months they did not participate, unless they or their spouses are actually employed and covered by an employer-sponsored group medical insurance plan. Those who receive Social Security, Railroad Retirement, or disability benefits are automatically enrolled in Medicare Part A and Part B.

Those who qualify for full Medicare benefits under Part A (hospital insurance) may also elect to take Medicare Part B (outpatient coverage). Medicare Part B recipients pay premiums to the SSA which may increase annually. Some pay a Medicare surtax on federal income tax payments. This premium may be automatically deducted from the patient's monthly Social Security check if he or she wishes. Those individuals not eligible for Medicare Part A at age 65 may purchase Part B from the SSA.

Enrollment for Aliens

An alien may be eligible for Part A and/or Part B Medicare coverage if he or she has lived in the United States as a permanent resident for 5 consecutive years. When billing Medicare, it is usually not necessary to state on the HCFA-1500 form that the patient is an alien.

Enrollment Status

A telephone hotline or, in some states, a modem is available to verify the enrollment status of a Medicare patient. This is useful because patients can switch coverage to a senior managed care plan on a month-to-month basis and still retain possession of their Medicare card. The patient's Medicare claim number and date of birth are entered into the telephone system and the digital response indicates the enrollment status. In some states it may also indicate how much of the deductible has been satisfied. Contact the Medicare fiscal agent in your location for information about this service.

Enrollment for Retirement Benefits

Social Security retirement benefits may be applied for at age 62 (partial benefits) or age 65 (full benefits). In the year 2000, the retirement age gradually increased for people born in the year 1938 or later. For people born after 1959, the full-benefits retirement age will be 67. Benefits may increase if retirement is delayed beyond full benefit retirement age. As of this edition, Medicare may still be applied for at age 65.

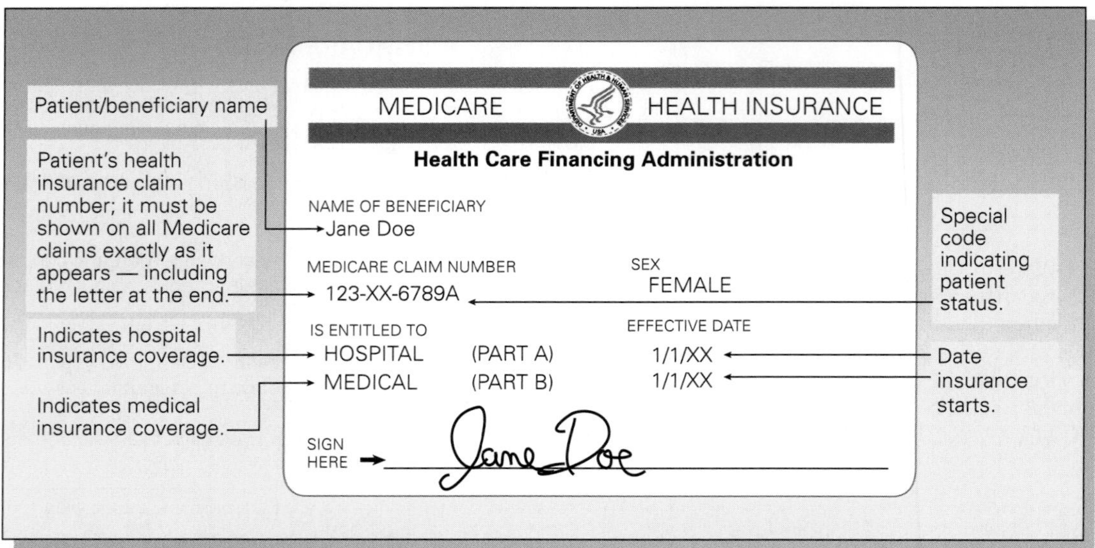

Figure 11–2. Medicare Health Insurance Identification card.

Identification Card

The Medicare patient should present his or her red, white, and blue health insurance card (Fig. 11–2). The insurance identification number on the card is the Social Security number of the wage earner and is referred to as the **insurance claim number.** Note that the claim number has an alpha suffix added which indicates the patient's status, or how he or she became eligible for benefits (see Fig. 11–2 and Example 11–1). The card also indicates hospital benefits (Part A), and/or medical coverage (Part B), along with the date the insurance became effective.

A patient whose Medicare card claim number ends in "A" will have the same Social Security and claim numbers. A patient whose Medicare card claim number ends in "B" or "D" will have different Social Security and claim numbers. When a husband and wife both have Medicare, they receive separate cards and claim numbers. A quick check between Social Security numbers and Medicare claim numbers may identify a submission error and forestall a claim rejection.

There may be letters preceding the insurance claim number on the identification card which represent *railroad retirees* (see Example 11–2).

Example 11–1

Medicare Identification Card Alpha Suffixes (Sample—123-XX-6789-A)

A	=	Wage earner
B	=	Husband's number (wife 62 years old or older)
D	=	Widow
HAD	=	Disabled adult
C	=	Disabled child
M	=	Part B benefits only
T	=	Uninsured and entitled only to health insurance benefits

Note: This is only a partial list.

Example 11–2

Railroad Retirees' Prefix Identification Letters (Sample—A123-XX-6789)

A	=	Retired railroad employee
MA	=	Spouse of retired railroad employee
WA	=	Widow of deceased employee (by age or disability)
WD	=	Widower of deceased employee (by age or disability)
CA	=	Child or student
WCA	=	Widow of retiree with child in her care
WCD	=	Disabled child of deceased employee
PA/PD	=	Parent of deceased employee
H	=	Railroad Retirement Board pensioner before 1937
MH	=	Wife of Railroad Retirement Board pensioner before 1937
WH	=	Widowed wife of Railroad Retirement Board pensioner before 1937
WCH	=	Widow of Railroad Retirement Board pensioner with child in her care
PH	=	Parent of Railroad Retirement Board pensioner before 1937
JA	=	Widow receiving a joint and survivor annuity
X	=	Divorced spouse's annuity, for use on forms AA-3 and AA-7 only

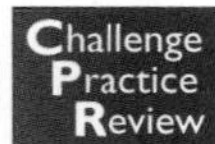

Pause and Practice CPR

REVIEW SESSIONS 11–1 AND 11–2

Directions: *Complete the following questions as a review of information you have just read.*

11–1 Briefly list the six categories of individuals who qualify for Medicare.

(a) ______________________________

(b) ______________________________

(c) ______________________________

(d) ______________________________

(e) ______________________________

(f) ______________________________

11–2 What do the alpha suffixes that follow the Medicare identification number on the Medicare identification card represent? ______________________________

____

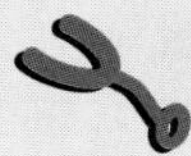

CHECK YOUR HEARTBEAT! Turn to the end of the chapter for answers to these review sessions.

Coverage and Benefits

Medicare Part A—Hospital Benefits

Medicare Part A is hospital insurance which provides benefits for the aged, disabled, and blind. Funds for this health service come from special contributions made by employees and self-employed persons, with employers matching contributions. These contributions are collected along with regular Social Security contributions from wages and self-employment income earned during a person's working years.

A **benefit period** begins the day a patient enters a hospital and ends when the patient has not been a bed patient in any hospital or nursing facility for 60 consecutive days. It also ends if a patient has been in a nursing facility but has not received skilled nursing care for 60 consecutive days.

A **nursing facility (NF)** (formerly called skilled nursing facility) offers nursing and/or rehabilitation services that are medically necessary to a patient's recovery. Services provided are not custodial. Custodial services are those that assist the patient with personal needs (i.e., dressing, eating, bathing, and getting in and out of bed). Hospital insurance protection is renewed every time the patient begins a new benefit period. There is no limit to the number of benefit periods a patient can have for hospital or nursing facility care.

Medicare Part A provides benefits to applicants in any of the following situations:

1. A bed patient in a hospital: up to 90 hospital days in each benefit period.
2. A bed patient in a nursing facility: up to 100 extended care days for each benefit period. Patients who become inpatients at an NF after a 3-day acute hospital stay and who also meet Medicare's qualified diagnosis and comprehensive treatment plan requirements pay nothing for the first 20 days.
3. A patient receiving home healthcare services.
4. A patient receiving care in a psychiatric facility: up to 190 days in a lifetime.
5. A terminally ill patient diagnosed as having 6 months or less to live who needs hospice care. A **hospice** is a public agency or private organization that is primarily engaged in providing pain relief, symptom management, and supportive services to terminally ill people (and their families) in their own homes or in a homelike hospice center. Medicare limits hospice care to 210 days if the patient is not certified terminally ill. All other Medicare benefits stop with the exception of physician services and any other treatment for conditions not related to the patient's terminal diagnosis.
6. A terminally ill patient in need of respite care: limited to inpatient stays of no more than 5 consecutive days for each respite period. **Respite care** is a short-term inpatient hospital stay provided for the terminally ill patient to give temporary relief to the patient's primary caregiver.

For a comprehensive look at five major classifications of inpatient hospital services and a breakdown of the cost-sharing benefits, refer to Figure 11–3.

Medicare Part B—Medical Coverage

Medicare Part B is referred to as supplementary medical insurance (SMI), which provides benefits for the aged, disabled, and blind. It is called "supplementary" because it supplements Part A. Funds for this come equally from those who sign up for it and from the federal government. A medical insurance premium is automatically deducted from monthly checks for those who receive Social Security benefits, Railroad Retirement benefits, or a civil service annuity. Others pay the premium directly to the SSA.

For a comprehensive look at six major classifications of outpatient services and a breakdown of the cost-sharing benefits, refer to Figure 11–4.

Practitioners and Related Services

The following is a list of practitioners and services covered under Medicare Part B:

- Chiropractor (DC)—Physical manipulation of the spine demonstrated by an x-ray.
- Doctor of Dental Surgery (DDS)—Fractures or surgery of the jaw.
- Doctor of Medicine (MD)—Office examinations, surgery, diagnostic testing, supplies.
- Doctor of Osteopathy (DO)—Office examinations, surgery, diagnostic testing, supplies.
- Doctor of Podiatric Medicine (DPM)—Limited foot care given at specific time intervals.
- Nurse Practitioner, Certified Nurse-Midwife, Clinical Nurse Specialist, Certified Registered Nurse Anesthetist, Physician Assistant, Clinical Psychologist, Certified Social Worker—Variety of medical services provided as physician extenders, that is, non-

Medicare (Part A): Hospital Insurance-Covered Services For 2002

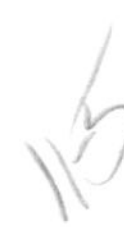

Services	Benefit	Medicare Pays	Patient Pays
HOSPITALIZATION Semiprivate room and board, general nursing and miscellaneous hospital services and supplies. (Medicare payments based on benefit periods.)	First 60 days	All but $812	$812 deductible
	61st to 90th day	All but $203 a day	$203 a day
	91st to 150th day (60-reserve-days benefit[1])	All but $406 a day	$406 a day
	Beyond 150 days	Nothing	All costs
NURSING FACILITY CARE Patient must have been in a hospital for at least 3 days and enter a Medicare-approved facility generally within 30 days after hospital discharge.[2] (Medicare payments based on benefit periods.)	First 20 days	100% of approved amount	Nothing
	21st to 100th day	All but $101.50 a day	Up to $101.50 a day
	Beyond 100 days	Nothing	All costs
HOME HEALTH CARE Part-time or intermittent skilled care, home health aide services, durable medical equipment and supplies, and other services.	Unlimited as long as Medicare conditions are met and services are declared "medically necessary".	100% of approved amount; 80% of approved amount for durable medical equipment.	Nothing for services; 20% of approved amount for durable medical equipment.
HOSPICE CARE Pain relief, symptom management, and support services for the terminally ill.	If patient elects the hospice option and as long as doctor certifies need.	All but limited costs for outpatient drugs and inpatient respite care.	Limited cost sharing for outpatient drugs and inpatient respite care.
BLOOD	Unlimited if medically necessary.	All but first 3 pints per calendar year.	For first 3 pints.[3]

1 This 60-reserve-days benefit may be used only once in a lifetime.
2 Neither Medicare nor private Medigap insurance will pay for most long-term nursing home care.
3 To the extent the blood deductible is met under Part B of Medicare during the calendar year, it does not have to be met under Part A.

Figure 11–3. Five major classifications of Medicare Part A benefits. (Modified from *Medicare & You 2002*, Washington, D.C., U.S. Government Printing Office.)

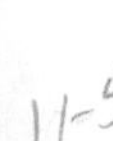

Medicare (Part B): Medical Insurance-Covered Services for 2002

Services	Benefit	Medicare Pays	Patient Pays
MEDICAL EXPENSES Physicians' services, inpatient and outpatient medical and surgical services and supplies, physical and speech therapy, ambulance, diagnostic tests, and other services.	Unlimited if medically necessary.	80% of approved amount (after $100 deductible). Reduced to 50% for most outpatient mental health services.	$100 deductible,[1] plus 20% of approved amount or limited charges.[2]
CLINICAL LABORATORY SERVICES Blood tests, urinalyses, and more.	Unlimited if medically necessary.	100% of approved amount.	Nothing for services.
HOME HEALTH CARE Part-time or intermittent care, home health aide services, durable medical equipment and supplies, and other services.	Unlimited as long as patient meets conditions and benefits are declared medically necessary.	100% of approved amount; 80% of approved amount for durable medical equipment.	Nothing for services; 20% of approved amount for durable medical equipment.
OUTPATIENT HOSPITAL TREATMENT Services for the diagnosis or treatment of illness or injury.	Unlimited if medically necessary.	Medicare payment to hospital based on hospital cost.	$100 deductible, plus 20% of whatever the hospital charges.
BLOOD	Unlimited if medically necessary.	80% of approved amount (after $100 deductible and starting with 4th pint).	First 3 pints plus 20% of approved amounts for additional pints (after $100 deductible).[3]
AMBULATORY SURGICAL SERVICES	Unlimited if medically necessary.	80% of predetermined amount (after $100 deductible.	$100 deductible plus 20% of predetermined amount.

[1]Once the patient has had $100 of expenses for covered services in the year, the Part B deductible does not apply to any further covered services received for the rest of the year.

[2]See Figure 11–8 for an explanation of approved amount for participating physicians and limited charges for nonparticipating physicians.

[3]To the extent the blood deductible is met under Part A of Medicare during the calendar year, it does not have to be met under Part B.

Figure 11–4. Six major classifications of Medicare Part B benefits. (Modified from *Medicare & You 2002*, Washington, D.C., U.S. Government Printing Office.)

physician practitioners providing services under the direction of a physician.

- Occupational Therapist—Therapy for activities of daily living.
- Physical Therapist—Physical therapy modalities.
- Registered Dietitian—Nutrition therapy.

Preventive Services

Preventive care benefits covered by Medicare are:

- Ambulance service meeting medical necessity requirements.
- Bone mass measurements (bone density) for women age 65 and older at high risk for osteoporosis.
- Colorectal cancer screening for people age 50 and older. Type of test is dependent on risk factors and time lapsed from last screening.
- Durable medical equipment (DME) for home use; rental or purchase (e.g., wheelchair, prosthetic devices, braces and supports).
- Glucose monitoring equipment (home devices) and testing strips for people with diabetes.
- Mammograms (annual) for women age 40 or older, plus a one-time baseline mammogram for women age 35 to 39.
- Nutrition therapy to assist in managing diabetes and kidney disease (beginning January 1, 2002).
- Papanicolaou test (Pap smear) every 3 years, and for women at high risk, annual examinations.

- Prostate cancer screening (annual), including digital rectal examinations and prostate-specific antigen (PSA) blood tests for men older than age 50.
- Vaccines: influenza, pneumococcal pneumonia, and hepatitis B.

Nonbenefit Services

Nonbenefit services consist of routine physical examinations, routine foot care, eye or hearing examinations, and cosmetic surgery unless due to injury or performed to improve functioning of malformed part. A physician may bill a patient separately for noncovered services.

There are many other benefits and nonbenefits too numerous to list. To find out whether a particular procedure qualifies for payment, refer to Medicare newsletters or contact your Medicare carrier.

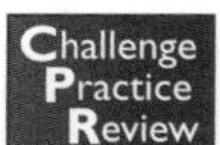

Pause and Practice CPR

CHALLENGE SESSIONS 11–3 THROUGH 11–5

Directions: *Refer to Medicare Coverage and Benefits for Part A and Part B in the manuscript and Medicare-covered services and payment amounts in Figures 11–3 (for Part A) and 11–4 (for Part B). Read all three exercises first, then use critical thinking skills when completing the questions.*

11–3 Luke Winston has Medicare Part A and Part B and has returned home from a 3-day (2-night) stay at College Hospital. His wife calls College Clinic and asks to speak to the insurance specialist. She states that their son has offered to help them with their medical bills and would like to know approximately how much of the $2,500 hospital bill they will be responsible for (the deductible has not been met). ____________________

11–4 Dr. Practon has ordered a visiting nurse to see Mr. Winston daily for wound care and to monitor his IV. What percent will Medicare pay for these services? ____________________

11–5 Dr. Practon charges the Medicare allowed amount and his fees total $250.62 for Mr. Winston's hospital care. Mr. Winston has not met his deductible. How much of this amount will Mr. Winston be responsible for? ____________________

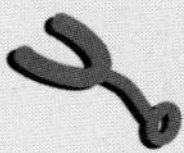

CHECK YOUR HEARTBEAT! Turn to the end of the chapter for answers to these challenge sessions.

Medicare Part C—Medicare Plus (+) Choice Program

Medicare Part C—Medicare + Choice plans were created to offer a number of healthcare options in addition to those available under Medicare Part A and Part B. These plans receive a fixed amount of money from Medicare to spend on their Medicare members. Some plans may require members to pay a premium similar to the Medicare Part B premium. If the patient chooses coverage under Part C, he or she will not need coverage under Part A and Part B.

Plans available under this program may include the following:

- Health Maintenance Organization (HMO)
- Point-of-Service (POS) Plan
- Private Fee-for-Service (PFFS) Plan
- Provider-Sponsored Organization (PSO)
- Religious Fraternal Benefit Society (RFBS)
- Medicare Medical Savings Account (MSA)—pilot program

Prior discussion in Chapters 2 and 9 covered a number of these plans. Following are descriptions of those not yet mentioned.

Provider-Sponsored Organization

A *Provider-Sponsored Organization (PSO)* is a risk-bearing managed care organization, made up of providers that contract directly with CMS for Medicare enrollees. They may be licensed by the state, or directly from CMS.

Religious Fraternal Benefit Society

A *Religious Fraternal Benefit Society (RFBS)* is a managed care option that is associated with a church, group of churches, or convention. Membership is restricted to church members and is allowed regardless of the person's health status.

Medicare Medical Savings Account

In a Medicare Savings Account (MSA), the patient chooses a catastrophic insurance policy approved by Medicare that has a high annual deductible. Medicare pays the premiums for this policy and deposits the dollar-amount difference between what it pays for the average beneficiary in the patient's area and the cost of the premium into the patient's MSA. The patient uses the MSA money to pay medical expenses until the high deductible is reached. If the MSA money becomes depleted, the patient pays out of pocket until reaching the deductible. Unused funds roll over to the next calendar year.

Medicare Managed Care Plans

Medicare enrollees have the right to join and assign their Medicare benefits to a managed care plan, often referred to as a senior plan or senior HMO. Upon doing so, the Medicare patient is sent an insurance card from the managed care plan (Fig. 11–5); however, the patient's Medicare card is not forfeited. An elderly patient may forget or become confused and show the Medicare card instead of the managed care card, or show two cards, leading to confusion about coverage and who to bill.

For patients enrolled in a Medicare HMO plan, Medicare makes payments on a monthly basis directly to the HMO for all enrollees. Enrollees pay the HMO a monthly premium, which is an estimate of the coinsurance amounts for which the enrollee would be responsible plus the Medicare deductible. The Medicare patient then pays a fixed copayment amount for medical services (e.g., $15). It appears that HMOs contracting to provide services for Medicare patients will be converted to a Medicare + Choice plan on their contract renewal dates.

Expressions from Experience

I believe the more knowledge and experience you have, the more you have to offer. . . . Knowledge is power.

Laura M. Garcia
President
LMG Medical Management

With a Medicare HMO, the patient does not need a Medicare supplementary insurance plan. Most HMOs provide services not usually covered by Medicare, such as eyeglasses, prescription drugs, and routine physical examinations.

If a Medicare patient has switched over to a managed care plan and wishes to disenroll, the patient must notify the plan in writing, complete a disenrollment form (Medicare form HCFA 566), and take a copy of the letter and the form to the Social Security office.

Many plans allow the patient to enroll and disenroll at any time during the year. It may take the plan 30 days for disenrollment, and Medicare may take as long as 60 days to reenroll a patient. Patients who disenroll may have to requalify for supplementary coverage at a higher cost.

There are two types of HMO plans that have Medicare Part B contracts: HMO risk plans and HMO cost plans.

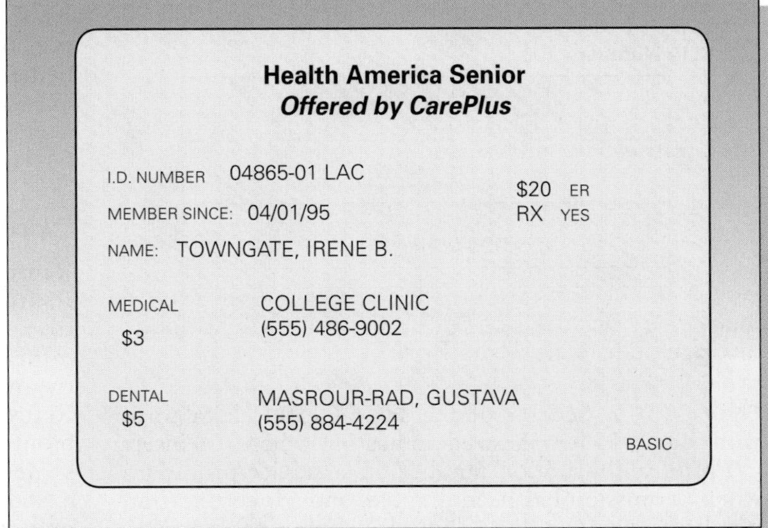

Figure 11–5. Example of a senior managed care card.

HMO RISK PLAN. In an HMO risk plan, beneficiaries agree to receive Medicare-covered services from contracted providers and facilities. Enrollees are referred to as "restricted beneficiaries." Services received "out-of-plan" are not covered when the same services are available through the HMO network unless prior authorization is obtained and medical necessity criteria are met, or the care is urgent or emergent. Enrollees choosing to go outside the network pay out of pocket. Claims for HMO risk plan beneficiaries must be sent directly to the organization.

Prior authorization is needed for referral to specialists, diagnostic tests, and surgical procedures. Some of the procedures requiring authorization are on a mandatory list, whereas others are chosen by the regional carrier.

Some carriers have an 800 toll-free line to call for authorization; some require the completion of a preauthorization form; and some require a letter only if there is a dispute over claims payment. Check with your local carrier regarding its policy for preauthorization.

The prior authorization number is used when billing the Medicare carrier and is entered on the HCFA-1500 claim form in Block 23 (Fig. 11–6A). If the request is not approved, the carrier sends a denial to the physician, the patient, and the hospital, if applicable. If the procedure is urgent or emergent, notify the carrier within the time frame designated by the insurance plan so an authorization can be arranged.

> *Expressions from Experience*
>
> *A quote by Louisa May Alcott sums up my journey as an entrepreneur: "I am not afraid of storms, for I am learning how to sail my ship."*
>
> Laura M. Garcia
> President
> LMG Medical Management

HMO COST PLAN. In an HMO cost plan, beneficiaries receive Medicare-covered services from sources in or outside of the HMO network. Enrollees are referred to as "unrestricted" beneficiaries. Claims for cost plan beneficiaries may be sent to the HMO plan or to the regular Medicare carrier.

NONCONTRACTED PHYSICIANS. If a noncontract physician treats a Medicare HMO patient, the services are considered "out-of-plan" services. The claim must be submitted to the managed care plan, which will determine whether it is responsible to pay for the services. Conditions that must be met are:

1. Service was an emergency, and the patient was not able to get to an HMO facility or member physician (out of HMO area).
2. Service was a Medicare-covered service.
3. Service was medically necessary.
4. Prior authorization or approval for referral was obtained.

The HMO reimburses according to the Medicare fee schedule's "Allowable Amount." The physician may not bill the patient for any balance. If the HMO denies the claim, the patient may be billed for an amount up to the Medicare fee schedule's "limiting charge." An appeal may be made using the HMO's appeal process.

Railroad Retirement Benefits

Railroad workers' beneficiaries apply to offices of the Railroad Retirement Board for Medicare benefits and to receive information about the program. Medical insurance premiums are automatically deducted from the monthly checks of people who receive Railroad Retirement benefits. Those who do not receive a monthly check pay their premiums directly, or, in some cases, have premiums paid on their behalf under a state assistance program. Benefits and deductibles under Parts A and B are the same as for other Medicare recipients.

Prior Authorization Number

20. OUTSIDE LAB? ☐YES ☐NO — $ CHARGES

22. MEDICAID RESUBMISSION CODE — ORIGINAL REF. NO.

23. PRIOR AUTHORIZATION NUMBER
1234567

F	G	H	I	J	K
$ CHARGES	DAYS OR UNITS	EPSDT Family Plan	EMG	COB	RESERVED FOR LOCAL USE

A

CLIA Number

20. OUTSIDE LAB? ☐YES ☐NO — $ CHARGES

22. MEDICAID RESUBMISSION CODE — ORIGINAL REF. NO.

23. PRIOR AUTHORIZATION NUMBER
07X0957214

F	G	H	I	J	K
$ CHARGES	DAYS OR UNITS	EPSDT Family Plan	EMG	COB	RESERVED FOR LOCAL USE

B

Figure 11–6. Section of the HCFA-1500 claim form with Block 23 emphasized indicating where to insert (*A*) prior authorization number for a service/procedure when permission has been granted, and (*B*) certification number issued by the Clinical Laboratory Improvements Amendment (CLIA) for waived tests.

Some railroad retirees are members of a railroad hospital association or a prepayment plan (HMO). These members pay regular premiums to the plan and then can receive health services the plan provides either without additional charge or with a small charge for specific services (e.g., drugs, home visits).

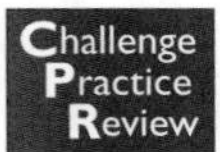

Pause and Practice CPR

REVIEW SESSIONS 11–6 THROUGH 11–10

Directions: *Match the following Medicare plans with their descriptions and fill in the blank with the appropriate letter.*

(a) Provider-Sponsored Organization (b) Medicare Medical Savings Account

(c) HMO risk plan (d) HMO cost plan (e) Medicare Managed Care

11–6 _______ Medicare "restricted beneficiaries" receive services from contracted providers and facilities.

11–7 _______ A risk-bearing managed care organization, made up of providers who contract directly with CMS.

11–8 _______ Medicare beneficiaries receive services from sources outside of the HMO network.

11–9 _______ A catastrophic insurance policy is purchased by the Medicare beneficiary and paid for by Medicare. Medicare deposits money into an account for the beneficiary to use for payment of the high deductible.

11–10 _______ A senior HMO.

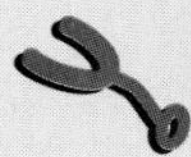

CHECK YOUR HEARTBEAT! Turn to the end of the chapter for answers to these review sessions.

MEDICARE AND ADDITIONAL INSURANCE PROGRAMS

Many Medicare recipients have Medicare in combination with other insurance plans. To know what additional benefits the patient might have and to distinguish whether Medicare is the primary or secondary payer, always ask to see the Medicare card as well as any other insurance cards. Make photocopies of both sides of all cards. If a patient carries a supplemental policy, determine whether he or she is still working, and if so, ask whether the policy was carried over (conversion policy) from his or her employer. If an accident occurred, determine the liability by asking if it was an automobile accident, or occurred on the job, or on the property of another person. Call the carrier if the type of plan or coverage is not clearly identified. The following section explains various types of other coverage and coverage combinations, as well as identifying primary and secondary payers.

Medicare and Medicaid

Medicare recipients with limited income may qualify for state assistance to help pay costs, such as deductibles and premiums. Those older than age 65 who qualify for assistance may be referred to as qualifying for *Old Age Security (OAS)* assistance benefits, *Qualified Medicare Beneficiary (QMB)*, or *Specified Low Income Medicare Beneficiary (SLMB)*. Patients qualifying for **Medicare/Medicaid** coverage are referred to as **"Medi-Medi"** patients. Medicaid is always the payer of last resort; therefore Medicare is the primary payer and Medicaid is the secondary payer.

Medicare and Medigap

A specialized insurance plan devised to supplement the traditional Medicare policy is called **Medigap (MG)** or *Medifill.* All Medigap policies are clearly marked "Medicare Supplement Insurance" and include basic benefits. Medigap plans are regulated by the federal government and offered to Medicare beneficiaries by private third party payers. Predefined minimum benefits for 10 Medigap standardized policies are categorized in Figure 11–7 by letters A through J. Basic benefits are found in Policy A and cover coinsurance amounts for Part A (days 61 to 150), coinsurance amounts for Part B (20% of allowed amount), 100% of charges for an extra 365 days in hospital, and benefits for additional blood supplies.

Other plans cover additional services such as preventive care, prescription drugs, skilled nursing coinsurance, and so forth. Each subsequent letter represents basic benefits plus other coverage, with the most

Ten Medigap Standardized Policies (Not all may be available in all states)

A	B	C	D	E	F	G	H	I	J
Basic Benefit	Basic Benefit	Basic Benefit	Basic Benefit	Basic Benefit	Basic Benefit	Basic Benefit	Basic Benefit	Basic Benefit	Basic Benefit
		Skilled Nursing Coinsurance	Skilled Nursing Coinsurance	Skilled Nursing Coinsurance	Skilled Nursing Coinsurance	Skilled Nursing Coinsurance	Skilled Nursing Coinsurance	Skilled Nursing Coinsurance	Skilled Nursing Coinsurance
	Part A Deductible	Part A Deductible	Part A Deductible	Part A Deductible	Part A Deductible	Part A Deductible	Part A Deductible	Part A Deductible	Part A Deductible
		Part B Deductible			Part B Deductible				Part B Deductible
					Part B Excess 100%	Part B Excess 100%		Part B Excess 100%	Part B Excess 100%
		Foreign Travel Emergency	Foreign Travel Emergency	Foreign Travel Emergency	Foreign Travel Emergency	Foreign Travel Emergency	Foreign Travel Emergency	Foreign Travel Emergency	Foreign Travel Emergency
			At-Home Recovery			At-Home Recovery		At-Home Recovery	At-Home Recovery
							Basic Drug Benefit ($1,250 Limit)	Basic Drug Benefit ($1,250 Limit)	Extended Drug Benefit ($3,000 Limit)
				Preventive Care					Preventive Care

Figure 11–7. Ten Medigap Standardized Policies.

comprehensive benefits in Policy J. Sales of all policies are not available in all states, so individuals in some states have fewer options than others.

Medicare Select is a variation of the Medigap policy which offers the same type of coverage. The difference is that beneficiaries must obtain medical care from a list of specified network providers.

Medicare Secondary Payer (MSP)

In some instances, people who have Medicare also have group health or other types of coverage and Medicare is not responsible for paying the claim first (primary payer). Such situations are classified as **Medicare Secondary Payer (MSP).**

Working Aged

There are a number of powerful laws that regulate health coverage for those age 65 and older who are employed. This population presents several scenarios which need to be studied to determine when Medicare is considered secondary coverage. Table 11–1 presents the act or law formed to protect and provide health coverage for the aged Medicare-eligible worker. The table also shows those to whom the act or law applies, lists employer eligibility requirements, indicates which insurance is primary and which secondary, and specifies factors that qualify an employer under the law or act.

Medicare and Managed Care Plans

Patients may be covered by a managed care plan and Medicare. When a patient's primary insurance is a managed care plan that requires fixed copayments, it is possible to obtain reimbursement from Medicare for those amounts. An assigned MSP claim must be filed with Medicare after the medical care organization (MCO) has paid its capitated amount. It may be necessary to include a signed statement by the patient regarding copayment requirements in lieu of an explanation of benefits. When Medicare's copayment reimbursement has been received, the provider must refund to the patient the copayment amount previously collected. A nonpar-

Table 11–1 **Elderly Employee Benefits (Medicare Secondary Coverage)**

Act/Law	Applies to	Employee Eligibility Requirements	Primary Insurance	Secondary Insurance (MSP)	Employer Qualifications
Omnibus Budget Reconciliation Act (OBRA) of 1981	Current employees; former employees; dependents younger than age 65 yr	Eligible solely because of end-stage renal disease	Employer group coverage (up to 12 mo)	Medicare	All employers regardless of number of employees
OBRA of 1986	Employee/dependent younger than age 65 yr	Eligible due to disability *other than* end-stage renal disease	Employer group coverage	Medicare	Employers having at least 100 full- or part-time employees (large groups)
Tax Equity and Fiscal Responsibility Act (TEFRA) of 1982	Employee/spouse age 65 to 69 yr	Entitled to same group health plan offered to younger employees and spouses	Employer group coverage	Medicare	Employers having 20 full- or part-time employees
Consolidated Omnibus Budget Reconciliation Act (COBRA) of 1985 (amendment to TEFRA)	Employee/spouse age 65 yr or older	Entitled to same group health plan offered to younger employees and spouses	Employer group coverage	Medicare	Employers having 20 full- or part-time employees

ticipating physician must file an unassigned MSP claim. The patient will be directly reimbursed by Medicare and no refund is necessary.

Automobile and Liability Insurance Coverage

Liability insurance is primary to Medicare because the contractural agreement exists between the injured party and the liability insurance company, not Medicare. The physician must bill the liability insurance company first, and if the payment is less than the Medicare allowed amount, the physician may file an assigned claim. The physician must accept as full payment the greater of either the Medicare-approved charge, or the sum of the liability insurance payment and the Medicare payment. A nonpar (nonparticipating) physician may file an unassigned claim to Medicare only if the payment by the liability insurance company is less than the Medicare limiting charge.

If the liability insurance company does not pay the claim promptly (e.g., within 120 days), and if the provided services are covered Medicare benefits, a par (participating) or nonpar physician may seek conditional payment from Medicare. However, if a claim is filed with Medicare, the provider must drop the claim against the liability insurer. All wrongful payments made by Medicare are subject to recovery.

Other situations may also occur where Medicare is the secondary payer. Study Table 11–2 which divides and illustrates events when Medicare is the primary payer and when Medicare is the secondary payer for a variety of insurance types and combinations.

Table 11–2 **A. Patients with Medicare and Other Insurance Coverage Secondary to Medicare**

Medicare Primary Payer			
Event	**Other Insurance Coverage**	**Primary Insurance**	**Secondary Insurance**
Illness or injury; any Medicare beneficiary	Medicaid	Medicare	Medicaid
Illness or injury; any Medicare beneficiary	Medigap	Medicare	Medigap
Illness or injury; *retired* employee with insurance through former employer	Employer supplemental health insurance conversion policy	Medicare	Employer supplemental insurance
Illness or injury; Medicare beneficiary younger than age 65 yr with Part A due to disability and Part B	TRICARE	Medicare	TRICARE
Illness or injury: Medicare beneficiary younger than 65 yr with Part A and Part B	CHAMPVA	Medicare	CHAMPVA

Table 11–2 B. Patients with Other Insurance Coverage Primary to Medicare

Medicare Secondary Payer (MSP)			
Event	**Other Insurance Coverage**	**Primary Insurance**	**Secondary Insurance**
Automobile accident	Automobile liability insurance/no-fault insurance	Liability policy	Medicare (MSP)
Accident on property belonging to someone else	Home owners/business liability insurance	Liability policy	Medicare (MSP)
Illness or injury; elderly employee/spouse; 65 yr of age or older	Employee Group Health Plan (EGHP)	EGHP	Medicare (MSP)
Illness related to black lung disease; coal miner or former coal miner	Federal Black Lung Act (FECA); workers' compensation provisions	FECA	Medicare does not apply
Injury/illness that is service-related	Department of Veterans Affairs	Department of Veterans Affairs	Medicare (MSP)
Injury or illness; dependent of active duty service person	TRICARE	TRICARE	Medicare (MSP)
Injury or illness occurring on the job	Workers' compensation	Workers' compensation	Medicare does not apply
End-stage renal disease; current or former employees	Employer group coverage	Employer group coverage	Medicare (MSP)
Disability (except end-stage renal disease); employee or dependent younger than age 65 yr	Employer group coverage	Employer group coverage	Medicare (MSP)
Laid-off employee with continuation coverage (COBRA)	COBRA coverage	COBRA	Medicare (MSP)
Spouse of employee who died—continuation coverage (COBRA)	COBRA coverage	COBRA	Medicare (MSP)

Challenge Practice Review

Pause and Practice CPR

REVIEW SESSIONS 11–11 THROUGH 11–14

Directions: *Complete the following questions as a review of information you have just read.*

11–11 Medicare beneficiaries who also have Medicaid coverage are referred to as ____________

____

11–12 If a Medicare patient has a Medigap policy, type G, will it pay for the Part A deductible? ____________ Will it pay for the Part B deductible? ____________

11–13 What is the term used when another insurance plan is the primary payer and Medicare pays second? ____

11–14 Under what circumstances should a participating physician file a claim to Medicare in a liability case? ____

____

____

CHALLENGE SESSIONS 11–15 AND 11–16

Directions: *Refer to Elderly Employee Benefits in Table 11–1 and use critical thinking skills to answer the following questions:*

11–15 (a) Bayshore Biscuit Company employs 35 full-time workers, including a 67-year-old. This elderly employee has Medicare benefits and is also on the company's group healthcare plan. Who is the primary insurer? ______

(b) What law/act determines primary/secondary coverage in this case? ______

11–16 (a) Leo Rutherford worked for Exact Copy Company along with 200 other employees. He became disabled due to an amputation and complications caused by juvenile diabetes mellitus. He continued his group coverage from his job and also has Medicare. Which coverage is primary? ______

(b) What act/law determines primary/secondary coverage in this case? ______

CHECK YOUR HEARTBEAT! Turn to the end of the chapter for answers to these review and challenge sessions.

MEDICARE FRAUD AND ABUSE PROTECTION

A number of federal laws and regulations have been passed to control the quality of medical services provided to Medicare patients and assure that all medical services are being utilized properly. Following are some measurements that have been put in place to satisfy those concerns.

Peer Review Organizations

A **peer review organization (PRO)** is a state-based group of physicians working under government guidelines who review cases to determine the appropriateness and quality of professional care. They also settle fee disputes. Using statistical data, they are involved in implementing an improvement plan for the quality of care that is given. Case reviews focus on hospital admission and discharge, invasive procedures, medical record documentation, extraordinarily high costs (outlier costs), and limitation of liability determinations.

A physician who receives a letter regarding quality of care should consult his or her attorney before responding. A photocopy of the patient's medical record can be used to substantiate the claim if there is detailed clinical documentation. If documentation is lacking, penalties can lead to fines, loss of staff privileges, and/or forfeiture of the physician's license.

Federal False Claims Amendment Act

The Federal False Claims Amendment Act was created to prevent overuse of services and to spot Medicare fraud. This act offers financial incentives of 15% to 25% of any judgment to informants who report physicians suspected of defrauding the federal government. Health insurance companies that process Medicare claims have a Medicare fraud unit whose job is to catch people who steal from Medicare. Fraud hotlines are in place for anonymous callers to report suspicious activity. For information on fraud and abuse, see Chapter 1, Tables 1–4 and 1–5.

Health Insurance Portability and Accountability Act

The *Health Insurance Portability and Accountability Act (HIPAA)* has a section that deals with the prevention of healthcare fraud and abuse of patients on Medicare and Medicaid. Physicians, insurance specialists, coders, and any individuals who knowingly and willfully break the law could suffer a penalty, a fine, and/or imprisonment. *Civil* monetary penalties are assessed for the following:

- Intentional incorrect coding that will result in increased payment.
- A pattern of claims being submitted for a service or product that is not medically necessary.
- Offering remuneration (kickback) to induce an individual to order from a particular provider or supplier who receives Medicare or state health funds.

The *federal* criminal sanctions of this act are established for those who:

- Knowingly embezzle, steal, or misapply a healthcare benefit program.
- Knowingly or willfully defraud a healthcare program.

Civil Monetary Penalties Law

The federal government passed the Civil Monetary Penalties Law (CMPL) to prosecute cases of Medicare and Medicaid fraud. The law carries three separate forms of sanction:

1. A penalty of up to $2,000 for each item or service wrongfully listed in a payment request to Medicare or Medicaid.

2. An assessment of up to twice the total amount improperly claimed.
3. Suspension from the program(s) for whatever period the Department of Health and Human Services determines.

A physician may be penalized when participating in the following violations:

- Billing for services that were not provided.
- Billing more than once for the same service to obtain greater reimbursement.
- Fragmenting billed services that could be accurately described by one procedural code.
- Upgrading (upcoding) the reported level or complexity of services, over those services actually furnished, to obtain greater reimbursement.

A physician who fails to practice due care to ensure the accuracy of Medicare and Medicaid claims prepared in his or her office risks enormous financial penalties. The CMPL makes no distinction between outright fraud and negligence in billing. Therefore, if an employee submits false billings that the physician knows nothing about, the physician may be held liable. Reckless disregard of federal and state regulations by the insurance billing specialist can affect the way claims are submitted, and possibly cause a physician to incur a civil monetary penalty.

Always document advice given by representatives of the fiscal agent or state welfare department. If the advice later proves to be erroneous, such records can support the physician's good faith. Notify the physician's attorney if the physician is advised that he or she is being investigated and do not release any documents without the attorney's approval.

Stark I and II Regulations

Stark I and II Regulations prohibit a physician (or immediate family member of the physician) who has a financial relationship with a designated health service (e.g., laboratory, medical equipment supply company, physical therapy facility, and so forth) from referring patients to that facility. It also prohibits the provider from billing for such designated health services and prohibits both Medicare and Medicaid from making payments to providers that result from such a referral.

Many states have passed laws and administrative rules that may apply the same principles to other private payers. Uncovered self-referral deceits or failure of a designated service provider to report financial information can lead to hefty fines, sanctions, payment denials, and exclusion from Medicare/Medicaid programs.

Clinical Laboratory Improvement Amendment

The Clinical Laboratory Improvement Amendment (CLIA) established federal standards, quality control, and safety measures for all laboratory testing (except testing performed for research and forensic purposes) for freestanding laboratories, including physician office laboratories (POLs). CLIA established categories for all laboratory procedures according to *complexity*. Each category level requires a yearly licensing fee to be paid by the physician; the more complex the level, the higher the fee and the stricter the quality control. The licensing certificate is then issued and must be posted in the laboratory. Tests are not exempt based on the qualifications of the person performing the test, whether tests are documented in the medical record, or whether the laboratory charges for the tests.

The lowest-level category (A) is referred to as "CLIA waived tests." Such tests must be simple to run and an erroneous result must not have a negative impact on the patient (e.g., blood sugar, dipstick urine, hematocrit). Tests approved for home use are usually waived. Tests in Category B are referred to as "physician-performed microscopy procedures," (e.g., microscopic urinalysis). Tests in Category C (nonwaived tests) require a microscope, specimen manipulation, calculations, or a judgment call. If the majority of the tests performed in the laboratory are waived tests (Category A), but one test from a higher category is performed (e.g., microscopic urinalysis—B), the higher level (Category B) dictates the level of certificate required by CLIA.

CLIA requires a written order for every laboratory test that is performed, including waived tests. The order may be written in the chart, on the encounter form, or on a separate requisition. A verbal order is acceptable; however, it must appear in writing within 30 days.

Waived laboratories are not routinely inspected but are required to follow the manufacturer's guidelines, including quality control measures. Fines may be levied if federal standards are not maintained. This has had an impact on POLs and, because of the strict requirements, many physicians have chosen to send patients to independent laboratories for tests (e.g., complete blood counts, cytology specimens, and cultures). Some physicians prefer to draw blood from patients, particularly if the patient has a history of difficult venous access, and send the blood to an outside laboratory for processing.

When submitting claims to Medicare fiscal intermediaries for laboratory services performed in a POL, the 11-digit CLIA certificate number needs to be entered in Block 23 of the HCFA-1500 claim form (see Fig. 11–6B). All laboratory services are exempt from deductible and coinsurance requirements in the Medicare program. Refer to Resources at the end of this chapter for information on where to obtain a list of CLIA categories and a complete list of waived tests.

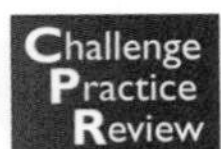

Pause and Practice CPR

REVIEW SESSIONS 11–17 THROUGH 11–20

Directions: *Complete the following questions as a review of information you have just read.*

11–17 What is the maximum monetary penalty for an item or service that is wrongfully listed on a Medicare claim? ______________________

11–18 If an employee submits fraudulent billing that the physician knows nothing about, can the physician be held liable? ______________________

11–19 What is the intention of Stark I and II regulations? ______________________

____

____

11–20 What is the name for the federal standards that outline quality control and safety measures for all physician-based laboratories? ______________________

CHECK YOUR HEARTBEAT! Turn to the end of the chapter for answers to these review sessions.

PAYMENT FUNDAMENTALS

Medicare Fee Schedule

Each fiscal intermediary within a region compiles fee data and annually sends a local Medicare fee schedule to each physician. Statistics on fees are kept in the Medicare Physician Fee Schedule Data Base (MPFSDB). The fee schedule consists of three columns of figures:

1. Participating amount—amount on which payment is based for participating physicians; providers agree to accept this amount, referred to as a **reasonable fee.**
2. Nonparticipating amount—amount on which payment is based for nonparticipating physicians.
3. Limiting charge—the highest amount (ceiling) which a nonparticipating physician can charge; established through the Omnibus Budget Reconciliation Act (OBRA) and referred to as the "maximum allowable actual charge" (MAAC) formula.

Fees are listed by code number for each approved procedure or service. Refer to the Mock Fee Schedule listed in Appendix B for an example of the Medicare fee schedule.

Deductible

A physician may choose to participate, or not participate in the Medicare program. Regardless, the patient must first satisfy the Medicare deductible of $100 per calendar year (January 1 through December 31) before payment can be calculated.

Multiple Procedure

Medicare has a standard payment rule for most multiple procedures and allows reimbursement of 100% of the fee schedule amount for the procedure of the highest value. The second most expensive procedure, and each additional procedure up to the fifth, is reimbursed at 50%. Each procedure after the fifth requires documentation and is subject to review. It is not necessary to use modifier -51 (multiple procedure) when billing Medicare.

Participating Physician

In a Medicare par agreement, the physician agrees to accept 80% of the approved charge from Medicare, and 20% of the approved charge from the patient, after the $100 deductible has been met (Fig. 11–8). The difference between the amount charged (actual charge) and the approved amount is credited (written off) and posted to the patient's account as a courtesy adjustment. This agreement is referred to as **accepting assignment.** The par physician may bill Medicare using the par-approved amount, the limiting charge, or usual and customary fees.

The physician must submit a claim electronically or manually (using the HCFA-1500 form) to the fiscal agent. The assignment of benefits located in Block 12 is signed by the patient. The physician indicates that assignment is being accepted by checking "Yes" in Block 27, and the payment goes directly to the physician (see Fig. D–6 in Appendix D). Certain services (e.g., influenza vaccine) are reimbursed at 100% of the allowable amount.

Nonparticipating Physician

A nonpar physician does not have a signed agreement with Medicare and has an option regarding assignment. The physician may not accept assignment for all services or may accept assignment for some services and collect from the patient for other services performed at the same time and place. An exception to this policy is clinical laboratory tests and services for which assignment is mandatory.

If a patient receives medical services from a nonpar physician, the patient is responsible for an annual deductible ($100), 20% of the nonpar-approved amount, and the difference between the nonpar-approved amount and the limiting charge. Medicare pays the physician 80% of the nonpar-approved amount (see Fig. 11–8). Usually a nonpar physician who is not accepting assignment collects the limiting charge from the patient at the time of service and Medicare sends the payment check to the patient. Certain services (e.g., influenza vaccine) are not subject to the limiting charge.

For assigned claims, nonpar physicians may bill using usual and customary fees. Nonpar physicians usually maintain two fee schedules, one with usual fees and one with limiting charges, because of these two situations. Some states have set limiting charges that are more restrictive than Medicare policies. These states are Connecticut, Massachusetts, New York, Ohio, Pennsylvania, Rhode Island, and Vermont. For state guidelines, contact the fiscal intermediary of those states.

New Patient versus Established Patient

The definition of a new patient has changed for Medicare patients. CMS states, "If no evaluation and

Payment Examples

Scenario	Actual charge	Medicare approved amount*	Deductible	Medicare pays	Beneficiary responsible for	Medicare courtesy adjustment**
Doctor A–accepts assignment	$480	$400	$100 already satisfied	$320 (80% of approved amount)	$80 (20% of approved amount)	$80 (difference between actual charge and approved amount)
Doctor B–does not accept assignment; charges the limiting amount	$437	$380	$100 already satisfied	$304 (80% of approved amount)	$133 20% of approved amount ($76) plus difference between limiting charge (actual charge) and approved amount ($57)= $133	None
Doctor C–accepts assignment; however the patient has not met the deductible amount	$480	$300 ($400 minus the deductible)	$100 has not been met	$240 (80% of approved amount determined after subtracting the deductible)	$60 (20% of the approved amount determined after subtracting the deductible	$80 difference between actual charge and approved amount

* The Medicare approved amount is less for non-participating physicians than for participating physicians.

** The courtesy adjustment is the amount credited to the patient's account in the adjustment column. The word "courtesy" implies that Medicare patients are treated well and is preferred to phrases like "not allowed."

Figure 11–8. Payment examples for three physicians showing a physician accepting assignment versus not accepting assignment, and the amounts the patient is responsible for paying with deductible satisfied and not met.

management service is performed, the patient may continue to be treated as a new patient." For example, if an established patient is not seen by the physician, but goes periodically to have blood tests for which the physician interprets and bills, the 3-year time period is not affected and the patient will be considered a new patient as long as he or she does not return to see the physician within that time frame.

Prepayment Screens

On some procedures, Medicare limits the number of times a given procedure can be billed (e.g., four office visits per month, one treatment every 60 days for routine foot care, one physical examination per year). These are known as Medicare Prepayment Screens. Refer to your local fiscal intermediary's Medicare newsletters/bulletins or request a complete list of the Medicare Prepayment Screens applicable to your area.

Correct Coding Initiative

Medicare's **Correct Coding Initiative (CCI)** is implemented by CMS in an attempt to eliminate unbundling or other inappropriate reporting of Current Procedural Terminology (CPT) codes. Coding conflicts are picked up and claims are reviewed, suspended, or denied when conflicts occur. Software is available to give physicians, private insurance companies, and billing services access to the same government database used in auditing physicians for improper use of CPT codes.

Denied Services

There are two situations, often confused, when Medicare does not pay for services. The insurance billing specialist needs to understand Medicare rules about these two scenarios in order to know when the physician is able to collect or not collect money from the Medicare patient.

Limitation of Liability Provision

The first situation is when a patient is to receive a service from a par physician that might be denied for **medical necessity.** Such services are found not to be covered because they are considered not reasonable or medically necessary for the diagnosis or treatment of an injury, illness, or condition as defined by Medicare. For example, the patient has been administered monthly vitamin B_{12} injections but would like another and it has only been 2 weeks since the previous injection. Medicare has a limitation on B_{12} injections and will only pay for one every 30 days. Inform the patient of the Medicare rule and if he or she agrees to pay for the service, instruct the patient to sign a waiver of liability agreement called an *Advance Beneficiary Notice (ABN)* (Fig. 11–9). The ABN cannot be signed *after* the patient has received the service and must *specifically state* what service or procedure is being waived. Keep this signed waiver with the patient's financial documents and not with the patient's medical record. If you do not know what the Medicare guidelines or parameters are for a certain procedure or service, refer to Medicare bulletins/newsletters or call the Medicare carrier and ask.

When sending in a claim, the HCPCS Level II modifier-GA (waived liability on file) must be added to pertinent codes to indicate a patient has signed the ABN. The Medicare carrier will inform the patient that he or she is responsible for the fee.

If no advance notice was given (no signed waiver of liability agreement), then append the code with modifier -GZ (item or service expected to be denied as not reasonable and necessary) and remember:

- You cannot collect from Medicare.
- You cannot collect from the patient (even the deductible or copayment amounts).
- If the patient has paid for the service, a full refund must be made to the patient.

If assignment is accepted and the physician and patient thought the service or procedure was covered under reasonable assumptions, then:

- Bill Medicare.
- The patient must pay the deductible and coinsurance.
- Medicare will not seek a refund of money already paid to the physician.

Nonpar physicians must refund any amounts collected from the beneficiary when services are later found to be not reasonable and necessary.

Noncovered Services

The second situation involves services that are not covered (noncovered) by Medicare. Such services are not a part of Medicare's benefit package and may *always* be billed to the patient. The patient should be notified prior to rendering services that are for noncovered benefits; however, it is not necessary to obtain a waiver of liability for this situation, although some physicians prefer to do so. A good rule is, whenever in doubt, get a waiver of liability.

Services denied as inclusive of another service (unbundled—and payment already made for the other service) are not considered a noncovered item and may not be billed to the patient.

If you need a formal denial to bill the patient or another insurer, send in a claim with a letter attached stating that you need the denial to bill another payer; otherwise, to bill for a noncovered service is inappropriate and may possibly be viewed by some as fraud.

Elective Surgery Estimate

A nonpar physician who does not accept assignment for an *elective surgery* for which the actual charge will

College Clinic

4567 Broad Avenue
Woodland Hills, XY
12345-0001
Tel (555) 486-9002
Fax (555) 487-8976

MEDICARE ADVANCE BENEFICIARY NOTICE

Medicare will only pay for covered items and services when Medicare rules are met. The fact that Medicare may not pay for a particular item or service does not mean that you should not receive it. There may be a good reason your doctor is recommending it. In your case, Medicare may deny payment for the following item, test, or service.

Item/Test/Service: **Approximate Cost:**

1.____________________ $__________

2.____________________ $__________

Reason Claim Will Be Denied:

☐ Not payable for listed diagnosis: ______________

☐ Routine items, services, and laboratory work usually denied.

☐ Test or service does not have FDA approval (payment approved for research or investigative use only).

☐ Exceeds time limitation on number of times this item/test/service can be ordered/performed.

☐ Not a Medicare benefit.

☐ Other:____________________

Beneficiary Agreement:

It is our responsibility to notify you that this item, test, or service may not be covered by Medicare. In the event Medicare denies payment, you will be billed for this item, test, or service. You have the right to decide whether or not to receive this item, test, or service.

☐ I have been notified that, in my case, Medicare is likely to deny payment for the above-named item, test, or service for the reason indicated. I choose to receive the above-named item, test, or service and I agree to be personally and fully responsible for the payment.______ (initials)

☐ I choose not to receive the item, test, or service named above and acknowledge this refusal may compromise my health care.______ (initials)

Patient Caution:

DO NOT sign a blank form. The item, test, or service must be clearly marked along with the reason it is believed that Medicare may deny payment and the approximate cost. You should receive a copy of this completed form; please indicate here _____(initials) that you have received a copy. You have a right to have a claim submitted to Medicare for this item, test, or service.

____________________ Beneficiary Signature acknowledges understanding

__________ Date

____________________ Provider or Provider's Representative Signature

__________ Date

Your health information collected on this form will be kept confidential in our facility. If a claim is submitted to Medicare, your health information on this form may be shared with Medicare. Medicare will keep confidential health information which has been shared with them on this form.

Figure 11–9. Example of a Medicare Advance Beneficiary Notice (ABN) waiver of liability agreement.

be $500 or more must provide the beneficiary, in writing, with (1) the estimated fee for the procedure, (2) the estimated Medicare-approved allowance for the procedure, and (3) the difference between the physician's actual charge (limiting amount) and the allowed amount (Fig. 11–10). *Elective surgery* is a surgical procedure that can be scheduled in advance, is not an emergency, is discretionary on the part of the physician and the patient, and does not pose a mortality threat if the patient does not have it done. Document the patient's acknowledgment by obtaining the Medicare patient's signature at the bottom of the estimation letter. Give a copy of the letter to the patient and keep the original for your files.

Hospital Reimbursement

Hospital Inpatient

In a hospital setting, Medicare payments were originally based, similar to payments for outpatient services, on reasonable fees (i.e., 80% of the Medicare-approved charge). The important development of the **prospective payment system (PPS)** changed the way payments were structured for hospitals and today hospital inpatient services are reimbursed according to preestablished rates for each type of illness based on diagnosis. Payments to hospitals for Medicare services are classified according to 503 diagnosis-related group

ESTIMATED MEDICARE PAYMENT FOR ELECTIVE SURGERY
Worksheet

A

1. Physician's actual fee (limiting charge) .... $ 1248.03
2. Medicare approved or allowed amount .... $ 1085.24
3. Difference between physician's actual fee and Medicare approved or allowed amount (1 - 2 = 3) .... - 162.79
4. Twenty per cent coinsurance (0.20 X 2 = 4) .... + 217.05
5. Beneficiary's out-of-pocket expense (3 + 4 + 5) .... $ 379.84
   Assume the $100 deductible has been met

Items 1, 2, and 5 must be included in the letter to the beneficiary

B

Beneficiary Letter

Dear Patient:

Because I do not accept assignment for elective surgery, Medicare requires that I give you certain information before surgery when my charges are $500 or more.

The following information concerns the surgery we have discussed. These estimates assume that you have already met the $100 deductible.

Type of surgery .... Osteotomy, proximal left tibia
Limiting charge $ 1248.03
Medicare estimated payment $ 868.19
Patient's estimated payment $ 379.84

This estimate is based upon our present expectations of what surgical procedure(s) will be required. Please remember that this is only an estimate of charges, we cannot be sure that additional procedures will or will not be necessary.

Sincerely,

Gerald Practon, M.D. 126XX5479
Medicare Provider Number

I understand the foregoing physician charges and my financial responsibility with respect to those estimated charges.

Patient's Signature .... Jane Doe .... Date 5-18-20XX
Jane Doe

Figure 11–10. *A*, Worksheet, and *B*, sample beneficiary letter for estimated Medicare payment for elective surgery.

(DRG) numbers. Beneficiaries (patients) cannot be billed beyond the preestablished DRG rate except for *outliers* (unusual circumstances or complications), normal deductible, and copayment amounts. Physicians providing services to inpatients bill according to the Medicare fee schedule, as discussed earlier.

Hospital Outpatient

An *ambulatory payment classification* (APC) system is used to bill for hospital outpatient services. Services are categorized into approximately 451 APCs and these will probably expand in subsequent years. The procedure code is the primary axis of classification, not the diagnostic code. An APC group may have a number of services or items packaged within it so that separate reimbursement cannot be obtained.

The reimbursement methodology is based on median costs of services and facility cost to determine charge ratios and copayment amounts. There is also an adjustment for the area wage difference. Some Medicaid programs and private payers have embraced this system because of the escalation of outpatient costs.

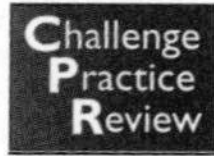

Pause and Practice CPR

REVIEW SESSIONS 11–21 THROUGH 11–23

Directions: *Match the following Medicare plans with their descriptions and fill the blank with the appropriate letter.*

a) participating amount b) nonparticipating amount c) limiting charge

11–21 ______ Amount on which payment is based for physicians who do not participate in the Medicare program.

11–22 ______ The highest amount which a physician who does not participate in the Medicare program can charge a patient.

11–23 ______ Amount on which payment is based for physicians who participate in the Medicare program.

PRACTICE SESSIONS 11–24 AND 11–25

Directions: *Refer to the section on participating and nonparticipating physicians and Figure 11–8. Read the following scenarios and calculate the correct amounts.*

11–24 Landon Russell saw Dr. Practon for a new patient level 5 evaluation and management service. The Medicare participating fee is $121.08; nonparticipating fee, $115.03; and limiting charge, $132.38. Dr. Practon participates in Medicare and the patient's deductible has been met.

(a) What is the amount Medicare pays? $ ______

(b) What is the amount the patient pays? $ ______

(c) What is the courtesy adjustment? $ ______

11–25 Myron Bailey saw Dr. Feelgood for a new patient level 5 evaluation. Dr. Feelgood does not accept the assignment and charges the Medicare limiting fee (see above).

(a) What is the amount Medicare pays? $ ______

(b) What is the amount the patient pays? $ ______

(c) What is the courtesy adjustment? $ ______

CHECK YOUR HEARTBEAT! Turn to the end of the chapter for answers to these review and practice sessions.

HEALTH CARE FINANCING ADMINISTRATION COMMON PROCEDURE CODING SYSTEM (HCPCS)*

As mentioned in Chapter 5, the federal government developed the Health Care Financing Administration Common Procedure Coding System (HCPCS) for the Medicare program. Up to this point you have primarily been working with HCPCS Level I (CPT) procedure codes. HCPCS Level II codes are used to bill for medication, durable medical equipment (DME), and a variety of services which may be reviewed in Chapter 5. As mentioned, Level II codes are national codes used to identify new procedures or specific supplies for which there are no Level I codes.

To obtain correct payment for a Medicare procedure or service, a code number must be selected from Level I, II, or III of the HCPCS coding system. When submitting a claim, be sure to use the Level II HCPCS national alphanumeric codes rather than CPT codes for certain appliances and procedures as indicated. Also check HCPCS Level II modifiers to see if they apply to the billing scenario. When using CPT modifiers, refer to Appendix C for a complete list of modifiers. A comprehensive list, which includes *Medicare Payment Rules*, can be found at the Worktext web site http://www.wbsaunders.com/MERLIN/Fordney/insurance/.

The HCPCS Level II codebook is arranged with codes grouped according to services (Table 11–3). Most codes have an alpha letter listed first followed by four digits (e.g., J0120) and a description of the item or service. Refer to Appendix C of the worktext for an abbreviated list of HCPCS Level II codes and modifiers.

Table 11–3 HCPCS Level II Codebook Contents

Section	Code Range
Transportation services	A0021–A0999
Medical and surgical supplies	A4206–A7509
Administrative, miscellaneous and investigational	A9150–A9901
Enteral and parenteral therapy	B4034–B9999
Hospital outpatient PPS codes (temporary)	C1000–C9711
Dental procedures	D0120–D9999
Durable medical equipment (DME)	E0100–E2101
Procedures and professional services (temporary)	G0001–G9016
Rehabilitative services	H0001–H1005
Drugs administered other than oral method*	J0120–J8999
Chemotherapy drugs*	J9000–J9999
K Codes: for durable medical equipment regional carriers (DMERC) use only	K0001–K0551
Orthotic procedures	L0100–L4398
Prosthetic procedures	L5000–L9900
Medical services	M0064–M0301
Pathology and laboratory services	P2028–P9615
Temporary codes	Q0035–Q9940
Diagnostic radiology services	R0070–R0076
Temporary national codes (nonmedicare)	S0009–S9999
Vision services	V2020–V2799
Hearing services	V5008–V5364
Appendix A—modifiers	E.g., -AA/-F1
Appendix B—summary of additions, changes, and revisions	Listed by code
Appendix C—table of drugs	E.g., Abbokinase (see urokinase)
Index	Alphabetical order of agent, item, or service with code listing, e.g., Back support, L0500–L0960

*National Drug Codes (NDCs) will be used instead of HCPCS codes effective 10/2002. Note: Appendices vary from book to book and may also include coverage issues, Medicare manual references, payer directory, Medicare carriers, intermediaries, and contacts.

Coding Regulations

The allowance for office supplies is incorporated into procedures as part of the overall practice expense. As discussed in Chapter 6, supplies may not be billed separately unless they are above and beyond the usual supplies provided for the service/procedure. An exception to this is the separate reimbursement for the cost of a surgical tray (HCPCS Level II code A4550) when billing for procedures which appear on a list published by Medicare (e.g., 19101 open, incisional biopsy of breast). The bill would be sent to the Medicare Fiscal Intermediary, not the Durable Medical Equipment Regional Carrier (DMERC).

*Since the change of HCFA to CMS, HCPCS may be referred to as Healthcare Common Procedure Coding System.

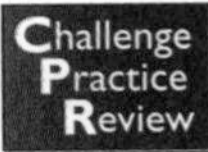

Pause and Practice CPR

REVIEW SESSION 11–26

Directions: *Refer to the section on HCPCS Level II codes and Table 11–3 to answer the following questions.*

11–26 HCPCS Level II codes for the following services would fall under which *section* and start with what *alpha letter?*

SERVICE/SUPPLY/PROCEDURE	SECTION	ALPHA
Example: Ambulance service	**Transportation Services**	**A**
(a) Cochlear implant	______	______
(b) Commode chair	______	______
(c) Injection, testosterone (chemo)	______	______
(d) Contact lens	______	______
(e) Foam dressing	______	______

CHECK YOUR HEARTBEAT! Turn to the end of the chapter for answers to this review session.

MEDICARE CLAIM SUBMISSION

Fiscal Intermediaries and Fiscal Agents

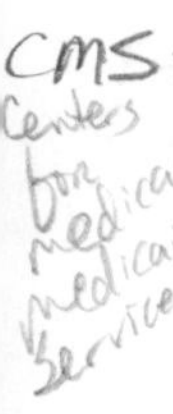

A **fiscal intermediary (FI)** is an organization under contract with the government that handles claims under Medicare Part A and/or Part B. The National Blue Cross Association holds the fiscal intermediary contract for Medicare Part A; it in turn subcontracts with member agencies in various regions. The fiscal intermediary handles Part A claims from hospital facilities, nursing facilities (NFs), **intermediate care facilities (ICFs),** and long-term care facilities (LTCFs).

Organizations handling Part B claims from physicians, chiropractors, physical therapists, nutritionists, and other suppliers of services are usually referred to as *fiscal agents, fiscal carriers*, or a *claims processor*. Private insurance companies contract with the government to handle Part B payments. Areas are divided into regions across the United States and a fiscal agent may handle more than one region. To determine where to send a claim, bill the carrier who covers the area where the service occurred or was furnished, NOT the carrier who services the physician's office.

All physicians and suppliers (par and nonpar) must file Part B claims on behalf of their Medicare patients, whether the claim is assigned or unassigned, with four exceptions:

1. Services covered by Medicare for which the patient has other insurance that is primary to Medicare (MSP) and the office does not have the information to file the claim to the primary carrier.
2. Services provided outside the United States.
3. When DME is purchased from a private source.
4. The physician does not have to file a patient's claim for a service not covered by Medicare unless the patient (or his/her representative) requests a formal ruling from CMS.

Under other circumstances, physicians, practitioners, and suppliers who fail to submit claims are subject to civil monetary penalties up to $2,500 for each claim.

Provider Identification Numbers

The Tax Reform Act established several types of identification numbers for each physician and nonphysician practitioner providing services paid by Medicare. Because there are so many numbers, they are easily confused and when completing the HCFA-1500 claim form, they end up being the source of many errors. You have already used many of these numbers when completing Billing Break scenarios for private carriers. For a review, refer to Figure 8–4 and the Medicare templates (Figures D–6 through D–9 in Appendix D).

For Medicare claims, College Clinic bills using its regular group identification number (3664021CC) for physician services. Although Medicare requires a Performing Physician Identification Number (PPIN) in Block 24J–K for providers billing under a group, use the Medicare National Provider Identifier (NPI) for all Billing Break cases. College Hospital has its own Medicare provider number (HSP43700F) for services provided at the hospital facility. If DME were supplied from either College Clinic or an independent supplier, each would have a separate DME number to bill for such services.

Protect your practice from fraud by protecting your physician's Provider Identification Number (PIN). It is like an unlimited credit card and if it falls into the wrong hands, claims may be paid under it and you will be responsible. If a physician leaves, closes, or relocates a practice, be sure to write the Provider Enrollment Unit and revoke the reassignment agreement to bill Medicare and close his or her Medicare account so that the PIN can be deactivated in Medicare's computer system.

Patient's Signature Authorization

The Medicare patient's signature authorization for (1) release of medical information, and (2) assignment of government benefits is recorded in Block 12 of the HCFA-1500 claim form. This block needs to be signed regardless of whether the physician is a par or nonpar physician because all patients need to sign to release medical information. The signed authorization may be obtained and kept on file in the patient's medical record for an episode of care or for a designated time frame (e.g., 1 year or lifetime). Subsequent claims may then indicate "Signature on file" or the abbreviation "SOF" in Block 12 of the claim form. The example of a lifetime beneficiary claim authorization and information release form shown in Figure 11–11 can be used for assigned Medicare claims and kept in the patient's medical record. An original copy of the HCFA-1500 claim form may also be used to obtain a lifetime signature authorization by writing across the top of the form "Lifetime Signature Authorization" and filling it in as described.

Signature requirements for various situations that may occur in a medical practice are:

- *Patients confined in a facility*, such as a nursing facility, hospital, or home, should have a lifetime signature authorization on file.
- *Patients who are deceased* have special signature requirements which are discussed later in this chapter.
- *Patients who are illiterate or physically handicapped and sign using an "X"* require a witness who signs his or her name next to the mark.
- *Patients who do not sign the form, but instead have another person sign it* should have the other person sign the patient's name, write "by" and sign his or her own name (with address), indicate their relationship to the patient, and state why the patient cannot sign.
- *Medicare/Medicaid (Medi-Medi) claims* do not require the patient's signature.
- *Medicare/Medigap claims* must fulfill the two signature requirements for Medicare, and contain an assignment of benefits for the Medigap carrier, which appears in Block 13 on the HCFA-1500 claim form or may be obtained and kept on file.

Further information on this topic may be found in Chapters 1, 2, and 3.

Physician's Signature Requirement

As mentioned in Chapter 8, there are a number of ways for the provider to sign the HCFA-1500 claim form in Block 31. Medicare prefers one of the following methods:

- Physician's original signature.
- Physician may authorize an employee to enter the physician's signature either manually, by stamp-facsimile, or by computer.
- Physician may authorize a nonemployee (e.g., billing service) to enter his or her name, as mentioned above.
- Physician signs a one-time certification letter for electronic claims.

For Billing Break exercises, you will be typing or printing the physician's name and signing it as if you were the physician.

Time Limit

The time limit for sending in Medicare claims is the end of the calendar year following the fiscal year in which services are furnished. The fiscal year for claims begins October 1 and ends September 30 (see Example 11–3).

4567 Broad Avenue
Woodland Hills, XY
12345-0001
Tel (555) 486-9002
Fax (555) 487-8976

LIFETIME BENEFICIARY CLAIM AUTHORIZATION AND INFORMATION RELEASE

Patient's Name ____Jane Doe____ Medicare I.D. number ____540-XX-8755A____

I request that payment of authorized Medicare benefits be made either to me or on my behalf to (name of physician/supplier) for any services furnished me by that physician/supplier. I authorize any holder of medical information about me to release to the Center for Medicare and Medicaid Services and its agents any information needed to determine these benefits or the benefits payable to related services.

I understand my signature requests that payment be made and I consent to the release of medical information necessary to pay the claim. If other health insurance is indicated in Item 9 of the HCFA-1500 claim form or elsewhere on other approved claim forms or electronically submitted claims, my signature authorizes release of the information to the insurer or agency shown. In Medicare assigned cases, the physician or supplier agrees to accept the charge determination of the Medicare carrier as the full charge, and the patient is responsible only for the deductible, coinsurance, and noncovered services. Coinsurance and the deductible are based upon the charge determination of the Medicare carrier.

Jane Doe
Patient's Signature

January 3, 20XX
Date

Figure 11–11. Lifetime Assignment of Benefits and Release for Medical Information agreement.

Example 11-3

Time Limit for Filing Medicare Claims

For services furnished on:		The time limit is:
Oct. 1, 2001–Sept. 30, 2002	⟶	December 31, 2003
Oct. 1, 2002–Sept. 30, 2003	⟶	December 31, 2004

EXAMPLE:

Dr. Cutler performed surgery on Mrs. Carver on April 2, 2002; however, the claim was held up because the hospital failed to send the operative report and it came to the insurance biller's attention on December 28, 2002. What is the deadline for filing this claim? **Answer: December 31, 2003**

On assigned claims, the provider may file without penalty up to 27 months after providing service if reasonable cause for the delay is shown to the insurance carrier. Otherwise, there is a 10% reduction in the reimbursement. On unassigned claims, the provider may be fined for delinquent claim submission up to $2,000 and/or lose his or her right to bill Medicare. When submitting a late claim ask the fiscal intermediary for the guidelines that CMS considers reasonable cause for delay.

Manual Claim Submission

The HCFA-1500 insurance claim form is used to submit claims to the Medicare fiscal agent. Refer to Appendix D for a complete block-by-block description of information required by Medicare on the claim form. The reference templates for Medicare with other coverage shown at the end of Appendix D are:

Medicare—no secondary coverage (Fig. D–6)
Medicare/Medicaid—crossover claim (Fig. D–7)
Medicare/Medigap—crossover claim (Fig. D–8)
Other insurance/Medicare—MSP (Fig. D–9)

Medicare claim status is explained in detail in Chapter 8 (i.e., clean, incomplete, rejected, invalid, dirty, dingy, and other claims).

Electronic Claim Submission

Electronic submission of Medicare claims is quick and easy compared to paper submission. Medicare requests that providers submit all claims electronically. Electronic transmission formats for Medicare claims are scheduled to be standardized by the use of ANSI ASCX12N Version 4010 837. Refer to the section on Electronic Data Interchange in Chapter 8 for information on electronic claims. Vendors who represent Medicare-compatible software are usually present at all Medicare seminars and will be glad to demonstrate their software and answer questions regarding electronic submission.

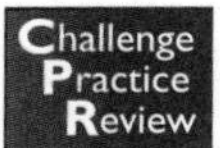

Pause and Practice CPR

REVIEW SESSIONS 11–27 THROUGH 11–31

Directions: *Complete the following questions as a review of information you have just read.*

11–27 When billing for a Medicare patient who is seen at College Clinic, what identification number is entered in Block 33? ____________________

11–28 When billing for DME, where are the claims sent? ____________________

11–29 When a Medicare patient's signature is on file for the release of medical information and assignment of benefits, what abbreviation may be used in Block 12 of the HCFA-1500 claim form? ____________

11–30 For Medicare Billing Break exercises, how will the physician's signature requirement be handled in Block 31 of the HCFA-1500 claim form? ____________________

____

11–31 Refer to the Medicare time limit for filing claims and Example 11–3. Determine what the deadline is for filing a claim, DOS May 4, 2003. ____________

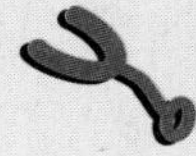

CHECK YOUR HEARTBEAT! Turn to the end of the chapter for answers to these review sessions.

Medicare/Medicaid Claim Submission

Medi-Medi patients qualify for the benefits of Medicare as well as Medicaid (Medi-Cal in California). Submit electronically, or use the HCFA-1500 claim form and check "Yes" for the assignment of benefits in Block 27. If the physician does not accept assignment, then payment goes to the patient and Medicaid will not pick up the residual. If filled out correctly, the HCFA-1500 claim form will be automatically transferred (crossed over) from Medicare to

9. OTHER INSURED'S NAME (Last Name, First Name, Middle Initial)
JOHNSON KATHRYN
a. OTHER INSURED'S POLICY OR GROUP NUMBER
b. OTHER INSURED'S DATE OF BIRTH
MM | DD | YYYY SEX M☐ F☐
c. EMPLOYER'S NAME OR SCHOOL NAME
d. INSURANCE PLAN NAME OR PROGRAM NAME
10. IS PATIENT'S CONDITION RELATED TO:
a. EMPLOYMENT? (Current or Previous)
☐YES ☒NO
b. AUTO ACCIDENT? Place (State)
☐YES ☒NO
c. OTHER ACCIDENT?
☐YES ☒NO
10d. RESERVED FOR LOCAL USE
MCD016745289

Figure 11–12. Section of the HCFA-1500 claim form with Blocks 9, 9a–d, and Block 10d emphasized to show placement of Medicaid information for a Medi-Medi claim.

Medicaid after processing is completed by Medicare. The fiscal agent may refer to this as a **crossover claim** or *claims transfer.* It is not necessary to submit another form. Claims should be sent by the time limit designated by the Medicaid program in your state, not by the Medicare time limit. Medicaid time limits are usually shorter so claims need to be expedited to ensure reimbursement.

See the Medi-Medi template (Fig. D–7) in Appendix D for a visual example of block-by-block completion. Refer to block-by-block instructions in Appendix D for specific guidelines. Figure 11–12 illustrates key blocks (Blocks 9, 9b, and 10d) where information is entered on the claim form for a Medi-Medi patient. Requirements vary from state to state regarding placement of crossover information.

Generally, the Medicare payment exceeds the Medicaid fee schedule and little or no payment is received. Two exceptions to this are (1) when the patient has not met his or her annual deductible, and (2) when Medicaid pays for services that are not covered by Medicare.

In some states the fiscal agent for a Medi-Medi claim may have a different address from that used for the processing of a patient who is on Medicare only. Write or call your nearest Medicare fiscal agent for the guidelines pertinent to your state.

Medicare/Medigap Claim Submission

In most states, Medicare has streamlined the processing of Medicare/Medigap claims. Whether claims are submitted electronically (the preferred method) or manually, Medicare carriers transmit Medigap claims electronically to the Medigap carrier after they have processed them for participating physicians. This is also called a *crossover* claim and the need to file an additional claim, referred to as a secondary claim, is eliminated. Medigap payments go directly to the participating physician, and a Medicare Summary Notice (MSN) is sent to the patient that states "This claim has been referred to your supplemental carrier for any additional benefits."

To assure automatic crossover of the Medicare/Medigap claim, complete Blocks 9 through 9d of the HCFA-1500 claim form and list the PAYERID number of the Medigap plan in Block 9d (Fig. 11–13). The PAYERID for Medigap plans is referred to as the "Other Carrier Name and Address" (OCNA) number,

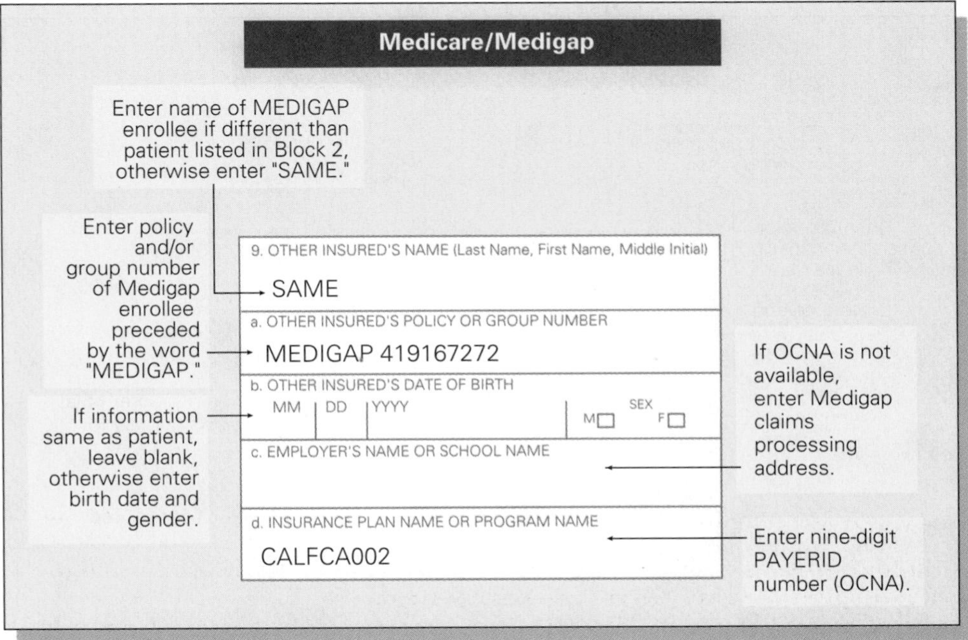

Figure 11–13. Blocks 9 and 9a–d of the HCFA-1500 claim form illustrating placement of information and description of entries for a Medicare patient who has Medigap insurance.

and a list of all OCNA numbers is published in the Medicare newsletter.

If automatic crossover capabilities are not offered in your state, attach the Medicare Remittance Advice to the claim form after Medicare has paid, and submit a claim to the Medigap plan separately.

Par physicians may not collect copayments or deductibles from patients covered by Medigap when processing a Medicare/Medigap claim. Collect copayments after receiving the Medicare/Medigap payment with the remittance advice document. Nonpar physicians may collect copayments and deductibles from patients at the time of service up to their limiting charge, unless state law forbids collection of more than the allowed amount.

Refer to Figure D–8 in Appendix D for a visual example when billing a Medicare/Medigap claim. Study block-by-block instructions for specific directions.

MSP Claim Submission

Before submitting an MSP claim, make sure that Medicare is the secondary payer. Identify the primary payer and follow directions on what should be entered in each block of the HCFA-1500 claim form according to the primary insurance plan guidelines, or follow MSP guidelines. Figure 11–14 illustrates key blocks (Blocks 11, 11a–c) where information is entered on the claim form for an MSP claim. For all MSP claims, the beneficiary's Medicare claim number is entered in Block 1a instead of the primary insurance company. Refer to the MSP template (Fig. D–9) in Appendix D for a visual example of an MSP claim. Refer to block-by-block instructions in Appendix D for specific directions.

After the primary insurance plan pays, attach a copy of the front and back sides of the primary insurance Explanation of Benefits to the claim form and bill Medicare. For MSP claims, Medicare will reimburse the par physician up to the *primary insurer's* allowable fee, as long as the secondary amount is not greater than what Medicare would have paid as a primary payer. In other words, if the physician's charge is $500, and the primary insurer's allowable amount is $500, of which they pay 80% ($400), Medicare will pay the remaining $100 even though the Medicare allowable for this service is only $400.

Deceased Patient Claim Submission

Rules for submitting a claim for a patient who has died will depend on whether the physician participates in the Medicare program and are as follows:

1. *Participating physician*—accepts assignment on the claim form to expedite payment. No signature is needed in Block 12; instead type "Patient died on [*indicate date*]."
2. *Nonparticipating physician*—does not accept assignment. Bill Medicare, and submit the following:
   a. A statement or the HCFA-1500 claim form itemizing all services provided.
   b. A signature in Block 12 of the HCFA-1500 claim form by the estate representative who is responsible for the bill.
   c. Name and address of the responsible party (estate representative).
   d. Provider's statement, signed and dated, refusing to accept assignment.

Nothing can be done about the open balance on the patient's account until the estate is settled. At that time Medicare will pay. If a family member of a deceased Medicare patient requests reimbursement for services for which they have already paid, the person(s) who paid the bill should complete Form HCFA-1660, available from the CMS web site (see Internet, Centers for Medicare and Medicaid Services under Resources at the end of this chapter).

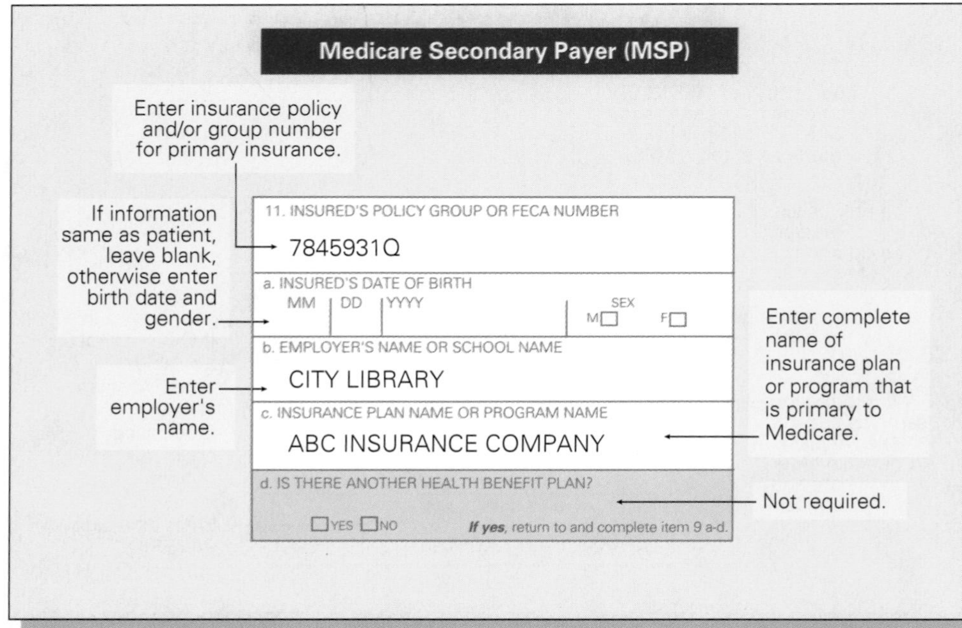

Figure 11–14. Blocks 11 and 11a–d of the HCFA-1500 claim form illustrating placement of information and description of entries for a Medicare patient who has another primary insurance plan; Medicare is secondary payer (MSP).

Physician Substitute Claim Submission

There are many times that special substitute coverage arrangements are made between physicians (e.g., on-call, vacation, unavailable due to another commitment). These arrangements are referred to as either reciprocal for on-call situations, or *locum tenens* for physician's covering and billing for a vacationing doctor. Specific modifiers are used to distinguish these situations and special billing guidelines are stated as follows:

- *Reciprocal arrangement*—When submitting Medicare claims, the *regular* physician must identify the service provided by the substitute doctor by listing the modifier -Q5 after the procedure code.
- *Locum tenens arrangement*—When submitting Medicare claims, the *regular* physician must identify the service provided by the substitute doctor by listing the modifier -Q6 after the procedure code.

When the claim for reciprocal or locum tenens arrangements is submitted by the "absentee" physician, enter the UPIN/NPI of the substitute physician in Block 23 (prior authorization number).

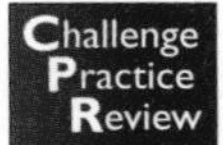

Pause and Practice CPR

REVIEW SESSIONS 11–32 THROUGH 11–34

Directions: *Complete the following questions as a review of information you have just read.*

11–32 Claims for patients who have both Medicare and Medicaid are referred to as ______________________________ claims.

11–33 What is the document called that is sent to the *patient* by the Medicare carrier which explains how the claim was processed? ______________________________

11–34 What additional blocks on the HCFA-1500 form need to be filled in when processing a Medicare/Medigap claim? ______________________________

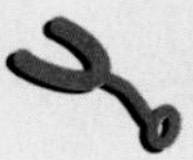

CHECK YOUR HEARTBEAT! Turn to the end of the chapter for answers to these review sessions.

SUMMATION AND PREVIEW

You now know the basics of Medicare, which is a major building block to be placed on the insurance foundation you have constructed. Once you are working with the Medicare program, you can concentrate on specific rules and regulations that apply to the type of practice you are billing for. If you like a challenge and learning new things, you will never be disappointed working in the complicated and ever-chang-

ODE TO MEDICARE

I've written and faxed, called and waited,
My claim remains unpaid.

Oh where, oh where has my claim gone?
Where could it possibly have strayed?

I called again, numerous times,
I think I need a breather.

Help me I ask, I don't know what's wrong,
Relax—we don't either!

It's my lot, to bear this load and I'm trying to get it straight.
But you must know, with Medicare, it's they who hold your fate.

Figure 11–15. "Ode to Medicare." (Permission granted by Sharon LaScala, NCICS.)

ing world of federal regulations. Read the "Ode to Medicare" in Figure 11–15 as a reminder to keep a good sense of humor when dealing with Medicare matters.

Next, you will be learning about two additional federal programs, TRICARE and CHAMPVA. If you have a military base near your area, this information will be of particular interest to you.

GOLDEN RULE

Stay current! Read your Medicare newsletters.

Chapter 11 Review and Practice

Study Session

Directions: *Review the objectives, key terms, and chapter information before completing the following study questions.*

298 11–1 Who administers the Medicare program? Centers for Medicare & Medicaid Services (CMS) formerly known as HCFA

298 11–2 Where do you go to apply for the Medicare program? local Social Security Administration offices

11–3 What is the premium penalty for qualifying individuals who miss the enrollment period for the Medicare program? will be assessed 10% Part B premium penalty for each 12 months they did not participate.

299

11–4 Define the Medicare Part A benefit period. begins the day the patient enters hospital & ends when patient has not been in a bed in a hospital or nursing facility for 60 consecutive Days.

301

Hospital Services 11–5 Basic benefits covered by Medicare Part A are Hospitalization, Nursing Facility, Home Health Care, Hospice Care, Blood

302/303 and by Medicare Part B are Med. Expenses, Clinical Lab Expenses, Home Health Care, Outpatient Hosp. Treatment, Blood, Ambul. Surg Services

Outpatient Services

11–6 Define physician extenders and give three examples.

302-303

11–7 What is a PRO and how does it function? Peer Review Organization Involved in implementing an improvement plan for the quality of care that is given using statistical data.

311

11–8. What three federal legislations are in place to assure that Medicare fraud is kept to a minimum?

311/312

(a) Federal False Claims Amendment Act

(b) Health Insurance Portability & Accountability Act

(c) Civil Monetary Penalties Law

11–9 Medicare pays 100 % for the first procedure, 50 % for the second procedure, and 50 % for the third procedure when multiple procedures are billed at the same operative setting.

314

11–10 The Medicare annual deductible is $100.

315 11–11 What is Medicare's Correct Coding Initiative? to eliminate unbundling or other inappropriate reporting of Current Procedural Terminology (CPT)

11–12 In order to collect from a Medicare patient for a service that Medicare deems "not medically necessary," what procedure must be followed? ______________________________

____

____

____

11–13 In order to collect from a Medicare patient for noncovered services, what procedure must be followed? ______________________________

____

11–14 A nonparticipating physician who does not accept assignment and performs an elective surgery in the amount of $ 500 or more must provide the beneficiary with a written document stating (1) estimated fee,

(2) estimated, and

(3) difference.

11–15 Physicians who participate in the Medicare program must submit claims to the regional

______________________________.

11–16 What time limit should be honored when submitting a Medi-Medi claim?

medicaid time limit for your state

11–17 What is the name for the number of the Medigap plan that is included on the HCFA-1500 claim form and allows the claim to be automatically crossed over?

____

11–18 For participating physicians, what is the rule about collecting deductibles and copayments from patients who have both Medicare and Medigap coverage? ______________________________

____

11–19 What additional blocks on the HCFA-1500 form need to be filled in when processing an MSP claim? 11a – c

11–20 When billing for an on-call physician, use modifier Q5. When billing for a physician who is covering for a doctor on vacation, use modifier Q6.

Billing Break

Time Started
Time Finished
Total Time

Case 11–1 Nina E. Fong

Directions: *Follow these steps to complete the HCFA-1500 insurance claim form for a Medicare case using OCR guidelines.*

1. Copy the HCFA-1500 insurance claim form found in Appendix F (Form 09).

2. Refer to the Patient Information form for Case 11–1 and abstract information to complete the top portion of the HCFA-1500 claim form.

3. Refer to the Medical Record for Case 11–1 to abstract information for the bottom portion of the HCFA-1500 claim form.

4. Copy the Medical Record Coding Worksheet found in Appendix F (Form 12) to use when abstracting information from the chart note.

5. Use the "HCFA-1500 Claim Form Block-by-Block Instructions" for Medicare patients found in Appendix D and the Medicare (no secondary coverage) template (Fig. D–6) for guidance and block help.

6. Use your procedure codebook to determine the correct code number(s) and modifier(s) for each professional service/procedure rendered.

7. Refer to the fee schedule in Appendix B for mock fees.

8. Use your diagnostic codebook to determine the correct diagnoses.

9. Address the claim to the "Medicare Fiscal Agent" and date the claim 07/26/20XX.

10. Copy and prepare the ledger card found in Appendix F (Form 07) for the patient. Complete the ledger by posting each transaction in this case and indicating when you have billed the insurance carrier.

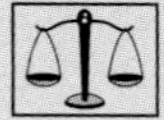

WEIGH YOUR PROGRESS. Turn to the Assignment Score Sheet in Appendix F and enter the information to track your success. Your instructor may ask that you include a Performance Evaluation Checklist, and if so, copy Form 11 found in Appendix F and attach it to your insurance claim.

4567 Broad Avenue
Woodland Hills, XY
12345-0001
Tel (555) 486-9002
Fax (555) 487-8976

REGISTRATION
(PLEASE PRINT)

Account # 0874 Today's Date: 07/14/XX

PATIENT INFORMATION

Name: Fong (Last Name) Nina (First Name) E. (Initial) Soc. Sec. # 352-XX-1410

Address 84506 Pine Mountain Road Home Phone (555) 985-4486

City Meadowridge State XY Zip 12345

Single___ Married___ Separated___ Divorced ✓ Sex M___ F ✓ Birthdate 02/12/1936

Patient Employed by Retired Occupation Factory Worker

Business Address N/A Business Phone___

Spouse's Name N/A Employed by:___ Occupation___

Business Address___ Business Phone___

Reason for Visit Face rash, Chest pain If accident:___ Auto___ Employment___ Other___

By whom were you referred? Friend

In case of emergency, who should be notified? Kuang Fang (Name) Friend (Relation to Patient) Phone (555) 985-5037

PRIMARY INSURANCE

Insured/Subscriber Fong (Last Name) Nina (First Name) E. (Initial)

Relation to Patient Self Birthdate___ Soc. Sec.#___

Address (if different from patient's) Same

City___ State___ Zip___

Insurance Company Ace Insurance Company (Medicare Fiscal Intermediary)

Insurance Address 1414 Crown Street San Bruno, XY 12345

Insurance Identification Number 352-XX-1410A Group #___

ADDITIONAL INSURANCE

Is patient covered by additional insurance? Yes___ No ✓

Subscriber Name___ Relation to Patient___ Birthdate___

Address (if different from patient's)___ Phone___

City___ State___ Zip___

Subscriber Employed by___ Buisness Phone___

Insurance Company___ Soc. Sec. #___

Insurance Address___

Insurance Identification Number___ Group #___

ASSIGNMENT AND RELEASE

I, the undersigned, certify that I (or my dependent) have insurance coverage with Medicare (Name of Insurance Company(ies)) and assign directly to Dr. Perry Cardi insurance benefits, if any, otherwise payable to me for services rendered. I understand that I am financially responsible for all charges whether or not paid by insurance. I hereby consent for the doctor to release all information necessary to secure the payment of benefits. I authorize the use of this signature on all insurance submissions.

Responsible Party Signature: Nina Fong Relationship: self Date: 07/14/xx

ORDER # 58-8426 @BIBBERO SYSTEMS, INC. •PETALUMA, CALIFORNIA• TO REORDER CALL TOLL FREE (800)242-9330

Medical Record

Account number: 0874
Patient's name: Fong, Nina E.
Date of birth: 02/12/36

Date	Progress Notes
	07/26/XX Patient returns to office for yearly examination of systemic lupus erythematosus (SLE) disease. She states she has been relatively symptom free except for occasional bouts of fatigue and mild chest pain; sometimes accompanied with heart palpitations. She has not experienced any episodes of severe chest pain (pericarditis) which she had last year. She states she noticed a small spot of vaginal blood in her underwear last week (bright red) but indicates that it only appeared one time. No other new complaints.
	Performed a D HX/PX with 12-lead ECG and urinalysis (UA - automated with microscopy). Abnormal ECG has not changed since last visit. UA indicates slight bacterial infection (UTI). She has no butterfly rash, as previously noted in visit of July 14 last year. On vaginal exam, inner vaginal labia, as well as vaginal canal appears red and irritated. M/MDM.
	Generally, patient appears in good condition. Prescribed vaginal cream for postmenopausal atrophic vaginitis, sulfa medication for UTI. She is cautioned about sun exposure and activities which induce fatigue. She has a standing order for an erythrocyte sedimentation rate test to be done at first sign of SLE flair. Return to office in 1 week for follow-up (F/U) UA.
	Perry Cardi, MD

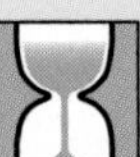

Billing Break

Time Started
Time Finished
Total Time

Case 11–2 Everett G. Edwards

Directions: *Follow these steps to complete the HCFA-1500 insurance claim form for a Medicare/Medigap case using OCR guidelines.*

1. Copy the HCFA-1500 insurance claim form found in Appendix F (Form 09).
2. Refer to the Patient Information form for Case 11–2 and abstract information to complete the top portion of the HCFA-1500 claim form.
3. Refer to the Medical Record for Case 11–2 to abstract information for the bottom portion of the HCFA-1500 claim form.
4. Copy the Medical Record Coding Worksheet found in Appendix F (Form 12) to use when abstracting information from the chart note.
5. Use the "HCFA-1500 Claim Form Block-by-Block Instructions" for Medicare/Medigap patients found in Appendix D and the Medicare/Medigap template (Figure D–8) for guidance and block help.
6. Use your procedure codebook to determine the correct code number(s) and modifier(s) for each professional service/procedure rendered.

7. Use your HCPCS Level II codebook or Appendix C to apply appropriate modifier(s).

8. Follow all Medicare global surgical rules.

9. Refer to the fee schedule in Appendix B for mock fees.

10. Use your diagnostic codebook to determine the correct diagnoses.

11. Address the claim to the "Medicare Fiscal Agent" and date the claim 04/27/20XX.

12. The PAYERID number for United American Insurance is UAIC00295.

13. Copy and prepare the ledger card found in Appendix F (Form 07) for the patient. Complete the ledger by posting each transaction in this case and indicating when you have billed the insurance carrier.

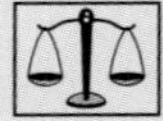

WEIGH YOUR PROGRESS. Turn to the Assignment Score Sheet in Appendix F (Form 10) and record the information to track your success. Your instructor may ask that you include a Performance Evaluation Checklist, and if so, copy Form 11 found in Appendix F and attach it to your insurance claim.

4567 Broad Avenue
Woodland Hills, XY
12345-0001
Tel (555) 486-9002
Fax (555) 487-8976

REGISTRATION
(PLEASE PRINT)

Account # 3989 Today's Date: 03/05/XX

PATIENT INFORMATION

Name Edwards (Last Name) Everett (First Name) G. (Initial) Soc. Sec. # 220-XX-4976

Address 205 Ojai Avenue Home Phone (555) 985-8512

City Meadowridge State XY Zip 12345

Single ✓ (widowed) Married___ Separated___ Divorced___ Sex M ✓ F___ Birthdate 07/02/1935

Patient Employed by Retired Occupation Utility Company Worker

Business Address ___ Business Phone ___

Spouse's Name N/A Employed by: ___ Occupation ___

Business Address ___ Business Phone ___

Reason for Visit Hip pain If accident: ___ Auto ___ Employment ___ Other ___

By whom were you referred? Gerald Practon MD

In case of emergency, who should be notified? Robert Edwards (Name) Son (Relation to Patient) Phone (555) 985-2945

PRIMARY INSURANCE

Insured/Subscriber Edwards (Last Name) Everett (First Name) G. (Initial)

Relation to Patient Self Birthdate 07/02/1935 Soc. Sec.# 220-XX-4976

Address (if different from patient's) Same

City ___ State ___ Zip ___

Insurance Company Ace Insurance Company (Medicare Fiscal Intermediary)

Insurance Address 1414 Crown Street San Bruno, XY 12345

Insurance Identification Number 220-XX-4976A Group # ___

ADDITIONAL INSURANCE

Is patient covered by additional insurance? Yes ✓ No ___

Subscriber Name Edwards, Everett G. Relation to Patient Self Birthdate 07/02/1935

Address (if different from patient's) Same Phone ___

City ___ State ___ Zip ___

Subscriber Employed by Retired Buisness Phone ___

Insurance Company United American Insurance Company Soc. Sec. # 220-XX-4976

Insurance Address 900 Freedom Way Santa Tierra, XY 12345

Insurance Identification Number 220XX4976UA Group # ___

ASSIGNMENT AND RELEASE

I, the undersigned, certify that I (or my dependent) have insurance coverage with Medicare/United American (Name of Insurance Company(ies)) and assign directly to Dr. Raymond Skeleton insurance benefits, if any, otherwise payable to me for services rendered. I understand that I am financially responsible for all charges whether or not paid by insurance. I hereby consent for the doctor to release all information necessary to secure the payment of benefits. I authorize the use of this signature on all insurance submissions.

Everett G Edwards (Responsible Party Signature) self (Relationship) 03/05/xx (Date)

Medical Record

Account number: 3989
Patient's name: Edwards, Everett G.
Date of birth: 07/02/35

Date	Progress Notes

03/05/XX NP referred by Gerald Practon MD for evaluation of painful left hip. Patient has walked approximately 3 miles a day for the past 10 years but has had to shorten walks and discontinue altogether the last 3 months due to increased hip pain.

D HX/PX performed. Patient indicated that he was a gymnast in his youth and jogged and played golf regularly throughout his mid-life. Patient has had occasional joint flares over the last 20 years, especially in neck, knees (bilateral), and hips but has been able to handle the pain with use of over-the-counter antiinflammatory medication. Left hip pain started increasing about 2 years ago.

Range of motion decreased in left hip. Increased pain in buttocks and upper thigh upon movement. Patient walks hesitantly to avoid pain. Left hip x-ray (2-views) reveals osteoarthritic changes with severe erosion of cartilage on head of femur. Recommend total hip replacement for primary osteoarthrosis localized in left hip. Advised patient of risks and benefits from surgical intervention. Patient will consider this option and return as necessary or call if he decides to schedule surgery. In the meantime, advise patient to reduce stress on the joint and rest it adequately. Prescribed antiinflammatory medication on a trial basis for hip pain. Patient advised that this is not a cure; medication is recommended for short term only for temporary relief. MDM/L.

Raymond Skeleton, MD

04/21/XX Patient calls stating that he would like to schedule hip replacement surgery as soon as possible. Dr. Skeleton is advised and indicates patient's chart should be given to Karen, the surgical scheduler to proceed.

Mary Guymer, CMA-C

04/24/XX Preoperative visit (PF HX/PX SF/MDM). Patient appears well and has no complaints of ill health. BP 150/86, T 98.6. Went over risks and complications; signed consents for surgery. Patient to go to College Hospital for preoperative laboratory work; will be admitted the day after tomorrow at 5:30 a.m.

Raymond Skeleton, MD

04/26/XX Admit patient to College Hospital for surgery (C HX/PX M/MDM). Total left hip replacement performed (see operative report).

Raymond Skeleton, MD

04/27/XX HV (EPF HX/PX M/MDM), patient tolerated surgery well and will proceed to regular diet. Ordered physical therapy (PT) to start this afternoon.

Raymond Skeleton, MD

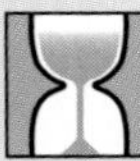

Billing Break

Time Started
Time Finished
Total Time

Case 11–3 Mildred V. Glaves

Directions: *Follow these steps to complete the HCFA-1500 insurance claim form for a Medicare/Medicaid case using OCR guidelines.*

1. Copy the HCFA-1500 insurance claim form found in Appendix F (Form 09).
2. Refer to the Patient Information form for Case 11–3 and abstract information to complete the top portion of the HCFA-1500 claim form.
3. Refer to the Medical Record for Case 11–3 to abstract information for the bottom portion of the HCFA-1500 claim form.
4. Copy the Medical Record Coding Worksheet found in Appendix F (Form 12) to use when abstracting information from the chart note.
5. Use the "HCFA-1500 Claim Form Block-by-Block Instructions" for Medicare/Medicaid patients found in Appendix D and the Medicare/Medicaid template (Fig. D–7) for guidance and block help.
6. Use your procedure codebook to determine the correct code number(s) and modifier(s) for each professional service/procedure rendered.
7. Refer to the fee schedule in Appendix B for mock fees.
8. Use your diagnostic codebook to determine the correct diagnoses.
9. Address the claim to the "Medicare Fiscal Agent" and date the claim 04/11/20XX.
10. Copy and prepare the ledger card found in Appendix F (Form 07) for the patient. Complete the ledger by posting each transaction in this case and indicating when you have billed the insurance carrier.

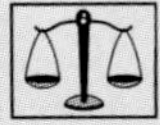

WEIGH YOUR PROGRESS. Turn to the Assignment Score Sheet in Appendix F (Form 10) and record information to track your success. Your instructor may ask that you include a Performance Evaluation Checklist, and if so, copy Form 11 found in Appendix F and attach it to your insurance claim.

4567 Broad Avenue
Woodland Hills, XY
12345-0001
Tel (555) 486-9002
Fax (555) 487-8976

REGISTRATION
(PLEASE PRINT)

Account # 2670 Today's Date: 01/12/XX

PATIENT INFORMATION

Name Glaves (Last Name) Mildred (First Name) V. (Initial) Soc. Sec. # 709-XX-3460

Address 683 Karin Court Home Phone (555) 985-1266

City Meadowridge State XY Zip 12345

Single ✓ (widowed) Married___ Separated___ Divorced___ Sex M___ F ✓ Birthdate 05/20/1934

Patient Employed by N/A Occupation ___

Business Address ___ Business Phone ___

Spouse's Name Jerry - Deceased Employed by: ___ Occupation ___

Business Address ___ Business Phone ___

Reason for Visit Relocating with new doctor If accident: ___ Auto___ Employment___ Other___

By whom were you referred? Daughter

In case of emergency, who should be notified? Paige Croix (Name) Daughter (Relation to Patient) Phone (555) 985-6700

PRIMARY INSURANCE

Insured/Subscriber Glaves (Last Name) Jerry (First Name) T. (Initial)

Relation to Patient Husband Birthdate 12/29/1930 Soc. Sec.# 159-XX-3407

Address (if different from patient's) ___

City ___ State ___ Zip ___

Insurance Company Ace Insurance Company (Medicare Fiscal Intermediary)

Insurance Address 1414 Crown Street San Bruno, XY 12345

Insurance Identification Number 159-XX-3407B Group # ___

ADDITIONAL INSURANCE

Is patient covered by additional insurance? Yes ✓ No ___

Subscriber Name Glaves, Mildred Relation to Patient Same Birthdate 05/20/1934

Address (if different from patient's) Same Phone ___

City ___ State ___ Zip ___

Subscriber Employed by N/A Buisness Phone ___

Insurance Company Medicaid Soc. Sec. # ___

Insurance Address 8100 Main Street Springville, XY 12345

Insurance Identification Number 01489625901129 Group # ___

ASSIGNMENT AND RELEASE

I, the undersigned, certify that I (or my dependent) have insurance coverage with Medicare/Medicaid (Name of Insurance Company(ies)) and assign directly to Dr. Gerald Practon insurance benefits, if any, otherwise payable to me for services rendered. I understand that I am financially responsible for all charges whether or not paid by insurance. I hereby consent for the doctor to release all information necessary to secure the payment of benefits. I authorize the use of this signature on all insurance submissions.

Mildred V Glaves — Responsible Party Signature Self — Relationship 01/12/xx — Date

ORDER # 58-8426 @BIBBERO SYSTEMS, INC. •PETALUMA, CALIFORNIA• TO REORDER CALL TOLL FREE (800)242-9330

Medical Record

Account number: 2670
Patient's name: Glaves, Mildred V.
Date of birth: 05/20/34

Date	Progress Notes
	04/08/XX Received a call from Dr. Cliff Rising (UPIN/NPI 34560202XX), the Emergency Room physician at College Hospital stating my patient, Mrs. Glaves arrived with severe abdominal pains localized in left lower quadrant (LLQ). She has noticed blood in her feces (melena) for the last month, on and off. No sign of blood on rectal exam. Hard, distended abdomen, BP 180/96, temp. 99.6. After examination and a complete general health panel showing leukocytosis and low hemoglobin (see lab report), Dr. Rising recommends admitting her for further tests to rule out colon cancer. Patient is in acute distress and has not responded to pain medication.
	I admitted the patient to room #503 of College Hospital. Performed a C HX/PX. Ordered upper gastrointestinal studies, air-contrast barium enema, and abdominal ultrasound. Started patient on antihypertensive medication for essential hypertension MDM/M. Gerald Practon, MD
	04/09/XX HV (7:00 a.m.) patient still in distress, nauseated this a.m., awaiting test results. BP 180/90 on BP medication, temp. 99.9. Will see patient again at lunch hour. 1:00 p.m.–no abnormalities seen in Upper G.I. or abdominal ultrasound. Barium enema shows several locations of diverticula, one especially large and inflamed in distal wall of sigmoid colon. No perforation seen. Ordered special diet. Patient to start on anticholinergic drugs for diverticulitis. EPF interval HX/PX with M/MDM. Gerald Practon, MD
	04/10/XX HV 7:00 a.m.–patient less nauseated this a.m. but still having some pain. BP 178/88. temp. 99.8. If she continues to improve will discharge her tomorrow. PF interval HX/PX SF/MDM. Gerald Practon, MD
	04/11/XX HV 7:00 a.m.–patient feeling much better. Abdomen not distended, BP 160/86, temp 98.9. Patient discharged home (discharge management 30 min.) Return to office in 1 week. Gerald Practon, MD

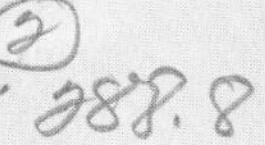

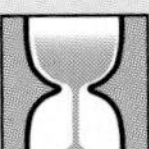

Billing Break

Time Started
Time Finished
Total Time

Case 11–4 Delbert K. Fillmore

Directions: *Follow these steps to complete the HCFA-1500 insurance claim form for a Medicare Secondary Payer case using OCR guidelines.*

1. Copy the HCFA-1500 insurance claim form found in Appendix F (Form 09).

2. Refer to the Patient Information form for Case 11–4 and abstract information to complete the top portion of the HCFA-1500 claim form.

3. Refer to the Medical Record for Case 11–4 to abstract information for the bottom portion of the HCFA-1500 claim form.

4. Copy the Medical Record Coding Worksheet found in Appendix F (Form 12) to use when abstracting information from the chart note.

5. Use the "HCFA-1500 Claim Form Block-by-Block Instructions" for Medicare Secondary Payer (MSP) patients found in Appendix D and the MSP template (Fig. D–9) for guidance and block help.

6. Use your procedure codebook to determine the correct code number(s) and modifier(s) for each professional service/procedure rendered.

7. Use your HCPCS Level II codebook or Appendix C to apply HCPCS Level II modifiers when applicable.

8. Refer to the fee schedule in Appendix B for mock fees (use private fees when billing MSP claims).

9. Use your diagnostic codebook to determine the correct diagnoses.

10. Address the claim to the other insurance carrier and date the claim 02/24/20XX.

11. Copy and prepare the ledger card found in Appendix F (Form 07) for the patient. Complete the ledger by posting each transaction in this case and indicating when you have billed the insurance carrier.

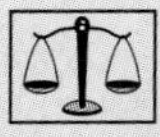

WEIGH YOUR PROGRESS. Turn to the Assignment Score Sheet in Appendix F and record the information to track your success. Your instructor may ask that you include a Performance Evaluation Checklist, and if so, copy Form 11 found in Appendix F and attach it to your insurance claim.

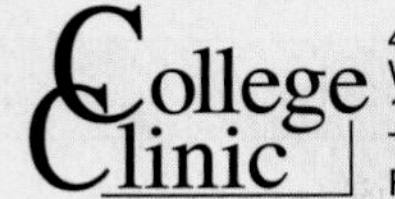

4567 Broad Avenue
Woodland Hills, XY
12345-0001
Tel (555) 486-9002
Fax (555) 487-8976

REGISTRATION
(PLEASE PRINT)

Account # 3012 Today's Date: 02/10/XX

PATIENT INFORMATION

Name Fillmore (Last Name) Delbert (First Name) K. (Initial) Soc. Sec. # 712-XX-3445

Address 182 Moonglow Street Home Phone (555) 985-3632

City Meadowridge State XY Zip 12345

Single___ Married ✓ Separated___ Divorced___ Sex M ✓ F___ Birthdate 08/29/1938

Patient Employed by Sandstone, Inc. Occupation Engineer

Business Address 5924 Shell Drive, Meadowridge, XY Business Phone (555) 985-7835

Spouse's Name Eleanor Employed by: N/A Occupation ______

Business Address ______ Business Phone ______

Reason for Visit Skin Examination If accident:___ Auto___ Employment___ Other___

By whom were you referred? Dr. Clarence Cutler

In case of emergency, who should be notified? Eleanor Fillmore (Name) Wife (Relation to Patient) Phone (555) 985-3632

PRIMARY INSURANCE

Insured/Subscriber Fillmore (Last Name) Delbert (First Name) K. (Initial)

Relation to Patient Self Birthdate 08/29/1938 Soc. Sec.# 712-XX-3445

Address (if different from patient's) Same

City ______ State ______ Zip ______

Insurance Company Atlantic Insurance Company

Insurance Address PO Box 1200 Manhatten, XY 12345

Insurance Identification Number 4007986 Group # Sand

ADDITIONAL INSURANCE

Is patient covered by additional insurance? Yes ✓ No ___

Subscriber Name Fillmore, Delbert Relation to Patient Self Birthdate 08/29/1938

Address (if different from patient's) Same Phone ______

City ______ State ______ Zip ______

Subscriber Employed by See above Buisness Phone ______

Insurance Company Ace Insurance Company (Medicare F.I.) Soc. Sec. # ______

Insurance Address 1414 Crown Street San Bruno, XY 12345

Insurance Identification Number 712-XX-3445A Group # ______

ASSIGNMENT AND RELEASE

I, the undersigned, certify that I (or my dependent) have insurance coverage with Atlantic/Medicare (Name of Insurance Company(ies)) and assign directly to Dr. Vera Curtis insurance benefits, if any, otherwise payable to me for services rendered. I understand that I am financially responsible for all charges whether or not paid by insurance. I hereby consent for the doctor to release all information necessary to secure the payment of benefits. I authorize the use of this signature on all insurance submissions.

Delbert K Fillmore (Responsible Party Signature) Self (Relationship) 02/10/XX (Date)

ORDER # 58-8426 ©BIBBERO SYSTEMS, INC. •PETALUMA, CALIFORNIA• TO REORDER CALL TOLL FREE (800)242-9330

Medical Record

Account number: 3012
Patient's name: Fillmore, Delbert K.
Date of birth: 08/29/1938

Date	Progress Notes
	02/10/XX NP referred by Dr. Clarence Cutler for full body skin examination and evaluation of multiple lesions. Patient had wide excision to remove Stage 1 melanoma from right calf 2 months ago. No other history of skin disease. Performed a C HX/PX which reveals actinic keratosis on face (2 lesions) and trunk (2 lesions–all in upper left back region). Recommend laser destruction of all of these premalignant lesions. Patient also has other multiple benign lesions on back and abdomen which I am not recommending to remove at this time. Schedule in-office surgery when convenient. MDM/M. Vera Cutis, MD
	02/24/XX Patient presents for laser removal of premalignant skin lesions (actinic keratosis). Surgical consents are signed and lesions are removed as follows: 0.4 cm lesion on mid-forehead, 0.2 cm lesion on right nostril, and 2 lesions on upper left back (0.6 cm and 0.2 cm). Patient questions 3 warts on right anterior wrist. They are identified as vulgaris (flat) warts and are removed with chemical cauterization. All specimens sent to outside laboratory. Patient will be called with pathology report. Return in 6 months for recheck. Vera Cutis, MD

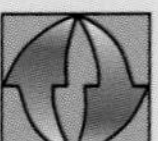

Exercise Exchange

11–1 Calculate Medicare Fees.

Directions

1. Refer to the section on Payment Fundamentals and Figures 11–4 and 11–8 for guidance.
2. Read the following scenarios, code the services/procedures, and calculate fees based on the rules for Medicare reimbursement.
3. Apply the appropriate Medicare fees found in Appendix B.
4. All physicians in College Clinic are participating physicians and accept assignment. All other physicians are nonparticipating physicians and do not accept assignment.

CASE #1

Tracy Olivena returns to see Dr. Practon for an EPF HX/PX with M/MDM for which Dr. Practon charges $60. Her Medicare deductible has been met.

a. What is the Medicare allowed amount? $ 56.31
b. How much will Medicare pay? $ 45.05 (56.31 x 80%)

c. What is the patient's responsibility? $ 11.26 (56.31 x 20 %)

d. What is the courtesy adjustment? $ 3.69 (61.51 − 56.31)

CASE #2

Roxanne Barney is a new patient. Dr. Practon performs a C HX/PX with H/MDM and charges $145. Her Medicare deductible has not been met. 99203

a. What is the Medicare allowed amount? $ 121.08

b. How much will Medicare pay? $ 16.86 (21.08 x 80%)

c. What is the patient's responsibility? $ 104.22 (100. + (21.08 x 20%))

d. What is the courtesy adjustment? $ 23.92 (145 − 121.08)

CASE #3

(Non Par physician)

Rex Yardley sees Dr. Joe Gentle for an office consultation (C HX/PX M/MDM) and the charge is $145.05. His Medicare deductible has been met.

a. What is the Medicare limiting charge? $ 145.05

b. What is the Medicare allowed amount? $ 126.13

c. How much will Medicare pay? $ 100.90 (126.13 x 80%)

d. What is the patient's responsibility? $ 44.15 (126.13 x 20%) + (145.05 − 126.13) (25.23 + 18.92)

e. What is the courtesy adjustment? $ ∅

11–2 **Complete an Advance Beneficiary Notice.**

Directions

1. Read the following scenario.
2. Complete the top portion of the Medicare Advance Beneficiary Notice for Mrs. Blair using the information provided.

Scenario: Mrs. Lucille Blair presents in Dr. Practon's office and insists on having an electrocardiogram. She had a complete physical examination last week, her ECG was normal, and Dr. Practon diagnosed her with anxiety-hysteria. Dr. Practon advises the clinical medical assistant to perform another 12-lead ECG and to "process the necessary paperwork so that we can bill the patient if Medicare does not pay."

College Clinic

4567 Broad Avenue
Woodland Hills, XY
12345-0001
Tel (555) 486-9002
Fax (555) 487-8976

MEDICARE ADVANCE BENEFICIARY NOTICE

Medicare will only pay for covered items and services when Medicare rules are met. The fact that Medicare may not pay for a particular item or service does not mean that you should not receive it. There may be a good reason your doctor is recommending it. In your case, Medicare may deny payment for the following item, test, or service.

Item/Test/Service: **Approximate Cost:**

1. ______________________ $ ____________
2. ______________________ $ ____________

Reason Claim Will Be Denied:

☐ Not payable for listed diagnosis: ____________
☐ Routine items, services, and laboratory work usually denied.
☐ Test or service does not have FDA approval (payment approved for research or investigative use only.)
☐ Exceeds time limitation on number of times this item/test/service can be ordered/performed.
☐ Not a Medicare benefit.
☐ Other: ____________

11–3 Code Using HCPCS Level II.

Directions

1. Use an HCPCS Level II codebook or refer to the partial listing of HCPCS codes in Appendix C of this worktext.
2. Locate the service, item, or procedure in the alphabetical index.
3. Insert the correct code.

Service/Item/Procedure	Code
a. rib belt, elastic	____________
b. blood testing supplies	____________
c. hallux valgus dynamic splint	____________
d. crutches, underarm, wood, pair	____________
e. swabs, Betadine or iodine	____________
f. alcohol wipes	____________
g. toilet seat, raised	____________
h. walker, wheeled, without seat	____________
i. Dextrostix	____________
j. Garamycin, injection	____________

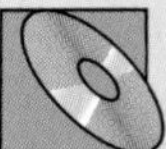

Computer Session—Cases 8, 9, and 10

Directions: *Insert the CD-ROM into the computer, locate and complete: Case 8—Medicare case, Case 9—Medicare/Medigap case, and Case 10—Medicare/Medicaid case.*

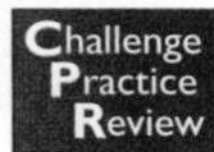

CPR Session: Answers

REVIEW SESSIONS 11–1 AND 11–2

11–1 (a) People age 65 or older who are retired or eligible for Social Security.
(b) People age 65 or older who are retired from the railroad or civil service.
(c) Blind individuals.
(d) Certain disabled individuals who are eligible for Social Security disability benefits.
(e) Children/adults with chronic renal disease (dialysis) or end-stage renal disease (transplant).
(f) Kidney donors (transplant expenses).

11–2 The patient's status, or how he or she became eligible for benefits.

CHALLENGE SESSIONS 11–3 THROUGH 11–5

11–3 $812 (deductible for Part A—first 60 days)
11–4 100% of all medically necessary charges
11–5 $130.12 ($250.62 − $100 deductible) = (150.62 × 20%) = ($30.12 + $100)

REVIEW SESSIONS 11–6 THROUGH 11–10

11–6 (c) HMO risk plan
11–7 (a) Provider Sponsored Organization
11–8 (d) HMO cost plan
11–9 (b) Medicare Medical Savings Account
11–10 (e) Medicare Managed Care

REVIEW SESSIONS 11–11 THROUGH 11–14

11–11 Medi-Medi (Medicare/Medicaid) patients
11–12 yes, no
11–13 Medicare Secondary Payer (MSP)
11–14 When the liability insurance company pays an amount less than the Medicare-allowed amount, or if the liability company does not pay the claim promptly for Medicare-covered benefits.

CHALLENGE SESSIONS 11–15 AND 11–16

11–15 (a) employer group coverage
(b) Tax Equity and Fiscal Responsibility Act (TEFRA) of 1982 and Consolidated Omnibus Budget Reconciliation Act (COBRA) of 1985

11–16 (a) employer group coverage
(b) Omnibus Budget Reconciliation Act (OBRA) of 1986

REVIEW SESSIONS 11–17 THROUGH 11–20

11–17 $2,000 (each line of service)
11–18 yes
11–19 to prevent referral of patients to facilities (e.g., laboratory, physical therapy practice, medical supply company) that a physician has a financial interest in, thereby receiving financial gain
11–20 Clinical Laboratory Improvement Amendment (CLIA)

REVIEW SESSIONS 11–21 THROUGH 11–23

11–21 (b)
11–22 (c)
11–23 (a)

PRACTICE SESSIONS 11–24 AND 11–25

11–24 (a) $96.86 (121.08 × .80)
(b) $24.22 (121.08 × .20)
(c) none

11–25 (a) $92.02 (115.03 × .80)
(b) $40.36 (115.03 × .20) + (132.38 − 115.03) = (23.01 + 17.35)
(c) none

REVIEW SESSION 11–26

11–26 (a) Orthotic Procedures—L
(b) Durable Medical Equipment—E
(c) Chemotherapy Drugs—J
(d) Vision Services—V
(e) Medical and Surgical Supplies—A

REVIEW SESSIONS 11–27 THROUGH 11–31

11–27 3664021CC (College Clinic group identification number)
11–28 regional DME carrier
11–29 SOF
11–30 type or print the physician's name and sign as if you are the physician
11–31 12/31/2004

REVIEW SESSIONS 11–32 THROUGH 11–34

11–32 crossover
11–33 Medicare Summary Notice
11–34 Blocks 9, 9a–d

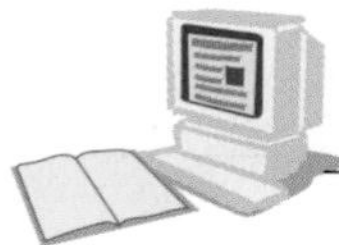

Resources

The insurance billing specialist should periodically attend Medicare training workshops. This is critical in order to keep up-to-date and gain a better understanding of federal claim requirements and specific regional rules. As you read your Medicare newsletters, mark important sections, copy and distribute information to office staff as needed, and cross-reference information for future reference. File all newsletters in a loose-leaf binder. Medicare manuals should be kept up-to-date and accessible. A loose-leaf format allows for easy insertion of updates, whether it be from newsletters or downloads from the computer system. For further information and booklets, pamphlets, and the annual *Medicare and You* handbook for beneficiaries, contact your nearest Social Security office.

Internet

Centers for Medicare and Medicaid Services (24-hour hotline 7 days a week [800] 633-4227), provide up-to-the-minute regulation changes, explanation of regulations, news releases, and more. To locate the HCFA-1660 form, go to the search feature and insert HCFA-1660, then click the search button.

Web site: www.hcfa.gov
Web site: www.cms.gov

- CLIA waived tests
  Web site: www.hcfa.gov key term "CLIA."
- Federal Register
  Web site: www.nara.gov/fedreg
- Medicare Publications
  Web site: www.medicare.gov
- Social Security Online
  Web site: www.ssa.gov

Reference Books

St. Anthony's Medicare Correct Coding and Payment Manual for Procedures and Services (includes unbundling information). St. Anthony/Ingenix Publishing Group, P.O. Box 96561, Washington, DC 20044-4212, (800) 632-0123

Education and Training

Medicare established a free Internet training program that details filing Medicare claims correctly. This web site will educate the staff who work in physician offices. The program also covers various other topics vital to the management of a doctor's office. Available courses are designed for both the beginner and advanced physician office worker. Once downloaded from the Medicare web site, they can be stored on your computer to use as a training module for staff members. The courses are 45 to 60 minutes in length and begin and end with a test so that the knowledge levels of participants can be checked. A certificate can be printed by the participant. Also, free computer training modules and satellite broadcasts are offered by CMS.

Web site: www.medicaretraining.com

NOTES

Objectives

After reading this chapter and completing the exercise sessions, you should be able to:

Learning Objectives:

- ✔ State who is eligible for TRICARE and CHAMPVA.
- ✔ Define pertinent TRICARE and CHAMPVA terminology and abbreviations.
- ✔ Explain how to access the Defense Enrollment Eligibility Reporting System (DEERS).
- ✔ Determine circumstances when a nonavailability statement is required.
- ✔ Describe a "catchment" area.
- ✔ Enumerate the difference between TRICARE Standard, Extra, and Prime programs.
- ✔ Give examples of other TRICARE programs and the beneficiaries they cover.
- ✔ List criteria for a TRICARE-certified provider, authorized provider, network provider, and non-network provider.
- ✔ Explain the referral and preauthorization process and name the healthcare professionals and representatives involved.

Performance Objectives:

- ✔ Demonstrate how to process claims for individuals who are covered under TRICARE.
- ✔ Complete claims for CHAMPVA patients.

Key Terms

active duty service member (ADSM)
authorized provider
beneficiary
catastrophic cap
catchment area
CHAMPVA
cooperative care
cost-share
Defense Enrollment Eligibility Reporting System (DEERS)
Health Benefits Advisor (HBA)
Health Care Finder (HCF)
military retiree (service retiree)
military treatment facilities (MTFs)
nonavailability statement (NAS)
other health insurance (OHI)
partnership program
point-of-service (POS) option
primary care manager (PCM)
service benefit program
sponsor
total, permanent, service-connected disabilities
TRICARE Extra
TRICARE For Life (TFL)
TRICARE Prime
TRICARE Service Center (TSC)
TRICARE Standard
veteran

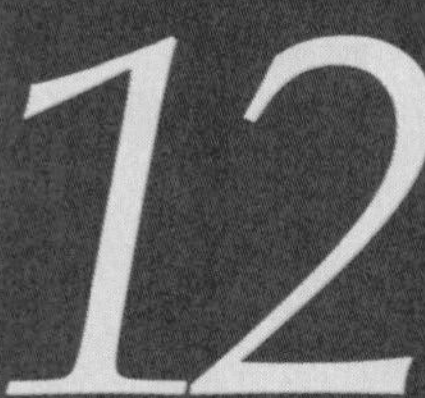

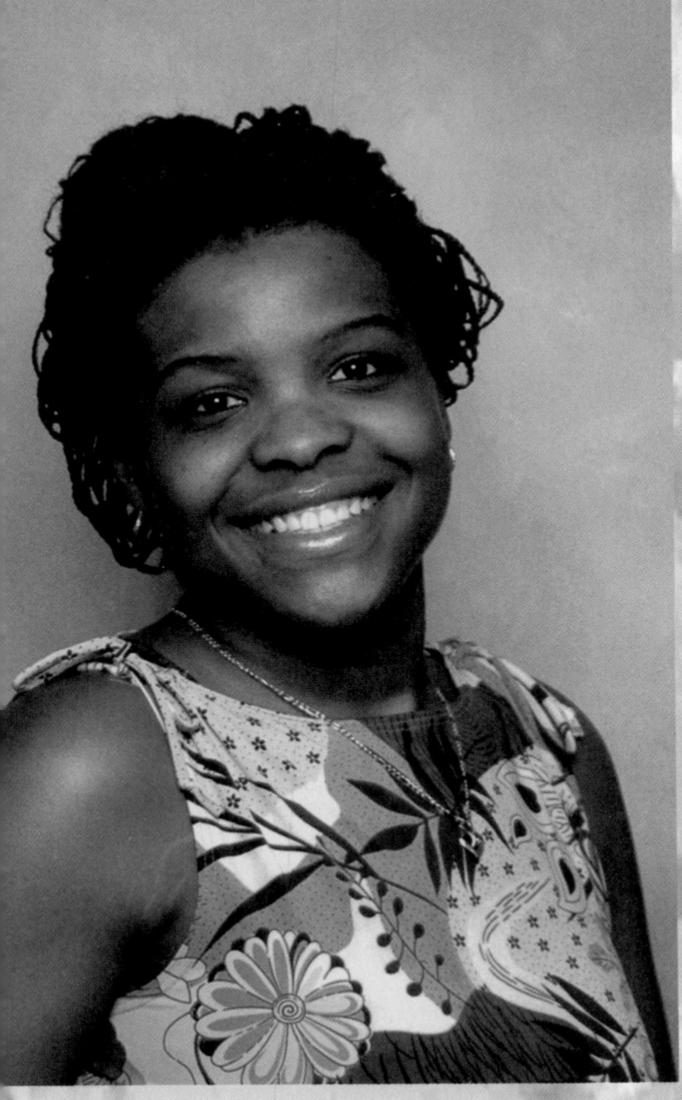

I am a multiskilled health practitioner working as a medical insurance billing specialist. My background in customer service and data entry really helped me secure this job. I work for a billing company that services over 25 hospitals and doctors' offices.

My job duties include inputting patient demographics, reviewing and coding physician's radiology reports, entering codes and charges for services, and processing and reviewing claims. Upon receipt of payment or denial, I review explanation of benefits data, process payments, and appeal denials.

One of the things I like best about my job is the diversity in my work. Nothing is the same from one day to the next. When questions arise, coworkers share their opinions, and this allows me to look at the situation from a different perspective. I feel that hearing other opinions and problem-solving techniques has allowed me to grow professionally.

Jimetria Smith
Insurance Billing Specialist
Radiology—Billing Service

The TRICARE and CHAMPVA Programs

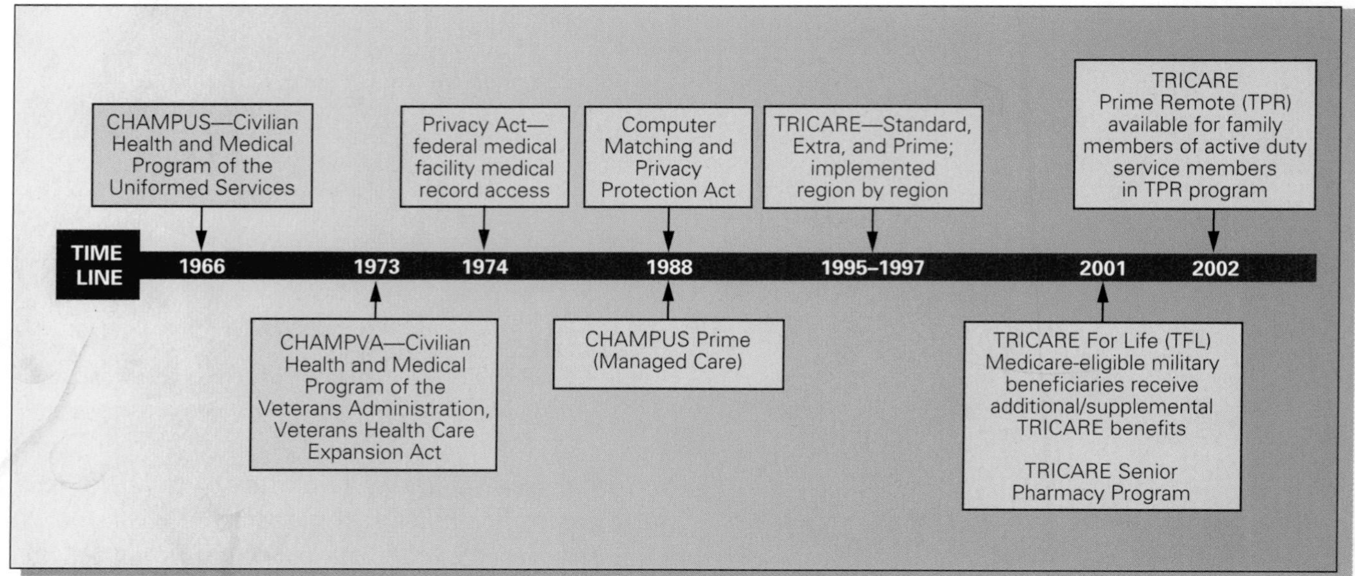

UNDERSTANDING TRICARE PROGRAMS

TRICARE is a comprehensive health benefits program offering three (TRI) types of plans for dependents of men and women in the Uniformed Services (military). Under the basic TRICARE program, individuals have the following three options:

- TRICARE Standard—fee-for-service cost-sharing plan.
- TRICARE Extra—preferred provider organization plan.
- TRICARE Prime—health maintenance organization plan with a point-of-service option.

TRICARE evolved from the original benefit plan, CHAMPUS, whose name still appears on the HCFA-1500 insurance claim form. CHAMPUS is an acronym for Civilian Health and Medical Program of the Uniformed Services. It was created because individuals in the military were finding it increasingly more difficult to pay for medical expenses incurred by their families. CHAMPUS branched into the three-choice program (TRICARE) as a means of controlling escalating medical costs and standardizing benefits for recipients.

Eligibility

An individual who qualifies for TRICARE is known as a **beneficiary,** and the **active duty service member (ADSM)** is called the **sponsor.** A person who is retired from a career in the armed forces, after serving approximately 20 years or more, is known as a **military retiree** or **service retiree.** Retirees receive retirement pay and can remain in a TRICARE health benefit program for life. In the event that an active duty military person served one term (from 2 to 6 years), then chose to leave the armed services, no further family benefits are provided. Those who are entitled to medical benefits under TRICARE are:

- Spouse and unmarried children up to age 21 (or 23 if full-time student) of Uniformed Service members who are in (1) active duty, (2) the United States Coast Guard, (3) Public Health Service, or (4) the National Oceanic and Atmospheric Administration.
- Eligible children over age 21 with disabilities.
- Uniform Service retirees and their eligible family members.
- Unremarried spouses and unmarried children of deceased, active, or retired service members.
- Former spouses of Uniformed Service personnel who meet certain length-of-marriage criteria and other requirements.
- Physically or emotionally abused spouses, former spouses, or dependent children of Uniformed Service personnel who were found guilty and discharged for the offense.
- Spouses and children of North Atlantic Treaty Organization (NATO) nation representatives (outpatient services only).
- Disabled beneficiaries younger than 65 years of age who have Medicare Parts A and B.

Those NOT eligible for TRICARE are:

- Medicare-eligible beneficiaries age 65 and over *not* enrolled in Medicare Part B.
- CHAMPVA beneficiaries.
- Uniformed Service member parents or parents-in-law (unless eligible under Supplemental Health Care Program).
- Secretarial designees who are entitled to care at a military treatment facility (MTF), or from a civilian provider.

Defense Enrollment Eligibility Reporting System

It is the responsibility of the sponsor to ensure that all TRICARE-eligible persons enroll in the **Defense Enrollment Eligibility Reporting System (DEERS)** computerized database. The sponsor's Social Security number (SSN) is used to access DEERS and file claims. TRICARE claims processors check DEERS before processing claims to verify beneficiary eligibility.

Providers can verify eligibility of TRICARE beneficiaries by using the *Voice Response Unit (VRU)* system. This system is manned 24 hours a day. Call the 800 number and follow the commands and it will connect you to DEERS and provide the requested eligibility information.

Nonavailability Statement

Active duty service personnel and their TRICARE-eligible dependents receive many of their healthcare services from **military treatment facilities (MTFs).** An MTF is a Uniformed Services hospital, sometimes referred to as a military hospital. If the military hospital is not able to provide the care needed by the beneficiary, a **nonavailability statement (NAS)** is required for TRICARE Standard and Extra beneficiaries in the following situations:

- Nonemergency inpatient services.
- Maternity care (valid from entry into prenatal program until 42 days postpartum).
- Transfer of beneficiary to another hospital.
- Beneficiaries referred to a civilian provider due to care requirements that exceed the capability of a Specialized Treatment Services (STS) facility at which their care began.

The NAS certification allows treatment by a civilian provider and is valid for 30 days. If this certification is not obtained, TRICARE may not pay.

The **catchment area** is defined by ZIP codes and is based on an area of approximately 40 miles in radius surrounding each United States MTF. Individuals whose home address ZIP code falls outside the local military hospital's service area do not need an NAS before they seek civilian healthcare under TRICARE.

An NAS is *not needed* for an outpatient procedure. An NAS is not needed for inpatient care in the following situations:

- Beneficiaries residing outside the MTF catchment area
- Life-threatening emergencies
- Partial Hospitalization Programs (PHPs)
- Psychiatric emergencies
- TRICARE Prime beneficiaries using network providers or the point-of-service option
- TRICARE Prime Remote (TPR) enrollees
- Residential Treatment Centers (RTCs), Skilled Nursing Facilities (SNFs), and Substance Use and Disorder Rehabilitation Facilities (SUDRFs)
- Student infirmaries
- Those who have **other health insurance (OHI)**

Automated NAS System

The Uniformed Service medical facility enters the NAS electronically into the DEERS computer files, thereby eliminating the need to send a paper copy of the NAS with the TRICARE or CHAMPVA insurance claim. Electronically filed statements are the only ones accepted for processing claims.

Fiscal Year

The TRICARE fiscal year begins October 1 and ends September 30. It is different from most programs so office staff need to be alert to collect deductibles during the fall months.

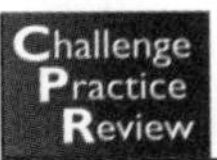

Pause and Practice CPR

REVIEW SESSIONS 12–1 THROUGH 12–5

Directions: *Complete the following questions as a review of information you have just read.*

12–1 TRICARE is a comprehensive health benefit program which offers how many types of plans?

____

12–2 The active duty service member (ADSM) is referred to as the ____________________ of the health benefit program.

12–3 The ADSM's dependent is referred to as the ____________________ of the health benefit program.

12–4 What is the acronym for the computerized database that is used to verify eligibility of TRICARE beneficiaries? ____________________

12–5 What is an MTF? ____

____

CHECK YOUR HEARTBEAT! Turn to the end of the chapter for answers to these review sessions.

TRICARE STANDARD

The **TRICARE Standard** program is available to all TRICARE beneficiaries who seek care from MTFs or civilian TRICARE-certified providers (Fig. 12–1). Patients are not limited to using contracted network providers.

Enrollment

Those entitled to medical benefits under TRICARE are automatically enrolled in the TRICARE Standard program.

Identification Card

Dependents and survivors (age 10 years or older) of active duty personnel and retirees carry a Uniformed Services (military) identification card (Fig. 12–2). Dependents younger than 10 years of age are not normally issued military identification cards so information for their claims should be obtained from either parent's card. Essential information must be abstracted from the front and back of the card, so photocopy both sides and retain it in the patient's medical record.

The sponsor's rank, pay grade, and status listed on the front of the card help determine the copayment, cost-share, and deductible amounts for the beneficiary. The status is either active or retired. The rank and pay grade are grouped as follows:

- Enlisted rank E-1 to E-4
- Enlisted rank E-5 to E-9
- Officer rank 0-1 to 0-10
- Warrant Officer rank W-1 to W-4

Refer to the back of the card under "medical" to ensure that the card authorizes civilian medical benefits. An expiration date is listed for dependents of ADSMs and retirees (e.g., 2001OCT09).

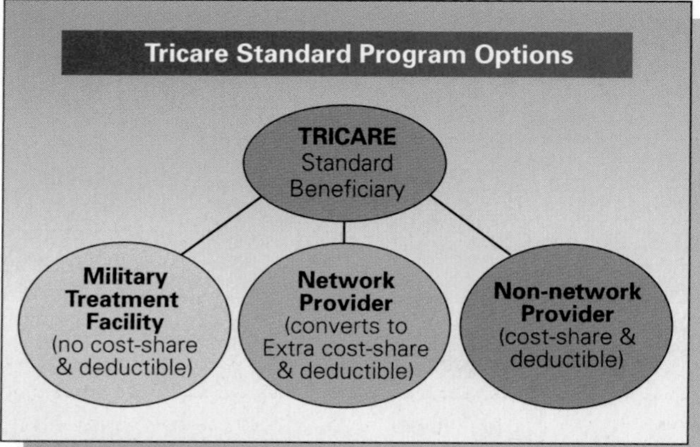

Figure 12–1. Illustration showing where a TRICARE Standard Program patient seeks care.

Benefits

In the TRICARE Standard program, beneficiaries may receive a wide range of civilian healthcare services, with a significant portion of the cost paid by the federal government. Benefits include medical and psychological services or supplies that are generally accepted by qualified professionals to be reasonable and adequate (*medically or psychologically necessary*) for the diagnosis and treatment of illness, injury, pregnancy, and mental disorders, or that are reasonable and adequate for well-baby care. Beneficiaries may also receive urgent care and emergency care services. To see the overall picture of TRICARE benefits, which includes cost sharing, deductibles, and copayments, read carefully through Figure 12–3 for outpatient benefits, and Figure 12–4 for inpatient benefits.

Noncovered Benefits

A list of services and procedures that are excluded or limited in the TRICARE program are published in the *TRICARE Handbook* which is issued to the beneficiary. In order for the provider to bill for noncovered services, TRICARE beneficiaries must be informed in advance and in writing of services and procedures that are not covered under TRICARE. A waiver of liability agreement, known in the TRICARE program as a "Request For Non-Covered Services Form" (Fig. 12–5), must be filled out and signed by the beneficiary. If the waiver of liability form is not obtained and the service is not authorized by the Health Care Finder (HCF), the service is considered unauthorized and the provider is expected to accept full financial liability. Keep a copy of the signed document with the patient's medical record. If there is a question about covered benefits, call the TRICARE 800 telephone number.

Treatment Facilities

Ordinarily, TRICARE Standard patients seek care from a military hospital near their home. If the MTF that is managing the patient cannot provide a particular service or medical supply, the military physician may refer the patient to a civilian source. When these services or supplies are cost-shared by TRICARE Standard, this is referred to as **cooperative care.**

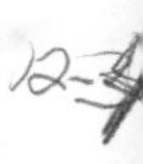

Another option that lets TRICARE Standard–eligible persons receive inpatient or outpatient treatment from civilian providers in a military hospital, or from uniformed providers in a civilian facility, is called a **partnership program.** Whether a partnership program is instituted at a particular military hospital depends on the facility's commander, who makes the decision based on economics.

In addition, there are times when there is no service hospital in the area and a TRICARE Standard beneficiary may seek care through a private physician's office or hospital. Delivery of care through the private physician will be emphasized in this chapter.

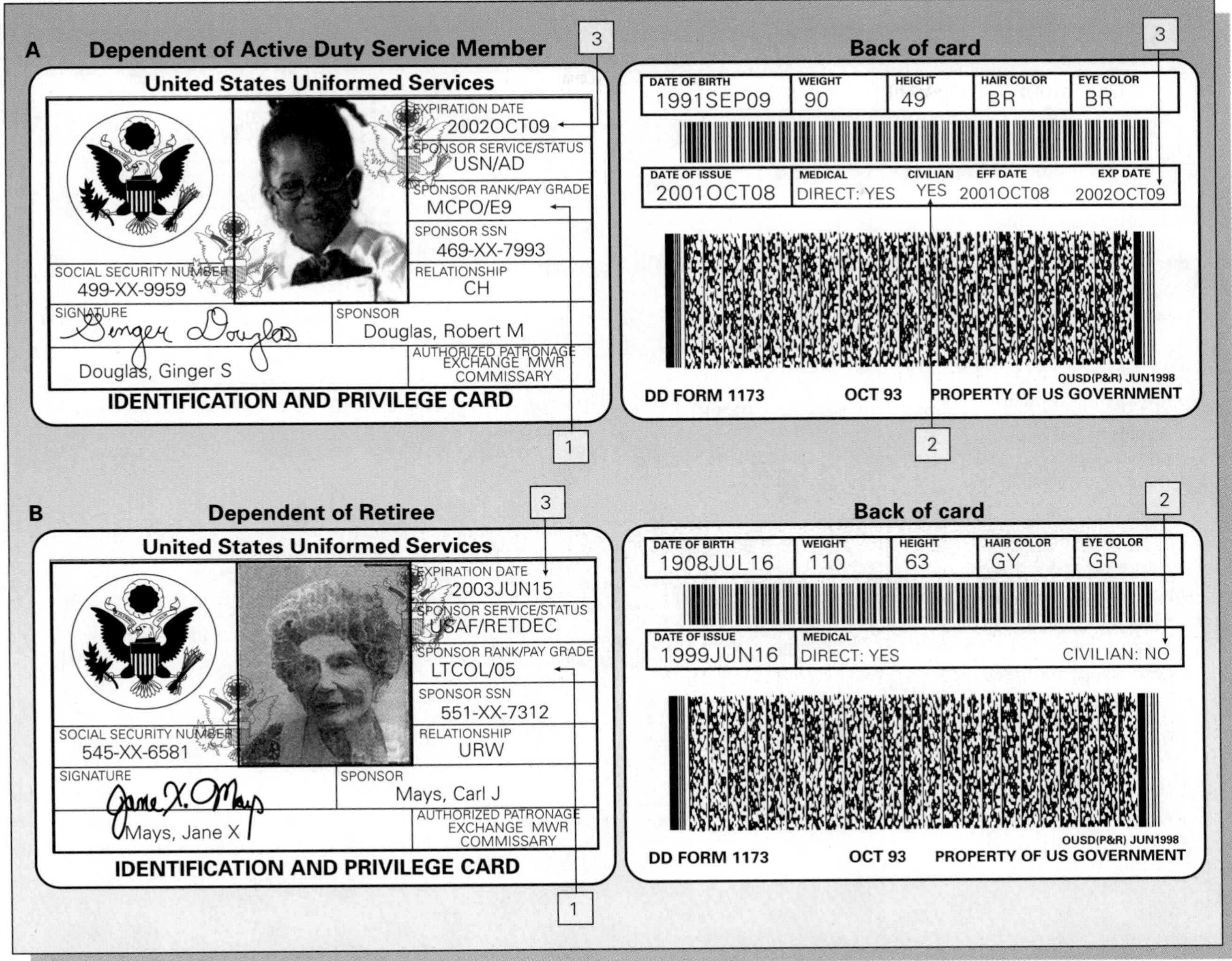

Figure 12–2. *A*, Sample TRICARE Standard active duty dependent's identification card (DD Form 1173) from which essential information must be abstracted. *B*, Sample identification card (DD Form 1173) for a retiree's widowed spouse. Cards indicate (1) sponsor's status and rank, (2) authorization status for treatment by a civilian provider, and (3) expiration date.

Authorized Providers of Healthcare

Providers must pass a credentialing process to become "TRICARE-certified providers." The certification means that they are qualified to treat TRICARE patients and are then "authorized" by TRICARE. The following types of healthcare professionals may be **authorized providers:**

- Doctor of Chiropody (DSC)
- Doctor of Dental Medicine (DDM)
- Doctor of Dental Surgery (DDS)
- Doctor of Medicine (MD)
- Doctor of Optometry (DO)
- Doctor of Osteopathy (DO/MD)
- Doctor of Podiatric Medicine (DPM)
- Psychologist (PhD)

Other authorized nonphysician providers include audiologists, certified nurse-midwives, clinical social workers, licensed practical/vocational nurses, psychiatric social workers, registered nurses, registered physical therapists, and registered speech therapists.

Referral and Preauthorization

In the TRICARE program, a *referral* is a process of sending a patient to another provider for services or consultation which the referring source is not prepared or qualified to provide (Fig. 12–6). Authorized referrals are valid for 60 days and the number of visits specified. When it is determined that services are not available at the MTF, the HCF refers the patient to a network or non-network provider.

ADFM = active duty family members
RFMS = retirees, family members and survivors

Benefit and Coverage Chart

Outpatient Services	Programs and Beneficiary Costs					
Program and Classification	**Tricare Prime**		**Tricare Extra**		**Tricare Standard**	
	ADFM	**RFMS**	**ADFM**	**RFMS**	**ADFM**	**RFMS**
Annual Enrollment Fee* (per fiscal year)	None	$230/person $460/family	None →		None →	
Annual Deductible (per fiscal year 10/1 to 9/30) (applied to outpatient services before cost-share is determined)	None (except when using Point-of-Service option)		E-4 and below $50/person $100/family E-5 and above $150/person $300/family	$150/person $300/family	E-4 and below $50/person $100/family E-5 and above $150/person $300/family	$150/person $300/family
Physician Services	None	$12	15% of contracted fee ↓	20% of contracted fee ↓	20% of maximum allowable charge ↓	25% of maximum allowable charge ↓
Ancillary Services (certain radiology, laboratory, & cardiac services)	None → (RFMS may have $12 copay if test provided independent of office visit)		↓	↓	↓	↓
Ambulance Services	None	$20	↓	↓	↓	↓
Home Health Services	None	$12	↓	↓	↓	↓
Family Health Services	None	$12	↓	↓	↓	↓
Durable Medical Equipment (greater than $100)	None	20% cost-share	↓	↓	↓	↓
Emergency Services (network and non-network)	None	$30 copayment	↓	↓	↓	↓
Outpatient Behavioral Health (limitations apply)	None	$25 copayment $17 group visits	↓	↓	↓	↓
Immunizations (for required overseas travel)	None	Not covered	↓	Not covered	↓	Not covered
Ambulatory Surgery (same day)	None	$25 copayment (applied to facility charges only)	$25 copayment for hospital charges	20% of contracted fee	$25 copayment for hospital charges	*Professional:* 25% of maximum allowable charge *Facility:* 25% of maximum allowable charge OR billed charges, whichever is less
Eye Examinations (limitations apply)	None	Clinical Preventive Service	15% of contracted fee	Not covered	20% of maximum allowable charge	Not covered
Prescription Drugs–Network Pharmacy	$3 copayment for each 30-day supply of **generic** medication $9 copayment for each 30-day supply of **brand name** medication					
Prescription Drugs–National Mail Order Pharmacy	$3 copayment for each 90-day supply of **generic** medication $9 copayment for each 90-day supply of **brand name** medication (Note: if the beneficiary has primary insurance that covers presciption medication, the beneficiary is not eligible for the mail order pharmacy benefit)					
Prescription Drugs–Non-network Pharmacy	$9 or 20% of total cost (whichever is greater) plus deductible					

*No enrollment fee for those who are eligible for Medicare (enrolled in Part B) on the basis of disability or end-stage renal disease

NOTE: TRICARE Prime Remote–benefits are similar to TRICARE Prime program; however, ADSMs have no copayment costs-share or deductible

Program for Persons with Disabilities–no deductible; monthly cost-share varies from $25 to $250, depending on sponsor's rank

Figure 12–3. TRICARE Prime, Extra, and Standard Outpatient Services Benefits and Coverage Chart.

ADFM = active duty family members
RFMS = retirees, family members and survivors

Benefit and Coverage Chart

Inpatient Services	Programs and Beneficiary Costs					
Program and Classification	**Tricare Prime**		**Tricare Extra**		**Tricare Standard**	
	ADFM	**RFMS**	**ADFM**	**RFMS**	**ADFM**	**RFMS**
Hospitalization* including **Maternity Benefits***	No copayment	$11.45/day; civilian care $11/day or $25 min charge per/admission, whichever is greater	$11.45/day; civilian care $11/day or $25 min charge per/admission, whichever is greater	$11.45/day; civilian care $250/day or 25% cost-share (contracted fee) whichever is less, plus 20% cost-share for separately billed professional charges	$11.45/day; civilian care $11/day or $25 min charge per/admission, whichever is greater	$11.45/day; civilian care $401/day or 25% cost-share (contracted fee) whichever is less, plus 25% cost-share (maximum allowable charge) for separately billed professional charges
Skilled Nursing Care	↓	↓	↓	↓	$25/admission, or $11.45/day whichever is greater	25% cost-share (billed charges), plus 25% cost-share (maximum allowable charge) for separately billed professional charges
Mental Ilness Hospitalization* and **Substance Use Treatment*** (inpatient, partial hospital program)	None	$40/day (no copayment or cost-share for separately billed professional charges)	$20/day	20% cost-share (contracted fee), plus 20% cost-share (contracted fee) for separately billed professional charges	$20/day	25% cost-share (max allowable charge), for separately billed professional charges plus: 25% of (1) per diem, (2) fixed daily amount or billed charges, or (3) 25% of allowed amount (RTC & partial hospitalization)
Partial Hospitalization* (mental illness)	None	$40/day or $25/admission, whichever is greater	$20/day	20% cost-share (contracted fee), plus 20% cost-share for separately billed professional charges	$20/day	25% of allowed amount, plus 25% maximum allowable charge for separately billed professional charges
Hospice Care	Available in lieu of other TRICARE benefits (provided by Medicare approved program).					

*Preauthorization required

Figure 12–4. TRICARE Prime, Extra, and Standard Inpatient Services Benefits and Coverage Chart.

When specialty care or hospitalization is required, the MTF must be used if services are available. If services are not available, the **Health Care Finder (HCF)** assists with the preauthorization process (Fig. 12–7). The request may be made via telephone or fax (Fig. 12–8). An HCF is a healthcare professional, usually a registered nurse, who acts as a liaison between military and civilian providers, verifies eligibility, determines availability of services, coordinates care, facilitates the transfer of records, and performs first-level medical review.

For TRICARE Standard beneficiaries, they may self-refer to any TRICARE-certified provider. All inpatient and certain outpatient services require preauthorization.

College Clinic 4567 Broad Avenue
Woodland Hills, XY
12345-0001

Phone: 555/486-9002 Fax: 555/487-8976

TRICARE
REQUEST FOR NON-COVERED SERVICES

I am hereby requesting that the following services be provided to me by Concha Antrum MD
(name of physician)

Service(s) (list all)	Frequency Limitations	Proposed Date(s) of Service	Estimated Cost of Service
hearing exam	non-covered	6/15/XX	$56

In making this request, I acknowledge that these services are not a benefit of my health plan coverage under TRICARE and that I will not receive the benefit of the TRICARE Hold Harmless Policy (defined below), which otherwise might apply to me. In addition, I acknowledge that if I have obtained services more frequently than authorized by TRICARE policy, I may be responsible for that professional service.

I also understand that if authorization for this care has been denied by TRICARE, or if reimbursement is denied upon submittal of a claim form, I may appeal the written notification of the denial issued by ______________________
(name of managed care contractor)

Unless the decision to deny is overturned as a result of an appeal or dispute, I agree that I will be personally responsible for the payment IN FULL of the billed charges for these services.

Stella Ryan
Signature of patient

6/15/XX
Date

TRICARE Hold Harmless Policy: A network provider may not require payment from the beneficiary for any excluded or excludable services that the beneficiary received from the network provider (i.e., the beneficiary will be held harmless) unless the beneficiary has been properly informed that the services are excluded or excludable and has agreed in advance in writing to pay for the services.

Figure 12–5. Illustration of a completed form for a patient who is to receive services listed as non-covered by TRICARE.

HCFs are found at a **TRICARE Service Center (TSC),** which is an office staffed by beneficiary service representatives. All admissions, ambulatory surgical procedures, and other selected procedures require preauthorization. Procedures and services requiring prior approval from TRICARE health contractors are listed according to procedure code number and may be obtained from the nearest TRICARE support office.

Payment

For TRICARE patients, acceptance of assignment means not only that the check will be sent directly to the physician but also that the physician will accept what the federal program designates as the "maximum allowable charge." The patient will pay a fixed amount (copayment) or a percentage of the allowed amount (cost-share), and the federal program will pay the remaining coinsurance up to the allowed amount.

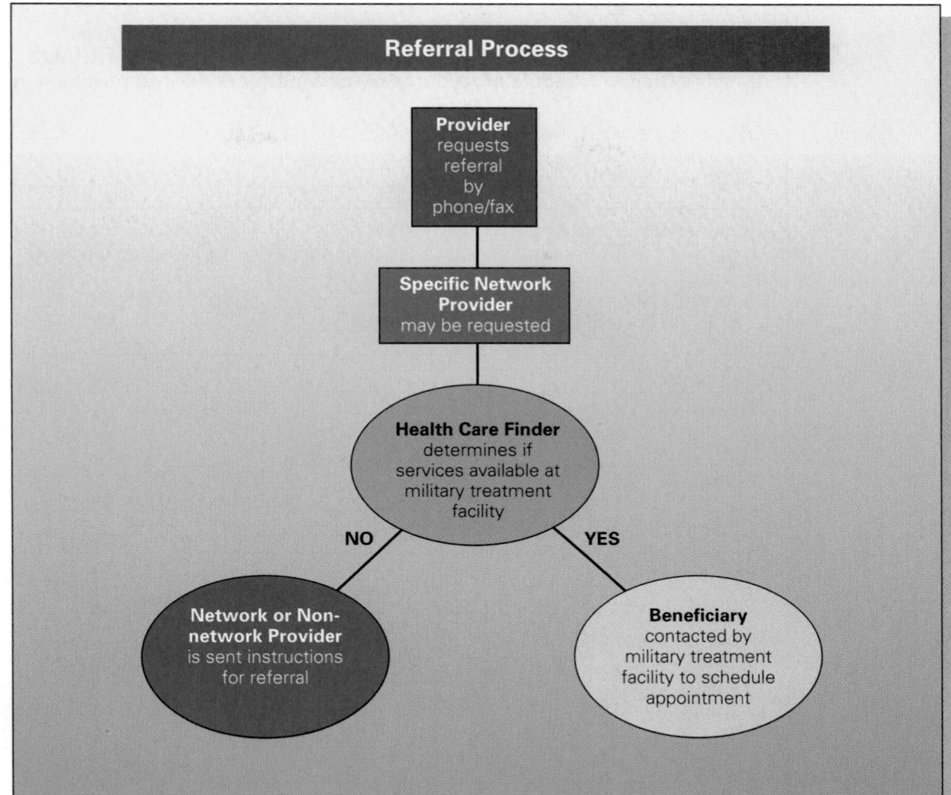

Figure 12–6. Flow of the referral process from the request by the provider, to approval or denial by the Health Care Finder (HCF).

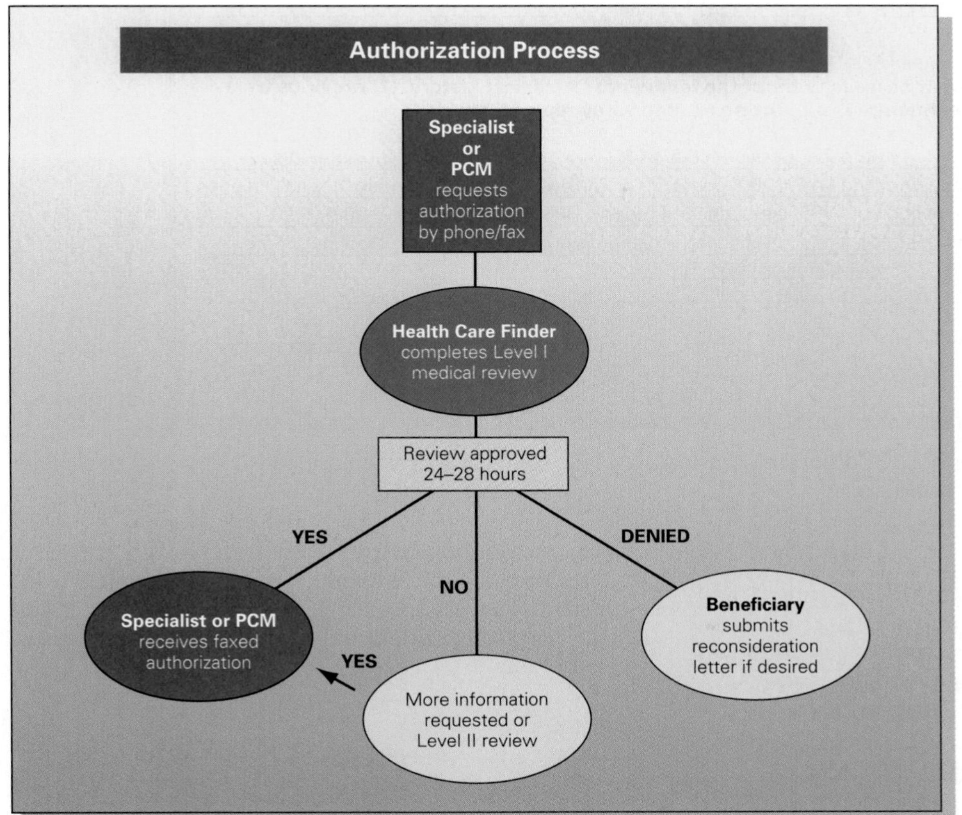

Figure 12–7. Flow of the preauthorization process from the request by the provider or primary care manager (PCM), to approval or denial by the Health Care Finder (HCF).

TRICARE PREAUTHORIZATION/REFERRAL REQUEST FORM
Do not schedule procedures or appointments prior to receiving authorization.

TRICARE Service Center Point Mugu, CA Fax No. (555)869-7200

HCF/CRN Seth Crouch Telephone No. (800) XXX-1255

Request is: ☐ Emergent ☑ Urgent ☐ Routine
☐ Referral/consult ☑ Preauthorization ☐ Second Opinion

Sponsor's Name Jacqueline Peterson Sponsor's SSN 269-XX-4913
Sponsor's Date of Birth 5 - 12 - 81 Sex: ☐ Male ☑ Female

Peterson	Dennis	T.	(555) 485-1926
Patient's Last Name	First Name	Middle Initial	Telephone No.

1219 Vista Point	Pont Hueneme,	CA	12345	10-1-80
Address	City	State	ZIP Code	Date of Birth

Plan: ☐ Prime ☐ Extra ☑ Standard ☐ TSP ☐ TPR ☐ SHCP
Other Insurance ☐ Yes ☑ No If yes, specify: ____

Requesting MD/MO (if not PCM): ____ TIN No. ____
Contact person: Eric Davidson Phone No. (555)484-1212 Fax No. (555)484-1213
Refer to facility (name): College Hospital Phone No. (555)487-6789
Refer to provider (name): Clarence Cutler MD Specialty: Surgeon
Provider phone No. (555)486-9002 TIN# 71-57372XX Suffix XXX
Place of service: ☑ Inpatient ☐ Outpatient Anticipated date(s) of service 9/14/XX–9/15/XX
PCM: Dr. Carlos Newcomb Telephone no. (555)869-7234
Diagnosis (description): Choledocholithiasis ICD-9-CM Code 574-31

CPT Code: 47564 Units: 1 Description: Laparoscopic cholecystectomy with exploration of common bile duct
CPT Code: ____ Units: ____ Description: ____
CPT Code: ____ Units: ____ Description: ____

Request CANNOT be processed without the following: (1) Clinical history, (2) previous treatment, (3) plan of treatment, (4) supporting lab and X-ray reports, etc.

Pt seen at Point Mugu MTF outpatient clinic on 8/5/XX. CC: two episodes of RUQ pain with severe indigestion, nausea and vomiting on 7/27/XX and 8/3/XX. PX reveals tender left margin of gall bladder. CBC indicates sight elevation of WBC (see attached report). BP elevated 180/90, T 98.9, P 90. Abdominal ultrasound confirms cholelithiasis (see attached report). Stones are lodged in common bile duct. Recommend immediate laparoscopic cholecystectomy with exploration of common duct.

FOR OFFICE USE ONLY: Auth/Referral # ____ Effective date ____
NAS (if required) ____ Effective date ____

Figure 12–8. Sample TRICARE Preauthorization/Referral Request Form completed and ready to fax to the managed care contractor.

Deductible and Copayment

A beneficiary may use both TRICARE Standard and TRICARE Extra to satisfy the annual deductible. Deductibles and copayments are determined according to two groups: (1) active duty family members, and (2) retirees, their family members, and survivors.

Outpatient Care

The sponsor's pay grade (noted on the military identification card) determines the deductible amount. For outpatient (nonhospitalized) care, refer to Figure 12–3 to determine (1) the individual or family deductible for each fiscal year (October 1 through September 30), and (2) the percentage of allowable charge the patient is responsible for.

Inpatient Care

For inpatient (hospitalized) care for active duty spouses and children, the beneficiary pays the first $25 of the hospital charge or a small fee for each day, whichever is greater. TRICARE pays the remainder of the allowable charges for authorized care.

For inpatient (hospitalized) care for retirees, family members, and survivors, the beneficiary pays $401 per day or 25% of the billed charges, whichever is less, plus 25% of the allowable charge for professional services. TRICARE pays the remaining hospital charges.

Participating Provider

For a TRICARE Standard case, if the physician agrees to *accept assignment*, then the participating (par) provider agrees to accept the TRICARE-determined allowable amount as payment in full. Par providers file claims and receive reimbursement directly from TRICARE. Providers may choose to accept TRICARE assignment on a case-by-case basis. To avoid collection problems, always accept assignment in cases when the service member is transferring within 6 months.

Cost-Share

The provider may bill the patient for his or her **cost-share** or coinsurance (20% or 25% of the allowable charge after the deductible has been met), and for any noncovered services or supplies when the patient has signed a "request for noncovered services" notice. The provider may not bill for the difference between the provider's usual charge and the allowable amount. This amount has to be written off of the books as an adjustment.

Catastrophic Cap

There is a limit to the amount that TRICARE enrollees pay each fiscal year or enrollment period for their cost-share. This amount is known as the **catastrophic cap.** After this cap is reached, TRICARE pays 100% of the allowable charges for the rest of the year. For active duty family members, the cap is $1,000. For uniformed service retirees and their family members and survivors, the cap is $3,000.

To help expedite claims processing and payment, enclose a note with the claim stating the patient has met the catastrophic cap. After completing the claim and sending it to the fiscal intermediary, the payment will go directly to the physician.

Nonparticipating Provider

A healthcare provider who chooses not to participate in TRICARE is called a nonparticipating (nonpar) provider and may not bill the patient more than 115% of the TRICARE allowable charge. For example, if the TRICARE allowable charge for a procedure is $100, providers who decide not to participate in TRICARE may charge the TRICARE patient no more than $115 for that procedure ($100 × 1.15% = $115). When the physician does not accept assignment, the patient pays the deductible, 20% or 25% of the allowable charge, and any amount over the allowable charge up to 115%.

TRICARE beneficiaries generally file their own claims for care obtained from a nonpar provider. TRICARE pays its portion of the allowable charges directly to the beneficiary.

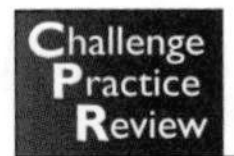

Pause and Practice CPR

REVIEW SESSIONS 12–6 THROUGH 12–9

Directions: *Complete the following questions as a review of information you have just read.*

12–6 Who are issued a Uniformed Services (military) identification card? ______________________

____

12–7 What are three things listed on the Uniformed Services identification card that determine the copayment, cost-share, and deductible amounts?

(a) ______________________

(b) ______________________

(c) ______________________

12–8 Providers that pass a credentialing process become ______________________ and are qualified and ______________________ by TRICARE to treat TRICARE patients.

12–9 When it is determined that a service or procedure is not available at an MTF, the ______________________ refers the patient to a network or non-network provider and assists with the ______________________ process.

CHECK YOUR HEARTBEAT! Turn to the end of the chapter for answers to these review sessions.

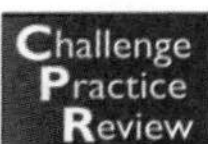

Pause and Practice CPR

PRACTICE SESSIONS 12–10 THROUGH 12–12

Directions: *Refer to the section on "Payment" and Figures 12–3 and 12–4 to interpret the following scenarios and compute the answers.*

12–10 The spouse of an Active Duty Service Member (ADSM) rank E-4 sees a participating physician for outpatient care using TRICARE Standard. The deductible has been met and the physician charges $75. The TRICARE maximum allowed amount is $69.

(a) What is the amount that TRICARE pays? ____________

(b) What is the amount the beneficiary pays? ____________

(c) What is the amount of the courtesy adjustment? ____________

12–11 The spouse of an ADSM (E-4) sees a participating physician for outpatient care using TRICARE Standard. The deductible *has not been met* and the physician charges $75. The TRICARE maximum allowed amount is $69.

(a) What is the amount that TRICARE pays? ____________

(b) What is the amount the beneficiary pays? ____________

(c) What is the amount of the courtesy adjustment? ____________

12–12 A military retiree sees a participating physician for outpatient care using TRICARE Standard. The deductible has been met and the physician charges $75. The TRICARE maximum allowed amount is $69.

(a) What is the amount that TRICARE pays? ____________

(b) What is the amount the beneficiary pays? ____________

(c) What is the amount of the courtesy adjustment? ____________

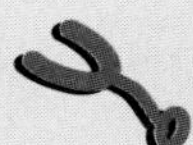

CHECK YOUR HEARTBEAT! Turn to the end of the chapter for answers to these practice sessions.

TRICARE EXTRA

TRICARE Extra is a preferred provider organization option where network providers receive a contract rate for giving care (Fig. 12–9).

Enrollment

Qualified TRICARE individuals do not have to enroll or pay an annual fee to enter the TRICARE Extra program. Enrollment is automatic when a TRICARE beneficiary seeks care from a network provider. If a beneficiary seeks care from a non-network TRICARE-certified provider, the services received are covered under TRICARE Standard. Therefore, a beneficiary may bounce back and forth between network and non-network providers on a visit-by-visit basis and receive benefits from both TRICARE Standard and TRICARE Extra options. The discounted services offered through TRICARE Extra provide the beneficiary reduced cost-share, so it is advantageous to seek care from TRICARE Extra network physicians.

Identification Card

A TRICARE beneficiary (older than 10 years of age) must present a military identification card when receiving care. Children younger than 10 years of age may use the sponsor's card. Active duty and retiree dependents and survivors carry a military identification card as shown in Figure 12–2. The active-duty retirees' card is light blue in color.

Benefits

See Figure 12–3 for outpatient and Figure 12–4 for inpatient benefits, including cost-sharing, deductible, and copayment amounts.

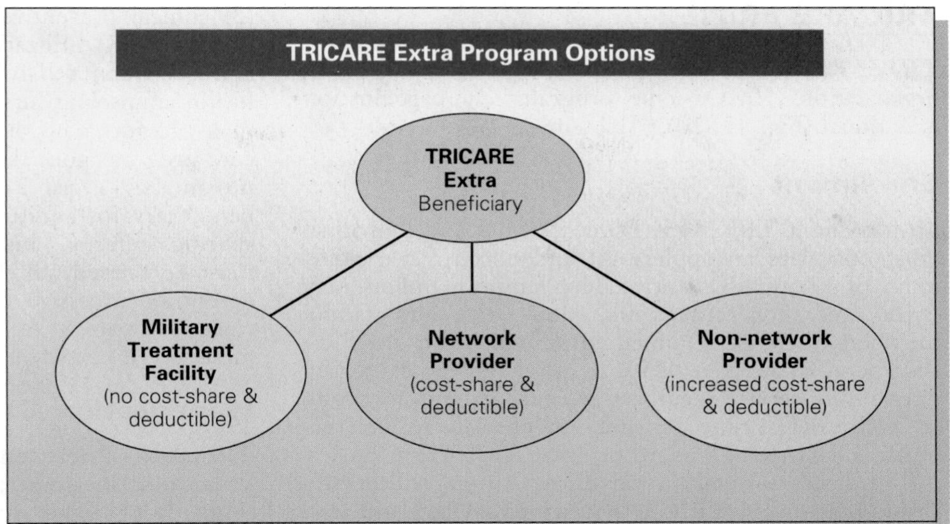

Figure 12–9. Illustration showing where a TRICARE Extra program patient seeks care.

Network Providers

Network providers are participating providers that have discount agreements with the TRICARE program. They are required to file claims and receive reimbursement directly from TRICARE.

Referral and Preauthorization

As with TRICARE Standard, TRICARE Extra beneficiaries can self-refer to any TRICARE network provider. All inpatient hospital stays and certain outpatient services require preauthorization from an HCF.

Payment

Deductible and Copayment

As stated in TRICARE Standard, a beneficiary may use both TRICARE Extra and TRICARE Standard to satisfy the annual deductible. Deductibles and copayments are determined according to two groups: (1) active duty family members, and (2) retirees, their family members, and survivors. Refer to Figure 12–3 (outpatient) and 12–4 (inpatient) to determine the (1) deductible amounts, (2) percentage of allowable charge, and/or (3) cost share.

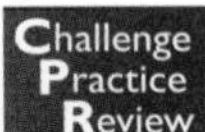

Pause and Practice CPR

REVIEW SESSIONS 12–13 AND 12–14

Directions: *Complete the following questions as a review of information you have just read.*

12–13 A beneficiary may bounce back and forth between network and non-network providers on a visit-by-visit basis and receive benefits from both TRICARE Standard and TRICARE Extra options.

(a) True

(b) False

12–14 What are three stipulations of a TRICARE network provider?

(a) ______________________

(b) ______________________

(c) ______________________

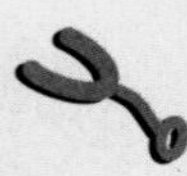

CHECK YOUR HEARTBEAT! Turn to the end of the chapter for answers to these review sessions.

TRICARE PRIME

TRICARE Prime is a voluntary health maintenance organization (HMO)–type program and participation is optional (Fig. 12–10).

Enrollment

To become a TRICARE Prime member, an individual must complete an application and enroll for a minimum of 12 months. Active duty family members may enroll free. For retirees and non–active duty family members, there is an annual enrollment fee charged either per person (i.e., $230) or per family (i.e., $460). Active duty service members are enrolled automatically in TRICARE Prime and are not eligible for benefits under TRICARE Standard or TRICARE Extra.

Enrollees normally receive care from within the Prime network of TRICARE-certified civilian and military providers. The beneficiary has the option of choosing or being assigned a primary care manager (PCM) for each family member.

The TRICARE Prime member may also choose the point-of-service option and seek care from any TRICARE-certified civilian provider at a much higher out-of-pocket cost.

Primary Care Manager

The **primary care manager (PCM)** is a physician who is responsible for coordinating and managing all the beneficiary's healthcare in TRICARE Prime, including referrals to specialists. The beneficiary must seek care from the PCM except for (1) emergencies, (2) clinical preventive services provided by a network physician, (3) utilization of a point-of-service option, and (4) when self-referring for outpatient behavioral health counseling (first eight sessions).

A provider who decides to participate in a managed care program goes through a credentialing process approximately every 2 years. The PCM may refer the beneficiary for additional services, when necessary, but specific referral and preauthorization requirements must be carried out. Referral patterns are evaluated to determine excessive or inappropriate referrals to specialists. A pattern of such referrals could result in termination of participation in TRICARE Prime.

Identification Card

TRICARE Prime enrollees are issued a TRICARE Prime identification card which lists the PCM selected (Fig. 12–11). This card does not guarantee TRICARE eligibility. Providers must also check the TRICARE Uniformed Services military identification card for the effective date and call an automated Voice Response Unit (VRU) system to verify eligibility. Copy both the military identification card and the TRICARE Prime card and retain them in the patient's file. Check both cards at every visit.

Benefits

Covered services are the same as those for TRICARE Standard patients plus additional preventive and primary care services. For example, periodic physical examinations are covered at no charge under TRICARE Prime, but are not covered under TRICARE

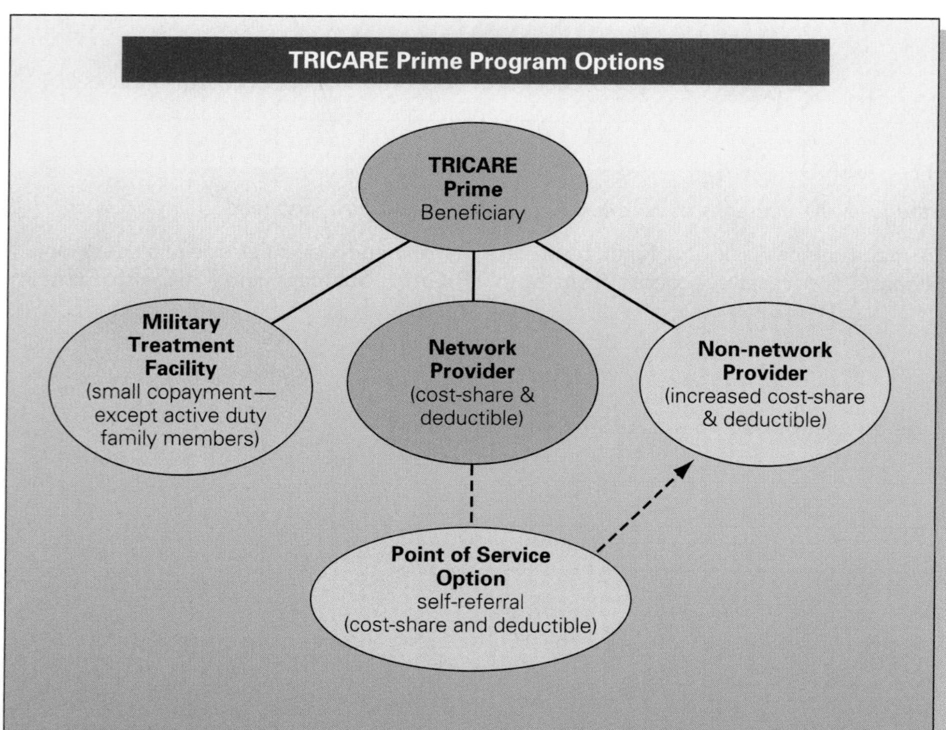

Figure 12–10. Illustration showing where a TRICARE Prime program patient seeks care.

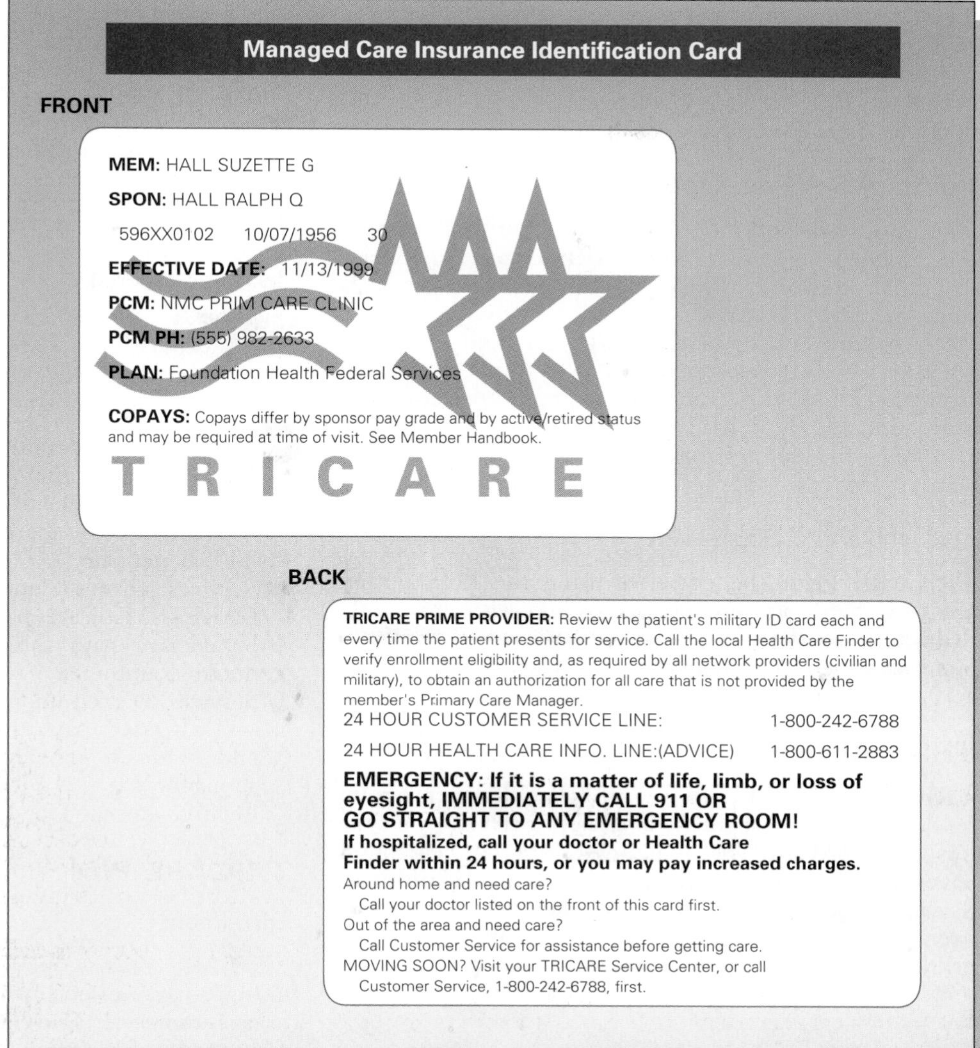

Figure 12–11. Sample TRICARE Prime identification card. A new TRICARE Prime identification card has been redesigned to incorporate essential contact information to help enrollees access healthcare. This card will gradually appear on the scene.

Standard or TRICARE Extra. Other, additional benefits Prime covers are certain immunizations and annual eye examinations for dependent children of retirees. A dental plan is available for an additional monthly premium. An NAS is required for certain inpatient services at a civilian hospital if the beneficiary resides within the designated MTF catchment area. See Figure 12–3 for outpatient and Figure 12–4 for inpatient benefits.

Referral and Preauthorization

The primary care manager must initiate all referrals of TRICARE Prime beneficiaries for services that are beyond the scope of primary care. Requests must be submitted to the HCF prior to services being rendered. If the services meet the criteria, the HCF will enter a preauthorization number into the system and communicate the number to the provider. The provider notifies the beneficiary and the service is scheduled.

All TRICARE programs require preauthorization for nonemergency inpatient and certain outpatient services. A list of approved surgeries is located in the TRICARE Policy Manual available on the Internet. See Resources at the end of this chapter for the web site address.

Payments

Deductible and Copayment

There is no deductible for the TRICARE Prime option. Copayments are determined according to two groups: (1) active duty family members, and (2) retirees, their family members, and survivors. Refer to Figures 12–3 (outpatient) and 12–4 (inpatient) to determine copayment and cost share amounts.

Catastrophic Cap

For active duty family members in TRICARE Prime, the catastrophic cap is $1,000 per *fiscal year*. All other

TRICARE Prime beneficiaries have a catastrophic cap of $3,000 per *enrollment period.* This only applies to enrollment fees, outpatient and inpatient cost-shares, and copayments. Point-of-service cost-shares and deductibles are not applied to this limit.

Point-of-Service Option

The **point-of-service (POS) option** for outpatient services allows the TRICARE Prime beneficiary maximum flexibility by providing the ability to self-refer for any TRICARE-covered nonemergency services to any civilian TRICARE-certified provider, whether in network or not. No referral is needed from the PCM; however, certain preauthorization requirements apply. TRICARE Prime beneficiaries may also self-refer to network providers for clinical preventive services.

Deductible and Copayment

TRICARE Prime beneficiaries using the POS option are responsible for a $300 per person or $600 family deductible per fiscal year (October 1 through September 30). The beneficiary is also responsible for a 50% cost-share of allowable charges.

TRICARE For Life

TRICARE For Life (TFL) is a healthcare program funded by the Department of Defense (DOD) that offers additional TRICARE benefits as a supplementary payer to Medicare. This program is for Uniformed Service retirees, their spouses, and survivors age 65 and over. In most cases, under TFL, Medicare will be the primary and TRICARE the secondary payer.

Enrollment

Most beneficiaries must be eligible for Medicare Part A and enrolled in Medicare Part B to qualify for TFL. An exception is Uniformed Services Family Health Plan (USFHP) members. Prospective TFL beneficiaries do not have to sign up or enroll for the program; however, they do need to be enrolled in DEERS.

Identification Card

Beneficiaries who qualify for TFL do not need a TRICARE enrollment card.

Benefits

Each beneficiary receives a matrix comparing Medicare benefits to TRICARE benefits. Refer to Resources at the end of this chapter for the TRICARE Management Activity web site address to download this information. Certain benefits (e.g., prescription medications) are covered under the TRICARE Senior Pharmacy Program and are not a benefit under Medicare. Pharmacy benefits provide Medicare-eligible retirees of the Uniformed Service, their family members, and survivors the same pharmacy benefit as retirees who are under age 65. This includes access to prescription drugs at MTFs, retail pharmacies, and through the National Mail Order Pharmacy. Medicare Part B enrollment is not mandatory in order to receive TRICARE Senior Pharmacy Program benefits.

Referral and Preauthorization

There are no preauthorization requirements for the TFL program. All services and supplies must be a benefit of the Medicare and/or TRICARE programs in order to be covered.

Payment

The following three scenarios represent most cases and explain the payment mechanism:

1. Services covered under Medicare and TRICARE—Medicare pays the Medicare rate and TRICARE covers the beneficiary's cost-share and deductible. No copayment, cost-share, or deductible is paid by the TFL beneficiary.
2. Services covered under Medicare, but not TRICARE—Medicare pays the Medicare rate and the beneficiary pays the Medicare cost-share and deductible amounts.
3. Services covered under TRICARE, but not Medicare—TRICARE pays the TRICARE allowed amount and Medicare pays nothing. The beneficiary is responsible for the TRICARE cost-share and the deductible amounts.

TRICARE Plus

Enrollment

TRICARE Plus is open to persons eligible for care in military facilities and not enrolled in TRICARE Prime or a commercial HMO. TRICARE Plus allows some Military Health System (MHS) beneficiaries to enroll with a military primary care provider. There is no enrollment fee.

Identification Card

Persons enrolled in TRICARE Plus will be issued an identification card and identified in the DEERS.

Benefits

The TRICARE Plus program is designed to function in the following ways:

- Enrollees use the military treatment facility as their source of primary care; it is not a comprehensive health plan.
- Enrollees may seek care from a civilian provider, but are discouraged from obtaining nonemergency primary care from sources outside the MTF.
- Enrollees are not guaranteed access to specialty providers at the MTF.
- Enrollees may not use their enrollment at another facility.
- The military treatment facility's commander determines the enrollment capacity at each MTF.

Payment

TRICARE Plus offers the same benefits as TRICARE Prime when using an MTF. It has no effect on the enrollees' use or payment of civilian healthcare benefits; therefore, TRICARE Standard, TRICARE Extra, or Medicare may pay for civilian healthcare services obtained by a TRICARE Plus enrollee.

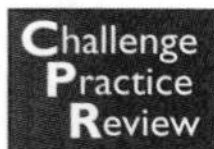

Pause and Practice CPR

REVIEW SESSIONS 12–15 THROUGH 12–19

Directions: *Complete the following questions as a review of information you have just read.*

12–15 Enrollment in TRICARE Prime is for a minimum of ____________________.

12–16 The ____________________ is a physician who is responsible for coordinating and managing all the beneficiary's healthcare needs in the TRICARE Prime program.

12–17 The ____________________ initiates all referrals of TRICARE Prime beneficiaries for services beyond basic primary care and submits requests to the ____________________ for preauthorization.

12–18 The deductible for the TRICARE Prime option is ____________________ and the copayment amount for active duty spouses and children is ____________ except for prescription drugs.

12–19 The TRICARE Prime point-of-service option allows the beneficiary maximum flexibility by ____

____

____

CHECK YOUR HEARTBEAT! Turn to the end of the chapter for answers to these review sessions.

TRICARE PRIME REMOTE PROGRAM

TRICARE Prime Remote (TPR) is a program designed for ADSMs who work and live more than 50 miles or 1 hour from an MTF. Family members of ADSMs in the TPR program will also become eligible for this program in 2002. This will allow service personnel and their families who live in remote areas to reduce or eliminate out-of-pocket costs.

Enrollment

ADSMs must enroll in this program, which enables them to receive care from any civilian provider.

Identification Card

Active duty service members must present their military identification card to receive care from providers (Fig. 12–12). Photocopy both sides of the card and retain it in the patient's medical record so that information will be available for reference when completing the insurance claim form.

Benefits

TPR program benefits are similar to TRICARE Prime, plus additional necessary medical care related to fitness-for-duty requirements. A PCM must be selected, if available in the area. If an MTF or a PCM is not available, services may be received from any TRICARE-certified civilian provider.

Referral and Preauthorization

Routine primary care does *not* require prior authorization (e.g., office visits and preventive healthcare). The PCM must initiate all specialty referrals and coordinate requests through the **Health Benefits Advisor (HBA)** for certain outpatient services, all inpatient surgical/medical services, maternity services, physical therapy, orthotics, hearing appliances, family planning, transplants, and inpatient/outpatient behavioral health services. The HBA is a government employee who is responsible for helping all Military Health System (MHS) beneficiaries to obtain medical care.

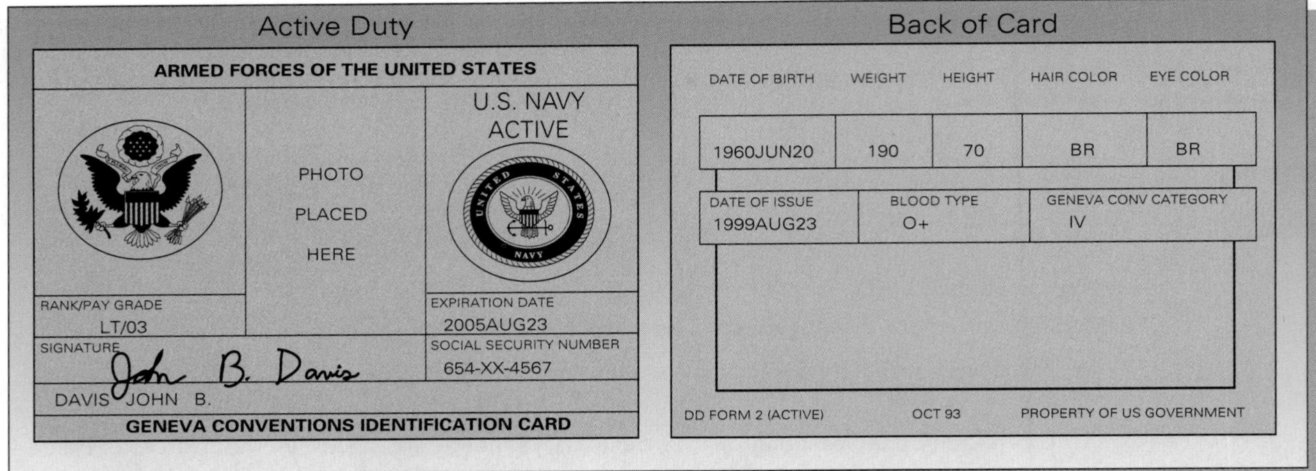

Figure 12–12. Sample military identification card for an active duty individual in the Armed Forces. It is used as the identification card for the TRICARE Remote program and is considered a sponsor identification card.

Payment

Those covered and receiving benefits under TPR are not responsible for *any* out-of-pocket costs. Active duty service member claims for services provided by a TRICARE network provider are paid at the same contracted rate as other TRICARE claims.

SUPPLEMENTAL HEALTH CARE PROGRAM

The MTF always administers routine care for ADSMs (e.g., routine office visits and preventive healthcare). The Supplemental Health Care Program (SHCP) was developed for ADSMs and other designated MTF patients who are referred from an MTF to civilian healthcare.

Enrollment

When ADSMs are not enrolled in a TPR program and are referred to civilian healthcare (e.g., ADSMs in travel status, assigned to deployable units, and so forth), a portion of SHCP covers the costs.

Non–TRICARE-eligible beneficiaries (e.g., eligible parents, parents-in-law) may be referred by an MTF for outpatient care with a civilian provider. Under this program, ADSMs and other MTF patients may be referred to a civilian hospital for specific inpatient services when they are not available at the MTF.

Identification Card

Active duty service members must present their military identification card to receive care from providers (see Fig. 12–12). Photocopy both sides of the card and retain it in the patient's medical record so information will be available for reference when completing the insurance claim form.

Benefits

SHCP offers benefits similar to TRICARE Prime, enabling beneficiaries to be referred to a civilian provider for care.

Referral and Preauthorization

The MTF will initiate all referrals for ADSMs and other designated patients to civilian specialists when needed.

Payment

Those covered and receiving benefits under SHCP are not responsible for *any* out-of-pocket costs. There is no deductible, copayment, or cost-share for services provided by a civilian provider. Active duty service member claims for services provided by a TRICARE network provider are paid at the same contracted rate as other TRICARE beneficiary claims.

OTHER TRICARE HEALTH BENEFITS

TRICARE offers additional health services such as:

- TRICARE Hospice Program
- Behavioral Health Services
- TRICARE Prime Clinical Preventive Services
- Specialized Treatment Services
- Program for Persons with Disabilities (PFPWD)
- Health Care Information Line

Go to the worktext web site at http://www.wbsaunders.com/MERLIN/Fordney/insurance/ for more information about these services and an exercise session to test your knowledge.

CHAMPVA PROGRAM

The Civilian Health and Medical Program of the Veterans Administration (CHAMPVA), now known as the Department of Veterans Affairs, is not an insurance program in that it does not involve a contract guaranteeing the indemnification of an insured party against a specified loss in return for a paid premium. It is considered a **service benefit program;** therefore, there are no premiums. It was created for veterans' spouses and children. A **veteran** is any person who has served in the armed forces of the United States, is no longer in the service, and has received an honorable discharge. Individuals who qualify for CHAMPVA are known as beneficiaries and the veteran is called the sponsor.

Eligibility

Determination of eligibility is the responsibility of the Department of Veterans Affairs. Not all veterans' spouses and children receive CHAMPVA benefits, only those related to a veteran who has **total, permanent, service-connected disabilities** or the surviving spouses and children of veterans who died as a result of a service-connected disability.

The following persons are eligible for CHAMPVA benefits as long as they are not eligible for TRICARE, and not eligible for Medicare Part A as a result of reaching age 65. The husband, wife, or unmarried child of a veteran

- with a total disability, permanent in nature, resulting from a service-connected injury;
- who died as the result of a service-connected disability or who, at the time of death, had a total disability, permanent in nature, resulting from a service-connected injury; or
- who died in the line of duty while on active service.

Children are those unmarried and younger than age 18 years regardless of whether dependent or not, or up to the age of 23 if enrolled in a course of instruction at an approved educational institution.

Examples of service-connected *total, permanent disability* are when an individual sustains an injury with paraplegic results, receives a bullet wound and suffers neurologic damage, loses a limb, and so on. This contrasts to a *chronic or temporary* service-connected disability, which might exist if an individual, while in the armed forces, improperly lifts a heavy object and suffers a back injury with ongoing sporadic symptoms which require continuing medical care after leaving the service. Both scenarios present service-connected disabilities, but the first example illustrates a person permanently disabled whereas the second example illustrates a chronic or temporary disability.

Enrollment

A Social Security number is required for enrollment in the CHAMPVA program and the veteran's dependents must claim dependency status to the veteran sponsor by contacting the local VA regional office. An application form is completed by telephone, fax, or downloading from the VA's web site (see Resources at the end of this chapter).

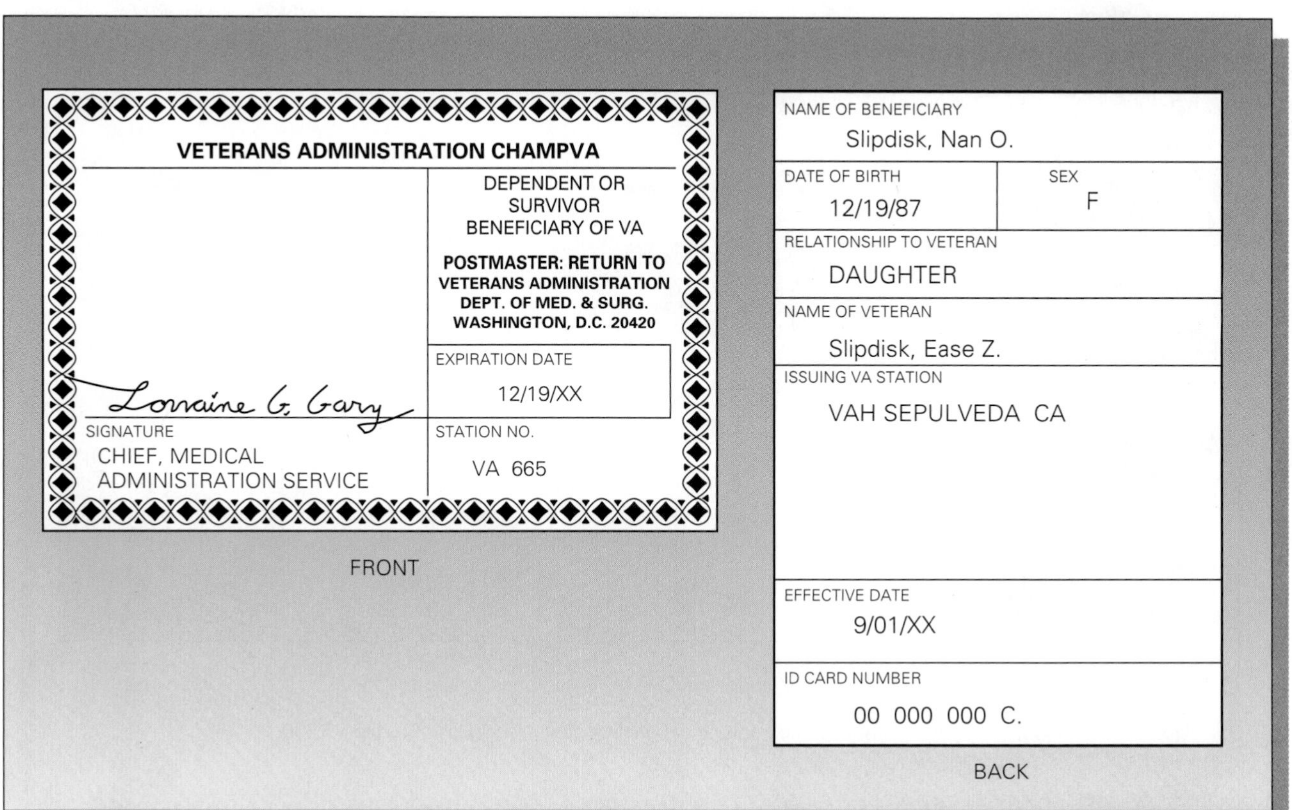

Figure 12–13. Sample CHAMPVA military identification card.

Identification Card

After enrollment is completed, the prospective beneficiary goes to the nearest VA medical center and, if eligible, receives a VA identification card. The issuing MTF's number appears on the identification card identifying the home facility where the beneficiary's case file is kept. The identification card number is the veteran's VA file number with an alpha suffix which is different for each beneficiary of a sponsor. All dependents 10 years of age or older are required to have a Uniformed Services (military) identification card for CHAMPVA, as shown in Figure 12–13 on preceding page.

Certain veterans may qualify for treatment at a VA Outpatient Clinic. In such cases, the veteran is issued a VA outpatient medical treatment information card.

Benefits

Benefits under the CHAMPVA program are similar to those provided for dependents of retired and deceased Uniformed Services personnel under TRICARE Standard; however, CHAMPVA beneficiaries over age 65 are not eligible for a senior plan or senior pharmacy plan. To see the overall picture of CHAMPVA benefits, which include deductibles and cost sharing, study Figure 12–14.

CHAMPVA Cost Share Summary

Benefit (Covered Services)	Beneficiary Pays [1,2]		CHAMPVA Pays
	Deductible ($50/individual or $100/family per calendar year)	**Cost Share**	
Outpatient services			
Ambulatory surgery ***Family services***	No	25% of allowable	75% of allowable
Professional services	Yes	25% of allowable	75% of allowable
Pharmacy services	Yes	25% of allowable	75% of allowable
Durable Medical Equipment (DME)			
Non–VA source	Yes	25% of allowable	75% of allowable
VA source	No	NONE	100% of VA cost
Inpatient services			
Facility services **DRG based**	No	Lesser of: 1) per day amt x number of inpatient days; 2) 25% of billed amount; or 3) DRG rate	DRG rate less beneficiary cost share
Non–DRG based	No	25% of allowable	75% of allowable
Mental health **High volume/RTC**	No	25% of allowable	75% of allowable
Low volume	No	Lesser of: 1) per day amt x number of inpatient days; 2) 25% of billed amount.	Balance of allowable AFTER beneficiary cost share
Professional services	No	25% of allowable	75% of allowable

1. Services received at VA healthcare facilities under the CHAMPVA Inhouse Treatment Initiative (CITI) program are exempt from beneficiary cost sharing.
2. Under catastrophic protection plan (Cat Cap), annual beneficiary cost sharing is limited to $7,500.

Figure 12–14. Summary of CHAMPVA Service Benefits and Cost Sharing amounts.

Provider

The beneficiaries of the CHAMPVA program have complete freedom of choice in selecting their civilian healthcare providers.

Referral and Preauthorization

CHAMPVA beneficiaries may self-refer to any civilian healthcare provider. Preauthorization is required for organ and bone marrow transplants, hospice services, all dental care, and DME with a purchase price or total rental cost of $300 or more. In addition, most mental health services and substance abuse care must be preauthorized.

Payment

For outpatient services the CHAMPVA deductible is $50 per person or $100 per family per calendar year (January 1 through December 31). CHAMPVA pays 75% of the allowed amount and the beneficiary is responsible for 25%. The catastrophic cap per calendar year is $7,500. For a detailed cost-share summary of outpatient and inpatient services, refer to Figure 12–14.

MEDICAL RECORDS

Medical Record Access

The Privacy Act of 1974 established an individual's right to review his or her medical record maintained by a federal medical care facility, such as a VA medical center or U.S. Public Health Service facility. Patients have the right to contest inaccuracies in such records. Each agency makes its own rules establishing access procedures and agencies are allowed to adopt special procedures when it is believed that direct access could be harmful to a person. The act requires that an individual from whom personal information is requested be informed of (1) the authority for the request, (2) the principal purpose of the information requested, (3) routine use of the information, and (4) the effect on an individual who does not provide the information.

The Computer Matching and Privacy Protection Act of 1988 was established to permit the government to verify information by way of computer matches. Both of these acts are mentioned on the back of the HCFA-1500 claim form.

It is important that TRICARE and CHAMPVA patients be made aware of this information by physicians who treat them, so that they are knowledgeable about routine use and disclosure of medical data. Patients may make a Privacy Act request in writing, in person, or by telephone.

Release of Patient Information

TRICARE-eligible beneficiaries must maintain a "Signature on File" (SOF) in the physician's office (1) to protect the patient's privacy, (2) for the release of important information, (3) to prevent fraud, and (4) to ensure that the proper beneficiary signature is submitted with claims.

If an inquiry is made by a beneficiary (including an eligible dependent, regardless of age), the reply should be addressed to the beneficiary, not the beneficiary's parent or guardian. Exceptions are:

- When a parent writes on behalf of a minor child (under 18).
- When a guardian writes on behalf of a physically or mentally incompetent beneficiary.

The Privacy Act of 1974 precludes disclosure of sensitive information which, if released, could have an adverse effect on the beneficiary. Providers must not provide information to parents/guardians of minors or incompetents when the services are related to acquired immunodeficiency syndrome (AIDS), alcoholism, abortion, drug abuse, or venereal disease.

Release of Medical Records

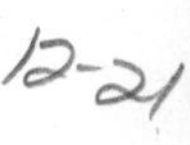

The TRICARE Prime beneficiary must sign a release of medical information at each site (including associated ancillary service sites) when receiving care from a specialty provider. For all routine referrals, specialty providers are required to then submit the medical records to the PCM and/or MTF commander within 14 days. If the care is urgent, the records should be given to the beneficiary at the time of the visit.

Active duty service members under the TPR program are instructed to sign annual medical release forms with their PCMs or TRICARE-certified providers to allow information to be forwarded to civilian and military providers. When the beneficiary is being reassigned to a new location, the PCM must provide complete copies of medical records and specialty and ancillary care documentation to the ADSM within 30 calendar days of a request.

Expressions from Experience

To improve my skills I have taken classes in medical terminology and am now taking medical insurance billing courses. My long-term goal is to pass a national insurance examination, receive my National Certification of Insurance and Coding Specialist certificate, and start my own billing company.

Jimetria Smith
Insurance Billing Specialist
Radiology—Billing Service

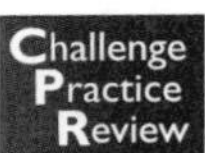

Pause and Practice CPR

REVIEW SESSIONS 12–20 THROUGH 12–24

Directions: *Complete the following questions as a review of information you have just read.*

12–20 CHAMPVA is not considered an insurance program but a ________________ program.

12–21 The first place to contact to enroll in the CHAMPVA program is the ________________ ________________.

12–22 What is the

(a) deductible for a CHAMPVA patient? ________________

(b) percent that CHAMPVA pays for the allowed amount? ________________

(c) catastrophic cap per calendar year? ________________

12–23 Name two acts mentioned on the back of the HCFA-1500 insurance claim form that were established to (a) give an individual rights to review his or her medical record, and (b) permit the government to verify information by way of computer match.

(a) ________________

(b) ________________

12–24 Providers must not provide information to parents or guardians of minors or incompetents when services are related to:

(a) ________________

(b) ________________

(c) ________________

(d) ________________

(e) ________________

CHECK YOUR HEARTBEAT! Turn to the end of the chapter for answers to these review sessions.

CLAIM PROCEDURES

Network providers are required to file all claim forms on behalf of TRICARE beneficiaries. Most "clean claims" (without clerical errors) are processed within 30 days. Generally, if a claim is not processed within 30 days, providers will pay interest on the claim. If a claim is submitted without obtaining required preauthorization, payment is reduced unless extenuating circumstances exist.

The Voice Response Unit (VRU) system can be used to obtain the following information regarding claims and claim submission:

- Benefits overview for TRICARE Standard
- Benefit changes (overview)
- Claim forms for TRICARE
- Claim status
- Customer service representative
- Information pamphlets
- Rates and procedures codes

TRICARE pays 100% for the first major procedure in a multiple procedure situation. Additional procedures occurring at the same operative session are paid at 50%; subsequent surgical procedures involving fingers and toes will be reimbursed at 25% of the contracted rate.

Claim Processing Areas

States are divided into regions, as shown in Figure 12–15, and assigned to a *Claims Processing Area.*

Claim Form Requirements

When using the HCFA-1500 claim form, the following requirements are emphasized. Some are unique to the TRICARE program.

- Emergency services—Include medical documentation to substantiate all emergency services.
- Provider identification number—Include the provider's Tax Identification Number in the bottom left portion of Block 33 regardless of whether the doctor

Figure 12–15. Map illustrating states divided into TRICARE regions for operational purposes and claim submission. Telephone numbers will assist in contacting the appropriate region where a beneficiary resides.

is a solo physician or practicing in a group (Fig. 12–16).

- Provider signature—Include the provider's original signature or use a signature stamp (must be on file with HNFS/PGBA).
- Referring "outside" physician—Include the referring physician's full name (address optional) and medical degree in Block 17, and the Tax Identification Number in Block 17a.
- Referring military physician—Include the MTF identification number in Block 19 for patients referred from an MTF provider.
- Services provided on behalf of another provider—Indicate "ON CALL" in a prominent place on the HCFA-1500 claim form (may use Block 19). Do not use red ink stamps.

Electronic Claim Submission

Professional and institutional claims may be submitted electronically to the TRICARE claims processing center. TRICARE advocates electronic submission to lower claim preparation costs, speed claim submission, and reduce claim errors. Electronic transfer can be done via physicians' offices (using system vendors), billing services, and claim clearinghouses. Most claims processing centers also accept other health insurance (OHI) information in electronic format. It is the provider's responsibility to secure and submit the EOB document from the primary insurance carrier with secondary TRICARE claims.

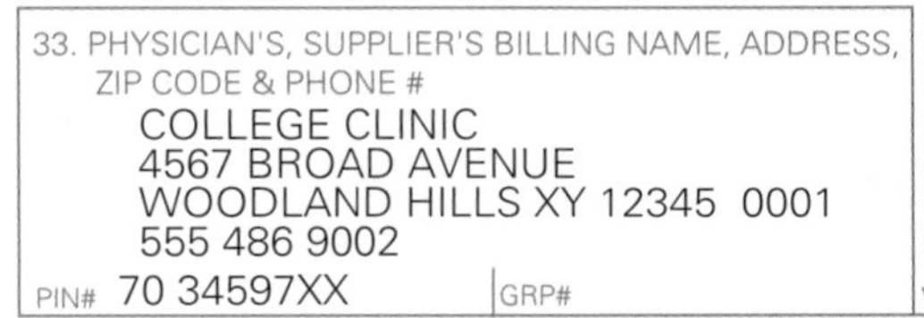

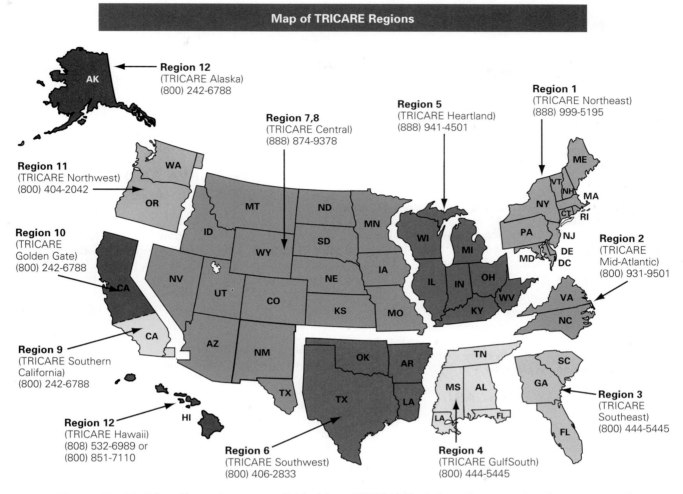

33. PHYSICIAN'S, SUPPLIER'S BILLING NAME, ADDRESS, ZIP CODE & PHONE #
COLLEGE CLINIC
4567 BROAD AVENUE
WOODLAND HILLS XY 12345 0001
555 486 9002
PIN# 70 34597XX GRP#

Figure 12–16. Block 33 of the HCFA-1500 claim form showing where the TRICARE provider's federal tax identification number is entered.

TRICARE Standard and CHAMPVA Claims

TRICARE Standard and CHAMPVA claims for participating physicians and nonparticipating physicians who accept assignment must be billed on the HCFA-1500 claim form and submitted to the claims processor. Refer to TRICARE or CHAMPVA block instructions in Appendix D for completing the HCFA-1500 claim form. Turn to Appendix D and refer to the template of a completed TRICARE case with no other insurance illustrated in Figure D–10. Refer to Figure D–11 for the template of a completed CHAMPVA case.

If the physician is nonparticipating and *does not accept assignment*, the patient completes the top portion of the HCFA-1500 claim form, attaches the physician's itemized statement or encounter form, and submits the claim. Alternatively, the patient may use the white TRICARE claim, Patient's Request for Medical Payment, DD Form 2642.

Time Limit

Claims must *arrive* at the processing center within 60 days from the date a service is provided, or, for inpatient care, within 60 days from the patient's date of discharge from the inpatient facility.

TRICARE Extra and TRICARE Prime Claims

TRICARE Extra and TRICARE Prime claims must be billed on the HCFA-1500 claim form and submitted to the claims processing center. Include the referral number from the MTF in Block 19 and the preauthorization numbers in Block 23 when applicable. The *beneficiary* does not file any claim forms under TRICARE Extra or TRICARE Prime programs when using network providers.

Time Limit

The following time limits are set for TRICARE Extra and TRICARE Prime claims to be *received* by the TRICARE contractor:

- Outpatient claims—60 days from the date of service.
- Inpatient claims—60 days from the date the patient was discharged from an inpatient facility.

A contractor may grant exemptions from filing deadlines. Submit a request including a complete explanation of the circumstances of the late filing and all available documentation supporting the request, along with the claim.

TRICARE Prime Remote and Supplemental Health Care Program Claims

Outpatient professional services are submitted using an HCFA-1500 claim form to the claims processing center. For specialty medical or surgical care and for behavioral health counseling and therapy sessions, a referral number provided by the HCF must be included on the claim form in Block 19. The POS options and NAS requirements do not apply to TPR and SHCP claims.

Time Limit

A claim must arrive at the processing center within 60 days from the date of service for outpatient care, and for inpatient care, within 60 days from the patient's date of discharge from the inpatient facility.

TRICARE/CHAMPVA AND OTHER INSURANCE COVERAGE

By law, TRICARE/CHAMPVA is second payer when a beneficiary is enrolled in **other health insurance (OHI).** OHI may be a civilian health plan, a health maintenance organization (HMO), or a preferred provider organization (PPO). There are three exceptions: (1) Medicaid, (2) coverage that is specifically designed to supplement TRICARE benefits, and (3) Indian Health.

When the patient has OHI that is primary, submit the claim following the primary insurance company's guidelines, using the HCFA-1500 claim form.

After payment (or a denial) is received from the primary carrier, attach the EOB that accompanies the check (or the denial letter), and bill TRICARE/CHAMPVA. The EOB must reflect the original amount billed, the patient's copayment amount, the allowed amount, and/or any discounts. The charges on the EOB must match the charges on the HCFA-1500 claim form. Mark "Yes" in Box 11d to indicate that there is another insurance plan. Enter the primary payer in Block 9, and indicate the amount paid by the other carrier in Block 29.

If the patient is submitting his or her claim to the primary insurance carrier, take these steps:

1. Use the other primary insurance carrier's claim form, if available.
2. After receiving payment from the primary carrier, bill TRICARE/CHAMPVA by completing the top section of the HCFA-1500 claim form.
3. Attach the physician's itemized statement or encounter form, which must include:
   a. Provider's name.
   b. Date the service/supply was provided.
   c. Place of treatment.
   d. Description of each service/supply.
   e. Procedure code number for each service/supply.
   f. Number/frequency of each service/supply.
   g. Fee for each service/supply.
   h. Diagnostic code number or description of condition for which treatment is being received.

Note: Canceled checks, cash register receipts, or billing statements showing only total charges are not acceptable.

4. Attach a photocopy of the EOB from the primary insurance carrier.

5. Send the TRICARE/CHAMPVA claim to the local claims processor (fiscal intermediary).

A coordination of benefits (COB) is necessary so that in double coverage situations there is no duplication of payment. Indicate this on the claim form by marking an "X" in Block 24J (COB). In such situations, TRICARE will pay the lower of:

1. The amount of TRICARE allowable charges remaining after the primary insurance carrier has paid its benefits, or
2. The amount TRICARE would have paid as a primary payer.

If payment by the primary insurance is greater than the amount allowed by TRICARE, no payment will be made by TRICARE and no cost-share can be collected from the beneficiary.

HMO Coverage and TRICARE

TRICARE considers HMO coverage to be the same as any other primary health insurance coverage. After the HMO has paid all it is going to pay, TRICARE shares the cost of care (including the HMO's user fees) under the following conditions:

- The physician must meet TRICARE provider certification standards.
- The type of care must be a TRICARE benefit and medically necessary.

TRICARE will not pay for emergency services received outside the HMO's normal service area. TRICARE will not cost-share services an individual obtains outside the HMO if the services are available through the HMO. For example, if an HMO provides psychiatric services but the patient does not like the HMO's psychiatrist and obtains services outside the HMO, then TRICARE will not pay anything on the claim.

Medicaid and TRICARE/CHAMPVA

File TRICARE/CHAMPVA claims first if the beneficiary is a recipient of the Medicaid program. File the claim to Medicaid second, if the amount paid by TRICARE/CHAMPVA is below the Medicaid fee schedule, or when services are not covered by TRICARE/CHAMPVA and covered by Medicaid.

Medicare and TRICARE

When a beneficiary becomes eligible for Medicare Part A, he or she must also purchase Part B in order for the professional services to be covered by TRICARE. TRICARE is considered secondary to Medicare for persons younger than age 65 who have Medicare Part A as a result of a disability and who have enrolled in Medicare Part B. If a beneficiary is over age 65 and does not qualify for Medicare, he or she must have a Social Security Notice of Disallowance on file in order for TRICARE to pay as the primary insurer.

TRICARE For Life

TRICARE For Life (TFL) claims are filed with the Medicare fiscal intermediary who will electronically transfer the claim to TRICARE for appropriate copayment, cost-share, and/or deductible payment. The physician's office will receive an EOB and RA (remittance advice) from both Medicare and TRICARE. All other health insurance plans that the beneficiary has in addition to Medicare and TRICARE must be billed prior to TRICARE. If a service/supply is normally a benefit of both Medicare and TRICARE, but Medicare denies payment due to "medical necessity" not being met, TRICARE will also deny payment.

Medicare and CHAMPVA

CHAMPVA is secondary payer to Medicare for persons younger than age 65 who are enrolled in Medicare Parts A and B and who are otherwise eligible for CHAMPVA. Submit claims to Medicare first and after receiving payment, attach a copy of the RA and submit a claim to CHAMPVA indicating how much Medicare paid in Block 29.

Third Party Liability and TRICARE/CHAMPVA

If the patient is in an automobile accident or receives an injury that may have third party involvement, the following two options are available for reimbursement:

Option 1. The patient completes TRICARE Form DD 2527 (Statement of Personal Injury—Possible Third Party Liability) and it is sent with the regular claim form. This form allows TRICARE to evaluate the circumstances of the accident and the possibility that the government may recover money for medical care from the person who injured the patient. Claims submitted with ICD-9-CM diagnosis related group (DRG) codes between 800 and 999 (Injury and Poisoning) trigger the suspicion that there might be third party litigation,

Expressions from Experience

As a 23-year-old single parent, working in a flexible medical billing office is definitely a great convenience. I enjoy a career as a medical insurance billing specialist that gives me the opportunity to exercise knowledge I already have, as well as learn more and more each day. Medical billing offers creativity, opportunity, and a chance to make decisions that will affect outcome.

Jimetria Smith
Insurance Billing Specialist
Radiology—Billing Service

and the claims processor may request the completion of DD Form 2527 if not included.

Option 2. The provider can submit claims exclusively to the third party liability carrier for reimbursement.

Workers' Compensation and TRICARE/CHAMPVA

If a TRICARE/CHAMPVA beneficiary sustains a work-related injury or illness, this becomes a workers' compensation case. The claim must be filed with the compensation insurance carrier. When all workers' compensation benefits have been exhausted, then TRICARE/CHAMPVA can be billed.

In some cases, it can happen that a determination has not been made as to whether the case is work-related and the claim is sent to the TRICARE/CHAMPVA claims processor. In those instances, the claims processor may file a lien with the workers' compensation carrier for recovery when the case is settled.

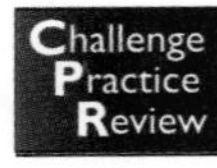

Pause and Practice CPR

REVIEW SESSIONS 12–25 THROUGH 12–31

Directions: *Complete the following questions as a review of information you have just read.*

12–25 What is the average time that it takes for a TRICARE claim to be processed? ____________

12–26 In a multiple surgical situation, what does TRICARE pay for the first major procedure? __________ And for the second procedure? __________

12–27 Does TRICARE accept electronic claims? __________

12–28 What is the time limit for submitting outpatient TRICARE claims? ________________
____

12–29 When a patient has other health insurance (OHI), is TRICARE considered the primary or secondary payer? __________

12–30 What are the three insurance types that are the exceptions to the above rule?

(a) ________________________________

(b) ________________________________

(c) ________________________________

12–31 When a patient has TRICARE and HMO coverage, who is the primary payer? ____________

CHECK YOUR HEARTBEAT! Turn to the end of the chapter for answers to these review sessions.

SUMMATION AND PREVIEW

Now that you have waded through the federal government's military service benefits programs, you can place the final building block for federal programs on your insurance foundation. When a patient presents in the physician's office who is a dependent of an active duty or retired military person, or a spouse or child of a veteran who is disabled, follow the guidelines you have just learned and you will have success in processing his or her insurance claims. Simple solutions to questions regarding military benefit programs may be found in the worktext or by contacting one of the references mentioned in Resources at the end of this chapter.

In the next chapter you will be learning the individual guidelines for processing insurance claims for workers' compensation patients. Such patients are seen in primary care physicians' offices (general practitioners, family practitioners, internists), as well as orthopedic offices, physical rehabilitation offices, and offices of a number of other specialists who may need to be consulted to provide care for an injured worker or person with an industrial illness.

GOLDEN RULE

Salute the military dependent program by complying with all regulations.

Chapter 12 Review and Practice

Study Session

Directions: *Review the objectives, key terms, and chapter information before completing the following study questions.*

12–1 Name the three plans in the TRICARE program.

(a) TRICARE Standard

(b) TRICARE Extra

(c) TRICARE Prime

12–2 What are the healthcare benefit options for a person who is retired from a career in the armed forces?

Retirees receive retirement pay & can remain in a TRICARE health Benefit Program for Life

12–3 Explain what DEERS is. ______________________________

12–4 If an MTF is unable to provide care for a pregnant TRICARE Standard beneficiary who lives inside a catchment area, what form is needed that allows the beneficiary to receive civilian care?

NAS

12–5 The status of a sponsor may be either active or retired.

12–6 In order to bill for noncovered services in the TRICARE program, the beneficiary needs to be informed in advance and in writing using the ______________________________ form.

12–7 Authorized referrals are valid for 60 days.

12–8 What are the referral and preauthorization requirements for TRICARE Standard patients in the following situations?

(a) Referral to TRICARE-certified providers: self referred

(b) Referral for all inpatient care: pre authorization

(c) Referral for certain outpatient services: pre authorization

12–9 What is the name of the office where the Health Care Finder (HCF) can be located?

TFC

12–10 The limit that the Uniformed Service family member enrolled in TRICARE pays each fiscal year is called the catastrophic cap. After the cap has been reached, TRICARE pays 100 % of the allowable charges for the rest of the year.

12–11 For a TRICARE Extra beneficiary, preauthorization requirements must be met for all inpatient hospital stays.

12–12 State the deductible for a TRICARE Extra beneficiary receiving *outpatient care* for a:

(a) Family member of an active duty E-3 service member. $__________

(b) Family member of a retired service member. $__________

(c) Family member of an active duty E-6 service member. $__________

(d) Maximum family deductible for an active duty E-6 service member with three family members. $__________

12–13 Providers who give care to TRICARE Prime beneficiaries must call the ______________ ______________ to verify eligibility.

12–14 What additional benefits are provided for TRICARE Prime beneficiaries who are not included in the TRICARE Standard program? ________________________________

____

____

12–15 To quality for TRICARE For Life, most beneficiaries must be eligible for ______________ and enrolled in ______________________.

12–16 For TRICARE Prime Remote specialty referrals, requests must be made through the ________________________________.

12–17 Why was the Supplemental Health Care Program (SHCP) developed and what benefits does it offer? ________________________________

____

____

____

12–18 TRICARE beneficiaries may self-refer to a network behavioral health provider for the first ______ outpatient counseling sessions per ______________ for TRICARE Prime, and per ______________ for TRICARE Extra and Standard.

12–19 Generally speaking, CHAMPVA was created to cover ________________________ ______________.

12–20 In order for spouses and children to receive CHAMPVA benefits, the veteran has to be either (a) or (b):

(a) ____

(b) ____

12–21 When the TRICARE Prime beneficiary receives care from a specialty provider, what is the rule about obtaining written release of information? ______________________

____

12–22 In Block 33, what is the provider number that the physician uses to report services in this block? ________________________________

12–23 Who are TRICARE For Life claims filed with? ________________________

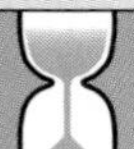

Billing Break

Time Started
Time Finished
Total Time

Case 12–1 Shannon L. Rochester

Directions: *Follow these steps to complete the HCFA-1500 insurance claim form for a TRICARE case using OCR guidelines.*

1. Copy the HCFA-1500 insurance claim form found in Appendix F (Form 09).
2. Refer to the Patient Information form for Case 12–1 and abstract information to complete the top portion of the HCFA-1500 claim form.
3. Refer to the Medical Record for Case 12–1 to abstract information for the bottom portion of the HCFA-1500 claim form.
4. Copy the Medical Record Worksheet found in Appendix F (Form 12) to use when abstracting information from the chart note.
5. Use the "HCFA-1500 Claim Form Block-by-Block Instructions" for TRICARE patients found in Appendix D and the TRICARE template (Fig. D–10) for guidance and block help.
6. Use your procedure codebook to determine the correct code number(s) and modifier(s) for each professional service/procedure rendered.
7. Refer to the fee schedule in Appendix B for mock fees.
8. Use your diagnostic codebook to determine the correct diagnoses.
9. Address the claim to the TRICARE fiscal intermediary and date the claim 03/28/20XX.
10. Copy and prepare the ledger card found in Appendix F (Form 07) for the patient. Complete the ledger by posting each transaction in this case and indicating when you have billed the insurance carrier.
11. Note: On 3/10/XX (per patient's medical record) a TRICARE preauthorization request is sent requesting surgery. If you would like to complete this form now, instructions may be found in Exercise Exchange 12–1.

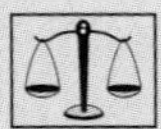

WEIGH YOUR PROGRESS. Turn to the Assignment Score Sheet in Appendix F (Form 10) and record the information to track your success. Your instructor may ask that you include a Performance Evaluation Checklist, and if so, copy Form 11 found in Appendix F and attach it to your insurance claim.

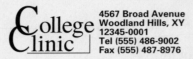

4567 Broad Avenue
Woodland Hills, XY
12345-0001
Tel (555) 486-9002
Fax (555) 487-8976

REGISTRATION
(PLEASE PRINT)

Account # 1884 — Today's Date: 01/26/XX

PATIENT INFORMATION

Name: Rochester (Last Name) Shannon (First Name) L. (Initial) — Soc. Sec. # 523-XX-9050

Address: 2984 Figuroa Street — Home Phone: (555) 487-7694

City: Woodland Hills — State: XY — Zip: 12345

Single___ Married ✓ Separated___ Divorced___ — Sex M___ F ✓ — Birthdate: 10/17/1970

Patient Employed by: Greatview National Bank — Occupation: Bank Teller

Business Address: 9523 Dolphin Way, Woodland Hills, XY — Business Phone: (555) 487-2550

Spouse's Name: David — Employed by: U.S. Army — Occupation: Missile Technician

Business Address: ______ — Business Phone: (555) 777-0070

Reason for Visit: Pregnancy — If accident: ___ Auto___ Employment___ Other___

By whom were you referred? TRICARE Office

In case of emergency, who should be notified? David Rochester (Name) Husband (Relation to Patient) — Phone: (555) 777-0070

PRIMARY INSURANCE

Insured/Subscriber: Rochester (Last Name) David (First Name) M. (Initial)

Relation to Patient: Husband — Birthdate: 10/01/1970 — Soc. Sec.#: 922-XX-4343

Address (if different from patient's) ______

City ______ State ______ Zip ______

Insurance Company: TRICARE Standard

Insurance Address: PO Box 5000 Sunset City, XY 12345

Insurance Identification Number: 922-XX-4343 — Group # ______

ADDITIONAL INSURANCE

Is patient covered by additional insurance? Yes___ No ✓

Subscriber Name ______ Relation to Patient ______ Birthdate ______

Address (if different from patient's) ______ Phone ______

City ______ State ______ Zip ______

Subscriber Employed by ______ Buisness Phone ______

Insurance Company ______ Soc. Sec. # ______

Insurance Address ______

Insurance Identification Number ______ Group # ______

ASSIGNMENT AND RELEASE

I, the undersigned, certify that I (or my dependent) have insurance coverage with TRICARE Standard (Name of Insurance Company(ies)) and assign directly to Dr. Caesar insurance benefits, if any, otherwise payable to me for services rendered. I understand that I am financially responsible for all charges whether or not paid by insurance. I hereby consent for the doctor to release all information necessary to secure the payment of benefits. I authorize the use of this signature on all insurance submissions.

Shannon L. Rochester — Self — 01/26/XX
Responsible Party Signature — Relationship — Date

ORDER # 58-8426 @BIBBERO SYSTEMS, INC. •PETALUMA, CALIFORNIA• TO REORDER CALL TOLL FREE (800)242-9330

Medical Record

Account number: 1884
Patient's name: Rochester, Shannon L.
Date of birth: 10/17/70

Date	Progress Notes

03/09/XX An established patient of Dr. Caesar's from Point Mugu Military Base, Mrs. Rochester presents complaining of urinary frequency, dribbling urine with exercise and/or coughing (stress incontinence), and pain during intercourse (dyspareunia). A D HX is taken–patient is gravida 5 para 6 (5 pregnancies with 6 viable deliveries). I delivered her twin girls approximately 6 months ago.

A D PX is performed and a pelvic examination reveals severe uterine prolapse. Both the anterior and posterior portions of her vagina are also prolapsed. A urine sample is collected for complete urinalysis (dip-stick and microscopy) which is negative for blood and bacteria. Surgical options are discussed and the patient decides to proceed with surgery as soon as possible; colporrhaphy with uterine suspension. Imp: cystocele, rectocele and uterine prolapse. Our surgical scheduler will call Mrs. Rochester with a date. Patient to return for preoperative appointment the week of surgery. M/MDM.

Bertha Caesar, MD

03/10XX TRICARE Preauthorization request sent for surgery scheduled on 03/24/XX–5 day stay; College Hospital.

Leigh Ray, Ins. Dept

03/22/XX Patient presents for preoperative appointment. BP 120/60, temp. 98.6, no colds, flu, or any other complaints. Patient to have preoperative laboratory work done at College Hospital this afternoon. Surgical consents signed (PF HX/PX SF/MDM).

Bertha Caesar, MD

03/24/XX Patient admitted to College Hospital (C HX/PX M/MDM). Performed a uterine suspension with anterior and posterior repair (colporrhaphy) to correct uterine prolapse and complete cystocele/rectocele. Operation went well. Patient will be off work for 6 weeks; return to work May 7, 20XX.

Bertha Caesar, MD

03/25/XX Hospital visit (EPF HX/PX M/MDM). Patient is ambulating well. Will remove catheter tomorrow.

Bertha Caesar, MD

03/26/XX Hospital visit (EPF HX/PX M/MDM). Patient is continuing to improve. Catheter removed.

Bertha Caesar, MD

03/27/XX Hospital visit (EPF HX/PX M/MDM). Patient is able to void without catheter. Discharge scheduled for tomorrow.

Bertha Caesar, MD

03/28/XX Patient discharged to home (discharge management 30 minutes). Return to office in 2 weeks.

Bertha Caesar, MD

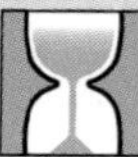

Billing Break

Time Started
Time Finished
Total Time

Case 12–2 Rodney L. Ramirez

Directions: *Follow these steps to complete the HCFA-1500 insurance claim form for a CHAMPVA case using OCR guidelines.*

1. Copy the HCFA-1500 insurance claim form found in Appendix F (Form 09).
2. Refer to the Patient Information form for Case 12–2 and abstract information to complete the top portion of the HCFA-1500 claim form.
3. Refer to the Medical Record for Case 12–2 to abstract information for the bottom portion of the HCFA-1500 claim form.
4. Copy the Medical Record Coding Worksheet found in Appendix F (Form 12) to use when abstracting information from the chart note.
5. Use the "HCFA-1500 Claim Form Block-by-Block Instructions" for CHAMPVA patients found in Appendix D and the CHAMPVA template (Fig. D–11) for guidance and block help.
6. Use your procedure codebook to determine the correct code number(s) and modifier(s) for each professional service/procedure rendered.
7. Refer to the fee schedule in Appendix B for mock fees.
8. Use your diagnostic codebook to determine the correct diagnoses.
9. Address the claim to CHAMPVA and date the claim 06/19/20XX.
10. Copy and prepare the ledger card found in Appendix F (Form 07) for the patient. Complete the ledger by posting each transaction in this case and indicating when you have billed the insurance carrier.

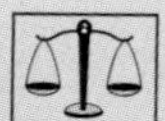

WEIGH YOUR PROGRESS. Turn to the Assignment Score Sheet in Appendix F and enter the information to track your success. Your instructor may ask that you include a Performance Evaluation Checklist, and if so, copy Form 11 found in Appendix F and attach it to your insurance claim.

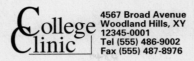

4567 Broad Avenue
Woodland Hills, XY
12345-0001
Tel (555) 486-9002
Fax (555) 487-8976

REGISTRATION
(PLEASE PRINT)

Account # 3992   Today's Date: 06/09/XX

PATIENT INFORMATION

Name Ramirez (Last Name) Rodney (First Name) L. (Initial)   Soc. Sec. # 450-XX-6713

Address 41 Sheridan Way   Home Phone (555) 486-9436

City Woodland Hills   State XY   Zip 12345

Single ✓ Married ___ Separated ___ Divorced ___   Sex M ✓ F ___   Birthdate 06/23/1933

Patient Employed by Retired Air Force   Occupation ___

Business Address ___   Business Phone ___

Spouse's Name N/A   Employed by: ___ Occupation ___

Business Address ___   Business Phone ___

Reason for Visit ___ If accident: ___ Auto ___ Employment ___ Other ___

By whom were you referred? ___

In case of emergency, who should be notified? Rodeen Ramirez (Name) Daughter (Relation to Patient) Phone (555) 486-2245

PRIMARY INSURANCE

Insured/Subscriber Ramirez (Last Name) Rodney (First Name) L. (Initial)

Relation to Patient Self   Birthdate ___   Soc. Sec.# ___

Address (if different from patient's) ___

City ___ State ___ Zip ___

Insurance Company CHAMPVA VA Station 067

Insurance Address PO Box 65024 Denver, CO 80206-9024

Insurance Identification Number 450-XX-6713   Group # ___

ADDITIONAL INSURANCE

Is patient covered by additional insurance? Yes ___ No ✓

Subscriber Name ___ Relation to Patient ___ Birthdate ___

Address (if different from patient's) ___ Phone ___

City ___ State ___ Zip ___

Subscriber Employed by ___ Buisness Phone ___

Insurance Company ___ Soc. Sec. # ___

Insurance Address ___

Insurance Identification Number ___ Group # ___

ASSIGNMENT AND RELEASE

I, the undersigned, certify that I (or my dependent) have insurance coverage with CHAMPVA (Name of Insurance Company(ies)) and assign directly to Dr. Cutler insurance benefits, if any, otherwise payable to me for services rendered. I understand that I am financially responsible for all charges whether or not paid by insurance. I hereby consent for the doctor to release all information necessary to secure the payment of benefits. I authorize the use of this signature on all insurance submissions.

Responsible Party Signature *Rodney L. Ramirez*   Relationship *Self*   Date 06/09/XX

Medical Record

Account number: 3992
Patient's name: Ramirez, Rodney L.
Date of birth: 06/23/33

Date	Progress Notes
	06/09/XX 69-year-old retired Navy Captain sent for surgical consultation from Castle Air Force base (authorization no. 60983321). Diagnostic ultrasound report sent which shows a mass (approximately 5 cm by 6 cm) in the left neck region. I performed a C HX/PX with M/MDM. Surgical risks and side effects are discussed and a decision is made for surgery. Patient taken off work (effective tomorrow) until surgery performed. 784.2 Clarence Cutler, MD
	06/12/XX Patient admitted to ambulatory surgical center at College Hospital for surgical removal of neck mass. An excision is made in the left neck. The 6 cm mass is located below the fascia and the tumor is completely dissected from the subfascia (connective tissue). On gross examination it appears benign. Closure of deep fascia with 3-0 Vicryl; skin closed with 4-0 Maxon. Steri-strips applied. Patient tolerated surgery well and will go home this afternoon. RTO in 3 days. CPT 21556 Clarence Cutler, MD
	06/15/XX Patient returns to office after outpatient surgery. Minimal swelling in left neck area. Patient feels well and would like to return to work. Recommend minimal activities at home until sutures are removed in 4 days and pathology report reviewed. PF HX/PX SF/MDM. Clarence Cutler, MD
	06/19/XX Patient returns to office for suture removal. Pathology confirms benign neoplasm of soft tissue. Sutures removed; wound healing well. Patient can return to work tomorrow (PF HX/PX SF/MDM). 215.0 Clarence Cutler, MD

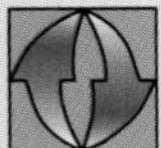

Exercise Exchange

12–1 **Complete a TRICARE Preauthorization/Referral Request Form.**

Directions

1. Refer to the Patient Registration form, Medical Record, and completed HCFA-1500 claim form from Billing Break exercise 12–1 for Shannon L. Rochester.
2. Use Form 14 in Appendix F (TRICARE Preauthorization/Referral Request Form) referring to Figure 12–9 for guidance and complete a routine TRICARE preauthorization request for Mrs. Rochester.
3. Dr. Caesar is the patient's Primary Care Manager and the contact person at the TRICARE Service Center is Pamela Long (telephone (555) 263-9000, fax (555) 263-9191).
4. You are faxing the request to Garth Lee, Health Care Finder at the Point Mugu Military Base (telephone (555) 263-9000, fax (555) 263-9191).
5. Be sure and include a summary of the patient's clinical history and supporting documentation abstracted from her progress notes.

12–2 **Edit a HCFA-1500 Claim Form prior to Electronic Submission for a TRICARE Case.**

Scenario: Brenda L. Belchere is an established patient with Bertha Caesar, MD, and her file indicates private insurance coverage through her parents. The insurance claim for her visit on 5/10/20XX was computer-generated on an HCFA-1500 claim form and sent to the private carrier. The claim was denied indicating that she is no longer covered. When telephoning Brenda, it was discovered that she married Air Force Lieutenant David A. Mercado last month (date of birth 9/22/75, Social Security number 456-XX-9018) and they now live at 1414 Seward Street, Orange Grove, XY 12345, telephone (555) 967-2843. She cancelled the private insurance policy she had through her parents on 4/18/XX and is a beneficiary for TRICARE Standard effective 5/01/XX.

Directions

1. Review TRICARE block instructions in Appendix D and the template for TRICARE patients (Fig. D–10).
2. Using TRICARE guidelines, mark all errors and/or omissions on the claim form with a highlighter pen in preparation for sending the claim electronically to the TRICARE Fiscal Intermediary.
3. Write a list (in numerical order according to blocks) indicating all of the changes that need to be made in the computer system before processing the insurance claim electronically to the TRICARE Fiscal Intermediary.

Top: ____________________

Block _____ ____________________

Block _____ ____________________

Block _____ ____________________

Block _____ ____________________

Block _____ ____________________

Block _____ ____________________

Block _____ ____________________

Block _____ ____________________

Block _____ ____________________

Block _____ ____________________

Block _____ ____________________

Block _____ ____________________

Block _____ ____________________

Block _____ ____________________

Block _____ ____________________

Block _____ ____________________

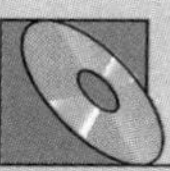

Computer Session—Case F

Directions: *Insert the CD-ROM into the computer and locate and complete Case 7—a TRICARE case.*

HEALTH EAST INSURANCE COMPANY
PO BOX 1212
MANCHESTER XY 12345

1. MEDICARE [ ] (Medicare #) MEDICAID [ ] (Medicaid #) CHAMPUS [ ] (Sponsor's SSN) CHAMPVA [ ] (VA File #) GROUP Health Plan [X] (SSN or ID) FECA BLK LUNG [ ] (SSN) OTHER [ ] (ID)

1a. INSURED I.D. NUMBER (FOR PROGRAM IN ITEM 1): 1234556 444

2. PATIENT'S NAME (Last Name, First Name, Middle Initial): BELCHERE BRENDA L

3. PATIENT'S BIRTH DATE MM DD YYYY: 06 16 1980 SEX M [ ] F [X]

4. INSURED'S NAME (LAST NAME, FIRST NAME, MIDDLE INITIAL): BELCHERE JOSEPH Q

5. PATIENT'S ADDRESS (No., Street): 173 C STREET

6. PATIENT RELATIONSHIP TO INSURED: Self [ ] Spouse [ ] Child [X] Other [ ]

7. INSURED'S ADDRESS (No, Street): SAME

CITY: ORANGE GROVE STATE: XY

8. PATIENT STATUS: Single [X] Married [ ] Other [ ]

CITY STATE

ZIP CODE: 12345 TELEPHONE (Include Area Code): (555) 967 4321

Employed [X] Full-Time Student [ ] Part-Time Student [ ]

ZIP CODE TELEPHONE (INCLUDE AREA CODE) ( )

9. OTHER INSURED'S NAME (Last Name, First Name, Middle Initial)

10. IS PATIENT'S CONITION RELATED TO:

11. INSURED'S POLICY GROUP OR FECA NUMBER

a. OTHER INSURED'S POLICY OR GROUP NUMBER

a. EMPLOYMENT? (CURRENT OR PREVIOUS) [ ] YES [X] NO

a. INSURED'S DATE OF BIRTH MM DD YYYY SEX M [ ] F [ ]

b. OTHER INSURED'S DATE OF BIRTH MM DD YY SEX M [ ] F [ ]

b. AUTO ACCIDENT? [ ] YES [X] NO PLACE (State)

b. EMPLOYER'S NAME OR SCHOOL NAME

c. EMPLOYER'S NAME OR SCHOOL NAME

c. OTHER ACCIDENT? [ ] YES [X] NO

c. INSURANCE PLAN NAME OR PROGRAM NAME

d. INSURANCE PLAN NAME OR PROGRAM NAME

10d. RESERVED FOR LOCAL USE

d. IS THERE ANOTHER HEALTH BENEFIT PLAN? [ ] YES [X] NO *If yes*, return to and complete item 9 a-d

READ BACK OF FORM BEFORE COMPLETING & SIGNING THIS FORM

12. PATIENT'S OR AUTHORIZED PERSON'S SIGNATURE. I authorize the release of any medical or other information necessary to process this claim. I also request payment of government benefits either to myself or to the party who accepts assignment below.

SIGNED SOF DATE

13. INSURED'S OR AUTHORIZED PERSON'S SIGNATURE. I authorize payment of medical benefits to the undersigned physician or supplier for services described below

SIGNED SOF

14. DATE OF CURRENT: MM DD YY ILLNESS (First symptom) OR INJURY (Accident) OR PREGNANCY

15. IF PATIENT HAS HAD SAME OR SIMILAR ILLNESS GIVE FIRST DATE MM DD YYYY

16. DATES PATIENT UNABLE TO WORK IN CURRENT OCCUPATION FROM MM DD YYYY TO MM DD YYYY

17. NAME OF REFERRING PHYSICIAN OR OTHER SOURCE: GERALD PRACTON MD

17a. I.D. NUMBER OF REFERRING PHYSICIAN: 46278897XX

18. HOSPITALIZATION DATES RELATED TO CURRENT SERVICES FROM MM DD YYYY TO MM DD YYYY

19. RESERVED FOR LOCAL USE

20. OUTSIDE LAB? [ ] YES [X] NO $ CHARGES

21. DIAGNOSIS OR NATURE OF ILLNESS OR INJURY. (RELATE ITEMS 1,2,3 OR 4 TO ITEM 24E BY LINE)

1. V2502
2.
3.
4.

22. MEDICAID RESUBMISSION CODE ORIGINAL REF. NO.

23. PRIOR AUTHORIZATION NUMBER

24. A DATE(S) OF SERVICE From MM DD YY	To MM DD YY	B Place of Service	C Type of Service	D PROCEDURES, SERVICES, OR SUPPLIES (Explain Unusual Circumstances) CPT/HCPCS	MODIFIER	E DIAGNOSIS CODE	F $ CHARGES	G DAYS OR UNITS	H EPSDT Family Plan	I EMG	J COB	K RESERVED FOR LOCAL USE
05 10 20XX		11		99212		1	28 55	1			43	056757XX
05 10 20XX		11		99070		1	25 00	1			43	056757XX

25. FEDERAL TAX I.D. NUMBER: 72 57130XX SSN [ ] EIN [X]

26. PATIENT'S ACCOUNT NO.: 4321

27. ACCEPT ASSIGNMENT? (For govt. claims, see back) [X] YES [ ] NO

28. TOTAL CHARGE $ 53 55

29. AMOUNT PAID $

30. BALANCE DUE $ 53 55

31. SIGNATURE OF PHYSICIAN OR SUPPLIER INCLUDING DEGREES OR CREDENTIALS (I certify that the statements on the reverse apply to this bill and are made a part thereof)

BERTHA CAESAR MD

SIGNED Bertha Caesar MD. DATE 051020xx

32. NAME AND ADDRESS OF FACILITY WHERE SERVICES WERE RENDERED (If other than home or office)

SAME

33. PHYSICIAN'S, SUPPLIER'S BILLING NAME, ADDRESS, ZIP CODE & PHONE #

COLLEGE CLINIC
4567 BROAD AVENUE
WOODLAND HILLS XY 12345 0001
555 486 9002

PIN# GRP# 3664021CC

reference initials

NOTES

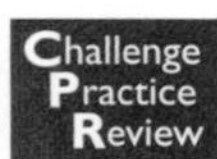

CPR Session: Answers

REVIEW SESSIONS 12–1 THROUGH 12–5

12–1 three
12–2 sponsor
12–3 beneficiary
12–4 DEERS
12–5 A military treatment facility is a Uniformed Services hospital where active duty service personal and their TRICARE-eligible dependents receive many of their healthcare services.

REVIEW SESSIONS 12–6 THROUGH 12–9

12–6 Dependents and survivors (age 10 years and older) of active duty personnel and retirees.
12–7 (a) sponsor's rank
(b) sponsor's pay grade
(c) sponsor's status
12–8 TRICARE-certified providers, authorized
12–9 Health Care Finder (HCF), preauthorization

PRACTICE SESSIONS 12–10 THROUGH 12–12

12–10 (a) \$55.20 (69 × .80)
(b) \$13.80 (69 × .20)
(c) \$6 (75 − 69)
12–11 (a) \$15.20 (69 − 50 = 19) (19 × .80 = 15.20)
(b) \$53.80 (19 × .20 = 3.80 + 50 = 53.80)
(c) \$6 (75 − 69)
12–12 (a) \$51.75 (69 × .75)
(b) \$17.25 (69 × .25)
(c) \$6 (75 − 69)

REVIEW SESSIONS 12–13 AND 12–14

12–13 (a)
12–14 (a) they are participating providers
(b) they have discount agreements
(c) they are required to file claims

REVIEW SESSIONS 12–15 THROUGH 12–19

12–15 12 months
12–16 primary care manager (PCM)
12–17 primary care manager (PCM), Health Care Finder (HCF)
12–18 zero, zero
12–19 providing the ability to self-refer for any TRICARE-covered nonemergency services to any civilian TRICARE-certified provider, whether in network or not.

REVIEW SESSIONS 12–20 THROUGH 12–24

12–20 service benefit program
12–21 VA regional office
12–22 (a) \$50 per person or \$100 per family per calendar year
(b) 75%
(c) \$7,500
12–23 (a) Privacy Act of 1974
(b) Computer Matching and Privacy Protection Act of 1988
12–24 (a) acquired immunodeficiency syndrome (AIDS)
(b) alcoholism
(c) abortion
(d) drug abuse
(e) venereal disease

REVIEW SESSIONS 12–25 THROUGH 12–31

12–25 30 days
12–26 100%, 50%
12–27 yes
12–28 must *arrive* in the claims processing center 60 days from the date of service
12–29 secondary
12–30 (a) Medicaid
(b) TRICARE supplemental insurance
(c) Indian Health
12–31 the HMO carrier

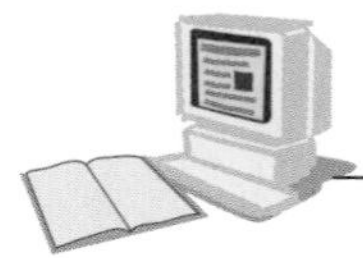

Resources

To improve your understanding of TRICARE programs, log onto the TRICARE University web site. The TRICARE (online) University provides an overview of TRICARE administration, offers an introduction to TRICARE options and benefits, reviews eligibility status and categories, and summarizes claim form requirements and submission policies. A "Course Objectives" button takes students through information related to objectives, prerequisites, and requirements. A "Navigation Tutorial" is available to learn how to navigate through various features and functions available in the course.

To obtain further information, a list of resources is provided that is available on the Internet and from TRICARE Management Activity (TMA).

Internet

- TRICARE Management Activity (TMA)—Following are some categories and subcategories listed under TRICARE's web site: www.tricare.osd.mil
  - Regional web sites
  - TRICARE acronyms and terms
  - TRICARE glossary
  - TRICARE provider information
    - Ambulatory surgeries
    - Claims
    - DRG weights and CMAC rates (allows download of pricing information for single CPT codes within a selected local)
    - Provider directory
    - Provider handbook
    - TRICARE manuals (policy manual, operational manual, automated data processing manual, and so forth).
    - TRICARE news releases (May 1995–current)
- CHAMPVA web site: www.va.gov/hac/champva

NOTES

Objectives

After reading this chapter and completing the exercise sessions, you should be able to:

Learning Objectives:

- ✔ State the purpose of workers' compensation laws.
- ✔ Enumerate who is covered under federal and state workers' compensation laws.
- ✔ Define terminology and abbreviations pertinent to workers' compensation cases and disability insurance programs.
- ✔ Compare workers' compensation insurance and employers' liability insurance.
- ✔ Define nondisability, temporary disability, and permanent disability claims.
- ✔ Describe benefits of workers' compensation and compare with benefits for disability income insurance.
- ✔ Discuss OSHA's role in protecting employees.
- ✔ Name federal disability benefit programs.
- ✔ Identify states that have state disability insurance programs.
- ✔ Explain voluntary disability insurance.

Performance Objectives:

- ✔ Complete a Doctor's First Report of Occupational Injury and Illness form.
- ✔ Complete a HCFA-1500 insurance claim form for a workers' compensation case.

Key Terms

accident
adjudication
benefit period
(BR) by report
case manager
claims examiner
coal miners
compromise and release (C and R)
deposition
disability income insurance
ergonomic
exclusion
extraterritorial
fee schedule
injury
insurance adjuster
lien
medical-legal (ML) evaluation
medical service order
nondisability (ND) claim
occupational illness
Occupational Safety and Health Administration (OSHA)
partial disability
permanent and stationary (P and S)
permanent disability (PD)
petition
second injury fund
Social Security Disability Insurance (SSDI)
State Disability Insurance (SDI)
sub rosa films
temporary disability (TD)
temporary disability insurance (TDI)
third party liability
third party subrogation
total disability
unemployment compensation disability (UCD)
voluntary disability insurance
waiting period (WP)
waiver of premium
work hardening
workers' compensation insurance

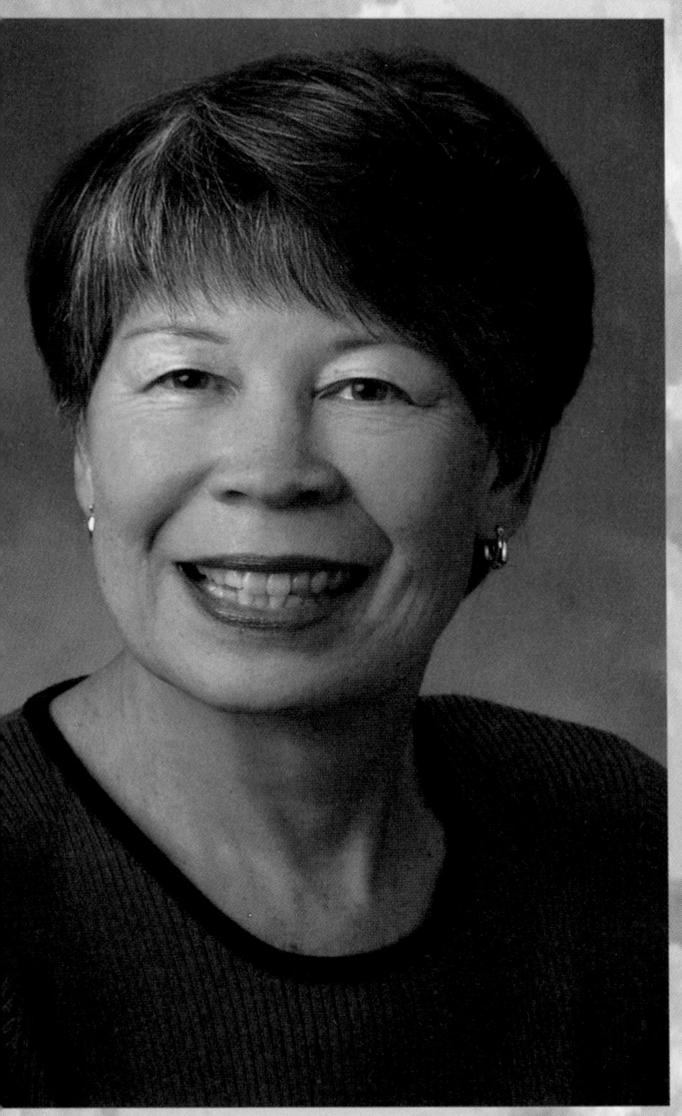

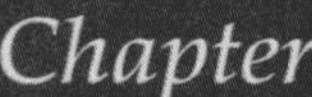

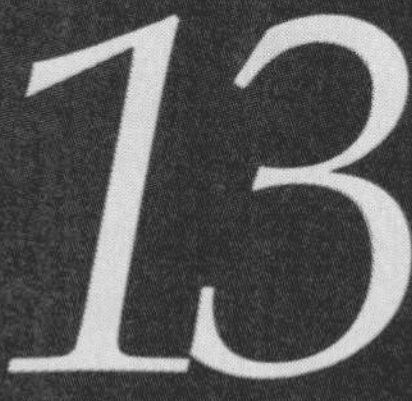

Chapter 13

I chose a profession in the medical field because I enjoy interacting with patients and working in a professional environment. I first worked as a receptionist for a family practice group. Next, I worked for a dermatology group and learned the importance of proper coding, insurance billing, and posting payments.

After seventeen years I went to work for a small orthopedic group and am now employed by fourteen orthopedic surgeons with six office locations. Due to the size of this practice, we have many employees in the billing department, each specializing in a specific area. I process all workers' compensation claims, appeal claims that are not reimbursed properly, and post payments. If reimbursement is not satisfactory, my job is to substantiate the reason I feel that the physician was not paid properly. The greatest satisfaction is when the bill reviewer is in agreement with the appeal and grants additional reimbursement.

Kara Chang
Workers' Compensation Specialist
Orthopedics

Workers' Compensation Coverage and Other Disability Programs

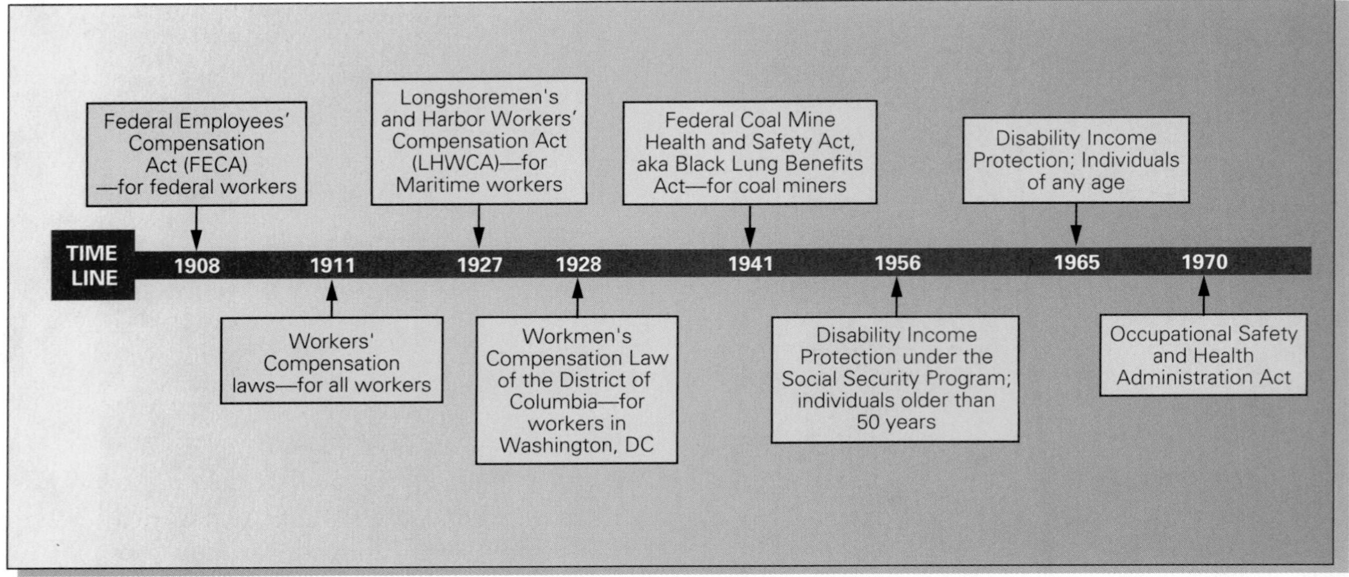

ORIGINS OF WORKERS' COMPENSATION

Beginning in the early 1900s, workers' compensation laws were gradually enacted allowing injured employees to receive medical care. An *employee* is considered an individual who works for another, generally providing labor or services in exchange for wages. A physician who is incorporated is also considered an employee under workers' compensation laws. Workers' compensation insurance is the most important coverage written to insure industrial accidents and illness. Today, all states have workers' compensation laws.

Workers' Compensation Reform

As compensation costs increased for insurance companies and employers, insurance carriers began to deny coverage, causing companies to close their doors. Some businesses began relocating in states which offered lower premiums. Soon widespread corruption evolved throughout the system, resulting in high medical costs and elevated legal expenses. An effort to reduce costs and minimize abuse of the system resulted in *workers' compensation reform laws.* These laws deal with the following:

- Antifraud legislation and increased penalties for workers' compensation fraud
- Antireferral provisions (i.e., restriction of the physician to refer patients for diagnostic studies to any sites where the physician has a financial interest)
- Preauthorization for major operations and expensive diagnostic tests
- Documented proof of medical necessity for tests or treatment
- Monetary limits on vocational rehabilitation
- Incorporation of managed care plans by employers, some with restriction of providers (e.g., HMOs)
- Increase in occupational safety measures
- Development of fee schedules
- Review of medical bills
- Use of mediators instead of lawyers to reach agreements between employers and employees
- Prosecution of physicians, lawyers, and employees who abuse the system
- Utilization of a disabled worker in another division of the company he or she was employed in so that the person may be gainfully employed while not using an injured body part.

Workers' Compensation Managed Care

An increasing number of employers are trying the managed care option instead of regular compensation contracts. Plans are not uniform and may limit the choice of providers, use fee schedule–based payments, require precertification for certain procedures, implement hospital and medical bill review, and incorporate utilization review of medical services. Some states have adopted laws authorizing managed care programs, and other states are conducting pilot programs to test the effectiveness of managed care networks.

WORKERS' COMPENSATION STATUTES

Workers' compensation statutes relieve the employer of liability for injury received or illness contracted by an employee in a work situation except in cases of gross negligence. They also enable the employee to be more easily and quickly compensated for loss of wages, medical expenses, and permanent disability. There are two kinds of statutes under workers' compensation described as follows.

Federal Laws

Federal compensation laws apply to:

- Government workers
- Miners
- Maritime workers

All employees who work for federal agencies are covered by a number of federal workers' compensation laws. Refer to the timeline at the beginning of this chapter for names of the laws and the dates they became effective.

State Laws

State compensation laws vary in each state and apply to:

- Private employees
- State employees

Workers not protected by federal statutes are covered by state laws. Federal law mandates that states set up laws to meet minimum requirements.

Self-Insurance

In 48 states and territories, large employers may qualify as self-insurers. If an employer does not purchase workers' compensation insurance from a private insurance company, the employer must self-insure and have enough cash in reserve to cover the cost of medical care for all workers who suffer work-related injuries or illness. A self-insuring company pays for medical expenses instead of insurance premiums. Benefits are variable from plan to plan and precertification of certain services may be required. Generally, the state insurance commissioner does not have jurisdiction over such plans. Some states may have laws that regulate self-insurers.

Compulsory and Elective Laws

Most state compensation laws are *compulsory laws*, meaning each employer must accept its provisions and provide for specified benefits.

The states of New Jersey and Texas have *elective laws*, where the employer may accept or reject the law. If the statute or the law is rejected, the employer loses the three common-law defenses, which are (1) assumption of risk, (2) negligence of fellow employee, and (3) contributory negligence.

Interstate Laws

If a worker's occupation takes him or her into another state, questions may arise as to which state's law determines payment of compensation benefits. Most compensation laws are **extraterritorial,** that is, effective outside of the state, by either specific provisions or court decision.

Provisions of Workers' Compensation Laws

Workers' compensation laws have been developed for the following reasons:

1. To provide the best available medical care necessary to achieve maximal recovery and ensure the prompt return to work of any injured or ill employee
2. To provide income to the injured or ill worker or to his or her dependents, regardless of fault
3. To reduce court delays, costs, and workloads arising out of personal injury litigation
4. To eliminate payment of fees to attorneys and witnesses, as well as time-consuming trials and appeals
5. To encourage maximal employer interest in safety and rehabilitation
6. To promote the study and causes of accidents and reduce preventable accidents and human suffering

Employer Liability Insurance

In addition to workers' compensation protection, statutes also require that employers have employers' liability insurance. The difference between workers' compensation insurance and employers' liability insurance is that the latter is coverage that protects the employer against claims arising out of bodily injury to others or damage to their property when someone is on the premises of the business. It is not considered insurance coverage for someone who is working at a business site. However, employers still occasionally use employers' liability coverage to protect themselves when their employees do not come within the scope of a compensation law.

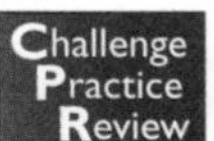

Pause and Practice CPR

CHALLENGE SESSIONS 13–1 AND 13–2

Directions: *Read the following two scenarios and use critical thinking skills to determine what type of insurance applies to each situation, employer liability insurance or workers' compensation insurance.*

13–1 Mary Beth works for Dr. Practon as an insurance billing specialist. She was carrying a box of files to the storage room and wrenched her back as she put them away.

____

13–2 Adel is a patient of Dr. Practon. She arrived at the office one rainy Monday morning and as she opened the door she slipped and fell, breaking her wrist.

____

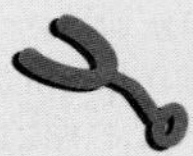

CHECK YOUR HEARTBEAT! Turn to the end of the chapter for answers to these challenge sessions.

FUNDING WORKERS' COMPENSATION

A number of states permit employers to purchase insurance from either a competitive state fund or a private insurance company. The employer pays the premiums for workers' compensation insurance. The amount of coverage varies, depending on the employee's job and the risks involved in job performance.

When a workers' compensation claim is filed, premiums may increase to help cover the injured or ill worker's benefits. In some instances, an employer may be reluctant to file a workers' compensation report with the state, preferring to pay medical expenses out of pocket to avoid premium rate increases. It is illegal for an employer to fail to report a work-related accident when it is required by state law. Some states consider it a misdemeanor and different penalties can be imposed, such as imprisonment or assessment of fines.

Second Injury Fund

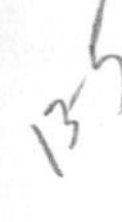

A **second injury fund,** also known as a *subsequent injury fund (SIF),* was established to meet problems arising when an employee has a preexisting injury or condition and is subsequently injured at work. The preexisting injury combines with the second injury to produce disability that is greater than that caused by the first alone.

Two functions of the fund are (1) to encourage hiring of the physically handicapped, and (2) to allocate equally the costs of providing benefits to such employees. Second injury employers pay compensation related primarily to the disability caused by the second injury, even though the employee receives benefits relating to the combined disability; the difference is made up from the subsequent injury fund (see Example 13–1).

Example 13–1

Second Injury Fund

Scenario: Bob Evans loses his *left index finger* while working a lathe. He files a workers' compensation claim and receives benefits based on the disability.

Two years later, Bob loses his *left thumb* in a *second work-related accident.* A question could arise of whether the *second injury* added to a preexisting condition or was related to the prior injury.

Conclusion: This case illustrates that the latter injury substantially increased (added to) the previous injury. The employer would pay compensation related to the second injury, and funds would come from a *second injury fund* to pay for the difference between the first and second injuries.

WORKERS' COMPENSATION REQUIREMENTS

Eligibility

Individuals entitled to workers' compensation insurance coverage are private business employees, state employees, and *federal employees* (e.g., postal workers, IRS employees, **coal miners,** maritime workers). **Workers' compensation insurance** coverage provides benefits to employees and their dependents if employees suffer work-related injury, illness, or death.

Minors

Minors are covered by workers' compensation, and in some states double compensation and legal benefits are provided. In some situations, there may be additional penalties for violations that include minors.

Volunteer Workers

Several states have laws to compensate civil defense and other volunteer workers, such as firemen who are injured in the line of duty.

Industrial Accident

An **accident** is an unplanned and unexpected happening traceable to a definite time and place causing **injury** (damage or loss). Industrial accidents do not necessarily occur at the work site. For example, the insurance specialist may be asked to obtain cash for the petty cash reserve during the lunch hour. While walking to the bank, he or she trips and suffers a fractured ankle. This person is considered to be working, although not at the work site, and the injury is covered under workers' compensation insurance.

Occupational Illness

Occupational illness is any abnormal condition or disorder caused by exposure to environmental factors associated with employment, including acute and

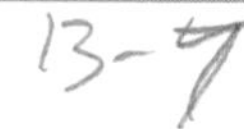

chronic illnesses or diseases that may be caused by inhalation, absorption, ingestion, or direct contact. Occupational diseases usually become apparent soon after exposure. However, some diseases may be latent for a considerable amount of time. Some states, therefore, have extended periods during which claims may be filed for certain slowly developing occupational diseases. These diseases might include:

- Cumulative trauma or repetitive motion disease (e.g., carpal tunnel syndrome)
- Loss of hearing
- Lung disease caused by inhalation of dust, fibers, or toxins (e.g., asbestosis, berylliosis, silicosis)
- Radiation exposure disability

Minimum Number of Employees

Table 13–1 shows the minimum number of employees required by each state and outlying U.S. areas before the workers' compensation law becomes effective. There are exemptions in many states for certain occupations such as domestic or casual employees, babysitters, charity workers, gardeners, laborers, and newspaper vendors or distributors. Some states do not require compensation insurance for farm laborers or may need a larger number of farm employees than the number shown in the table.

Referring the Injured or Ill Worker

Various routes may be used when referring the injured or ill worker for medical care.

On-Site Physician

Medical staff on-site may be the first to evaluate an injured worker. Even if this physician provides no treatment beyond the initial contact, the description of the incident, his or her work duties, and a documented observation of the functional capacity of this encounter are useful.

Predesignated Physician

In some states, at the time an employee is hired, the employee may "predesignate" his or her own doctor for treatment involving a future workers' compensation claim. If this is not done, the employer has the legal authority to select the treating physician for an employee with a work-related injury/illness.

Employer Referral

When the employer selects the treating physician for a workers' compensation injury or illness, he or she may refer the employee to an independent physician, industrial clinic, urgent care center, or emergency department.

Employee Self-Referral

Occasionally, a patient may present to the treating physician with a complaint that he or she thinks is work-related, without a referral from the employer. The treatment rendered may be considered *self-procured* and not payable, unless specific authorization has

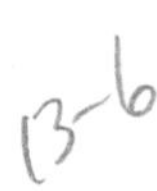

Table 13–1 Minimum Number of Employees Required by Workers' Compensation Laws

No. of Employees				
1	2	3	4	5
Alaska	Nebraska	American Samoa	Florida	Alabama
Arizona	Nevada	Arkansas	South Carolina	Mississippi
California	New Hampshire	Georgia		Missouri
Colorado	New Jersey	Michigan		Tennessee
Connecticut	New York	New Mexico		
Delaware	North Dakota	North Carolina		
District of Columbia	Ohio	Virginia		
Guam	Oklahoma			
Hawaii	Oregon			
Idaho	Pennsylvania			
Illinois	Puerto Rico			
Indiana	Rhode Island			
Iowa	South Dakota			
Kansas	Texas			
Kentucky	Utah			
Louisiana	Vermont			
Maine	Virgin Islands			
Maryland	Washington			
Massachusetts	West Virginia			
Minnesota	Wisconsin			
Montana	Wyoming			

been received from the employer. Telephone the employer to clarify the situation as soon as it becomes evident that it may be work-related, preferably before treatment is rendered. The following nine states hold the injured employee responsible for unauthorized care: Alabama, Alaska, Arkansas, New Jersey, North Dakota, Ohio, Washington, West Virginia, and Wisconsin.

Selecting a Treating Physician

If an employer designates a treating physician, most states have laws allowing the worker to request a one-time change of physicians, usually within the first 30 days of treatment.

There may be an additional provision that allows the worker who is being treated by an employer-assigned physician to select his or her own treating physician *after* 30 days from the date that the employer was notified of the injury or illness.

These two provisions occurring in states that allow for a change of physicians within the first 30 days and after the first 30 days may seem conflicting. This is because they went into effect at different times.

Waiting Period

Laws state that a **waiting period (WP)** must elapse before income benefits are payable. This waiting period affects only wage compensation because medical and hospital care is provided immediately. To find the waiting period in your state, refer to Table 13–2.

Medical Evaluator

Physicians who conduct medical-legal evaluations of injured workers must pass a complex medical examination. They are then certified by the Industrial Medical Council (IMC) and may be known by one of the following titles:

- Agreed Medical Evaluator (AME)
- Independent Medical Evaluator (IME)
- Qualified Medical Evaluator (QME)

The medical evaluator is hired by the insurance company or appointed by the referee or appeals board to examine an injured worker, independent of the attending physician, and render an unbiased opinion regarding the degree of disability. When the physician

Table 13–2 **Waiting Period for Income Benefits***

Jurisdiction	Waiting Period (days)	Jurisdiction	Waiting Period (days)
Alabama	3	Nebraska	7
Alaska	3	Nevada	5
Arizona	7	New Hampshire	3
Arkansas	7	New Jersey	7
California	3	New Mexico	7
Colorado	3	New York	7
Connecticut	3	North Carolina	7
Delaware	3	North Dakota	5
District of Columbia	3	Ohio	7
Florida	7	Oklahoma	3
Georgia	7	Oregon	3
Guam	3	Pennsylvania	7
Hawaii	3	Puerto Rico	3
Idaho	5	Rhode Island	3
Illinois	3	South Carolina	7
Indiana	7	South Dakota	7
Iowa	3	Tennessee	7
Kansas	0	Texas	7
Kentucky	7	Utah	3
Louisiana	7	Vermont	3
Maine	7	Virgin Islands	0
Maryland	3	Virginia	7
Massachusetts	5	Washington	3
Michigan	7	West Virginia	3
Minnesota	3	Wisconsin	3
Mississippi	5	Wyoming	3
Missouri	3	FECA	3
Montana	6	LHWCA	3

*Statutes provide that a waiting period must elapse during which *income benefits* are not payable. This waiting period affects only compensation, because medical and hospital care is provided immediately.

FECA, Federal Employees Compensation Act; LHWCA, Longshoremen's and Harbor Workers' Compensation Act.

performs an evaluation of an injured worker, the workers' compensation fee schedule may have specific procedure codes to bill for the examination. Evaluation and Management (E/M) consultation codes, or the CPT code for work-related evaluation by "other" physician, 99456, may be used.

Medical-Legal Evaluation

A **medical-legal (ML) evaluation** is an evaluation of an employee which results in the preparation of a narrative medical report prepared and attested to in accordance with the labor code. The evaluation and any applicable procedures must be performed by a QME, AME, or primary treating physician for the purpose of proving or disproving a contested claim. Reimbursement of ML expenses are obtained by following strict guidelines presented in the workers' compensation fee schedule. The schedule sets forth a section of reasonable charges for ML evaluation reports and ML testimony. A single fee includes reimbursement for the examination, review of records, preparation of a medical-legal report, and overhead expenses. The complexity of the evaluation is the dominant factor determining the appropriate level of service. Check your state workers' compensation fee schedule to verify if billing for such services involves use of special codes (see Example 13–2) and modifiers.

Example 13–2

Medical-Legal Evaluation

CODE	DESCRIPTION OF SERVICES
ML100	Missed appointment for a comprehensive or follow-up ML evaluation
ML101	Follow-up ML evaluation
ML102	Basic comprehensive ML evaluation
ML103	Complex comprehensive ML evaluation
ML104	Comprehensive ML evaluation involving extraordinary circumstances; ML testimony; supplemental ML evaluations

MODIFIER	DESCRIPTION
-92	Performed by a primary treating physician
-93	Interpreter needed at time of examination (or other circumstances which impair communication)
-94	Evaluation and ML testimony performed by an AME
-95	Evaluation performed by a panel-selected QME
-96	ML testimony
-97	Supplemental ML evaluations

Benefits

Workers' compensation insurance coverage provides benefits to employees and their dependents if employees suffer work-related injury, illness, or death. Five principal types of state compensation benefits may apply.

1. *Medical treatment*—Treatment that is reasonable and necessary to cure or relieve the worker from the effects of an industrial injury or illness. This includes hospital, medical, and surgical services, medications, and prosthetic devices. Treatment may be rendered by a licensed physician, osteopath, dentist, or chiropractor.
2. *Temporary disability indemnity*—Weekly cash payments made directly to the injured or ill person.
3. *Permanent disability indemnity*—This may consist of either cash payments (weekly or monthly) or a lump sum award based on a rating system that determines the percentage of permanent disability.
4. *Vocational rehabilitation benefits*—These benefits are provided to restore the severely injured worker to suitable gainful employment.
5. *Death benefits for survivors*—Cash payments to dependents of employees who are fatally injured or die because of an industrial accident or illness. In some states, a burial allowance is also given.

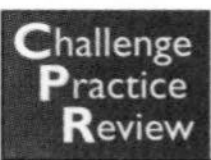

Pause and Practice CPR

REVIEW SESSIONS 13–3 THROUGH 13–7

Directions: *Complete the following questions as a review of information you have just read.*

13–3 It is ______________________ for an employer to fail to report a work-related accident when it is required by state law.

13–4 If an employee suffers work-related ______________________, ______________________, or ______________________, workers' compensation laws provide benefits.

13–5 Are minors covered under workers' compensation laws? ________________

13–6 Are there provisions for an employee to change his or her treating physician, and if so, when may this be done? ____

____

13–7 Write the meanings of the following acronyms which represent types of physicians who conduct medical-legal evaluations of injured workers.

(a) QME ______________________

(b) IME ______________________

(c) AME ______________________

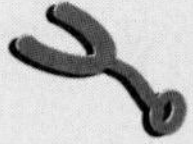

CHECK YOUR HEARTBEAT! Turn to the end of the chapter for answers to these review sessions.

TYPES OF WORKERS' COMPENSATION CLAIMS

There are three types of state workers' compensation claims: (1) nondisability claims, (2) temporary disability claims, and (3) permanent disability claims. Each type will be discussed in detail for a clear definition and an understanding of the determination process.

Nondisability Claim

A **nondisability (ND) claim** usually involves a minor injury in which the patient is seen by the doctor but is able to continue working. This is the simplest type of claim. Medical benefits would be paid and there would be no need for weekly temporary disability payments.

Temporary Disability Claim

Temporary disability (TD) occurs when a worker has a work-related injury or illness and is unable to perform all or part of his or her work duties for a period of time. The TD can be total or partial and may or may not result in permanent disability in the future. The time period of TD can extend from the date of injury until the worker (1) returns to modified work, (2) returns to full duty, or (3) fails to improve because of a residual disability that the physician states is *permanent and stationary*, thus qualifying the patient for partial or total permanent disability.

If an injured or ill worker cannot return to full work, the patient is sometimes released to modified work to effect a transition between the period of inac-

Table 13–3 Work Limitations, Types of Pain, and Frequency of Symptoms

Type of Disability, Pain, and Frequency of Symptoms	Disability Limitation and Type of Pain	Definition and Example
Disabilities related to abdominal weakness, heart disease, pulmonary disease, or spinal problems	Limited to light work	Patient is capable of working in a standing position or walking that demands minimal effort
	Precludes heavy work	Loss of approximately 50% capacity to perform bending, stooping, lifting, pushing, pulling, and climbing activities
	Precludes heavy lifting, repeated bending and stooping	Loss of approximately 50% capacity to perform heavy lifting and repeated bending and stooping
	Precludes heavy lifting	Loss of approximately 50% capacity for lifting
Disabilities related to extremities	Limitation to sedentary work	May work while sitting with minimal demands for physical effort; may do some standing and walking
	Limitation to semisedentary work	May work at a position that allows for half-time sitting and half-time standing or walking, with minimal demand for physical effort while sitting, standing, or walking
Disabilities related to pain (types of pain)	Minimal pain (mild)	Pain is annoying, but will not handicap the performance of the individual's work
	Slight pain	Pain is tolerable; there may be some limitations in performance of assigned duties
	Moderate pain	Pain is tolerable, but there may be a marked handicap of performance
	Severe pain	Pain precipitates precluding the activity causing the pain
Frequency of symptoms	Occasional	Occur approximately 25% of the time
	Intermittent	Occur approximately 50% of the time
	Frequent	Occur approximately 75% of the time
	Constant	Occur 90%–100% of the time

tivity due to disability and return to full duty, especially when heavy work is involved. Other times an employee is returned to the company and placed in a different department or division so he or she is gainfully employed while not using the injured body part. Various types of limitations can be placed on the worker according to what the injury or illness prevents the worker from doing. Terms used to define work limitations, types of pain, and the frequency of symptoms are presented in Table 13–3.

Permanent Disability Claim

In a **permanent disability (PD)** claim, the disability (impairment of the normal use of a body part) is expected to continue for the lifetime of the injured worker and the person cannot return to his or her occupation, thereby impairing his or her earning capacity. The patient or injured party is usually on TD benefits for a time and does not continue to improve to the state of health that he or she enjoyed prior to the illness or injury. The physician states in the report that the worker has residual disability that will hamper his or her opportunity to compete in the open job market. Examples of residual disability include loss of a hand, an eye, or a leg, or neurologic problems. Each case is rated according to the severity of the injury, the age of the injured person, and the patient's occupation at the time of the injury. The older the person, the greater the PD benefit. One might think that a younger person deserves higher compensation because he or she will be disabled for a longer portion of his or her working career. However, workers' compensation laws assume that a young person has a better chance of being rehabilitated into another occupation.

COMMON WORKERS' COMPENSATION TERMINOLOGY

Insurance Adjuster

An **insurance adjuster** is the person at the workers' compensation insurance carrier that oversees the industrial case and *adjusts the industrial claim.* This means that the insurance adjuster must evaluate the injury or illness, predict in advance the amount of money needed to cover medical expenses, and accurately calculate a reserve for weekly payments to the injured party. This is frequently a difficult task, because a seemingly minor back strain may ultimately require fusion or a small cut may become gangrenous and lead to an amputation. The adjuster keeps in contact with the physician's office regarding the patient's ongoing progress and grants permission for diagnostic testing and procedures.

Case Manager

If a case is complicated, a registered or licensed vocational nurse may be assigned as a **case manager.** The case manager's job is to supervise the administration of medical or ancillary services provided to the patient and act as a liaison between the patient, the physician, and the insurance company. He or she attends all appointments with the patient and if diagnostic testing is required, helps with the authorization process. Case managers are assigned to expedite the patient's care and help resolve the claim quickly. By law, some states require that case managers be assigned to all injured or ill workers.

Permanent and Stationary

To state that an injured or ill worker has a PD, the physician must first determine that the patient's condition is **permanent and stationary (P and S).** This phrase, which must be stated in the final report, means that damage from the injury or illness is permanent, the patient has recovered to the fullest extent possible, the physician is unable to do anything more for the patient, and the patient will be hampered by the disability to some extent for the rest of his or her life. It is sometimes referred to as *maximum medical improvement.*

The P and S examination is usually a comprehensive examination. Depending on the fee schedule used, a level 5 CPT code (e.g., 99215), or code 99455 (work-related disability examination by the treating physician) would be appropriate. The fee schedule may supply a modifier that indicates that the E/M service is a P and S examination.

Compromise and Release

Once the case is rated PD, a settlement is made called a **compromise and release (C and R).** This is an agreement between the injured or ill party and the insurance company on a total benefit sum. The case can then be closed.

Rating

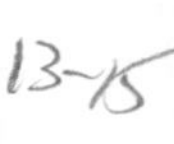

Final determination of the issues involving settlement of an industrial accident or illness is known as **adjudication,** or the *rating* of a case. A physician does not rate the disability but renders a professional opinion on whether the injured individual has temporary or permanent disability that prevents him or her from gainful employment. Rating itself is carried out by the state's industrial accident commission or workers' compensation board. Wage loss, earning capacity, and physical impairment are three categories that may be taken into consideration to rate permanent partial and total disability. The physician determines the impairment and a schedule for rating permanent disability is used by the disability rating specialist to then determine the level (percentage) of disability. Following are definitions for permanent partial and permanent total disability:

- *Permanent partial disability*—A disability to a part of the injured or ill worker's body that has some degree of irreversible anatomic loss or physiologic dysfunction. In some cases, the injured worker will not be able to resume his or her original job. The injury is declared permanent and stationary, that is, will not improve. The worker is qualified to be rated in or-

Example 13–3

Permanent Partial Disability

Scenario: Patient injured his back at work. He had a lumbar fusion (L4–5) and received physical therapy to strengthen his back muscles. He fails to improve and the injury is declared permanent and stationary.
Physician's Determination: The individual has lost approximately 50% of his preinjury capacity for lifting, bending, and stooping.
Rating: This impairment translates into a partial permanent disability rating of 25%.

der to determine the percentage of disability according to the diminished capacity to compete in the open job market (see Example 13–3).

- *Permanent total disability*—An impairment that is expected to continue for the lifetime of the injured or ill worker. The injury or illness inhibits the worker from engaging in *any* gainful or substantial employment.

If an injured person is dissatisfied with the rating after the case has been declared P and S, he or she may appeal the case by **petition** (formal written request) to the Workers' Compensation Appeals Board (WCAB) or the Industrial Accident Commission.

Surveillance

In rating a case, **sub rosa films** are sometimes provided to document the extent of a patient's permanent disability. *Sub rosa* means "under the rose." In ancient times, the rose was a symbol of silence or secrecy. Videotapes are made over a period of 2 to 3 days without the patient's knowledge. This surveillance is expensive and is used as a last resort, especially in cases when a person receiving workers' compensation benefits is suspected of making exaggerated complaints. It is also used in cases when a worker has been off work for a long period of time and is supposedly unable to perform any work activity, not even light duty.

Investigators have been known to carry a camera in a gym bag and videotape a supposedly disabled claimant bench-pressing at the gym. Patients have also been videotaped going into the physician's office for an appointment wearing a neck brace and removing the brace upon returning to their car.

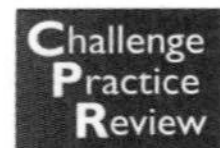

Pause and Practice CPR

REVIEW SESSIONS 13–8 THROUGH 13–10

Directions: *Complete the following questions as a review of information you have just read.*

13–8 Name and give a brief description of the three types of workers' compensation claims.

(a) ND ______________________________

____

(b) TD ______________________________

____

(c) PD ______________________________

____

3–9 What are three factors that influence the rating of permanent disability?

(a) ______________________________

(b) ______________________________

(c) ______________________________

3–10 Who is the person at the workers' compensation insurance company that the physician's office receives permission from for diagnostic testing and procedures? ______________________________

____

CHECK YOUR HEARTBEAT! Turn to the end of the chapter for answers to these review sessions.

EMPLOYEE'S CLAIM FOR WORKERS' COMPENSATION BENEFITS

There are laws that clearly state that the injured person must promptly report the industrial injury or illness to his or her employer or immediate supervisor. Some states require that a form be filed with the employer to obtain workers' compensation benefits. Information on the employee's section of the form usually includes the injured/ill party's name and address, the date and time of injury or when the illness first presented, a description of where the injury happened or where exposure occurred, and what body part was injured or how the illness manifested, along with the Social Security number and employee's original signature.

The employer then completes his or her portion of the form, including the name and address of the employer, the date the employer first knew of the injury, the date the claim form was given to the employee and the date returned, the insurance carrier's name, and the address, telephone number, and policy number, along with the original signature of the employer or the employer's representative and his or her title.

Fraud and Abuse

Because of increases in fraudulent workers' compensation claims involving employers, employees, insurers, medical providers, and lawyers, an increasing number of states have enacted some kind of antifraud legislation and stiffened penalties for workers' compensation fraud, making it a felony. Some states require reporting suspected insurance fraud and have forms to incorporate wording in regard to fraudulent statements.

Physicians are responsible for determining the legitimacy of work injuries and reporting findings accurately. If a report is prepared with the intent to use it in support of a fraudulent claim, or if a fraudulent claim is knowingly submitted for payment under an insurance contract, the physician may be subject to fines and/or imprisonment and the revocation or suspension of a medical license.

It is the responsibility of all individuals who deal with workers' compensation cases to notify the insurance carrier of any suspicious situation. By doing so, action can be taken to have the case investigated further by personnel from the fraud division or referred to the district attorney's office. Perpetrators and signs of workers' compensation fraud and abuse are listed in Table 13–4.

Table 13–4 Perpetrators and Signs of Workers' Compensation Fraud and Abuse

EMPLOYEE

- Misses the first physician's visit.
- Cannot describe the pain or is overly dramatic, such as an employee who comes into the physician's office limping on the left leg, suddenly starts limping on the right leg, and then goes back to limping on the left leg.
- Delays in reporting the injury.
- Does not report Friday's injury until Monday morning.
- First reports an injury to a legal or regulatory agency.
- Reports an injury after missing several days of work.
- Changes physicians frequently.
- Is a short-term worker.
- Has a curious claim history.
- Fabricates an injury.
- Exaggerates a work-related injury to obtain larger benefits, such as an injured employee who has back pain and claims inability to bend over or lift. Surveillance cameras capture the individual at work on weekends repairing cars in the driveway at home—a task he or she is supposedly unable to perform.
- Blames an injury that occurred off the job on the employer.

EMPLOYER

- Misrepresents the annual payroll to get lower premium rates.
- Misrepresents the number of workers employed.
- Gives a false address with the least expensive premium rates.
- Falsely classifies the job duties of workers (as not hazardous), such as stating the job title as clerical worker when, in fact, the employee is using a lathe every day.

INSURER

- Refuses to pay valid medical claims.
- Forces the injured worker to settle by using unethical tactics. An insurance agent told an employee that he had a back sprain. Relying on that information, the worker settled the case. Later, a myelogram revealed a herniated intervertebral disk. The patient was left with a permanent partial disability.

MEDICAL PROVIDER

- Orders or performs unnecessary tests.
- Renders unnecessary treatment.
- Charges the insurance carrier for services never rendered.
- Participates in a provider mill scheme (see explanation under Lawyer).
- Makes multiple referrals from a clinic practice regardless of type of injury.
- Sends medical reports that look photocopied with the same information typed in (e.g., employer's address, description of injury) or that read almost identical to other reports.
- Sends in many claims in which injuries are of a subjective nature, such as stress, emotional distress, headaches, inability to sleep.
- Sends in claims from one employer showing several employees with similar injuries, using the same physicians and/or attorneys.

LAWYER

- Overbills clients.
- Participates in a medical provider mill scheme. An individual is solicited while in the unemployment line by a recruiter known as a "capper." The capper tells the worker it is possible to obtain more money on disability than through unemployment. The worker is referred to an attorney and a "provider mill" clinic, which helps the individual fabricate a claim by claiming stress or an on-the-job injury. In some states, such acts may be considered a public offense and punishable as a misdemeanor or felony.

For further information on fraud and abuse in the medical setting, see Chapters 1, 10, and 11.

Payment of Benefits

Usually, workers' compensation weekly TD payments are based on the employee's earnings at the time of the injury. Compensation benefits are not subject to income tax.

MEDICAL REPORTS

Confidentiality

There is a difference in how confidential information is treated in industrial cases as opposed to private insurance cases and federal programs. In most states, insurance claims adjusters have unlimited access to the injured employee's medical records, pertaining to the industrial case only. This means that information can be shared over the telephone and reports sent to the insurance company without the patient's signed consent. Some states allow employers similar access. Check with your state's laws to see if the employer must sign an authorization to release records before giving them to a third party.

Documentation

Documentation must always show the necessity for procedures performed. If there is not an accurate diagnostic code to explain the patient's condition, a report should be sent describing the details of the diagnosis. The physician may list the total time spent in reviewing records, face-to-face time with the patient, preparation of a report, and other relevant activities. CPT code 99080 may be used to bill for workers' compensation reports if the report is not included in the E/M service. The monetary value assigned to the code is usually determined by the number of pages in the report. If medical records are reviewed before or after consulting or treating a workers' compensation patient, submit a bill for this service using an appropriate code from the workers' compensation fee schedule, or code 99358 (prolonged E/M service before and/or after direct face-to-face patient care).

Medical Record Keeping

Never mix a private medical record with a workers' compensation record because there are separate disclosure laws for each. If a private patient comes to the office with an industrial injury, set up a separate medical record (chart) and financial record (ledger) for the work-related injury/illness. Some medical practices use colored file folders or colored tabs to distinguish the industrial medical record from the patient's private medical record. If two charts are maintained, it is easy to identify which record is needed and it may be pulled quickly without having to dig through the patient's unrelated medical documents.

Appointments

It is preferable never to schedule a patient to see the physician for a workers' compensation follow-up examination and an unrelated complaint during the same appointment time. Separate appointments (back to back, if necessary) need to be arranged. This allows for separate dictation without intermixing the required documentation for each chart. It also allows for separate charges to be made to the workers' compensation carrier and private insurance company or patient.

If an appointment was arranged by the employer or insurance company for a workers' compensation patient and was not canceled 72 hours before the appointment time, a charge can often be made. Check individual state laws to verify if such charges can be applied in your state.

If a translator is needed for a workers' compensation patient, contact the insurance adjuster handling the case. He or she will make arrangements for an official translator to be present for all appointments. Do not allow a member of the patient's family or a friend of the patient to serve as a translator because if information is miscommunicated leading to a bad outcome, there may be no legal recourse for the physician.

Reporting Requirements

Reporting requirements vary from state to state. To obtain instructions and proper forms for your state, contact the state bureau of individual insurance carriers.

Employer's Report

In most states, reporting of the industrial injury or illness is required by law. To meet this requirement, and the requirement of the Federal Occupational Safety and Health Act of 1970, many employers have adopted the Employer's Report of Occupational Injury or Illness form (Fig. 13–1). This form is sent to the insurance company. The time limit on submission varies from state to state, anywhere from "immediately" to 30 days. Refer to Table 13–5 for the time limit in your state.

Medical Service Order

In addition to the employer's report, the employer may complete and sign a **medical service order,** giving this to the injured or ill employee to take to the physician's office (Fig. 13–2). This authorizes the physician to treat the injured employee. Photocopy the form, retaining the copy for the physician's file, and attach the original to the Doctor's First Report of Occupational Injury or Illness (preliminary report).

An employer may prefer to write the service order on his or her business letterhead or authorization may be obtained over the telephone. Written authorization is preferred in case of a claim dispute because the written documentation can be sent to collect payment.

State of California EMPLOYER'S REPORT OF OCCUPATIONAL INJURY OR ILLNESS	Please complete in triplicate (type, if possible). Mail two copies to: XYZ Insurance Company PO Box 5 Woodland Hills, XY 12345	OSHA Case No. # 18 ☐ Fatality

Any person who makes or causes to be made any knowingly false or fraudulent material statement or material representation for the purpose of obtaining or denying workers' compensation benefits or payments is guilty of a felony.

NOTICE: California law requires employers to report within **five days** of knowledge every occupational injury or illness which results in lost time beyond the date of the incident **OR** requires medical treatment beyond first aid. If an employee subsequently dies as a result of a previously reported injury or illness, the employer must file within **five days** of knowledge an amended report indicating death. In addition, every serious injury/illness, or death must be reported **immediately** by telephone or telegraph to the nearest office of the California Division of Occupational Safety and Health.

EMPLOYER

1. FIRM NAME: The Conk Out Company
1A. POLICY NUMBER: B12345
2. MAILING ADDRESS (Number and Street, City, ZIP): 45 South Gorman St. Woodland Hills, XY 12345
2A. PHONE NUMBER: 555-430-3488
3. LOCATION, IF DIFFERENT FROM MAILING ADDRESS (Number and Street, City, ZIP):
3A. LOCATION CODE:
4. NATURE OF BUSINESS, e.g., painting contractor, wholesale grocer, sawmill, hotel, etc.: Plumbing Repair
5. STATE UNEMPLOYMENT INSURANCE ACCT. NO.:
6. TYPE OF EMPLOYER: ☒ PRIVATE ☐ STATE ☐ CITY ☐ COUNTY ☐ SCHOOL DIST. ☐ OTHER GOVERNMENT - SPECIFY ______

EMPLOYEE

7. EMPLOYEE NAME: Ima B. Hurt
8. SOCIAL SECURITY NUMBER: 120-XX-6542
9. DATE OF BIRTH (mm/dd/yy): 3-4-66
10. HOME ADDRESS (Number and Street, City, ZIP): 300 E.Central Ave. Woodland Hills, XY 12345
10A. PHONE NUMBER: 555-476-9899
11. SEX: ☐ MALE ☒ FEMALE
12. OCCUPATION (Regular job title — NO initials, abbreviations or numbers): Clerk Typist
13. DATE OF HIRE (mm/dd/yy): 1-20-86
14. EMPLOYEE USUALLY WORKS: 8 hours per day; 5 hours per week; 40 total weekly hours
14A. EMPLOYMENT STATUS (check applicable status at time of injury): X regular full-time ___ part-time ___ temporary ___ seasonal
14B. Under what class code of your policy were wages assigned? 7219
15. GROSS WAGES/SALARY: $ 700.00 per week
16. OTHER PAYMENTS NOT REPORTED AS WAGES/SALARY (e.g. tips, meals, lodging, overtime, bonuses, etc.)? ☐ YES $ ______ PER ______ ☒ NO

INJURY OR ILLNESS

17. DATE OF INJURY OR ONSET OF ILLNESS (mm/dd/yy): 4-3-XX
18. TIME INJURY/ILLNESS OCCURRED: ______ A.M. 2:00 P.M.
19. TIME EMPLOYEE BEGAN WORK: 8:00 A.M. ______ P.M.
20. IF EMPLOYEE DIED, DATE OF DEATH (mm/dd/yy):
21. UNABLE TO WORK AT LEAST ONE FULL DAY AFTER DATE OF INJURY? ☒ YES ☐ NO
22. DATE LAST WORKED (mm/dd/yy): 4-3-XX
23. DATE RETURNED TO WORK (mm/dd/yy):
24. IF STILL OFF WORK, CHECK THIS BOX ☒
25. PAID FULL WAGES FOR DAY OF INJURY OR LAST DAY WORKED? ☒ YES ☐ NO
26. SALARY BEING CONTINUED? ☐ YES ☒ NO
27. DATE OF EMPLOYER'S KNOWLEDGE/NOTICE OF INJURY/ILLNESS (mm/dd/yy): 4-3-XX
28. DATE EMPLOYEE WAS PROVIDED: 4-3-XX
29. SPECIFIC INJURY/ILLNESS AND PART OF BODY AFFECTED, MEDICAL DIAGNOSIS, if available, e.g., second degree burns on right arm, tendonitis of left elbow, lead poisoning.: ankle injury swelling, possible fracture
30. LOCATION WHERE EVENT OR EXPOSURE OCCURRED (Number, Street, City): 45 South Gorman St. Woodland Hills, XY 12345
30B. ON EMPLOYERS PREMISES? ☐ YES ☒ NO
31. DEPARTMENT WHERE EVENT OR EXPOSURE OCCURRED, e.g., shipping department, machine shop.: stock room
32. OTHER WORKERS INJURED/ILL IN THIS EVENT? ☐ YES ☒ NO
33. EQUIPMENT, MATERIALS AND CHEMICALS THE EMPLOYEE WAS USING WHEN EVENT OR EXPOSURE OCCURRED, e.g., acetylene, welding torch, farm tractor, scaffold.: 6 foot ladder
34. SPECIFY ACTIVITY THE EMPLOYEE WAS PERFORMING WHEN EVENT OR EXPOSURE OCCURRED, e.g., welding seams of metal forms, loading boxes onto truck.: climbed ladder to remove a ream of paper from shelf; fell
35. HOW INJURY/ILLNESS OCCURRED. DESCRIBE SEQUENCE OF EVENTS. SPECIFY OBJECT OR EXPOSURE WHICH DIRECTLY PRODUCED THE INJURY/ILLNESS, e.g., worker stepped back to inspect work and slipped on scrap material. As he fell, he brushed against fresh weld, and burned right hand. USE SEPARATE SHEET IF NECESSARY.: worker climbed ladder to remove a ream of paper from top shelf in stock room. She was descending and mis-stepped falling to the floor. She tried to land upright, and her left leg took the brunt of the fall.
36. NAME AND ADDRESS OF PHYSICIAN (Number and Street, City, ZIP): Raymond Skeleton, MD 4567 Broad Ave., Woodland Hills, XY 12345
36A. PHONE NUMBER: 555-486-9002
37. IF HOSPITALIZED AS AN INPATIENT, NAME AND ADDRESS OF HOSPITAL (Number and Street, City, ZIP):
37A. PHONE NUMBER:

DO NOT USE THIS COLUMN: Case No. | Ownership | Industry | Occupation | Sex | Age | Daily Hours | Days per week | Weekly hours | Weekly wage | County | Nature of injury | Part of body | Source | Event | Sec. Source | Extent of injury

Completed by (type or print)	Signature	Title	Date
J.D. Hawkins	J. D. Hawkins	owner	4-3-XX

FILING THIS REPORT IS NOT AN ADMISSION OF LIABILITY

Figure 13–1. Employer's Report of Occupational Injury or Illness. This form complies with OSHA requirements as well as California State Workers' Compensation laws.

Table 13–5 Employers' and/or Physicians' Report of Accident*

Jurisdiction	Time Limit	Injuries Covered
Alabama	Within 15 days	Death or disability exceeding 3 days
Alaska	Within 10 days	Death, injury, disease, or infection
Arizona	Within 10 days	All injuries
Arkansas	10 days from notice of injury	Indemnity, injuries, or death; medical claims reported monthly
California	Immediately (employer)	Death or serious injuries**
	As prescribed	1-day disability or more than first aid
	Within 5 days of employer's notice	Occupational diseases or pesticide poisoning
Colorado	Immediately	Death
	Within 10 days	Injuries causing lost time of 3 days or more
	Immediately	Any accident in which 3 or more employees are injured
	10 days	Occupational disease cases
	10 days	Cases of permanent physical impairment
Connecticut	7 days or as directed	Disability of 1 day or more
Delaware	Within 48 hours	Death or injuries requiring hospitalization
	Within 10 days	Other injuries
	Upon termination of disability	Supplemental report
District of Columbia	Within 10 days	All injuries
Florida	Within 24 hours	Death
	Within 7 days of carrier receipt of notice	All injuries
	30 days after final payment	Supplemental report
Georgia	Within 21 days	All injuries requiring medical or surgical treatment or causing over 7 days of absence
	On 1st payment, suspension of payment, 30 days after final payment	Supplemental report
Guam	Within 10 days	Injury, illness, or death
Hawaii	Within 48 hours	Death
	Within 7 working days	All injuries
Idaho	As soon as practicable but not later than 10 days after the accident	All injuries requiring medical treatment or causing 1 day's absence
	After 60 days, upon termination of disability	Supplemental report
Illinois	Within 2 working days	Death or serious injuries
	Between 15th and 25th of month	Disability of over 3 days
	As soon as determinable	Permanent disability
Indiana	Within 7 working days	Disability of more than 1 day
	Within 10 days after termination of compensation period	Supplemental report
Iowa	Within 4 days	Disability of more than 3 days, permanent partial disability, death
Kansas	Within 28 days	Death
	Within 28 days	Disability of more than remainder of day or shift
Kentucky	Within 7 days	Disability of more than 1 day
	After 80 days or upon termination	Supplemental report
Louisiana	Within 10 days of employer's actual knowledge of injury	Lost time over 1 week or death
	Within 90 days	Death, any nonfatal occupational illness or injury causing loss of consciousness, restriction of work or motion, job transfer, or medical treatment other than first aid (employers with more than 10 employees)
Maine	Within 7 days	Only injuries causing 1 day or more of lost time
	30 days from date of diagnosis	Abestosis, mesothelioma, silicosis, exposure to heavy metals
Maryland	Within 10 days	Disability of more than 3 days
Massachusetts	Within 7 days, except Sundays and holidays	Disability of 5 or more calendar days
Michigan	Immediately	Death, disability of 7 days or more, and specific losses
Minnesota	Within 48 hours	Death or serious injury
	Within 14 days	Disability of 3 days or more
Mississippi	Within 10 days	Death or disability of more than 5 days
Missouri	Within 10 days	Death or injury
	1 mo after original notice	Supplemental report
Montana	Within 6 days	All injuries

Table 13–5 **Employers' and/or Physicians' Report of Accident* *Continued***

Jurisdiction	Time Limit	Injuries Covered
Nebraska	Within 48 hours	Death
	Within 7 days	All injuries
Nevada	Within 6 working days after report from physician	All injuries requiring medical treatment
	File notice of injury, retain 3 yr	Injuries not requiring medical treatment
New Hampshire	Within 5 calendar days	All injuries involving lost time or medical expenses
New Jersey	Immediately	All compensable injuries
New Mexico	Within 10 days of employer notification	Any injury or illness resulting in 7 or more days of lost time
New York	Within 10 days	Disability of 1 day beyond working day or shift on which accident occurred or requiring medical care beyond 2 first-aid treatments
North Carolina	Within 5 days	Disability of more than 1 day
	After 60 days, or upon termination	Supplemental report
North Dakota	Within 7 days	All injuries
Ohio	Within 1 week	Injuries causing total disability of 7 days or more
Oklahoma	Within 10 days or a reasonable time	All injuries causing lost time or requiring treatment away from work site
Oregon	Within 5 days	All injuries requiring medical treatment
	Within 21 days	Insurers to send disabling claims
Pennsylvania	Within 48 hours	Death
	After 7 days but not later than 10 days	Disability of 1 day or more
Puerto Rico	Within 5 days	All injuries
Rhode Island	Within 48 hr	Death
	Within 10 days	Disability of 3 days of more and all injuries requiring medical treatment
	Within 2 yr of injury	Any claim resulting in medical expense to be reported within 10 days
	Every 6 mo	Supplemental report
South Carolina	Within 10 days	All injuries requiring medical attention costing more than $500, more than 1 day disability or permanency
	After 60 days, every 6 mo, or upon termination	Supplemental report
South Dakota	Within 7 days	All injuries that require treatment other than first aid or that incapacitate employee 7 calendar days
Tennessee	Within 14 days	All injuries requiring medical attention
Texas	Within 8 days	Disability of more than 1 day, or occupational disease
	After 60 days or upon termination	Supplemental report
Utah	Within 7 days	All injuries requiring medical attention
Vermont	Within 72 hr	Disability of 1 day or more requiring medical care
	After 60 days or upon termination	Supplemental report
Virgin Islands	Within 8 days	Injury or disease
Virginia	Within 10 days	All injuries
	After 60 days or upon termination	Supplemental report
Washington	Within 8 hr	Death and accidents resulting in workers' hospitalizations or inability to work
West Virginia	Within 5 days	All injuries
Wisconsin	Within 14 days	Disability beyond 3-day waiting period
Wyoming	Within 10 days	Compensable injuries
FECA	Immediately	All injuries involving medical expenses, disability, or death
LHWCA	10 days	Injuries that cause loss of 1 or more shifts of work or death

*Federal Occupational Safety and Health Act of 1970 established uniform requirements and forms to meet its criteria for all businesses affecting interstate commerce to be used for statistical purposes and compliance with the act—12 U.S.C. §651.

**California. To Division of Occupational Safety and Health. Within 5 days of employer's notice or knowledge of employee death, employer must report death to the Department of Industrial Relations.

NOTE: FECA, Federal Employees Compensation Act; LHWCA, Longshoremen's and Harbor Workers' Compensation Act.

Physician's First Report

As soon as possible after the physician sees the injured or ill worker, he or she sends in a completed Doctor's First Report of Occupational Injury or Illness form (Fig. 13–3) or a First Treatment Medical Report, which may appear similar to the HCFA-1500 claim form.

If the physician prefers to submit a narrative letter, the medical report should include the same components listed in the form. Failure to file the report can

WORKERS' COMPENSATION
MEDICAL SERVICE ORDER

To: Dr./Clinic Raymond Skeleton, MD

Address 4567 Broad Avenue, Woodland Hills, XY 12345

We are sending Mrs. Ima Hurt

Address 300 East Central Ave., Woodland Hills, XY 12345

Social Security No. 120-XX-6542 Date of birth 3-4-1966
to you for treatment in accordance with the terms of the Worker's Compensation Laws. Please submit your report to the
XYZ Insurance Company
at once. Compensation cannot be paid without complete medical information.

Insurance carrier XYZ Insurance Company

Address P.O. Box 5, Woodland Hills, XY 12345 Telephone 555-271-0562

Employer The Conk Out Company

Address 45 S. Gorman St. Woodland Hills, XY 12345 Telephone 555-430-3488

Signature J. A. Hawkins Date 4-3-20XX
If patient is able to return to work today or tomorrow, please show date and time below — sign and give to patient to return to employer. If there are any work restrictions indicate on the back of this form. Please submit your usual first report in any case.

Date/Time ____________ By ____________

Figure 13–2. Medical Service Order authorization for treatment by College Clinic physician, Dr. Skeleton, of injured worker (Mrs. Ima Hurt).

be a misdemeanor. This form should be submitted as follows:

- Original to the insurance carrier (unless more copies are required)
- One copy to the state agency
- One copy to the patient's employer
- One copy retained for the physician's files in the patient's workers' compensation file folder

In some states, attending physicians may file a single report directly to the insurer or self-insured employer. The insurer or self-insured employer, in turn, is required to send a report to the state agency. The report is a legal document; therefore, each copy *must be signed in ink by the physician.* The insurance company waits for the physician's report and bill, then issues payment to the physician. If there is no further disability or treatment, the case can be closed.

Completing the Doctor's First Report of Occupational Injury or Illness

You may be abstracting information from the medical record to complete this report. Many items on the form are self-explanatory. Be sure all sections are filled out completely and all questions answered. The top of the form includes information regarding the insurance carrier, employer, and employee.

The bottom portion of the form contains the patient's account of the injury/illness and specific findings made by the physician. Further description and directions are given to clarify certain items:

Item 17—Have the patient complete this section if possible in *his or her own words* stating how the illness or injury occurred. If this is not possible, the physician may dictate this information after obtaining it from the patient.

Item 18—Enter the patient's *subjective complaints* or symptoms (e.g., pain, numbness, dizziness, weakness).

Item 19

a. Enter all *objective findings* from the physical examination (e.g., lump, redness, bruising, edema).

b. Enter all x-ray and laboratory results, or if none, state "none" or "pending."

Item 23—Enter a *full description* of what treatment was rendered.

Item 24—Enter an explanation if further treatment is required, and if so, specify the treatment plan. Indicate if physical therapy is required and its frequency and duration.

Item 26—Enter a check mark "yes" or "no" to indicate whether the patient is able to return to his or her regular work duties. If the answer is "no," give the date when it is *estimated* that the patient will be able to return to regular or modified work. A date *must* be entered. Specify any work restrictions. It is very important for the insurance company to anticipate how long the patient will be off work so that money may be set aside for TD benefits, medical benefits, and if necessary, PD benefits. If the estimated date of return to work should change after the form is submitted, a supplemental report or progress note

STATE OF CALIFORNIA

DOCTOR'S FIRST REPORT OF OCCUPATIONAL INJURY OR ILLNESS

Within 5 days of your initial examination, for every occupational injury or illness, send two copies of this report to the **employer's worker's compensation insurance carrier** or the **self-insured employer**. Failure to file a timely doctor's report may result in assessment of civil penalty. **In the case of diagnosed or suspected pesticide poisoning,** send a copy of this report to Division of Labor Statistics and Research, P.O. Box 420603, San Francisco, CA 94142-0603, and notify your local health officer by telephone within 24 hours.

		PLEASE DO NOT USE THIS COLUMN
1. **INSURER NAME AND ADDRESS** XYZ Insurance Company, P.O. Box 5, Woodland Hills, XY 12345		
2. **EMPLOYER NAME** The Conk Out Company Policy# B12345		Case No.
3. Address No. and Street City Zip 45 So. Gorman St. Woodland Hills, XY 12345		Industry
4. Nature of business (e.g., food manufacturing, building construction, retailer of women's clothes) plumbing repair		County
5. **PATIENT NAME** (first name, middle initial, last name) Ima B. Hurt / 6. Sex ☐ Male ☒ Female	7. Date of birth Mo. Day Yr. 3-4-1966	Age
8. Address: No. and Street City Zip 300 East Central Ave., Woodland Hills, XY 12345	9. Telephone number (555) 476-9899	Hazard
10. Occupation (Specific job title) clerk typist	11. Social Security Number 120-XX-6542	Disease
12. Injured at: No. and Street City 45 So. Gorman St., Woodland Hills, XY 12345	County Humbolt	Hospitalization
13. Date and hour of injury or onset of illness Mo. Day Yr. 4-3-20XX Hour ____a.m. 2:00 p.m.	14. Date last worked Mo. Day Yr. 4-3-20XX	Occupation
15. Date and hour of first examination or treatment Mo. Day Yr. 4-3-20XX Hour ____a.m. 4:00 p.m.	16. Have you (or your office) previously treated patient? ☐ Yes ☒ No	Return date/Code

Patient please complete this portion, if able to do so. Otherwise, doctor please complete immediately. Inability or failure of a patient to complete this portion shall not affect his/her rights to workers' compensation under the California labor Code.

17. **DESCRIBE HOW THE ACCIDENT OR EXPOSURE HAPPENED** (Give specific object, machinery or chemical. Use reverse side if more space is required.)
I climbed a ladder in the stock room and while I was coming down I missed a step, lost my balance, and fell hurting my left ankle.

18. **SUBJECTIVE COMPLAINTS** (Describe fully. Use reverse side if more space is required.)
Pain in left ankle.

19. **OBJECTIVE FINDINGS** (Use reverse side if more space is required.)
A. Physical examination
Swelling and discoloration of left ankle
B. X-ray and laboratory results (state if none or pending.) Ankle x-ray (left) 3 views

20. **DIAGNOSIS** (if occupational illness specify etiologic agent and duration of exposure.) Chemical or toxic compounds involved? ☐ Yes ☒ No
Trimalleolar ankle fracture (left) ICD-9 Code 824.6

21. Are your findings and diagnosis consistent with patient's account of injury or onset of illness? ☒ Yes ☐ No if "no", please explain.

22. Is there any other current condition that will impede or delay the patient's recovery? ☐ Yes ☒ No if "Yes", please explain.

23. **TREATMENT RENDERED** (Use reverse side if more space is required.)
Examination, x-rays, closed treatment of trimalleolar ankle fracture (left) without manipulation.

24. If further treatment required, specify treatment plan/estimated duration.
Return in one week for recheck.

25. If hospitalized as inpatient, give hospital name and location Date admitted Mo. day Yr. Estimated stay

26. WORK STATUS–Is patient able to perform usual work? ☐ Yes ☒ No
If "no", date when patient can return to: Regular work 5/17/20XX
Modified work ____ Specify restrictions ____

Doctor's signature Raymond Skeleton MD CA license number CO4561X
Doctor name and degree (please type) Raymond Skeleton MD IRS number 74-65412XX
Address 4567 Broad Avenue, Woodland Hills, XY 12345 Telephone number (555) 486-9002

FORM 5021 (REV. 4) 1992

Any person who makes or causes to be made any knowingly false or fraudulent material statement or material representation for the purpose of obtaining or denying worker's compensation benefits or payments is guilty of a felony.

reference initials

Figure 13–3. Doctor's First Report of Occupational Injury or Illness form, used in California.

should be sent to the insurance carrier advising them of the new estimated date.

Complete all required information (if not printed) on the bottom of the form. The insurance billing specialist should type his or her reference initials in the lower left-hand corner of the form. If the physician does not personally fill out this form it must be reviewed for accuracy. The form *must be signed in ink by the physician* with the date the report is submitted. Any copies of the report must also be signed in ink by the physician. A stamped signature will not be accepted. Only those documents considered as *original* medical records are acceptable. The initial report is usually not separately reimbursable. Its preparation is included in the E/M service.

Progress or Supplemental Report

In a TD case, a *supplemental report* is sent to the insurance carrier to provide a treatment plan that describes the course, scope, frequency, and duration of the treatment, along with an estimated date for return to work. In many cases, the initial report may cover this information and the supplemental report would then provide information on the current status of the patient. If there is a significant change in the prognosis, a detailed progress report (sometimes called a reexamination report) should be sent. Supplemental reports should be sent after each office visit or hospitalization to update the progress of a case. Individual states may have specific requirements, as seen in Table 13–5, regarding submission of supplemental reports.

Supplemental reports may be narrative and are sometimes a copy of the patient's medical record. They are usually not required to be submitted on special forms available in most states, but may be, if preferred. If the disability appears to be long-term, monthly progress reports should be submitted. A follow-up report must contain the following information:

1. Date of most recent examination
2. Present condition and progress since last report
3. Measurements of range of motion (ROM) and circumference dimensions of limbs if atrophy or swelling is involved
4. X-ray or laboratory report since last examination
5. Treatment (give type and duration, including medications)
6. Further testing if required to make an official diagnosis
7. Work status (patient working, work limitations, or estimated date of return to work)
8. Permanent disability to be anticipated

Final Report

Temporary disability ends when the physician tells the insurance carrier that the patient is able to return to work. A final report is submitted at the time of discharge and the insurance carrier closes the case. Any impairment or permanent disability should be stated and a statement listing *total expenses incurred* should accompany the report.

Electronic Reports

Because workers' compensation is operated under state laws, each state is required to report financial data, statistics on injuries and illnesses, and other required information to state insurance regulators. Some workers' compensation insurance companies use telephone reporting where employers report injuries occurring on the job by calling a toll-free number. Calls go to a regional center where service representatives document the first report of injury and transmit it electronically to the local claims office handling workers' compensation insurance. Paper processing costs are reduced and payments are expedited by prompt reporting.

Universal electronic injury report forms have been developed by the American National Standards Institute (ANSI) and the International Association of Industrial Accident Boards and Commissions (IAIABC). Texas is one of the first states to establish an insurance regulation requiring workers' compensation carriers to use universal electronic transmission for first report of injury forms and subsequent reports.

A coast-to-coast electronic claims processing and report-filing network, called Workers' Compensation Reporting Service, was developed by Electronic Data Systems, Inc. (EDS) and Insurance Value-Added Network Services (IVANS) to process all claims and follow-up reports. This system is operational in many states.

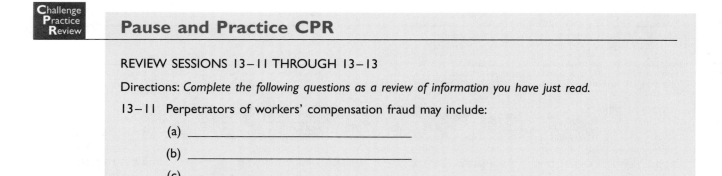

Pause and Practice CPR

REVIEW SESSIONS 13–11 THROUGH 13–13

Directions: *Complete the following questions as a review of information you have just read.*

13–11 Perpetrators of workers' compensation fraud may include:

(a) ______________________________

(b) ______________________________

(c) ______________________________

(d) ______________________________

(e) ______________________________

13–12 Use CPT code ____________ to bill for workers' compensation reports if the report is not included in the E/M service.

13–13 What is the name of the report that the physician must fill out, sign, and send to the insurance carrier after the initial visit and treatment of the injured/ill worker?

____

CHECK YOUR HEARTBEAT! Turn to the end of the chapter for answers to these review sessions.

TESTING AND TREATMENT

If the physician needs to send the patient for outside testing or treatment, obtain authorization over the telephone from the employer or the insurance company adjuster. Always state the name of the procedure or test and the medical necessity for it. Obtain the name and title of the person giving authorization and write this in the patient's medical record and on the order form, along with the date and time authorization was granted. No authorization numbers are issued in workers' compensation cases.

Vocational Rehabilitation

Many states provide rehabilitation in the form of retraining, education, job guidance, and placement to assist an injured individual to find work before temporary disability compensation benefits expire. In any successful rehabilitation program, the insurance carrier, physician, physical therapist, employer, supervisor, and personnel department must act as a team with the common goal of getting an injured employee back to work (or light duty) as soon as possible. It is believed that the longer a person remains out of work, the less chance there is that he or she will return to the workplace.

Physical Therapy

Various forms of physical therapy are used to strengthen the injured worker (e.g., sports medicine therapy, physical medicine rehabilitation). CPT code 97001 is used to report the initial physical therapy evaluation. Physical medicine/therapy CPT codes 97010 through 97140 are used to report various modalities and therapeutic procedures.

A type of therapy called **work hardening** is an individualized program that is sometimes used to help prepare the injured worker to return to work, especially if the job demands heavy lifting or requires fine motor skills of an injured body part. Patients often spend 6 to 8 hours in therapy programs which use conditioning regimens individually designed to simulate real work tasks in order to build up strength and improve the worker's endurance to take on a full day's work. CPT codes 97545 and 97546 are used to report work hardening conditioning.

Ergonomics

In some cases, an **ergonomic** evaluation of the work site is performed. This evaluation identifies modifications that may be instituted in the job or work site. Adjustments are made to lessen the possibility of future injury and to get the employee back to gainful employment as soon as possible. CPT code 97537 may be used to report a work site modification analysis.

LEGAL SITUATIONS

Depositions

A **deposition** is a discovery device by which one party asks questions of the other party or a witness for the other party. In a workers' compensation case, the questions are typically asked by an attorney representing the workers' compensation insurance company. The physician and/or injured worker answers the questions, under oath, outside the courtroom. The injured party's attorney may also be present. Direct and cross-examination may be done by both attorneys. This proceeding may take place in the attorney's office or in the physician's office.

The session may be recorded on a stenotype machine, in shorthand, or by audio- or videotape. The injured party or physician is allowed to read the transcript and make corrections or changes. The injured party or physician may be asked to sign the transcript but can waive signature if his or her attorney does not wish this to be done. The deposition may be used when the case comes to trial.

Medical Testimony

In a workers' compensation case, the physician may have to testify as an expert witness, take time to give a deposition, or attend a pretrial conference. It is important that there be a clear understanding of the terms of testimony and payment to eliminate any future misunderstandings. A written agreement from the patient's lawyer should be obtained stating exactly what compensation the physician will receive for research (preparation), time spent waiting to testify (if appointments must be canceled), and actual testimony time. In some cases, the physician may want to include an advanced partial payment clause in the agreement. If the physician is subpoenaed, he or she must appear in court regardless of whether an agreement exists. The correct CPT code for medical testimony is 99075.

Liens

The word **lien** is derived from the same origin as the world *liable.* The right of lien expresses legal claim on the property of another for the payment of a debt (Fig. 13–4). If a workers' compensation case is in dispute, a lien is sometimes placed by the injured party for medical expenses, which are to be paid after the case is settled and the injured party has obtained a monetary reward.

Many physicians do not want to take liens because payment is often delayed for many years, or, if the patient does not win the case, payment may not be received at all. The physician has to be sure that the patient has a legitimate case before taking a lien.

If the physician takes a case with no lien and the case goes to court, there is no legal documentation as far as collecting monies owed to the physician. A case could be settled, the attorney would get his or her fee, and the physician's fee may be placed last on the list for payment, or remain unpaid. Refer to Example 13–4 for a scenario in which a lien should have been obtained.

The patient/employee consents to the lien by his or her signature. Protect the physician's fee by also having the patient's attorney sign the lien, thereby indicating that he or she will pay the physician directly from any money received in a settlement. This makes the attorney responsible for the fee. The patient's file must be placed in a Hold for Settlement category until the case comes up in court. Call the office of the patient's attorney at least quarterly for an update.

A copy of the lien should be completed and sent to all concerned parties:

- Appeals board
- Employer of the patient
- Employee (the patient)
- Patient's attorney
- Insurance carrier
- Physician's file (lien claimant)

REQUEST FOR ALLOWANCE OF LIEN
ASSIGNMENT AND AUTHORIZATION

WHEREAS, I have a right or cause of action arising out of personal injury, to wit:

I, ____________________ hereby authorize ____________________,
patient's name physician's name

to furnish, upon request, to my attorney, ____________________, any and all medical records, or reports of examination, diagnosis, treatment, or prognosis but not necessarily limited to those items as set forth herein, in addition to an itemized statement of account for services rendered therefore or in connection therewith, which my attorney may from time to time request in connection with the injuries described above and sustained by me on the __________ day of __________, 20XX.

I, hereby irrevocably authorize and direct my said attorney set forth herein to pay to ____________________ all charges for attendance in court,
physician's name

if required as an expert witness whether he testifies or not; reports or other data supplied by him; depositions given by said doctor; medical services rendered or drugs supplied; and any other reasonable and customary charges incurred by my attorney as submitted by ____________________ and in
physician's name

connection with said injury. Said payment or payments are to be made from any money or monies received by my attorney whether by judgment, decree, or settlement of this case, prior to disbursement to me and payment of the amount as herein directed shall be the same as if paid by me. This authorization to pay the aforementioned doctor shall constitute and be deemed as assignment of so much of my recovery I receive. It is agreed that nothing herein relieves me of the primary responsibility and obligation of paying my doctor for services rendered, and I shall at all times remain personally liable for such indebtedness unless released by the aforementioned doctor or by payment disbursed by my attorney.
I accept the above assignment:
Dated: ____________________ Patient: ____________________

As the attorney of record for the above-named patient, I hereby agree to observe the terms of this agreement, and to withhold from any award in this case such sums as are required for the adequate protection of Dr. ____________________.

Date: ____________________ Attorney: ____________________

Figure 13–4. Patient's authorization to release information to an attorney and to grant lien to the physician against proceeds of settlement in connection with accident, industrial, or third party litigation cases.

Example 13–4

Filing a Lien

Scenario: Dr. Practon treated Katie Crest who was unable to pay for medical treatment except on legal monetary recovery. Katie was having a dispute with the insurance company over liability and the case was going to litigation. Dr. Practon testified on Ms. Crest's behalf in court. He had an oral agreement with the patient covering his fee for services and medical testimony. When Katie Crest settled her case, she forgot about Dr. Practon's bill and the fee for his medical testimony. The money was hers and she immediately moved from the area.

Comment: If a lien had been signed, then when the case was settled the money would be paid to Dr. Practon for his fee and expert medical testimony.

Check with your local division of industrial accidents for forms pertinent to filing a lien, instructions on the formalities, number of copies required, and where copies are to be sent.

Third Party Subrogation

The legal term **third party subrogation** means to substitute one person for another. When applied to workers' compensation cases, it means a transfer of the claims and rights from the original creditor (workers' compensation insurance carrier) to the third party liability carrier. In a compensation case involving third party subrogation, the participants are the patient, the workers' compensation insurance carrier, and a third party responsible for the injury who may also have insurance, sometimes referred to as **third party liability.** Refer to Example 13–5 for a scenario demonstrating third party subrogation.

Example 13–5

Third Party Subrogation

Scenario: Monica Valdez, a secretary, goes to the bank to deposit some money for her employer. While on the errand, Monica's car is rear-ended by another automobile and she is injured.

Rationale: In such a case there is no question of fault and no question of cause. Monica was hurt during the performance of her work, and the workers' compensation insurance carrier is liable. The carrier must adjust the claim, provide all medical treatment, and pay all TD and/or PD benefits.

Third Party Subrogation: Monica has a good subrogation case. She may seek the advice of an attorney, sue the third party (other automobile driver) in civil court, and when an award is made, the workers' compensation insurance carrier is reimbursed and Monica receives the balance of the reward. In some states, such as California, the patient is legally prevented from collecting twice.

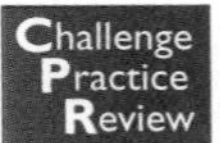

Pause and Practice CPR

REVIEW SESSIONS 13–14 THROUGH 13–16

Directions: *Complete the following questions as a review of information you have just read.*

13–14 A discovery device used in which one party asks questions of another party or witness outside of a courtroom is called a/an ______________________.

13–15 If the physician testifies in court, it is considered a ______________ testimony.

13–16 Who are the participants in a third party subrogation case? ______________

____

PRACTICE SESSIONS 13–17 THROUGH 13–21

Directions: *Use your procedure codebook and code the following services for a workers' compensation case as if you were working for a physical therapist.*

13–17 Application of a hot pack to the patient's back ______________

13–18 Manual traction to the patient's right leg (15 minutes) ______________

13–19 Whirlpool therapy for a decubitus ulcer (right heel) ______________

13–20 Physical therapy reevaluation ______________

13–21 Ultrasound on the patient's left calf (15 minutes) ______________

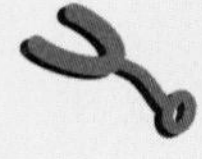

CHECK YOUR HEARTBEAT! Turn to the end of the chapter for answers to these review and practice sessions

CLAIM PROCEDURES

Financial Responsibility

Workers' compensation is the primary payer for services due to a work-related injury. Other insurance companies (e.g., Medicare) may pick up the residual when workers' compensation benefits have been exhausted or when services are not covered under workers' compensation.

Insurance Contract

As discussed in Chapter 2, in a workers' compensation case, the contract exists between the physician and the insurance company. This is because the patient's employer is providing medical services through a workers' compensation health insurance policy, and the patient is not financially responsible. The same is true when a business is self-insured. As long as treatment is authorized by the insurance carrier, the insurance company is responsible for payment.

Nonrelated Injury/Illness

Sometimes while examining an injured worker, the physician may discover a problem unrelated to the industrial injury or illness, for example, high blood pressure. Always obtain private health insurance information in case you need to bill for such services that are not work-related or if the injury or illness is declared nonindustrial. In this example, the physician may bill the workers' compensation carrier for the examination but the diagnostic code should indicate the injury as the reason for the examination. If treatment is initiated for the patient's high blood pressure, then that portion of the examination becomes the financial obligation of the patient and not the workers' compensation carrier. To assist in informing patients of financial responsibility for nonrelated illness, obtain a signed agreement for nonrelated medical expenses, as shown in Figure 13–5.

Fee Schedules

Some states have developed and adopted workers' compensation **fee schedules.** Other states may pay medical claims based on the Medicare fee schedule plus or minus a certain percentage. Workers' compensation fee schedules assist with the following:

1. They limit the fees providers can charge for standard medical procedures.

PATIENT AGREEMENT

Patient's Name James Doland Soc. Sec. # 431-XX-1942

Address 67 Blyth Dr., Woodland Hills, XY 12345 Tel. No. 555-372-0101

WC Insurance Carrier Industrial Indemnity Company

Address 30 North Dr., Woodland Hills Telephone No. 555-731-7707

Date of illness 2-13-20XX Date of first visit 2-13-20XX

Emergency Yes X No ____

Is this condition related to employment Yes X No ____

If accident: Auto ____ Other ____

Where did injury occur? Construction site

How did injury happen? fell 8 ft from scaffold suffering fractured right tibia

Employee/employer who verified this information Scott McPherson

Employer's name and address Willow Construction Company

Employer's telephone No. 555-526-0611

In the event the claim for worker's compensation is declared fraudulent for this illness or condition or it is determined by the Workers' Compensation Board that the illness or injury is not a compensable workers' compensation case, I James Doland, hereby agree to pay the physician's fee for services rendered.

I have been informed that I am responsible to pay any services rendered by Dr. Raymond Skeleton with regard to the discovery and treatment of any condition not related to the workers' compensation injury or illness. I agree to pay for all services not covered by workers' compensation and all charges for treatment and personal items unrelated to my workers' compensation illness or injury.

Signed James Doland Date 2-13-20XX

Figure 13–5. Patient agreement to pay the physician's fees if the case is declared not work-related.

2. They limit the amount that providers will be paid.
3. They make the allowable charges for procedures more consistent.
4. They provide follow-up procedures in case of a fee dispute.

Workers' compensation fee schedules may list maximum reimbursement levels for physicians and other nonhospital providers. Generally, a physician who agrees to treat a workers' compensation patient must agree to accept payment in full according to the workers' compensation fee schedule. There is no assignment of benefits. The workers' compensation carrier pays the fee for authorized services rendered according to its fee schedule and the check is automatically sent to the physician. The patient is not responsible for payment of any work-related injury or illness, including copayment amounts or amounts for noncovered services. It is best to note that the physician's compensation depends on workers' compensation rules. These rules cannot be changed or altered except by state laws.

Types of Fee Schedules

A *percentile-of-charge schedule* may be used that is designed to set fees at a percentile of the provider's usual and customary fee. For example, if the percentile was 70%, and the usual and customary fee was $100, the workers' compensation fee would be $70 ($100 × .70 = $70).

A *relative value scale (RVS) schedule* may be used which takes into account the time, skills, and extent of the service provided by the physician. Each procedure is rated on how difficult it is, how long it takes, the training a physician must have to perform it, and expenses the physician incurs, including the cost of malpractice insurance.

Many RVS fee schedules are similar to the CPT format as far as sections (i.e., E/M, Anesthesia, Surgery). To establish a reasonable maximum fee, a conversion factor that uses a specific dollar amount for each of the sections of the fee schedule is multiplied by the unit value for each procedure (see Example 13–6). Conversion factors may be adjusted to reflect regional differences and in some states are recalculated on an annual basis. Other states may update their fee schedule every 2 or 3 years.

Example 13–6

Conversion Factors for Workers' Compensation in California

$8.50/unit	Evaluation and Management section
$34.50/unit	Anesthesia section
$153.00/unit	Surgery section
$12.50/unit	Radiology section (total unit value)
$1.95/unit	Radiology section (professional component)
$1.50/unit	Radiology section (technical component)
$1.50/unit	Pathology section (technical component)
$6.15/unit	Medicine section

Expressions from Experience

Although the billing department is specialized and everyone has his or her own job, getting along with coworkers and helping each other is beneficial. Regardless of what position one has (receptionist, billing clerk, data entry, medical assistant), each plays an important role in having a successful practice.

Kara Chang
Workers' Compensation Specialist
Orthopedics

Helpful Billing Tips

The following are helpful hints for billing workers' compensation claims.

1. Ask whether the injury occurred within the scope of employment and verify insurance information with the benefits coordinator at the employee's workplace. This will assure filing initial claims with the correct insurance carrier.
2. Request that the patient obtain the claim number of his or her case prior to coming in for the initial visit. If no claim number has been assigned, ask for the insurance policy number.
3. Educate the patient with regard to the medical practice's billing policies for workers' compensation cases and have him or her complete the patient agreement form shown in Figure 13–5.
4. Document in a telephone log or patient's record all data for authorization of examination, diagnostic studies, or surgery (e.g., date, name of individual who authorizes, response).
5. Complete the Doctor's First Report of Occupational Injury or Illness form for your state and submit it within the time limit shown in Table 13–5.
6. Obtain a workers' compensation fee schedule for your state.
7. Use appropriate five-digit code numbers and modifiers to ensure prompt and accurate payment for services rendered (these may be codes and/or modifiers other than in CPT).
8. Submit an itemized statement after treatment, monthly or on termination of treatment for nondisability claims.
9. Clearly define any charges in excess of the fee schedule. Attach any x-ray reports, operative reports, discharge summaries, pathology reports, and so forth to clarify such excess charges. When using a workers' compensation codebook and a procedure code has **BR (by report)** next to the code, include the necessary report.  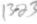
10. Itemize and send invoices for drugs and dressings furnished by the physician. Bill medical supplies on

a separate claim or statement because this may be routed to a different claims processing department.

11. Call the insurance carrier and talk with the **claims examiner** who is familiar with the patient's case, if you have a question regarding a fee.
12. Search the Internet for a web site or write to your state's workers' compensation office for booklets, bulletins, forms, and legislation information. See Resources at the end of this chapter for additional information.

Claim Submission

For efficiency in processing industrial claims, many insurance carriers have developed their own workers' compensation claim forms while others allow use of the HCFA-1500 claim form. Figure D–12 in Appendix D is an illustration of a completed workers' compensation case on a HCFA-1500 claim form.

Electronic Claim Submission

Check with individual carriers to see if they are equipped to receive electronic claims. If so, transmit according to their requirements. When electronic processing is possible, it is always more expedient to use it.

Out-of-State Claims

When billing for an out-of-state claim, insurance billing specialists must follow all workers' compensation regulations from the jurisdiction (state) in which the injured worker was *hired* and not the state where the injury occurred.

Companies that have employees that travel to other states are required to obtain workers' compensation insurance in those states. Obtain an out-of-state fee schedule to determine proper procedure codes, modifiers, and amounts for billing the claim. Ask whether the claimant's jurisdiction accepts electronic submission, the HCFA-1500 claim form, or another form.

Delinquent Claims

If a workers' compensation claim becomes 45 days' delinquent, the insurance billing specialist should send a letter to the insurance carrier (Fig. 13–6). For problem claims it may be wise to obtain and complete a

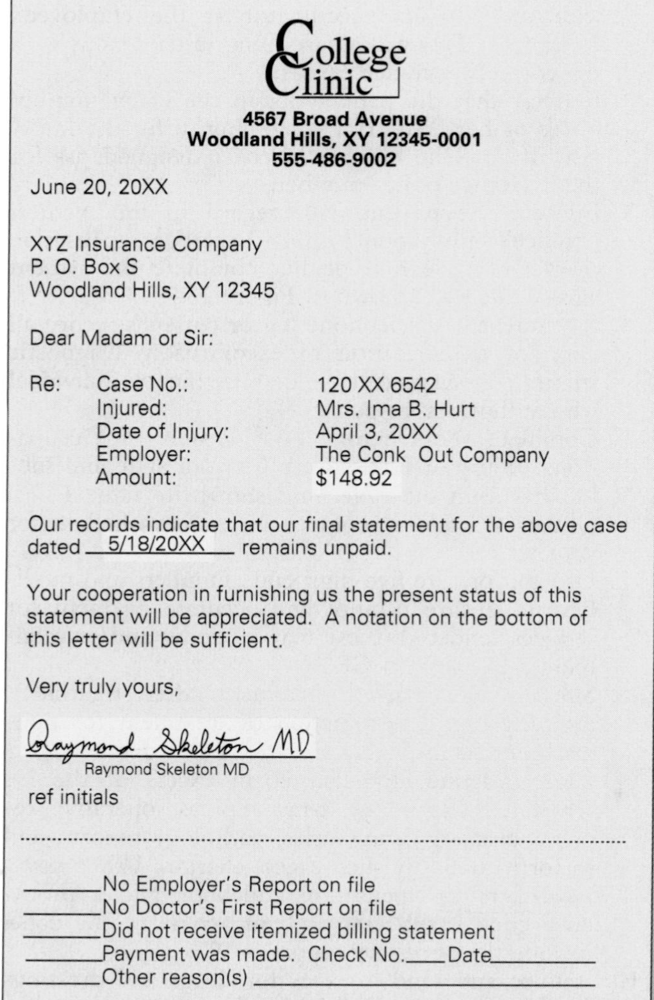

College Clinic
4567 Broad Avenue
Woodland Hills, XY 12345-0001
555-486-9002

June 20, 20XX

XYZ Insurance Company
P. O. Box S
Woodland Hills, XY 12345

Dear Madam or Sir:

Re: Case No.: 120 XX 6542
Injured: Mrs. Ima B. Hurt
Date of Injury: April 3, 20XX
Employer: The Conk Out Company
Amount: $148.92

Our records indicate that our final statement for the above case dated 5/18/20XX remains unpaid.

Your cooperation in furnishing us the present status of this statement will be appreciated. A notation on the bottom of this letter will be sufficient.

Very truly yours,

Raymond Skeleton MD
Raymond Skeleton MD
ref initials

______ No Employer's Report on file
______ No Doctor's First Report on file
______ Did not receive itemized billing statement
______ Payment was made. Check No.____ Date______
______ Other reason(s) ____________

Figure 13–6. Letter sent to the insurance carrier when a workers' compensation claim becomes 45 days delinquent.

Certificate of Mailing form from the U.S. Postal Service. The form is initialed and postmarked at the post office and returned to the insurance biller to be kept in the office file. Because the post office does not keep a record of the mailing, this certificate costs less than certified mail. It shows proof that a special communication was mailed or sent on a certain date.

OCCUPATIONAL SAFETY AND HEALTH ADMINISTRATION (OSHA)

Background

Congress has established an office known as the **Occupational Safety and Health Administration (OSHA)** to protect employees against on-the-job health and safety hazards. This program includes strict health and safety standards and a sensible complaint procedure enabling individual workers to trigger enforcement measures.

Work standards are designed to minimize exposure to on-the-job hazards such as faulty machinery, excess noise, dust, and toxic chemical fumes. Employers are required by law to meet these health and safety standards. Failure to do so can result in fines against the employer that could run into thousands of dollars.

Coverage

The act provides that if a state submits an OSHA plan and it is approved by the federal government, then the state may assume responsibility for carrying out OSHA policies and procedures and is excluded from federal jurisdiction.

The act applies to almost all businesses, large or small. It applies to heavy, light, and service industries; nonprofit and charitable institutions; farmers; retailers; and churches' secular activities in hospitals. Employees of state and local governments are also covered.

Federal employees, a farmer's immediate family, church employees engaged in religious activities, independent contractors, and household domestic workers are not covered.

Regulations

Specific regulations that affect the medical setting are those aimed at minimizing exposure to hepatitis B virus (HBV), human immunodeficiency virus (HIV), and other bloodborne pathogens. Any worker who comes in contact with human blood and infectious material must receive proper information and training on using universal precautions to avoid exposure. Vaccinations must be provided for those who are at risk for exposure to HBV, and comprehensive records must be maintained. Material safety data sheets (MSDS), which include the various components in chemicals and the risks and instructions for exposure, must be obtained for each hazardous chemical used on-site. Refer to Resources at the end of this chapter for details on where to obtain further information.

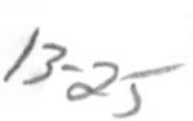

Filing a Complaint

To file a complaint, the proper form is obtained from the federal Division of Industrial Safety or a state OSHA office and completed by the employee. It is against the law for an employer to take any adverse actions against an employee who files such a complaint.

Record Keeping and Reporting

Employers must keep records of their employees' work-related injuries and illnesses on OSHA Form 200. This document must be on file at the workplace and available to employees and OSHA compliance officers on request. Form 200 must be retained in the file for 5 years. After 6 days, a case recorded on Form 200 must have a supplementary record, OSHA Form 101, completed and kept in the files. Some states have modified their workers' compensation forms so they may be used as substitutes for Form 101.

Companies with fewer than 11 employees must complete a safety survey using OSHA Form 200-S. Companies are also required to display OSHA posters to inform employees of their job safety rights. Federal law states that an accident that results in the death or hospitalization of five or more employees must be reported to OSHA.

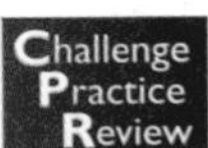

Pause and Practice CPR

REVIEW SESSIONS 13–22 THROUGH 13–28

Directions: *Complete the following questions as a review of information you have just read.*

13–22 *Multiple choice: Circle the best answer.* Generally, a physician who agrees to treat a workers' compensation patient

(a) must agree to accept the maximum amount of the workers' compensation fee schedule as payment in full;

(b) must agree to accept a percentage of the workers' compensation fee schedule;

(c) may submit his/her regular private fees and payment will be based on the private rate that the physician charges at the discretion of the workers' compensation carrier.

13–23 What percentage of the bill is the workers' compensation patient responsible for?

____

13–24 If no claim number has been assigned to a workers' compensation case, what number should the physician's office ask the employer for? ________________

13–25 If you have a question regarding a workers' compensation fee that was paid, whom do you call at the workers' compensation insurance carrier? ________________

13–26 What does the acronym OSHA stand for? ________________

____

13–27 What is the main function of OSHA? ________________

____

13–28 What must a medical practice do to inform employees of their job safety rights?

____

CHECK YOUR HEARTBEAT! Turn to the end of the chapter for answers to these review sessions.

OTHER DISABILITY INSURANCE PLANS

Accidents, injury, and illness may occur outside of the workplace that could cause an individual partial or total disability. There may be unusual circumstances that lead to such events. Example 13–7 illustrates some extraordinary situations where individuals were injured and needed medical attention.

There are various types of disability income insurance plans, as well as a number of disability benefit programs to cover non–work-related injury and illness. Because the definition of disability varies among policies, the critical issues are the content and wording on the claim form. Each plan may have its own claim form; a portion of the form is usually completed by the patient, and a portion by the attending physician.

In come cases, the physician may wish to dictate a medical report and attach it to the claim form instead of completing the physician's portion. The insurance billing specialist must be prepared to extract data from source documents, such as medical and financial records, to complete the claim form. Always ask the physician to read the information carefully before signing the document.

The following section explains private and federal disability plans, offers basic definitions for terms encountered when dealing with plans, and defines eligibility and benefits.

Example 13–7

Describe How Your Disability Occurred

- "I dislocated my shoulder swatting a fly."
- "A got a hernia from pulling the cork out of a bottle."
- "Getting on a bus, the driver started before I was all on."
- "While waving goodnight to friends, fell out of a two-story window."
- "Put tire patch on girdle and it caused an infection on right thigh."
- "Back injury received from jumping off a ladder to escape being hit by a train."

Disability Income Insurance

13-26

Disability income insurance is a form of health insurance providing periodic payments under certain conditions when the insured is unable to work because of illness, disease, or injury—not as a result of a work-related accident or condition. Disability income policies do not provide medical expense benefits. Income insurance is available from private insurance companies (individual policies) and employer-sponsored plans (group policies). To collect benefits, the individual must meet the policy's criteria of what constitutes partial, temporary, or total disability. The physician documents this information either on a form or in a report that is sent to the private insurance company.

Types of Disability

The definitions of the various types of disability vary from those defined in workers' compensation and also among different insurance carriers. General definitions are as follows:

- **Total disability**—The insured must be unable to perform the major duties of his or her specific occupation.
- **Partial disability**—When an illness or injury prevents an insured person from performing one or more of the functions of his or her regular job.

- **Temporary disability**—When a person cannot perform all the functions of his or her regular job for a limited period of time.

Benefit Period

A **benefit period** is the maximum amount of time that benefits will be paid to the injured or ill person for the disability (e.g., 2 years, 5 years, to age 65, or lifetime).

Benefits

Benefits paid to the insured disabled person are called *indemnity* and can be received daily, weekly, monthly, or semiannually depending on the policy. Premiums and benefits hinge on several risk factors, such as age, sex, health history and physical state, income, and occupational duties.

Waiver of Premium

A **waiver of premium,** if included in the insurance contract, means that, while the person is disabled, the policy pays all premiums and the employee does not have to pay.

Exclusions

Exclusions are provisions written into the insurance contract denying coverage or limiting the scope of coverage.

Federal Disability Programs

Social Security Disability Insurance Program

The term *disability* under Social Security has a strict definition: "Inability to engage in any substantial gainful activity by reason of any medically determinable physical or mental impairment which can be expected to result in death or which has lasted or can be expected to last for a continuous period of not less than 12 months."

Eligibility

The following is a list of individuals who meet eligibility requirements for **Social Security Disability Insurance (SSDI).**

- Disabled workers younger than age 65 and their families
- Individuals who become disabled before age 22 years, if a parent (or, in certain cases, a grandparent) who is covered under Social Security retirement becomes disabled or dies
- Disabled widows or widowers, age 50 years or older, if the deceased spouse worked at least 10 years under Social Security
- Disabled surviving divorced spouses older than age 50 years, if the ex-spouse was married to the disabled person for at least 10 years
- Blind workers whose vision in the better eye cannot be corrected to better than 20/200 or whose visual field in the better eye, even with corrective lenses, is 20 degrees or less.

Benefits

Monthly benefits are paid to qualified individuals. After 24 months of disability payments, the disabled individual also becomes eligible for Medicare. When an individual reaches age 65, the benefits convert to retirement benefits.

Supplemental Security Income

Eligibility

The Supplemental Security Income (SSI) program provides disability payments to needy people (adults and children) with limited income and few resources. No prior employment is needed. Many SSI recipients also qualify for Medicaid, a state assistance program. A strict disability determination process is undergone to establish disability. The following individuals qualify for SSI disability payments:

- Disabled persons younger than age 65 years who have very limited income and resources
- Disabled children younger than age 18 years, if the disability compares in severity with one that would keep an adult from working and has lasted or is expected to last at least 12 months or result in death
- Blind adults or children who, in the better eye, with the use of corrective lenses, have a visual acuity no better than 20/100, or a visual field of 20 degrees or less

Benefits

Social Security disability programs are designed to give long-term protection and benefits to individuals totally disabled who are unable to do any type of work in the national economy.

Civil Service and Federal Employees Retirement System Disability

Federal employees who work in civil service fall under the Civil Service Retirement System (CSRS). This system has provisions for those who become totally disabled. This program is a combination of federal disability and Social Security disability. Both portions of

Expressions from Experience

Establishing good rapport with workers' compensation adjusters and their bill reviewers is a must. Oral and written communication skills are important in all areas of the medical office.

Kara Chang
Workers' Compensation Specialist
Orthopedics

the program must be applied for by the worker. For a civil servant, the disability cannot be work-related, and 5 years of service are required before benefits are payable. Eighteen months of service are required under the Federal Employees Retirement System (FERS). Those who qualify are entitled to benefits that are payable for life.

Armed Services Disability

Individuals covered under this program must be members of the armed services on active duty. If a disability occurs or is aggravated while serving in the military service, monthly benefits are payable for life. Benefit amounts are based on years of service, base pay, and severity of disability, subject to review.

Veterans Affairs Disability

The Veterans Affairs (VA) is authorized by law to provide a wide range of benefits to those who have served their country in the armed forces and to their dependents. If a veteran who is honorably discharged files a claim for a *service-connected* disability within 1 year of sustaining that injury, he or she is eligible for outpatient treatment. Certain veterans with *non–service-connected disabilities* who are unable to travel to a VA facility owing to geographic inaccessibility are also eligible for treatment in an outpatient facility.

Numerous benefits are available; however, each benefit requires that certain criteria be met. These criteria are ever-changing and will not be mentioned here. A complete up-to-date booklet listing all the benefits is available (see Resources at the end of this chapter).

State Disability Insurance

State Disability Insurance (SDI) is a form of insurance that is part of an employment security program that provides temporary cash benefits for workers suffering a wage loss due to off-the-job illness or injury. It can be referred to as **unemployment compensation disability (UCD)** or **temporary disability insurance (TDI).**

For many decades only five states and one U.S. commonwealth have had state disability insurance: California, Hawaii, New Jersey, New York, Rhode Island, and Puerto Rico. Web sites for most of these programs can be found in the Resources section at the end of this chapter.

Funding

To fund state disability insurance, a small percentage of the wages is deducted from the employees' paychecks each month, or the employer may elect to pay all or part of the cost of the plan as a fringe benefit. The money is then sent in quarterly installments to the state and put into a special fund.

Eligibility

To receive state disability insurance benefits, an employee must be:

- Employed full- or part-time or actively looking for work when disability begins
- Suffering a loss of wages because of disability
- Eligible for benefits depending on the amount withheld during a previous period before disability began
- Disabled at least 7 calendar days, or hospitalized as an inpatient in Puerto Rico
- Filing a claim within the time limit

Benefits

Weekly benefits are determined by the wages earned in a base period or based on a percentage of average weekly wages. Benefits begin after the seventh consecutive day of disability. There is no provision under the law for hospital or other medical benefits except in Hawaii and Puerto Rico, where hospital benefits are payable under a prepaid healthcare program if the employee meets certain eligibility requirements.

Time Limits

A claim for state disability insurance should be filed within the time limit of the state laws (see Table 13–6). There is usually a grace period, and the claim is approved and benefits become payable after the waiting period, as stated under each state law.

State Disability Form

Forms vary among states and may be two or three pages long. Two important dates listed on all forms are (1) the date the employee last worked, and (2) the first date the employee was unable to perform job duties. Unlike workers' compensation, these two dates must *not* be the same. For example, if the patient went home sick on October 4, that would be considered the last

Table 13–6 State Disability Information Summary

State	Name of State Law	Maximum Benefit Period (wk)	Time Limit for Filing Claims
California	California Unemployment Insurance Code	52	49 days from disability
Hawaii	Temporary Disability Insurance Law	26	90 days from disability
New Jersey	Temporary Disability Benefits Law	26	30 days from disability
New York	Disability Benefits Law	26	30 days from disability
Puerto Rico	Disability Benefits Act	26	3 mo from disability
Rhode Island	Temporary Disability Insurance Act	30	1 yr from disability

day worked and October 5 becomes the first day the patient was unable to go to work.

State Disability and Workers' Compensation

If a recipient is collecting benefits from a workers' compensation insurance carrier and the amount that the compensation carrier pays is *less* than that allowed by the state disability insurance program, then the disability program will pay the balance.

Voluntary Disability Insurance

Persons residing and working in states that do not have state disability insurance programs may elect to contact a local private insurance carrier to arrange for coverage under a **voluntary disability insurance** plan. If these persons become ill or disabled, they receive a fixed weekly or monthly income, usually for approximately 6 months. If the disability or illness is permanent and the individual is unable to return to work, there is sometimes a small monthly income for the duration of the person's life. Some of the state laws provide that a "voluntary plan" may be adopted instead of the "state plan" if a majority of company employees consent to private coverage.

The insured (claimant) is always responsible for notifying the insurance company of the disability. The form submitted by the physician must indicate that the patient's disability meets the policy's definition of disability or benefits will be denied.

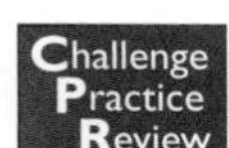

Pause and Practice CPR

REVIEW SESSIONS 13–29 THROUGH 13–32

Directions: *Complete the following questions as a review of information you have just read.*

13–29 Is disability income insurance

(a) a form of health insurance? ________

(b) an insurance plan that provides medical benefits? ________

(c) an insurance plan that provides periodic payments? ________

13–30 Are definitions the same in disability income insurance plans for "total disability," "partial disability," and "temporary disability" as in the workers' compensation program? __________

13–31 The acronym SSDI stands for ____,

which is a _______________ disability program.

13–32 Lists the state(s) and the commonwealth that have State Disability Insurance (SDI).

(a) ______________________________

(b) ______________________________

(c) ______________________________

(d) ______________________________

(e) ______________________________

(f) ______________________________

CHECK YOUR HEARTBEAT! Turn to the end of the chapter for answers to these review sessions.

SUMMATION AND PREVIEW

You have now completed the final program (workers' compensation) and can place this building block on the solid foundation that you have constructed. When working with workers' compensation claims, good communication tools are needed to speak with adjusters and claims examiners. Always be courteous and present your inquiries with respect for the job that they are trying to do. Learn the specific rules and regulations that apply to your state. Claims representatives will respect physicians' employees who are knowledgeable about workers' compensation laws.

Whether or not you work for the type of practice that handles workers' compensation claims, you will undoubtedly process some type of disability form. Be meticulous and detail-oriented when abstracting information and completing such forms. When the patient has a bona fide claim, his or her financial benefits depend on the submission and content of the form or report.

In the next chapter you will learn about billing practices, credit and collection laws, various credit arrangements, and the collection process. Communicating payment requirements and working within the laws that regulate collection are key to gaining maximum reimbursement for the physician's office.

GOLDEN RULE

Physician compensation depends on workers' compensation rules.

Chapter 13 Review and Practice

Study Session

Directions: *Review the objectives, key terms, and chapter information before completing the following study questions.*

13–1 Workers' compensation federal laws apply to:

(a) Government workers

391 (b) Miners

(c) Maritime workers

13–2 Workers' compensation state laws apply to:

391 (a) Private employees

(b) State employees

13–3 How many states qualify large employers as self-insurers? 48

13–4 Summarize the reasons that workers' compensation laws have been developed.

(a) provide Best care & to ensure prompt return to work

391 (b) provide income to ill worker or dependents, regardless of fault

(c) reduce court delays, costs, & workloads that arise from litigation

(d) eliminate payment of fees to attorneys & witnesses & time consuming trials & appeals

(e) to encourage employer interest in safety & rehabilitation

(f) promote the study of causes of accidents & reduce preventable accidents & suffering

392 13–5 What is the name of the fund that helps to encourage hiring of the physically handicapped?

Second Injury Fund

393 13–6 Refer to Table 13–1 and list the number of employees your state requires for workers' compensation laws. 3

13–7 List the various ways an employee may be referred to a physician after a work-related injury or illness has occurred.

(a) On Site Physician

(b) Predesignated Physician

(c) Employer Referral

(d) Employee Self-Referral.

394 13–8 Refer to Table 13–2 and list the waiting period required by your state before income benefits are payable. 7 days (ranges from 0–7)

394 13–9 What is the job of an AME, IME, or QME? Physicians who conduct medical-legal evaluations of injured workers. w/ unbiased

13–10 When a medical-legal (ML) evaluation is performed, what reimbursement is included in the fee?

395 (a) examination

(b) review of records

(c) preparation of medical-legal report

(d) overhead expenses.

13–11 Using the sample codes and modifiers listed in Example 13–2, what modifier would you use to append a code for an ML testimony? 96

13–12 If a worker is injured/ill and cannot return to full work, what other options are used to get the employee back to work? released to modified work OR placed in a different department or division.

13–13 A healthcare person who is assigned to a workers' compensation case to expedite the patient's care and help resolve the claim quickly is called the Case manager.

13–14 Define and describe P and S. Permanent + Stationary - damage from injury or illness is permanent, patient recovered to fullest extent possible, physician unable to do anything more for patient, patient will be hampered by disability to some extent for the rest of his or her life.

13–15 The process of making a final determination of the issues involving settlement of an industrial accident or illness is known as rating of a case, or adjudication.

13–16 In most states, insurance claims adjusters have unlimited access to the injured employee's medical records that pertain to the industrial case. Information [can, cannot] be shared over the telephone and reports [can, cannot] be sent to the insurance company without the patient's signed consent.

13–17 Why should a patient's private medical record and workers' compensation record be kept separate? Because there are seperate disclosure laws for each.

13–18 Complete the following sentence: "It is believed that the longer a person remains out of work, the less chance there is that he or she will return to the workplace."

13–19 A physical therapy program individualized to simulate real work situations and prepare an injured worker to return to work is called work hardening.

13–20 A/an ergonomic evaluation is performed on the work site to identify modifications that may be instituted in the job or work site to lessen the possibility of future injury to the employee.

13–21 What is an option for handling medical expenses when a workers' compensation case is in dispute and the employee/patient has no money to pay until after the case is settled? a lien is sometimes placed on the injured party

13–22 In a workers' compensation case, the contract exists between the physician and the insurance company.

13–23 What does BR stand for and what does it mean? "By Report" used next to a procedure code in worker's compensation codebook & means to include the necessary report.

412 13–24 How long should an insurance billing specialist wait to submit a letter inquiring about a workers' compensation insurance claim? 45 Days.

13–25 What is the purpose of "material safety data sheets?" Include various
413 components in chemicals & the risks & instructions for exposure.

13–26 Benefits for disability income insurance can be received Daily, weekly, monthly
414 OR semiannualy.

415 13–27 What period of time does an individual have to be on Social Security Disability Insurance (SSDI) before qualifying for Medicare? After 24 months.

13–28 A form of insurance which is part of an employment security program may be known as one of the following:

(a) State disability Insurance (SDI)

(b) Unemployment Compensation Disability (UCD)

(c) Temporary Disability Insurance (TDI)

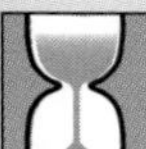

Billing Break

Time Started
Time Finished
Total Time

Case 13–1 Paige V. Ulwelling

Directions: *Follow these steps to complete the HCFA-1500 insurance claim form for a workers' compensation case using OCR guidelines.*

1. Copy the HCFA-1500 insurance claim form found in Appendix F (Form 09).
2. Refer to the Patient Information form for Case 13–1 and abstract information to complete the top portion of the HCFA-1500 claim form.
3. Refer to the Medical Record for Case 13–1 to abstract information for the bottom portion of the HCFA-1500 claim form.
4. Copy the Medical Record Coding Worksheet found in Appendix F (Form 12) to use when abstracting information from the chart note.
5. Use the "HCFA-1500 Claim Form Block-by-Block Instructions" for workers' compensation patients found in Appendix D and the workers' compensation template (Fig. D–12) for guidance and block help.
6. Use your procedure codebook to determine the correct code number(s) and modifier(s) for each professional service/procedure rendered.
7. Refer to the fee schedule in Appendix B for mock fees.
8. Use your diagnostic codebook to determine the correct diagnoses.
9. Address the claim to the workers' compensation insurance carrier and date the claim 10/28/20XX.
10. Copy and prepare the ledger card found in Appendix F (Form 07). Address it to the workers' compensation insurance company and indicate the injured workers' name and employer along with the other required information. Complete the ledger by posting each transaction in this case and indicating when you have billed the insurance carrier.

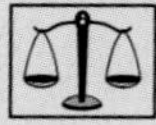

WEIGH YOUR PROGRESS. Turn to the Assignment Score Sheet in Appendix F (Form 10) and record the information to track your success. Your instructor may ask that you include a Performance Evaluation Checklist, and if so, copy Form 11 found in Appendix F and attach it to your insurance claim.

College Clinic
4567 Broad Avenue
Woodland Hills, XY
12345-0001
Tel (555) 486-9002
Fax (555) 487-8976

REGISTRATION
(PLEASE PRINT)

Account # 2542 Today's Date: 10/28/XX

PATIENT INFORMATION

Name Ulwelling (Last Name) Paige (First Name) V. (Initial) Soc. Sec. # 908-XX-7373

Address 336 Citrus Circle Home Phone (555) 967-3472

City Orange Grove State XY Zip 12345

Single ✓ Married ___ Separated ___ Divorced ___ Sex M ___ F ✓ Birthdate 01/25/1970

Patient Employed by CHEMCO Occupation Chemical Engineer

Business Address 2121 Lemonwood, Orange Grove Business Phone (555) 967-8000

Spouse's Name N/A Employed by: ___ Occupation ___

Business Address ___ Business Phone ___

Reason for Visit Shortness of breath If accident: ___ Auto ___ Employment ✓ Other ___

By whom were you referred? Concha Antrum MD

In case of emergency, who should be notified? Gail Ulwelling (Name) Mother (Relation to Patient) Phone (555) 967-9243

PRIMARY INSURANCE

Insured/Subscriber CHEMCO (Last Name) ___ (First Name) ___ (Initial)

Relation to Patient Employer Birthdate ___ Soc. Sec.# ___

Address (if different from patient's) Same

City ___ State ___ Zip ___

Insurance Company State Compensation Insurance Fund

Insurance Address 12 Chelan Lane, Surf City, XY 12345

Insurance Identification Number No claim no. or policy no. Group # ___

ADDITIONAL INSURANCE

Is patient covered by additional insurance? Yes ___ No ✓

Subscriber Name ___ Relation to Patient ___ Birthdate ___

Address (if different from patient's) ___ Phone ___

City ___ State ___ Zip ___

Subscriber Employed by ___ Buisness Phone ___

Insurance Company ___ Soc. Sec. # ___

Insurance Address ___

Insurance Identification Number ___ Group # ___

ASSIGNMENT AND RELEASE

I, the undersigned, certify that I (or my dependent) have insurance coverage with State Compensation Ins. Fund (Name of Insurance Company(ies)) and assign directly to Dr. Coccidioides insurance benefits, if any, otherwise payable to me for services rendered. I understand that I am financially responsible for all charges whether or not paid by insurance. I hereby consent for the doctor to release all information necessary to secure the payment of benefits. I authorize the use of this signature on all insurance submissions.

N/A
Responsible Party Signature ___ Relationship ___ Date ___

ORDER # 58-8426 @BIBBERO SYSTEMS, INC. •PETALUMA, CALIFORNIA• TO REORDER CALL TOLL FREE (800)242-9330

1.) 506.4 3.) 401.0
Diagnostic Codes 2.) 994.9

Medical Record

Account number: 2542
Patient's name: Ulwelling, Paige V.
Date of birth: 01/25/70

Date	Progress Notes
	10/28/XX Dr. Concha Antrum requests a consultation on inpatient, Paige Ulwelling in College Hospital who was admitted on 10/26/XX with severe dyspnea, no known cause. Patient experiences periods of tachypnea and has moist persistent cough. She states that this has been going on for the past "several" years but has recently gotten worse. A C HX reveals no history of smoking, drug use, or childhood respiratory infections other than the "common cold." The patient has been working the past 15 years at a chemical plant. Various chemicals are discussed and it appears that the patient has been exposed to sulfur dioxide on and off during these past 15 years.
	A C PX is performed. A pulmonary function test indicates increased tidal volume and a marked reduction in her ability to exhale carbon dioxide; consistent with chronic emphysema. PA and lateral chest x-ray shows increased heart size, depressed diaphragm, and translucent-appearing lungs. Patient is hypertensive with a BP of 200/96. Arterial blood gas indicates decreased arterial oxygen and increased carbon dioxide.
	Oxygen is administered and the patient is started on drug therapy which includes an inhalant. Antihypertensive medication is prescribed. M/MDM. Diagnosis: Chronic respiratory emphysema due to inhalation of chemical fumes (sulfur dioxide) and malignant hypertension. Possible lung biopsy to be performed. Employer and workers' compensation carrier to be advised of employee's condition and diagnosis. Request authorization to treat as a work comp illness. Patient will be off work from 10/26/XX to 11/26/XX.
	Brady Coccidioides, MD

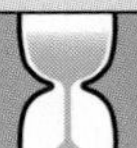

Billing Break

Time Started
Time Finished
Total Time

Case 13–2 Blair M. Hamashita

Directions: *Follow these steps to complete the HCFA-1500 insurance claim form for a workers' compensation case using OCR guidelines.*

1. Copy the HCFA-1500 insurance claim form found in Appendix F (Form 09).
2. Refer to the Patient Information form for Case 13–2 and abstract information to complete the top portion of the HCFA-1500 claim form.
3. Refer to the Medical Record for Case 13–2 to abstract information for the bottom portion of the HCFA-1500 claim form.
4. Copy the Medical Record Coding Worksheet found in Appendix F (Form 12) to use when abstracting information from the chart note.

5. Use the "HCFA-1500 Claim Form Block-by-Block Instructions" for workers' compensation patients found in Appendix D and the workers' compensation template (Fig. D–12) for guidance and block help.

6. Use your procedure codebook to determine the correct code number(s) and modifier(s) for each professional service/procedure rendered.

7. Refer to the fee schedule in Appendix B for mock fees.

8. Use your diagnostic codebook to determine the correct diagnoses.

9. Address the claim to the workers' compensation insurance carrier and date the claim 08/12/20XX.

10. Copy and prepare the ledger card found in Appendix F (Form 07). Address it to the workers' compensation insurance company and indicate the injured worker's name, date of injury, and employer, along with the other required information. Complete the ledger by posting each transaction in this case and indicating when you have billed the insurance carrier.

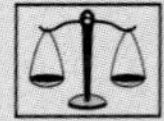

WEIGH YOUR PROGRESS. Turn to the Assignment Score Sheet in Appendix F (Form 10) and record the information to track your success. Your instructor may ask that you include a Performance Evaluation Checklist, and if so, copy Form 11 found in Appendix F and attach it to your insurance claim.

4567 Broad Avenue
Woodland Hills, XY
12345-0001
Tel (555) 486-9002
Fax (555) 487-8976

REGISTRATION
(PLEASE PRINT)

Account # 3996 Today's Date: 08/12/XX

PATIENT INFORMATION

Name Hamashita (Last Name) Blair (First Name) M. (Initial) Soc. Sec. # 623-XX-5180

Address 509 Rose Creek Road Home Phone (555) 967-1508

City Orange Grove State XY Zip 12345

Single ✓ Married ___ Separated ___ Divorced ___ Sex M ✓ F ___ Birthdate 12/01/1974

Patient Employed by Teloma Lakes Golf Course Occupation Greenskeeper

Business Address 3216 Teloma Street, Orange Grove Business Phone (555) 967-7112

Spouse's Name N/A Employed by: ___ Occupation ___

Business Address ___ Business Phone ___

Reason for Visit Accident If accident: ___ Auto ___ Employment ___ Other ___

By whom were you referred? Employer

In case of emergency, who should be notified? Mitch Tanaka (Name) Friend (Relation to Patient) Phone (555) 967-4321

PRIMARY INSURANCE

Insured/Subscriber Teloma Lakes Golf Course (Last Name / First Name / Initial)

Relation to Patient Employer Birthdate ___ Soc. Sec.# ___

Address (if different from patient's) Same

City ___ State ___ Zip ___

Insurance Company State Compensation Insurance Fund

Insurance Address 12 Chelan Lane, Surf City, XY 12345

Insurance Identification Number 9023500 (policy no.) Group # ___

ADDITIONAL INSURANCE

Is patient covered by additional insurance? Yes ___ No ✓

Subscriber Name ___ Relation to Patient ___ Birthdate ___

Address (if different from patient's) ___ Phone ___

City ___ State ___ Zip ___

Subscriber Employed by ___ Buisness Phone ___

Insurance Company ___ Soc. Sec. # ___

Insurance Address ___

Insurance Identification Number ___ Group # ___

ASSIGNMENT AND RELEASE

I, the undersigned, certify that I (or my dependent) have insurance coverage with State Compensation Ins. Fund (Name of Insurance Company(ies)) and assign directly to Dr. Skeleton insurance benefits, if any, otherwise payable to me for services rendered. I understand that I am financially responsible for all charges whether or not paid by insurance. I hereby consent for the doctor to release all information necessary to secure the payment of benefits. I authorize the use of this signature on all insurance submissions.

N/A
Responsible Party Signature Relationship Date

ORDER # 58-8426 @BIBBERO SYSTEMS, INC. •PETALUMA, CALIFORNIA• TO REORDER CALL TOLL FREE (800)242-9330

Diagnostic Codes
1) 813.04
2) 832.04
3) 813.43
4) 923.8

Medical Record

Account number: 3996
Patient's name: Hamashita, Blair M.
Date of birth: 12/01/74

Date	Progress Notes
	08/12/XX 4:00 p.m.—Mr. Blair Hamashita, was sent by his employer, Teloma Lakes Golf Course in Orange County for an emergent evaluation after an accident that occurred at the golf course at 3:30 p.m. this afternoon. While driving a golf cart, the 28-year-old employee drove down a slope near the lake and the cart flipped over on its side. The employee jumped from the cart as it began to roll and landed hard on the cart path. The patient complains of left elbow pain and pain in both wrists. I have not treated Mr. Hamashita prior to today. A C HX/PX are taken to evaluate the patient's condition. There are multiple contusions on upper limbs. The left elbow is very tender and extreme pain occurs when trying to move it so I am not able to evaluate the range of motion. The left wrist shows adequate ROM on flexion, extension, and circular rotation. Decreased ROM in the right wrist causing pain upon movement. X-rays are obtained of the left elbow (3-views) and both wrists (2-views). The x-rays show a fracture at the proximal end of the ulna with lateral dislocation of the radial head of the left elbow which is manipulated into place. A long arm plaster cast is applied. The right wrist shows an ulnar styloid fracture and a closed reduction is performed. A short arm fiberglass cast is applied. There is no fracture of the left wrist. Multiple contusions are cleaned and dressed and the patient is advised to withdraw from all activities for 1 week. Patient is taken off work for approximately 6 weeks. Estimated date of return to work, 9/23/XX. Return to office in 1 week for cast check. H/MDM. Raymond Skeleton, MD

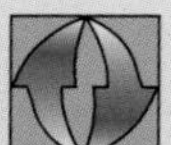

Exercise Exchange

13–1. Complete a Doctor's First Report of Occupational Injury and Illness Form

Directions

1. Refer to the Patient Registration form and Medical Record for Billing Break case 13–2 on Mr. Blair M. Hamashita.
2. Abstract information and complete the Doctor's First Report of Occupational Injury and Illness found in Appendix F (Form F–15).

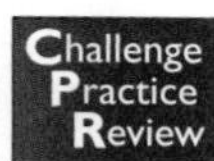

CPR Session: Answers

CHALLENGE SESSIONS 13–1 AND 13–2

13–1 workers' compensation insurance
13–2 employers' liability insurance

REVIEW SESSIONS 13–3 THROUGH 13–7

13–3 illegal
13–4 injury, illness, or death
13–5 yes
13–6 there may be two separate provisions: within the first 30 days and/or after the first 30 days
13–7 (a) Qualified Medical Evaluator
(b) Independent Medical Evaluator
(c) Agreed Medical Evaluator

REVIEW SESSIONS 13–8 THROUGH 13–10

13–8 (a) Nondisability claim involves a minor injury/illness; work is continued, and medical benefits apply.
(b) Temporary disability claim involves an injury/illness that renders the employee unable to perform all or part of his or her work duties for a period of time; medical benefits and wage compensation apply.
(c) Permanent disability claim involves a major injury/illness where the impairment/limitation is lifelong. Competition in the open job market is diminished; medical benefits and wage compensation (payments or lump sum) apply.
13–9 (a) severity of injury/illness
(b) age of injured person
(c) patient's occupation at time of injury/illness
13–10 insurance adjuster

REVIEW SESSIONS 13–11 THROUGH 13–13

13–11 (a) employees
(b) employers
(c) insurers
(d) medical providers
(e) lawyers
13–12 99080
13–13 Doctor's First Report of Occupational Injury; also called Illness or First Treatment Medical Report

REVIEW SESSIONS 13–14 THROUGH 13–16

13–14 deposition
13–15 medical
13–16 patient, workers' compensation insurance carrier, third party responsible for the injury

PRACTICE SESSIONS 13–17 THROUGH 13–21

13–17 97010
13–18 97140
13–19 97022
13–20 97002
13–21 97035

REVIEW SESSIONS 13–22 THROUGH 13–28

13–22 (a)
13–23 0% (none)
13–24 the policy number for the workers' compensation insurance plan
13–25 claims examiner
13–26 Occupational Safety and Health Administration
13–27 to protect employees against on-the-job health and safety hazards
13–28 display OSHA posters

REVIEW SESSIONS 13–29 THROUGH 13–32

13–29 (a) yes
(b) no
(c) yes
13–30 no
13–31 Social Security Disability Insurance, federal
13–32 (a) California
(b) Hawaii
(c) New Jersey
(d) New York
(e) Rhode Island
(f) Puerto Rico

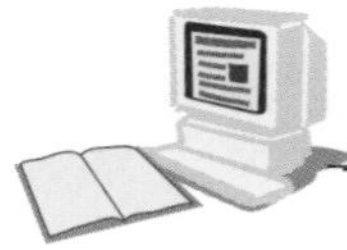

Resources

As an insurance billing specialist, from time to time you will need to locate answers to questions on state and federal laws governing workers' compensation and disability benefit programs. You may also need to obtain state workers' compensation forms. Very few seminars are offered which cover the topics discussed in this chapter. A web site gives quick access to up-to-date information and forms may be downloaded for certain states. In addition, booklets and books may be of value and a few are also listed in this resource section.

Internet

State Workers' Compensation

- Forms, statutes, news bulletins, links to all states
  Web site: www.workerscompensation.com

State Disability Insurance Programs

- State disability laws
  Web site: www.vpainc.com

Reference Books

- *Guide to the Evaluation of Permanent Impairment,* 2000, American Medical Association, Order Department, P.O. Box 930876, Atlanta, GA 31193-0876, (800) 621-8335

Booklets

- *Disability Income Insurance: An Overview of Income Protection Insurance,* Health Insurance Association of America, 1201 F Street NW, Suite 500, Washington, DC 20004-1204, (202) 824-1600
- *Federal Benefits for Veterans and Dependents,* Department of Veterans Affairs, Washington, DC (published annually), Superintendent of Documents, U.S. Government Printing Office, Mail Stop: SSOP, Washington, DC 20402-9328
- Occupational Safety and Health Administration (OSHA), OSHA Compliance Kit, Superintendent of Documents Publication Office, 200 Constitution Avenue NW, Room N3101, Washington, DC 20210
  Web site: www.osha.gov

NOTES

Objectives

After reading this chapter and completing the exercise sessions, you should be able to:

Learning Objectives:

- ✔ Execute formulas used to analyze the accounts receivable and determine the financial status of a medical practice.
- ✔ Explain aging analysis.
- ✔ Describe patient billing procedures in the medical office.
- ✔ Define credit and collection terminology.
- ✔ Enumerate payment and credit options available to patients.
- ✔ Summarize credit laws applicable to the physician's office.
- ✔ Perform oral and written communication collection techniques.
- ✔ State options for tracing a patient who has left the area with an unpaid account balance.

Performance Objectives:

- ✔ Complete a credit card voucher.
- ✔ Calculate dates for payment and fill out a financial agreement for a payment plan.
- ✔ Type a collection letter.

Key Terms

age analysis
bankruptcy
collection ratio
computer billing
credit card
cycle billing
debit card
debt
dun messages
insurance balance bill
itemized statement
manual billing
open accounts
skip
statute of limitations

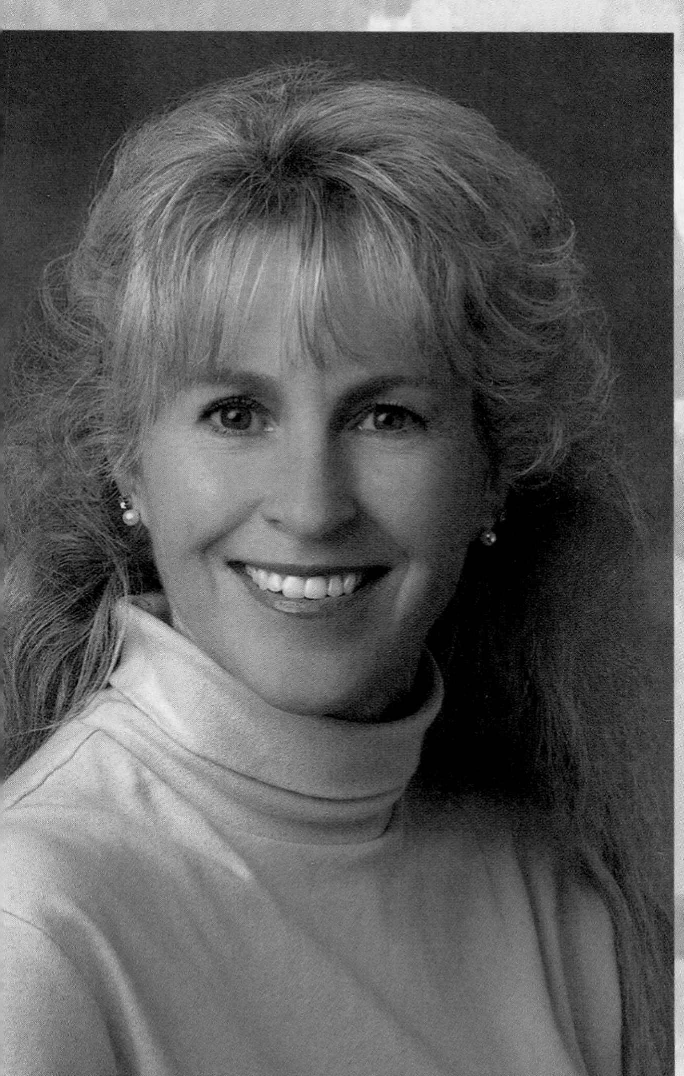

Chapter

14

I started in the medical field 17 years ago and now work for a family practice group with four physicians. I do the billing and collections, and as the years have passed I have seen many changes in billing procedures.

It is wonderful to work in a family practice because we treat grandparents, grandchildren, and everyone in between. It is to my advantage that I know my clientele because I am aware of the best personal approach to collect unpaid accounts.

I discovered over the years that follow-up is the key to success. If I am told I am to receive payment by the 10th and there is no payment on the 11th, I make another inquiry. This works successfully with private accounts and with outstanding insurance claims.

Those that know me, know I am a BIG coupon nut, maybe that's why I am so good at collections. I am either saving money or collecting money!

Tamra Hollins
Collection Specialist
Family Practice Group

Patient Billing: Credit and Collection Practices

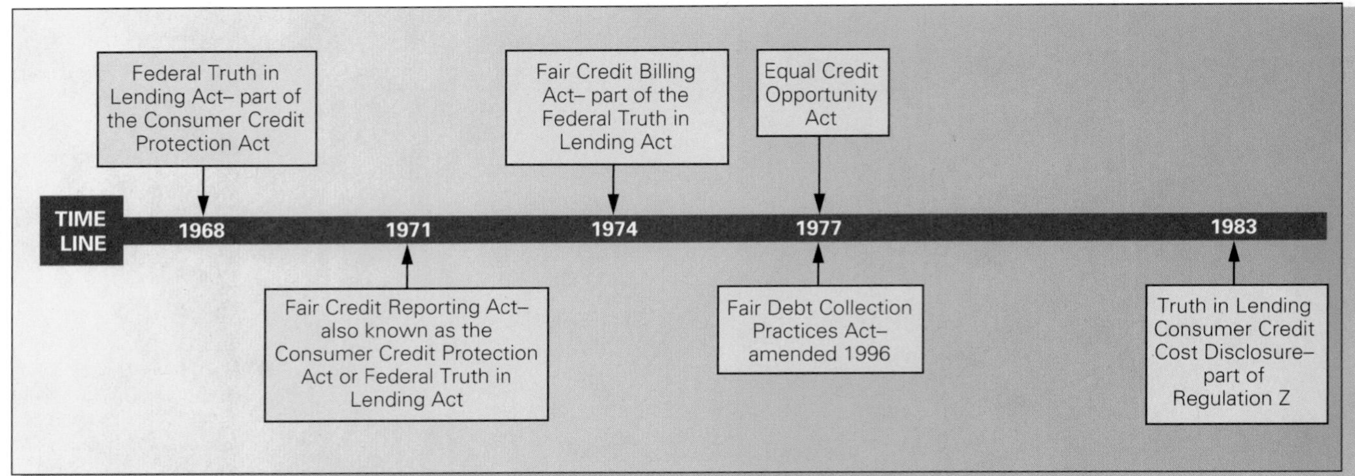

PATIENT PAYMENT RESPONSIBILITY

The individual responsible for payment of the medical bill was described in Chapter 2 under *guarantor.* The guarantor is often but not always the patient. Regardless of whether the patient has medical health insurance or not, the guarantor has a financial obligation to pay the physician for services and procedures performed. This chapter deals with the patient's responsibility for payment, billing routines and various methods of payment, credit arrangements, and the collection process. The bill that the patient is given or sent reflects the amount due and is referred to as a statement. When charges, payments, and adjustments are listed separately, it is called an itemized statement.

ITEMIZED STATEMENTS

From the first interaction a patient has with the practice to when he or she receives a statement, the billing/collection process poses opportunities for gain and loss. Every patient should receive an **itemized statement** (Fig. 14–1) of his or her account showing the dates of service, detailed charges, payments (copayments and deductibles), the date the insurance claim was submitted (if appropriate), applicable adjustments, and the account balance. These items will also be listed on the patient's ledger/account (see Chapter 3, Fig. 3–7). When sending itemized statements, timeliness, accuracy, and consistency have a significant effect on the cash flow and the collection process.

Professional bills are a reflection of the professionalism and efficiency of a medical practice. The billing statement should be patient-oriented and easy to read and understand. Avoid technical terms and abbreviations that might lead to confusion or misunderstandings. A return envelope with the statement "Forwarding Service Requested" must be included so the postal service can forward the mail and provide the physician's office with a notice of the patient's new address. When a postal notice is received in the physician's office, it should be circulated to all necessary departments to record the new information.

Patients can be oriented to the billing process when leaving the office by having the insurance specialist generate a printed statement explaining the pertinent information. When statements go out in the mail, the office is likely to experience an increase in telephone calls from inquiring patients. One person should handle all billing questions, ensuring a consistent response. A decision tree showing time frames for sending statements and telephone calls is presented later in this section (see Fig. 14–3).

Age Analysis

As mentioned in Chapter 3, the accounts receivable (A/R) is the total of all charges that have been posted to the general ledger/day sheet that have not yet been collected. **Age analysis** is a term used for the procedure of systematically arranging the A/R by age from the date of service. Accounts are usually aged in time periods of 30, 60, 90, and 120 days and older, as shown at the bottom of Figure 14–1. An aging analysis is automatically done in the computer using medical accounting software. This expedites collection follow-up by providing easy recognition of overdue accounts and allows the insurance specialist to determine which accounts need action in addition to a regular statement.

Each medical practice has a policy about handling the A/R. The effectiveness of this policy and its enforcement is reflected in the practice's cash flow. When charges are collected at the time of service, the A/R is zero. In an ideal situation, all outstanding balances are paid within 60 days; however, this is not always possible. The A/R is an important vital sign for the doctor's office because it is used to determine the medical practice's financial solvency. By monitoring the A/R the insurance billing specialist will be able to evaluate the effectiveness of the collection process.

The formula for determining the A/R ratio is to divide the month-end A/R balance by the monthly

College Clinic
4567 Broad Avenue
Woodland Hills, XY 12345-0001

NOTE: Insert this stub showing address in window and your payment; seal, stamp and drop in mail box. Thank You.

MO. DAY YR.
10 27 XX
0423M
ACCOUNT NO.

1. Reference account number and statement date

STATEMENT OF ACCOUNT

TO:

Eleanor Bassett
1619 Encina Ave
Woodland Hills, XY 12345-0001

AWAITING MEDICARE PAYMENT
FINAL BILL WILL FOLLOW

2. Dun message

☐ PLEASE CHECK IF ABOVE ADDRESS IS INCORRECT AND INDICATE CHANGE ON REVERSE SIDE. TO INSURE PROPER CREDIT TO YOUR ACCOUNT DETACH THIS PORTION AND RETURN WITH YOUR PAYMENT

$__________
AMOUNT ENCLOSED

DATE MO. DAY YR.	SERVICE CODE	DESCRIPTION	CHARGES OR DEBITS	PAYMENTS OR CREDIT
09 17 XX	99213	NP Office visit – Level 3	40.20	
09 17 XX	71020	Chest X-ray, 2 views	40.97	
09 17 XX	94010	Spirometry	38.57	
09 17 XX		Co-payment		10.00
10 24 XX	99212	Est Pt Office visit – Level 3	28.55	
10 24 XX		Co-payment		10.00

3. Itemized charges and payments shown line by line

OVER 120 DAYS	90–120 DAYS	60–90 DAYS	30–60 DAYS	CURRENT
			109.74	18.55

4. Aging analysis

AMOUNT DUE
128.29

5. Balance due

STATEMENT DATE	10 27 XX

CHARGES AND PAYMENT AFTER THIS DATE WILL APPEAR ON NEXT STATEMENT

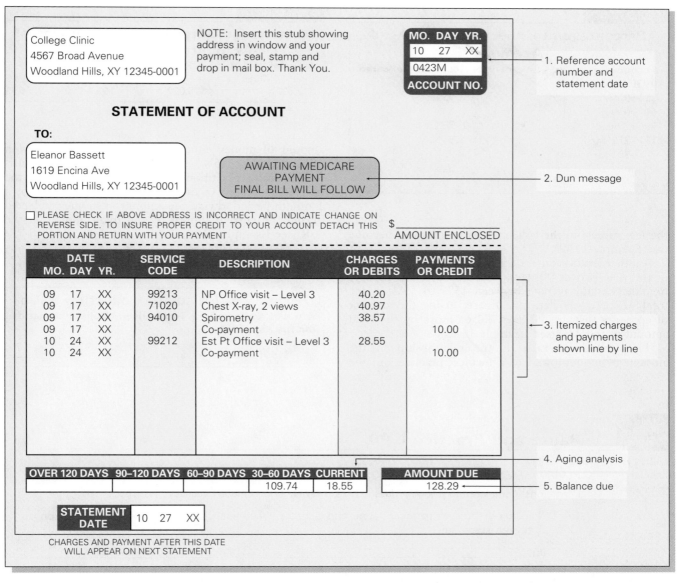

Figure 14–1. Computerized statement. (Courtesy of Bibbero Systems, Inc., Petaluma, CA, (800) 242-2376, web site: www.bibbero.com).

average charges for the prior 12-month period. An average total A/R (all monies not collected at the time of service) should equal one and one-half to two times the charges for 1 month of services (see Example 14–1).

As time passes, outstanding account balances become increasingly difficult to collect from patients. This is because patients do not have a sense of urgency about paying for healthcare services. Often, medical bills are placed at the bottom of the patient's payment priority list, partially because patients may weigh the consequences of nonpayment of medical bills versus nonpayment of other bills; with the former there is nothing tangible to return or repossess. Therefore, collection efforts within the first 30 days after services are rendered are most successful. The older the account,

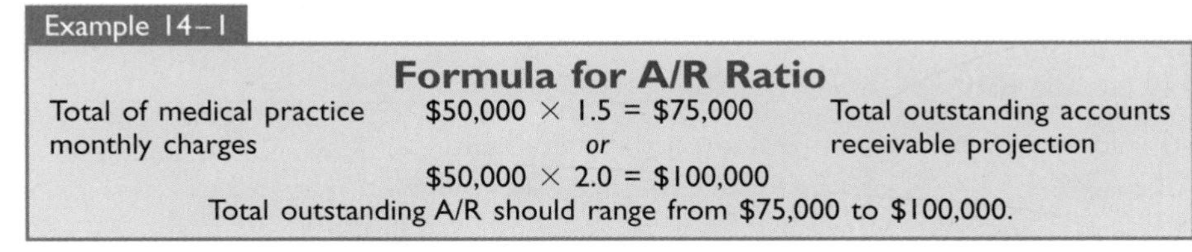

Example 14–1

Formula for A/R Ratio

Total of medical practice monthly charges — $\$50,000 \times 1.5 = \$75,000$ *or* $\$50,000 \times 2.0 = \$100,000$ — Total outstanding accounts receivable projection

Total outstanding A/R should range from $75,000 to $100,000.

14-6

Example 14–2

Percentage of Collectability on Aged Accounts

Account Age	Percent of Accounts Collected
0–30 days	98%
31–60 days	95%
61–90 days	84%
91–120 days	78%
181–210 days	58%
271–300 days	40%
1 year	22%
2 years	10%

the less successful the collection of monies will become (see Example 14–2).

Another evaluation tool is to determine how much of the A/R is over 90 days. Accounts that are 90 days or older should average between 15% to 25% of the total A/R. To calculate this figure, divide the amount of accounts that are 90 days old or more by the total amount of the A/R (see Example 14–3).

The **collection ratio** is the relationship of the amount of money owed to a medical practice and the amount of money collected on the A/R. A collection rate of 90% to 95% should be a goal for the multi-skilled health practitioner managing collections in the physician's office. To calculate the collection rate for a 1-month period, divide the amount of monies collected during the current month by the total amount of the A/R (see Example 14–4).

Example 14–3

Formula for Determining Percentage of Accounts Over 90 Days

Amount of A/R over 90 Days		A/R Total		Percentage of A/R over 90 Days
$12,000	÷	$75,000	=	16%

Example 14–4

Formula to Calculate Collection Ratio

Amount Collected for the Month of August		Total A/R		Collection Ratio
$15,963.53	÷	$17,589.53	=	91%

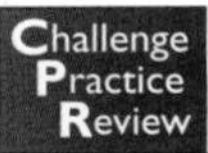

Pause and Practice CPR

REVIEW SESSIONS 14–1 AND 14–2

Directions: *Complete the following questions as a review of information you have just read.*

14–1 In addition to the patient's name and address, what financial information is included on an itemized statement?

(a) ____________________

(b) ____________________

(c) ____________________

(d) ____________________

(e) ____________________

(f) ____________________

14–2 When are collection efforts the most successful? ____________________

____

PRACTICE SESSIONS 14–3 THROUGH 14–6

Directions: *Refer to the section on itemized statements and determine the correct answers.*

14–3 Refer to Figure 14–1 and record how many dates of service this statement indicates?

____

14–4 List the dates of service. ____________________

14–5 How many services are listed on this statement? ____________________

14–6 Why is $109.74 aged at 30 to 60 days? ______________________________

____

____

CHECK YOUR HEARTBEAT! Turn to the end of the chapter for answers to these review and practice sessions.

Dun Messages

Dun messages are used on billing statements to promote payment (see Figs. 14–1 and 14–2). The best and most effective collection statements include a handwritten note; however, this is seldom possible. Dun messages can also be printed by the computer system or applied with brightly colored labels purchased via a medical office supplies catalogue.

Do not send intimidating, impatient, or threatening statements. These will only serve to antagonize patients. If possible, dun messages should be available in different languages and sent to patients who speak English as a second language. Example 14–5 illustrates some common dun messages.

Manual Billing

Small offices frequently use **manual billing.** Statements are generally typed on continuous form paper, separated, folded, and placed into billing envelopes. Photocopying the patient's ledger card and placing it in a window envelope is also a method occasionally used for manual billing. The ledger card then becomes the statement and should be neat and readable with no cross-outs or misspellings.

With manual billing, a coding system with metal clip-on tabs or peel-off labels placed on ledger cards can be used. Each time the account is billed, a different color tab or label is placed on the card. This shows, at a glance, how many times the account has been billed and provides aging of accounts, although a report, if desired, would have to be manually generated.

Computer Billing

Computer billing is the most widely used method and is made possible by installing software that controls the A/R. All charges, payments, and adjustments are input (posted) into the computer system and these figures can be used to generate a hard copy, that is, statements and various financial reports (see Fig. 14–1). The computer program usually offers choices of *billing types* which are assigned to various patients, for example, patient bill (monthly statement), **insurance balance bill** (statement after insurance has paid), discounted bill (reduced fee statement), and no bill. The insurance specialist can instruct the computer to print all billing statements of a specific type. The computer can also be instructed to print bills according to specific accounts, dates, and insurance types (e.g., all Medicare bills for 5/4/XX). Accounts are automatically aged and standard messages

Example 14–5

Dun Messages

- If there is a problem with your account, please call me at (555) 486-9002, Marlayn.
  Wenn es Probleme gibt mit deinem Vertrag (mit Rechnungen), bitte ruf mir an (555) 486-9002 Marlayn (German)
- This bill is past due. Please remit payment.
  (Chinese)

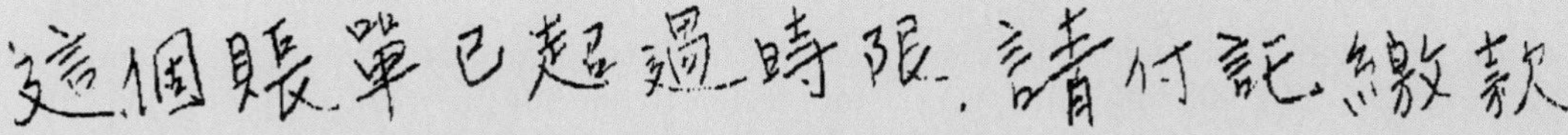

- This bill is now 60 days past due. Please send payment immediately.
  Ang iyong utang ay lampas na ng animnapung (60) araw. Kung maaari ay pakibayaran agad. (Tagalog)
- Your account is 90 days past due. Please remit payment now to avoid collection action.
  Khoân no tien bâo hiém y té côa quí vị dã quá hạn 90 ngày. Xin quí vị thanh toán, dê tránh khôi phâi chịu tiên phạt côa hãng chuyên dòi nọ. (Vietnamese)
- FINAL NOTICE: If we do not hear from you within 10 days, this account will be turned over to our collection agency.
  Aviso final: Si no se pone en contacto dentro de 10 dias, esta cuenta se pasará a una agencia de colección (Spanish)

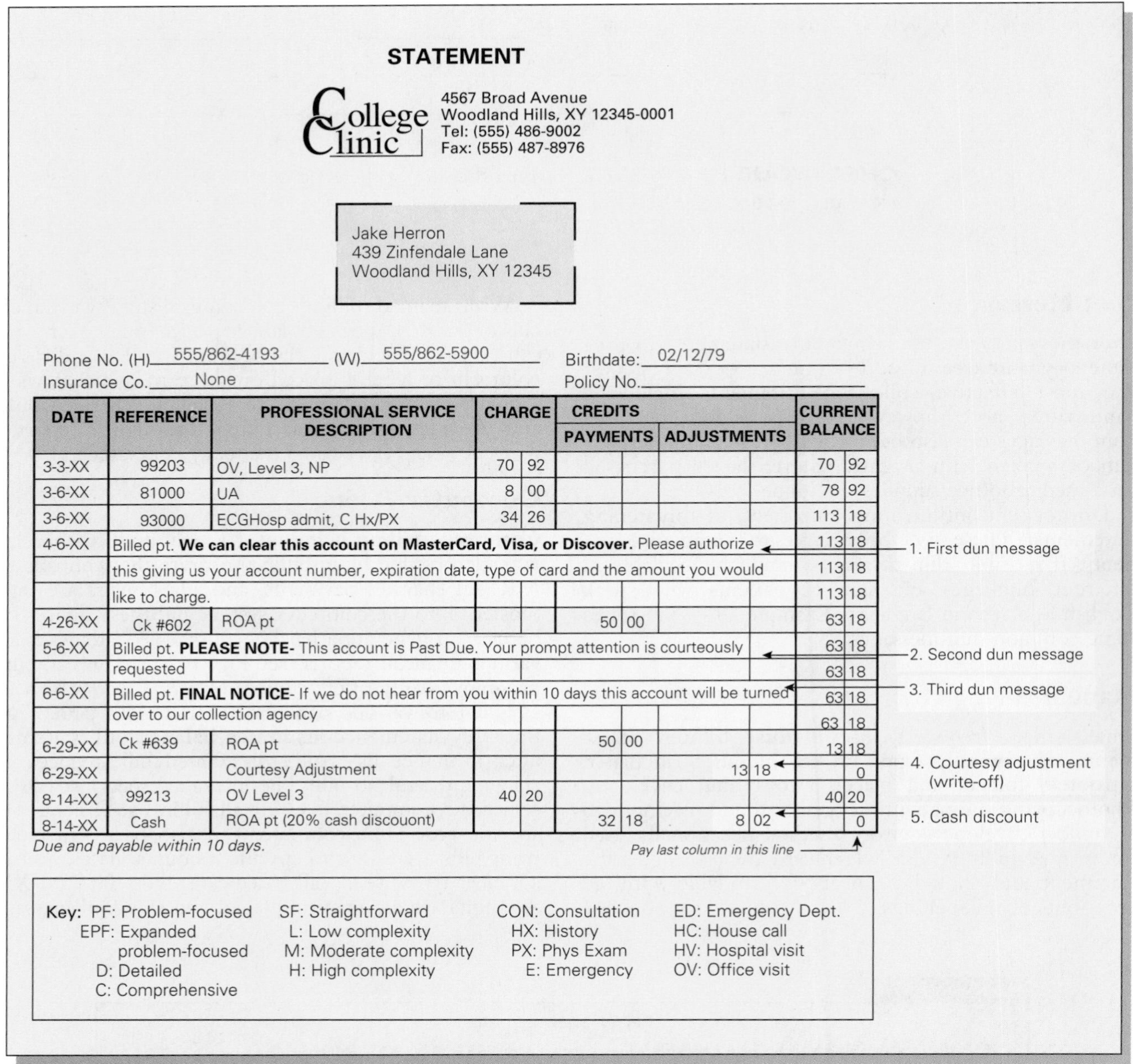

STATEMENT

College Clinic
4567 Broad Avenue
Woodland Hills, XY 12345-0001
Tel: (555) 486-9002
Fax: (555) 487-8976

Jake Herron
439 Zinfendale Lane
Woodland Hills, XY 12345

Phone No. (H) 555/862-4193 (W) 555/862-5900 Birthdate: 02/12/79
Insurance Co. None Policy No.

DATE	REFERENCE	PROFESSIONAL SERVICE DESCRIPTION	CHARGE	CREDITS		CURRENT BALANCE
				PAYMENTS	ADJUSTMENTS	
3-3-XX	99203	OV, Level 3, NP	70 92			70 92
3-6-XX	81000	UA	8 00			78 92
3-6-XX	93000	ECGHosp admit, C Hx/PX	34 26			113 18
4-6-XX	Billed pt. **We can clear this account on MasterCard, Visa, or Discover.** Please authorize					113 18
	this giving us your account number, expiration date, type of card and the amount you would					113 18
	like to charge.					113 18
4-26-XX	Ck #602	ROA pt		50 00		63 18
5-6-XX	Billed pt. **PLEASE NOTE-** This account is Past Due. Your prompt attention is courteously					63 18
	requested					63 18
6-6-XX	Billed pt. **FINAL NOTICE-** If we do not hear from you within 10 days this account will be turned					63 18
	over to our collection agency					63 18
6-29-XX	Ck #639	ROA pt		50 00		13 18
6-29-XX		Courtesy Adjustment			13 18	0
8-14-XX	99213	OV Level 3	40 20			40 20
8-14-XX	Cash	ROA pt (20% cash discouont)		32 18	8 02	0

Due and payable within 10 days. *Pay last column in this line*

Key: PF: Problem-focused
EPF: Expanded problem-focused
D: Detailed
C: Comprehensive
SF: Straightforward
L: Low complexity
M: Moderate complexity
H: High complexity
CON: Consultation
HX: History
PX: Phys Exam
E: Emergency
ED: Emergency Dept.
HC: House call
HV: Hospital visit
OV: Office visit

Figure 14–2. Ledger card showing dun messages, courtesy adjustment (write-offs), and cash discount.

can be printed on statements for each of the aged date groupings (e.g., over 30, 60, 90, or 120 days). Some systems allow personalized messages to be inserted, which override the standard message. Computer billing saves time, money, and guarantees quicker payment.

Billing Services

Billing services are employed by many medical practices to reduce administrative paperwork by taking over the task of preparing and mailing patient statements. This service may also be called a statement service, centralized billing, or outsourcing.

They may also prepare and send insurance forms (electronically or manually), and provide data entry of patient demographics, insurance information, charges, receipts, and adjustments. Other services offered are tracking of payments from patients and third party payers, production of management reports, purging of inactive accounts, and collection of accounts.

Billing services incorporate advanced technology and generate professional-looking statements. Experts answer all billing-related telephone inquiries, thus allowing the medical office to have fewer disruptions and freedom from worry about financial matters when trying to provide medical care. Employing a billing service avoids downtime in the billing process due to vacations, illness, or personal leave.

Billing Procedures

Billing procedures are determined by the specialty of the practice, the number of accounts, and the number of staff members assigned to the collection process. Adopt a specific method of handling accounts and decide which billing routine best fits the practice. Check insurance and managed care contracts carefully to determine which circumstances allow for patients to be billed. If there is a need to bill managed care patients, be sure to conform to federal guidelines.

Billing Routines

Monthly Billing

Using a monthly billing system, all statements are mailed at the same time during the month. Choose a mail-out day at the beginning of the month so patients will receive their bills near the 15th, or send statements near the end of the month so patients receive their bills by the 1st. These target times are chosen because it is likely the employed patient will receive his or her paycheck at those times.

Cycle Billing

A system of billing accounts at spaced intervals during the month is referred to as **cycle billing.** The breakdown of accounts is determined by either an alphabetical list of last names, or by account numbers, insurance types, or dates of first service. Cycle billing relieves the pressure of mailing all statements at one time and allows collection at a faster, more organized rate. It also allows continuous cash flow throughout the month and distributes the influx of incoming calls about problem accounts from patients. The number of cycles may be determined by how the collector wishes to divide the workload. Using *two cycles* per month, statements would be sent on the 25th to arrive by the 1st, and on the 10th to arrive by the 15th of the month. Using *four*

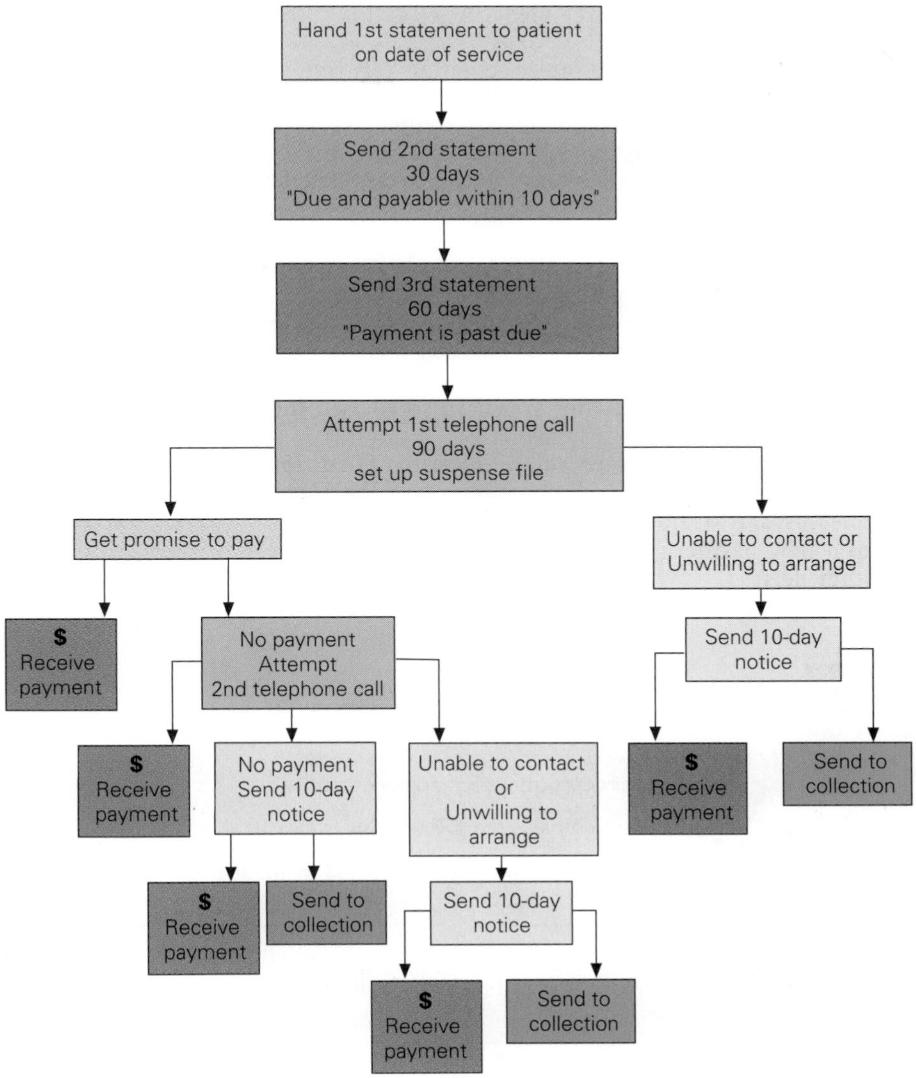

Hand 1st statement to patient on date of service
Send 2nd statement 30 days "Due and payable within 10 days"
Send 3rd statement 60 days "Payment is past due"
Attempt 1st telephone call 90 days set up suspense file
Get promise to pay
$ Receive payment
No payment Attempt 2nd telephone call
$ Receive payment
No payment Send 10-day notice
$ Receive payment
Send to collection
Unable to contact or Unwilling to arrange
Send 10-day notice
$ Receive payment
Send to collection
Unable to contact or Unwilling to arrange
Send 10-day notice
$ Receive payment
Send to collection

Figure 14–3. Collection decision tree. This quick reference may be used to help determine when to send statements, make telephone calls, and send accounts to a collection agency.

Example 14–6

Messages to Patients Awaiting Insurance Payment

- Your account is due and payable at the time of service. Your insurance company has been billed as a courtesy.
- We have received payment from your insurance company. The balance of $______ is your responsibility. Please remit today. Thank you.
- Your insurance company has paid its share of the bill. This statement is for the amount payable directly by you.
- Your insurance company has not responded. The account is due and payable. Please contact your insurance company about payment. Thank you for your assistance.

cycles per month, statements would be sent every Tuesday or Wednesday to arrive at the end of each week. If the cycle is established according to the first date of service, and the patient was first seen on the 11th of the month, then every month on the 11th he or she would receive a bill.

Seven-Step Billing and Collection Guidelines

1. Present the *first* statement at the time of service. This can be a formal statement or a multipurpose billing form.
2. Mail the *second itemized statement* within 30 days of treatment. The phrase "due and payable within 10 days" should be printed on each statement regardless of whether the patient has insurance or not.
3. Send the *third* statement 30 days after the second statement was sent, approximately 60 days from date of service. Indicate the payment is past due.
4. When the account has aged 90 days, place the *first telephone call* to the patient and ask if there is a problem. Ask for a payment commitment and set up a *suspense file*. Accounts are put in a suspense file for active follow-up. Action must be taken within the time frame mentioned, after you have so advised the patient.
5. Check for payment as promised allowing 1 day for mail delay. If not received, promptly place the *second telephone call* to the patient and ask for payment. Set up a new payment date allowing 5 days for mail or other delay.
6. Check for payment as promised. If no payment has been received, send a *10-day notice* advising the patient that unless payment is received in 10 days, the account will be turned over for legal action.
7. Check for payment when promised. If no payment is received, promptly surrender the account to a collection agency for legal action.

Figure 14–3 shows a collection decision tree to be used to determine when to send statements, make telephone calls, send 10-day notices, and send accounts to a collection agency.

Billing Patients with Insurance

Generally, if a bill has not been paid the physician's office rebills the patient every 30 days. It is important to bill patients on a regular (monthly) basis, even when insurance payment is expected. Clearly identify on the statement that the insurance specialist has submitted an insurance claim as well as what action is expected from the patient (see Example 14–6). If the patient has been billed regularly and collection becomes a problem, action can be referenced to the date of service instead of the date the insurance company paid.

Notify patients promptly when the insurance payment has been received. The remaining balance must be submitted immediately because, as indicated in the first and all subsequent statements, it was due and payable at the time of service. Ask patients to get involved in the insurance process or to pay the bill within 10 days if a problem exists.

Challenge Practice Review

Pause and Practice CPR

REVIEW SESSIONS 14–7 THROUGH 14–11

Directions: *Complete the following questions as a review of information you have just read.*

14–7 What are two methods used in manual billing?

(a) ______________________________

(b) ______________________________

14–8 How is it possible to perform computerized billing in the physician's office?

____

14–9 Patient billing statements can be generated using a computerized system by selecting according to:

(a) ______

(b) ______

(c) ______

14–10 What determines billing procedures in the physician's office?

(a) ______

(b) ______

(c) ______

14–11 What are two basic types of billing routines? ______

CHECK YOUR HEARTBEAT! Turn to the end of the chapter for answers to these review sessions.

CREDIT ARRANGEMENTS

Although payment at the time of service is ideal, many patients do not have funds available to pay when they need medical care. Alternative payment methods may be offered to help continuous cash flow and reduce collection costs.

Payment Options

Credit Card Billing

Credit card payment is an option that provides patients with an alternative to clear their account balances. Credit cards are issued by organizations that entitle the cardholder to credit at their establishments. This method of payment may be most useful as a down payment on uninsured or elective procedures. Credit cards can help manage the A/R by reducing billing costs, improving cash flow, and reducing the risk of bad debts.

If a practice accepts credit cards, advise all patients in the following ways: display a credit card acceptance sign, include an insignia or message on the statement, include the credit card policy in the new patient brochure, and have staff members tell patients that this option is available. Patients may prefer to clear a debt immediately and make monthly payments to the credit card company instead of owing money to their doctor.

Verifying Credit Cards

A small physician's office may have a simple credit card imprinter in the office. The insurance specialist should check credit card warning bulletins to make sure that the card has not been canceled or stolen.

Large practices may have an electronic credit card machine that allows the insurance specialist to swipe the card through the machine that is linked to the credit card company. Transactions are then approved, processed, and deposited into a bank account, usually in 2 working days. These machines may be rented or purchased.

Verifying Credit Cardholders

Always verify the cardholder by asking for a photo identification such as a driver's license. Examine the card carefully and observe the following guidelines:

- Accept the credit card only from the person whose name appears on the card.
- Match the name on the card with the patient's other identification and make sure the expiration date has not passed.
- Check the "hotline" for problem cards.
- Look on the back of the card for the word "void." This will alert you if the card has been heated, which is a method used to forge a signature.
- Verify all charges regardless of the amount and get approval from the credit card company.
- Complete the credit card voucher (Fig. 14–4) before asking for a signature.
- Compare the signature on the credit card voucher against the signature on the card.
- Record the credit card number in the patient's financial file for future use if the patient's account has to be traced or transferred to a collection agency.

Debit Cards

A **debit card** is a card permitting bank customers to withdraw cash at any hour from any affiliated automated teller machine (ATM). The holder may also make cashless purchases from funds on deposit without incurring revolving finance charges. A small fee is charged (debited) to the customer's checking account when the card is used; however, this fee is usually applied only once a month (if the debit card is used) regardless of how many times the card is used during the month. Medical practices offering credit card payment may use the same electronic credit card ma-

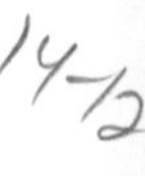

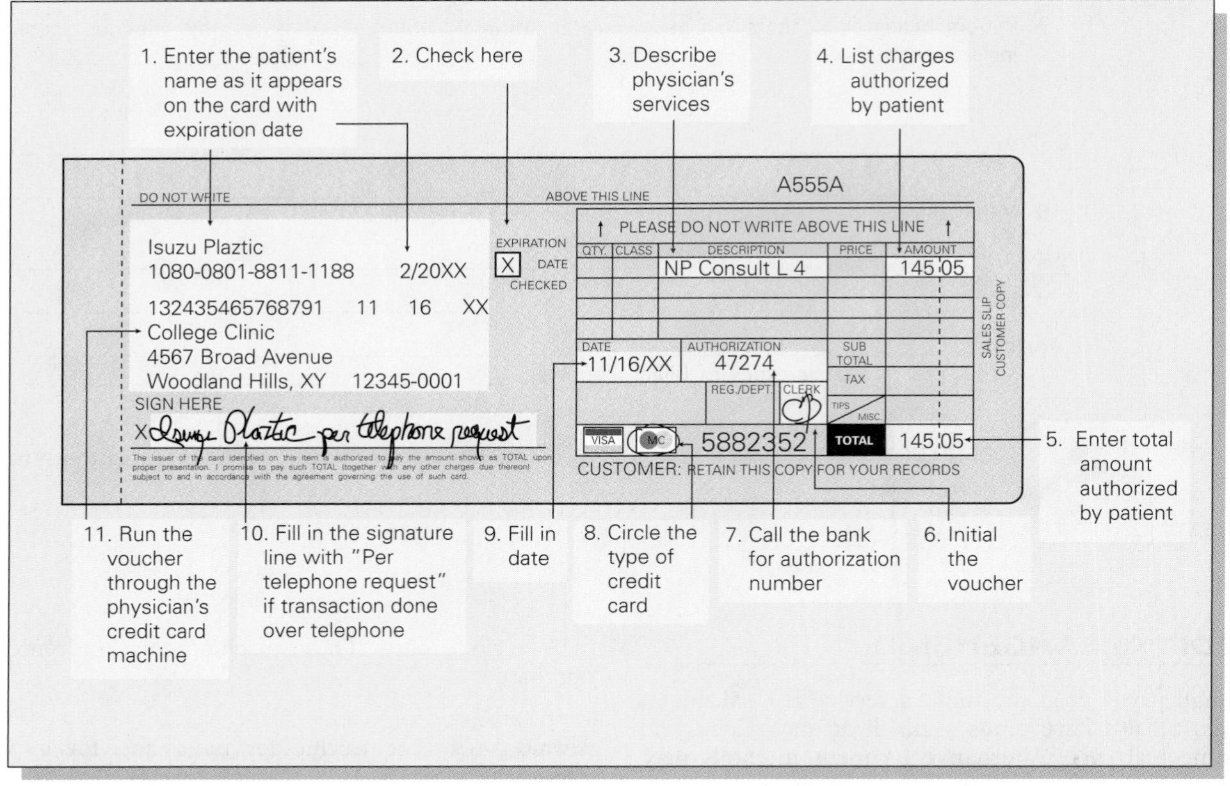

Figure 14–4. Example of a completed credit card voucher used in a physician's office.

chine to swipe the debit card for verification and approval. Separate debit card machines are also available for businesses that do not accept credit cards. Debit cards take the place of writing checks; however, once the debit card is approved for a certain amount, the bank which issued the debit card is responsible for paying the funds that were approved. There are no checks returned for nonsufficient funds with this method of payment. Since debit and credit cards look similar, always ask the patient what kind of card it is.

Payment Plans

Payment plans are another way of offering the patient a way of paying off an account by spreading out the amount due over a period of time. The Truth in Lending Consumer Credit Cost Disclosure Law (see Credit and Collection Laws), also referred to as Regulation Z, requires full written disclosure regarding the finance charges for large payment plans involving *four or more installments*, excluding a down payment. Refer to Figure 14–5 for an illustration of a financial agreement that adheres to Regulation Z. This regulation does not apply, however, if the patient agrees to pay in one sum or makes drawn-out partial payments. Patients often think that if they make any amount of payment, the physician is required to accept that payment and not take any additional action. This is incorrect. The physician can take action, including sending the account to a collection agency.

It is important to have a written payment plan schedule when working with accounts in which payment plans may be offered. Figure 14–6 illustrates sample guidelines that may be used or revised according to individual practice and management policies.

Payment plans can be negotiated over the telephone but the debtor needs to be present to sign the financial agreement. It is important to let the patient know that the practice is willing to help and that if he or she runs into further problems in making the payment, the debtor should inform the insurance specialist. This personal contact helps if renegotiation of the agreement is needed. A medical practice cannot refuse an immediate appointment of an established patient because of a **debt,** but the office staff should take advantage of asking the patient for payment while in the office. The physician ultimately must determine if he or she should continue treating the patient or terminate care (see Fig. 2–3 in Chapter 2).

FINANCIAL AGREEMENT

1. Total amount of the debt; wording "cash price" must be used according to Regulation Z
2. Amount of down payment
3. Finance charge; must be in capital letters and stand out
4. Interest rate expressed as an annual percentage; must be in capital letters and stand out
5. Amount of each payment
6. Date each payment is due
7. Date final payment is due; itemized payment record allows tracking of payments and balance owed
8. Signature of patient and physician with copies retained by both; narrative must be included

For professional SERVICES rendered or to be rendered to:

Patient Keenan Kellog Daytime phone 555-486-0132

Parent if patient is a minor ______

1. Cash price for services .... $ 5000.-
2. Cash down payment .... $ 300.-
3. Charges covered by insurance service plan .... $ 4000.-
4. Unpaid balance of cash price .... $ 700.-
5. Amount financed (the amount of credit provided to you) .... $ 700.-
6. FINANCE CHARGE (the dollar amount the credit will cost you) .... $ -0-
7. ANNUAL PERCENTAGE RATE (the cost of credit as a yearly rate) .... $ 0%
8. Total of payments (5 + 6 above – the amount you will have paid when you have made all scheduled payments) .... $ 700.-
9. Total sales price (1 + 6 above – sum of cash price, financing charge and any other amounts financed by the creditor, not part of the finance charge) .... $ 5000.-

You have the right at anytime to pay the unpaid balance due under this agreement without penalty. You have the right at this time to receive an itemization of the amount financed.

X I want an itemization ☐ I do not want an itemization

Total of payments (#8 above) is payable to Dr. Astro Parkinson in 7 monthly installments of $100. each and -0- installments of $ -0- each. The first installment being payable on Feb. 15 20 XX and subsequent installments on the same day of each consecutive month until paid in full.

NOTICE TO PATIENT

Do not sign this agreement if it contains any blank spaces. You are entitled to an exact copy of any agreement you sign. You have the right at any time to pay the unpaid balance due under this agreement.

The patient (parent or guardian) agrees to be and is fully responsible for total payment of services performed in this office including any amounts not covered by any health insurance or prepayment program the responsible party may have. See your contract documents for any additional information about nonpayment, default, any required prepayment in full before the scheduled date and prepayment refunds and penalties.

Signature of patient or one parent if patient is a minor:

X Keenan Kellog

Doctor's Signature Astro Parkinson MD

SCHEDULE OF PAYMENT

No.	Date due	Amount of installment		Ck #	Date paid	Amount paid		Balance owed	
	Total amount							700	–
1	2/15	100	–	572	2/10	100	–	600	–
2	3/15	100	–	598	3/13	100	–	500	–
3	4/15	100	–						
4	5/15	100	–						
5	6/15	100	–						
6	7/15	100	–						
7	8/15	100	–						
8									
9									
10									
11									
12									
13									
14									
15									
16									
17									
18									
19									
20									
21									
22									
23									

Figure 14–5. Financial Agreement Form (#1826) used for a financial payment plan. By completing this form the physician provides full disclosure of all information required by the Federal Truth in Lending Act, Regulation Z. (Reprinted with permission of SYCOM, a division of New England Business Service, Inc., Groton, MA, (800) 356-8141.)

Payment Plan Schedule

Balance due amount	Minimum monthly payment	Time frame for full payment
$0 – $200	$35	6 months
$201 – $500	$50	1 year
$500 – $1,000	$100	1 year
$1,001 – $3,000	$125	2 years
$3,001 – $5,000	$150	2 years
>$5,001*	$200	5 years

*Accounts over $5,000 must complete credit card application to certify minimum required payment and are subject to approval by office manager.

Figure 14–6. Schedule used in the physician's office to negotiate payment plans; it lists balance due amounts, minimum monthly payments, and payment time frames.

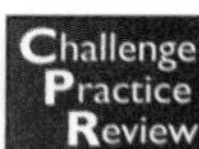

Pause and Practice CPR

REVIEW SESSIONS 14–12 THROUGH 14–14

Directions: *Complete the following questions as a review of information you have just read.*

14–12 When a medical practice accepts credit cards, patients should be advised in the following ways:

(a) ______________________________

(b) ______________________________

(c) ______________________________

(d) ______________________________

14–13 When setting up a payment plan according to Regulation Z, how many installments apply?

____

14–14 Can a patient who owes the doctor $2,500 and has not paid in 6 months be refused an appointment? Explain. ______________________________

____

____

____

CHECK YOUR HEARTBEAT! Turn to the end of the chapter for answers to these review sessions.

THE COLLECTION PROCESS

For collections to be handled effectively, staff members need to be informed and trained in collection techniques for the medical office. Most insurance specialists are trained to be efficient collectors; however, new collectors will need time to gain confidence, which is an important aspect of being a good collector.

Office Collection Techniques

Telephone Debt Collection

Telephone collections are made easier if the insurance billing specialist is convinced that he or she can collect before trying to convince the patient to pay. Important factors to consider are the insurance specialist's ability to contact and negotiate with the patient and the patient's ability to pay the bill. Contact the patient in a timely manner at the first sign of payment delay. Prepare before making a telephone collection call by reviewing the account and noting anything unusual. Determine where the patient is employed or if unemployed. Discuss with the physician the amount you can settle for if you cannot get payment in full. Make the first call count. Act in a calm, business-like manner and combine empathy with diligence. Be positive and persuasive. Listen to what the patient has to say, even if the patient becomes angry and raises his or her voice. Lower the volume of your voice and respond in a composed manner. Ask questions, show interest, and let the patient know that he or she is being listened to. Carefully word your reply. Your goal is to encourage the patient to pay, not agitate the patient. Use all resources and learn to negotiate. When the patient has agreed to pay a specific amount, follow up the telephone call with a letter verifying the amount of payment and the date that was agreed on (Fig. 14–7).

Organizing Overdue Accounts

Use an organized approach to determine which collection calls to make first. Print out the A/R by age and target the accounts that are in the 60- to 90-day category. If you use ledger cards, pull all cards with tabs or labels that indicate the patient has received two or three statements, depending on office protocol. Start with the largest amount owed and work the accounts in decreasing order according to dollar value. After this category has been completed, move on to the 90- to 120-day accounts. Finally, go after accounts that are more than 120 days old.

As you call, track the times you are able to contact the most patients and adjust your telephone schedule accordingly. The physician's office hours may need to be adjusted to include one evening a week or Saturday morning to make collection calls. Other options would

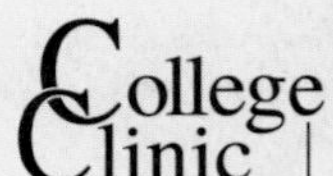

4567 Broad Avenue
Woodland Hills, XY
12345-0001
Tel (555) 486-9002
Fax (555) 487-8976

October 2, 20XX

Mr. Leonard Blabalot
981 McCort Circle
Woodland Hills, XY 12345-0001

Dear Mr. Blabalot:

I am glad we had an opportunity to discuss your outstanding balance with our practice during our phone conversation on October 1, 20XX. This will confirm and remind you that you agreed to pay $100 on your account on or before October 15, 20XX.

A return envelope is enclosed for your convenience.

Sincerely,

Charlotte Rose Routingham
Business Office

Enc. envelope

Figure 14–7. Telephone confirmation letter sent to remind patient of the payment terms agreed to in a telephone conversation.

include the use of flextime whereby the employee can choose his or her own working hours from within a broad range of hours approved by management, or take accounts home and place calls when the office is not open.

Use a private phone away from the busy operations of the office to eliminate interruptions. Patients may be embarrassed about not being able to pay their bills so privacy and patient confidentiality must be maintained. Follow the rules stated in the Fair Debt Collection Practices Act. Follow the steps listed in Table 14–1 to assist in making the first collection call.

Telephone collection calls are also effective the day before patients are due for their appointments. State the date and time of the appointment and then remind the patient of the balance owed and ask if he or she would please bring payment to the office.

Telephone Collection Scenarios

The most difficult part of one-on-one collection is preparing for the many situations you may encounter and the various responses that patients may make. Following are some statements patients make about not paying an account and examples of responses the insurance specialist can make.

Statement: *"I can't pay anything right now."*

Response: *"That's unfortunate. Are you employed? Are you receiving unemployment compensation, welfare, or Social Security benefits?"*

You are determining the patient's ability to pay.

"Are you able to pay some of your bills?"

You are uncovering the fact that the patient is paying certain bills. You can then tell the patient that your bill must also be taken care of, even if only a small amount at a time.

Statement: *"I can't pay the whole bill right now."*

Response: *"Okay, we can work together on this. Can you pay half of the amount?"*

Ask this instead of "How much can you pay?"

Statement: *"I will pay the bill, but not until next month."*

Response: *"All right. What date shall we expect payment? When do you get paid?"*

Ask for payment due the day after payday.

"Do you have a checking account?"

Inform the patient that he or she can take care of the debt with a postdated check.

Statement: *"How about $10 a month (on a $350 bill)?"*

Response: *"I'd like to accept that, but our office policy will not allow us to stretch out payments beyond 90 days."*

Table 14–1 Telephone Collection Call

1. Set the mood of the call by the manner in which you speak and the tone of your voice. The first 30 seconds of the call will set the scene for your relationship with the patient.
2. Identify the patient. Be certain you are talking to the debtor before revealing the nature of the call.
3. Identify yourself and your facility.
4. Verify the debtor's address and all telephone numbers.
5. State the reason you are calling.
6. Take control of the conversation and establish urgency by asking for full payment *now;* disclose the full amount owed.
7. Find out if the patient needs clarification of the bill.
8. Ask when payment will be made, how it will be made, and if it will be sent by mail or in person.
9. Pause for effect; this turns the conversation back to the patient to respond to the demand or to tell you why payment has not been made. If a patient does not respond, never assume it means no.
10. Ask if the patient has a problem and if the practice can be of assistance, especially when the patient is unable to give a reason for nonpayment.
11. Question the patient by asking "How much are you willing to pay?," and "Do you have a regular paycheck?," if the patient is reluctant to agree to an amount.
12. Obtain a promise to pay with an agreeable amount and a due date; be clear how and when payment is expected, but give the patient a choice of action.
13. Ask for half of the amount if full payment is not possible.
14. Discuss a payment plan if the patient is not able to pay half of the balance owed. Be realistic and reasonable. It is self-defeating to set up payment arrangements the patient cannot afford. Advise the patient that if the payment is even 1 day late, the entire balance becomes due and payable. Ask the patient to please call you before the due date with an explanation if any problems arise that prevent payment.
15. Restate the importance of the agreement.
16. Tell the patient to write down the amount and due date.
17. Document the agreement on the patient's ledger, in the computer system, or in a collection telephone log. Note the date and time you spoke to the patient.
18. Send confirmation of the agreement (see Fig. 14–7).
19. Check the account the day after the payment was due; allow 1 day for mail delay.
20. If the patient fails to make payment as promised, make another telephone call and ask the patient if there is still a problem. Get a new commitment to pay and confirm again. If the patient continues to avoid payment, advise the patient that the account will be turned over to a collection agency and follow through as stated.

This adheres to (Truth in Lending Law) regulations for collecting payment in installments without a written agreement. If the patient tries to cooperate, then compromise. If not, turn the account over to a collection agency.

Statement: *"I sent in payment."*

Response: *"Thank you. We appreciate it. When was the payment sent? To what address was it sent? Was it a check? On what bank was it drawn and for what amount? Did you receive the cancelled check? If so, what is the check number?"*

Investigate to see if the check was posted to a wrong account. If not, call the patient back and ask if he or she would call the bank to verify that it has cleared; if it has not, the patient should stop payment. Ask the patient to call you back and let you know the status of the check. If the patient is lying, he or she will not follow through. Ask for a new check to be sent and tell the patient a refund will be made if the other one shows up.

Statement: *"The check is in the mail."*

Response: *"That's great. May I have the check number and the date it was mailed so I can watch for it?"*

Call back in 3 days if not received.

Statement: *"I thought the insurance company was paying this."*

Response: *"Your insurance paid the portion that was allowed under your contract; the balance is your responsibility. Please send your payment before Friday to keep your account current."*

Explain why the insurance company paid as they did—deductible, allowed amount, coinsurance payment, benefit not covered under the insurance plan.

Statement: *"I'm not going to pay the bill because I was rushed in and out of the office. The doctor didn't spend any time with me."*

Response: *"That is unfortunate. I will confirm the day and time you were in and the doctor you saw. For what reason did you see the doctor? Do you still have the problem?"*

Get as much information as possible and research the office schedule for the day the patient was seen. Let the doctor know about the patient's complaint and inquire how he or she would like to handle the complaint.

Collection Letters

Collection letters are another method of reminding patients of their debt. Collection letters can reach a large number of patients rapidly and the cost is relatively low. However, letters may lie unopened by the patient, they are one-way communication, it takes time to prepare letters (especially if a decision has to be made about the account), and the response and recovery through letters is relatively poor.

The insurance billing specialist is often the one to compose collection letters and devise a plan for follow-up. A series of collection letters may be written using varying degrees of forcefulness, starting with a gentle reminder. When writing a collection letter use a friendly tone and ask why payment has not been made. Imply that the patient has good intentions and is just as anxious as you are to clear the debt. You may do this by suggesting that the patient has overlooked a previous statement. Communicate the doctor's interest in the patient. Always invite the patient to explain the reason for nonpayment, either in a letter, telephone call, or visit to the office.

Types of Collection Letters

There are several types of collection letters. An individual letter can be personalized and speak to the patient's situation. Form letters save time and can go out automatically at specific times during the billing cycle (Fig. 14–8). Letters with checklists are a type of form letter that makes it easier for the patient to choose a payment op-

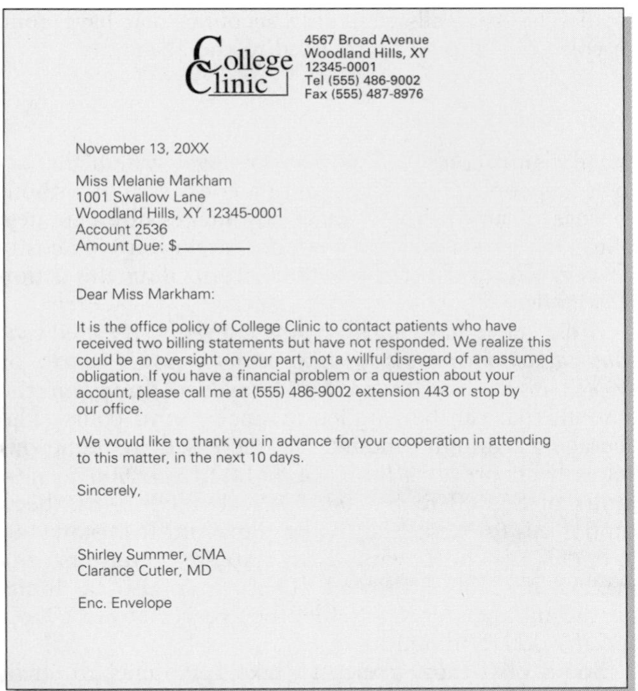

College Clinic
4567 Broad Avenue
Woodland Hills, XY
12345-0001
Tel (555) 486-9002
Fax (555) 487-8976

November 13, 20XX

Miss Melanie Markham
1001 Swallow Lane
Woodland Hills, XY 12345-0001
Account 2536
Amount Due: $________

Dear Miss Markham:

It is the office policy of College Clinic to contact patients who have received two billing statements but have not responded. We realize this could be an oversight on your part, not a willful disregard of an assumed obligation. If you have a financial problem or a question about your account, please call me at (555) 486-9002 extension 443 or stop by our office.

We would like to thank you in advance for your cooperation in attending to this matter, in the next 10 days.

Sincerely,

Shirley Summer, CMA
Clarance Cutler, MD

Enc. Envelope

Figure 14–8. Collection form letter sent to all patients who have not responded after two billing cycles.

tion (Fig. 14–9). Collection letters should be short and to the point. Always personalize the letter by addressing the patient by name and include the following information:

- Full amount owed
- What action the patient should take
- Time frame in which the patient should respond
- How and why the patient should take care of the bill (list payment options)
- Address to which patients send payment
- Contact person's name and telephone and extension number
- Signature, which can be listed as "Insurance Specialist," "Financial Secretary," "Assistant to Dr. ___________," or your name and title with the physician's name below

When pursuing collection, the insurance specialist should stay within the authorization of the physician. All letters sent should be noted on the back of the ledger, in the collection log, or in the computer comment area. Abbreviations can be used to indicate which letter was sent along with the date the letter was mailed. Letters can be sent in brightly colored envelopes to attract attention. All envelopes should include "Forwarding Service Requested" and a stamped self-addressed envelope. Refer to the worktext web site for a list of collection abbreviations.

Other Collection Options

Collection Agencies

Delinquent accounts should be turned over to a collection agency only after all reasonable attempts have been made by the physician's office to collect. The longer the unpaid balance remains in the physician's office, the less chance the agency has to collect the account, so the determination that an account is uncollectable needs to be made quickly. Some guidelines are:

- When a patient states that he or she will not pay or there is a denial of responsibility
- When a patient breaks a promise to pay and fails to contact the office with a legitimate reason for doing so
- When a patient makes partial payments and 60 days have lapsed without payment
- When a patient fails to respond to the physician's letters or telephone calls
- When a check is returned by the bank due to nonsufficient funds and the patient does not make an effort to rectify the situation within 1 week of notification
- When a patient is paid by the insurance company and does not forward the payment to the physician (this constitutes fraud and may be pursued with legal action)

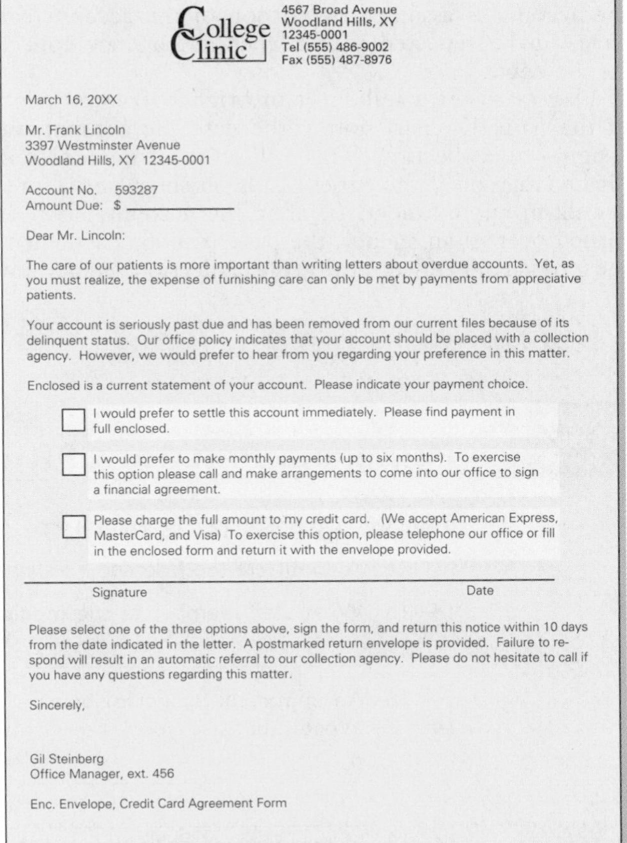

College Clinic
4567 Broad Avenue
Woodland Hills, XY
12345-0001
Tel (555) 486-9002
Fax (555) 487-8976

March 16, 20XX

Mr. Frank Lincoln
3397 Westminster Avenue
Woodland Hills, XY 12345-0001

Account No. 593287
Amount Due: $ ________

Dear Mr. Lincoln:

The care of our patients is more important than writing letters about overdue accounts. Yet, as you must realize, the expense of furnishing care can only be met by payments from appreciative patients.

Your account is seriously past due and has been removed from our current files because of its delinquent status. Our office policy indicates that your account should be placed with a collection agency. However, we would prefer to hear from you regarding your preference in this matter.

Enclosed is a current statement of your account. Please indicate your payment choice.

☐ I would prefer to settle this account immediately. Please find payment in full enclosed.

☐ I would prefer to make monthly payments (up to six months). To exercise this option please call and make arrangements to come into our office to sign a financial agreement.

☐ Please charge the full amount to my credit card. (We accept American Express, MasterCard, and Visa) To exercise this option, please telephone our office or fill in the enclosed form and return it with the envelope provided.

____
Signature Date

Please select one of the three options above, sign the form, and return this notice within 10 days from the date indicated in the letter. A postmarked return envelope is provided. Failure to respond will result in an automatic referral to our collection agency. Please do not hesitate to call if you have any questions regarding this matter.

Sincerely,

Gil Steinberg
Office Manager, ext. 456

Enc. Envelope, Credit Card Agreement Form

Figure 14–9. Multipurpose collection letter with checklist. Advises patient of a seriously past due account, offers the patient three payment options, and warns the patient that failure to respond will result in referral to a collection agency.

- When a patient gives false information
- When a patient moves and the office has used all resources to locate the patient

Not all accounts should go to a collection agency. Such accounts include those of personal friends, elderly widows or widowers living on pensions, and accounts with balances of less than $25. Many physicians prefer to adjust small bad debts off of the books rather than increase administrative costs. All disputed accounts should be reviewed and approved by the physician before going to collection. There should be a systematized approach to turning accounts over to a collection agency that still allows room for an exception, should one occur.

Agency Assigned Accounts

All patient accounts turned over to a collection agency should have a letter of withdrawal sent by certified mail (see Chapter 2, Fig. 2–3). Once an account has been assigned to a collection agency, it is illegal to send the patient a statement. To prevent future billing, a note should be placed on all such ledgers/accounts indicating the date the account was assigned. Financial management consultants usually recommend that the patient's balances be written off of the A/R at the time the account is assigned. A portion of the account balance can be reposted if and when the agency collects on the debt.

Flag or insert a full sheet of brightly colored paper in the patient's chart noting the date the account was assigned to collection. This will alert all medical staff of the situation if the patient calls on short notice or is a walk-in appointment. If, after the account has been turned over to an agency, the patient sends payment to the physician's office, notify the collection agency immediately. Any calls regarding accounts that have gone to collection should be referred to the agency.

Small Claims Court

Small claims court is a part of our legal system that allows laypeople to have access to a court system without the use of an attorney. Some advantages are a modest filing fee, minimal paperwork, exclusion of costly lawyers, and a short time frame from filing the action to trial date.

Most states have small claims courts, also called *conciliation*, *common pleas*, *general sessions*, *justice courts*, or *people's court*. Each state has monetary limits on the amount that can be handled in small claims court. The average maximum amount has increased in numerous states from previous limits of $2,000 to $3,000 to new limits of $5,000 to $10,000. A recent effort has been supported to raise the dollar limit in five states to $20,000, so check with your state to determine the maximum amount allowed. There may also be limits on the number of claims filed per year that are over a specific dollar amount.

Some physicians prefer to take bad debts to small claims court instead of turning the accounts over to a collection agency. Paperwork and directions on the court process can be obtained from the clerk's office located at the municipal or justice court.

When filing a claim, the person filing the petition (the physician's office) is referred to as the *plaintiff* and the party being brought to suit (the patient) is called the *defendant*. It is generally recommended that the plaintiff send a written demand to the defendant before filling a lawsuit to give the defendant a last opportunity to resolve the claim.

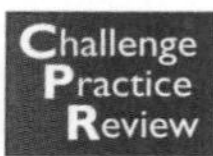

Pause and Practice CPR

REVIEW SESSIONS 14–15 THROUGH 14–19

Directions: *Complete the following questions as a review of information you have just read.*

14–15 What staff member in the medical office usually takes on the responsibility of collections?

____

14–16 An important aspect of being a good collector is having ______________________________.

14–17 What should be your response when a patient has agreed to pay a specific amount?

____

____

14–18 Name types of collection letters and reasons for their use.

(a) ______________________________

(b) ______________________________

(c) ______________________________

14–19 When an account is turned over to a collection agency, what other actions should be taken by the physician's office? ______________________________

____

____

CHECK YOUR HEARTBEAT! Turn to the end of the chapter for answers to these review sessions.

Credit and Collection Laws

The following laws are important because they provide the legal framework within which the insurance specialist must execute the physician's collection policy. In addition, each state may have specific collections laws that are necessary to research and comply with. Summaries of collection laws for individuals who handle healthcare accounts may be found in the book entitled *State-by-State Health Care Collection Laws and Regulations* (see Resources at the end of this chapter).

Statute of Limitations

A formal regulation or law setting time limits on legal action is known as a **statute of limitations.** In regard to collections, the statute of limitations is the maximum time during which a legal collection suit may be rendered against a debtor. For a lawsuit to be successful, a concerted effort should be made to collect on an account from the time services are rendered. The patient should receive regular statements indicating that if the insurer does not pay, the patient will be held responsible.

Statutes vary according to three kinds of accounts: (1) open book accounts, (2) written contract accounts, and (3) single-entry accounts. Physician accounts are usually **open accounts** to which charges are made from time to time. Payment is expected within a specific period but credit has been extended without a formal written contract. Accounts having a formal written agreement in which a patient signs to pay his or her bill in more than four installments is a *written contract account* (see Federal Truth in Lending Act).

Equal Credit Opportunity Act

The Equal Credit Opportunity Act is a federal law which prohibits discrimination in all areas of granting credit. If credit is offered, credit is to be available fairly and impartially to all patients who request it. Obtaining detailed credit information before performing services will prevent accusations of credit discrimination.

Fair Credit Reporting Act

Agencies who either issue or use reports on consumers (patients) in connection with the approval of credit are regulated by the Fair Credit Reporting Act. The act states that credit reporting agencies can only provide reports when:

- There is a legitimate business need for the information.
- A court order is issued.
- The report is requested by the consumer (patient) or instructions are given by the patient to provide the report.

If credit is refused, the physician must provide the name and address of the agency from which the report came and the reason credit was denied. The patient must have an opportunity to correct any inaccuracies. Specific information about what the report contains should not be given.

Fair Credit Billing Act

The Fair Credit Billing Act states that the patient has 60 days from the date a statement is mailed to complain about an error. The creditor must acknowledge the complaint within 30 days of receiving it. If an actual error occurred, the provider is required to correct the mistake within two complete billing cycles, or a maximum of 90 days. If the bill was correct, its accuracy must be explained to the patient.

Expressions from Experience

I love the challenge of collecting past due accounts or accounts that require an extra effort, such as sending additional reports. I also enjoy the thrill of an appeal. Often claims are not paid to the office's satisfaction, and the reimbursement needs to be reviewed. An appeal will need to be written, accompanied by additional information, and as always, follow-up will need to be done.

Tamra Hollins
Collection Specialist
Family Practice Group

Federal Truth in Lending Act

The Federal Truth in Lending Act, commonly referred to as the Truth in Lending Act (TILA), is a consumer protection act that applies to anyone who charges interest or agrees on payment of a bill in more than four installments, excluding a down payment. When a specific agreement is reached between patient and physician, Regulation Z of this act requires that a written disclosure of all pertinent information be made, regardless of the existence of a finance charge (see Fig. 14–5). This full disclosure must be discussed at the time the agreement is first reached between patient and physician and credit is extended. It is essential to include the following items:

1. Total amount of the debt
2. Amount of down payment
3. Finance charge
4. Interest rate expressed as an annual percentage
5. Amount of each payment
6. Date each payment is due
7. Date final payment is due
8. Signature of patient and physician with copies retained by both

According to the Federal Trade Commission (FTC), the truth in lending provision is not applicable and no disclosures are required if a patient decides on his or her own to pay in installments or whenever convenient.

Late Payment Charges

Medical practices that implement late payment charges that meet the criteria defined in the TILA as a finance charge must comply with a host of requirements that revolve around proper disclosure to patients.

Charges must meet the following criteria to qualify as late payment charges:

1. It must be stated that the account balance is required to be paid in full at the time of initial billing.
2. The account is treated as delinquent when unpaid.
3. The charge will be assessed to a patient's account only because of his or her failure to make timely payments.
4. Installments are limited to no more than three.
5. The creditor (physician/insurance specialist) makes a "commercially reasonable" effort to collect these accounts.

Truth in Lending Consumer Credit Cost Disclosure

The Truth in Lending Consumer Credit Cost Disclosure is part of Regulation Z of the Federal Truth in Lending Act. It requires businesses to disclose all direct and indirect costs and conditions related to the granting of credit. All interest charges, late charges, collection fees, finance charges, and so forth must be explained up front, prior to the time of service. To charge interest and bill the patient monthly, include the following on all statements:

- Amount of each payment
- Due date
- Unpaid balance at the beginning of the billing period

Fair Debt Collection Practices Act

The Fair Debt Collection Practices Act (FDCPA) was designed to address the collection practices of third party debt collectors and attorneys who regularly collect debts for others. Although this act does not apply directly to physician practices collecting for themselves, a professional healthcare collector must avoid the actions that are prohibited for collection agencies. The main intent of the act is to protect consumers from unfair, harassing, or deceptive collection practices. Refer to the guidelines in Table 14–2, which are taken from the FDCPA, to help avoid illegalities, enhance collections, and maintain positive patient relations.

When a physician continues to treat a patient with an overdue account, the courts have viewed this as continuation of care and an *extension of credit.* Patients who fall into this delinquent status should be referred elsewhere. See Chapter 2, Figure 2–3 (termination of

Table 14–2 Fair Debt Collection Practices Act Guidelines

1. Contact debtors only once a day; in some states, repeated calls in one day or in the same week could be considered harassment.
2. Place calls after 8 A.M. and before 9 P.M.
3. Do not contact debtors on Sunday or any other day that the debtor recognizes as a Sabbath.
4. Identify yourself and the medical practice you represent; do not mislead the patient.
5. Contact the debtor at work *only* if unable to contact the debtor elsewhere; no contact should be made if the employer or debtor disapproves.
6. Contact the attorney, if an attorney represents the debtor; contact the debtor only if the attorney does not respond.
7. Do not threaten or use obscene language.
8. Do not send postcards for collection purposes; keep all correspondence strictly private.
9. Do not call collect or cause additional expense to the patient.
10. Do not leave a message on an answering machine indicating that you are calling about a bill.
11. Do not contact a third party more than once, unless requested to do so by the party or the response was erroneous or incomplete.
12. Do not convey to a third party that you are calling about a debt.
13. Do not contact the debtor when notified in writing that a debtor refuses to pay and would like contact to stop, except to notify the debtor that there will be no further contact or that there will be legal action.
14. Stick to the facts; do not use false statements.
15. Do not prepare a list of "bad debtors" or "credit risks" to share with other healthcare providers.
16. Take action immediately when stating a certain action will be taken (e.g., filing a claim in small claims court or sending the account to a collection agency).
17. Send the patient written verification of the name of the creditor and the amount of debt within 5 days of the initial contact.

a case) for instructions on sending a letter of withdrawal. After the patient has paid the overdue amount, the patient can be taken back and treated on a cash-only basis. For more information about collection laws in your state, contact your state attorney general's office. If there is a conflict between state and federal laws, the stricter law prevails.

Office Collection Problem Solving

Tracing a Skip

A patient who owes a balance on his or her account and moves but leaves no forwarding address is called a **skip.** In these cases an unopened envelope will be returned to the office marked "Returned to Sender, Addressee Unknown." Be sure all outgoing mail has the words "Forwarding Service Requested" below the doctor's return address on the envelope so the post office will make a search and forward the mail to the new address. The physician's office will be informed of the new address for a nominal fee. Complete the Freedom of Information Act form at the post office if the address is a rural delivery box number, and the U.S. Postal Service will provide the location of the person's residence. When patients send payments by mail, precautions must be taken to avoid discarding envelopes with a change of address. Always match the address on the envelope, along with the check, against the patient's account. One staff person should have the responsibility for updating all patients' addresses in all locations to avoid this problem.

Skip-Tracing Techniques

Once it is determined that a patient is a skip, tracing should begin immediately. Office policy should be established stating how the skip should be traced, whether it is to be traced in the office, or at what point the account should be sent to a collection agency. Go to the worktext web site http://www.wbsaunders.com/MERLIN/Fordney/insurance/ for additional information on electronic skip tracing and to obtain techniques that can be used to initiate the search for the debtor.

If the physician decides to use an outside service for skip tracing, there are several from which to choose. Some agencies offer customized service with several levels of skip tracing available; each level is more extensive and more costly. A collection agency or credit bureau may also offer the services of skip tracing.

Refer to Resources at the end of this chapter for a listing of some of the larger directories used on the Internet.

> **Expressions from Experience**
>
> *I live by the rule "ask, and you shall receive, or all they can say is no!" By taking the extra time to appeal, I have found that most often I win, which means more money paid on the claim.*
>
> Tamra Hollins
> Collection Specialist
> Family Practice Group

Bankruptcy

Bankruptcy laws are federal laws applicable in all states that ensure equal distribution of the assets of an individual among all creditors. There are two kinds of bankruptcy petitions: voluntary and involuntary. A *voluntary petition* is one filed by a person asking for relief under the Bankruptcy Reform Act—the Code. An *involuntary petition* is one filed against a person by his or her creditors requesting that a person obtain relief under the Code.

When a patient files for bankruptcy, this indicates that he or she is declared unable to pay debts and becomes a ward of the court and has its protection. The patient is granted an *automatic stay* against creditors, which means that the physician may contact patients only for the name, address, and telephone number of their attorney. The insurance specialist should no longer send statements, make telephone calls, or attempt to collect the account. Notification of bankruptcy does not have to be in writing; oral communication is valid. Bankruptcy remains part of the debtor's permanent credit record for 10 years.

There are several types of bankruptcy. Patients most commonly file for Chapter 7 (straight petition in bankruptcy) or Chapter 13 (wage earner's bankruptcy). Under Bankruptcy Rules, an unsecured creditor must file proof of claim in Chapter 7 or Chapter 13 bankruptcies within 90 days after the first date set for the meeting of creditors. If the creditor fails to file the claim, the creditor will lose his or her right to any proceeds from the bankruptcy. A plan for payment will be approved by the court. The trustee may be contacted from time to time to check the status of the claim and the payments that should be expected.

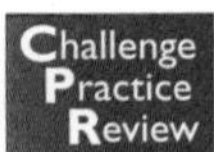

Pause and Practice CPR

REVIEW SESSIONS 14–20 THROUGH 14–23

Directions: *Complete the following questions as a review of information you have just read.*

14–20 What is the name of the law that stipulates terms for a payment plan?

____

14–21 What act lends guidance to the medical insurance billing specialist who is collecting on accounts? ______________________________

14–22 How do the courts view a physician who continues to treat a patient with an overdue account? ______________________________

14–23 A patient who moves but leaves no forwarding address is called a ______________.

CHECK YOUR HEARTBEAT! Turn to the end of the chapter for answers to these review sessions.

SUMMATION AND PREVIEW

The business operations of a medical practice should not conflict with the treatment of ill patients. It is because of this that many physicians leave the collecting of accounts and processing of insurance claims to the medical insurance billing specialist.

The patient's responsibility to pay for medical care is at the time of service. However, a medical practice is one of the few businesses that exist where services are received and credit is granted without a formal agreement, or payment is delayed while insurance claims are processed. It is therefore imperative to be knowledgeable about billing practices, credit and collection laws, various credit arrangements, and the collection process. The knowledge that you have gained in this chapter and the skills that you have learned can help you solve collection problems. Use your knowledge and skills wisely and you will be an asset to the medical practice.

The last chapter addresses what happens after claim submission. After insurance claim forms are sent to the insurance carrier, skills needed to handle payment and follow up after claim submission are presented.

GOLDEN RULE

Come up with knowledge-based solutions when facing collection problems.

Chapter 14 Review and Practice

Study Session

Directions: *Review the objectives, key terms, and chapter information before completing the following study questions.*

14–1 When sending itemized statements, name three things that have a direct effect on the collection process.

(a) ______________________

(b) ______________________

(c) ______________________

14–2 What statement should be included on all return envelopes to ensure forwarding of all billing statements should the patient move? ______________________

14–3 What is an advantage of having a printed statement generated and presented to patients when they leave the office? ______________________

____

14–4 Define the term "age analysis." ______________________

____

14–5 The financial solvency of a medical practice is determined by analysis of the accounts receivable.

14–6 Refer to Example 14–2 and state the average percentage of accounts collected in the 181- to 210-day range. 58%

14–7 Statements used on billing statements to promote payment are called Dun Messages.

14–8 Name common "billing types" that may be assigned to computerized patient accounts and state what the various types mean.

(a) ______________________

(b) ______________________

(c) ______________________

(d) ______________________

14–9 When setting up cycle billing, what are the various ways to select accounts?

____

____

14–10 How often should patients with insurance be billed? every 30 days

14–11 Why might patients like to choose the credit card option if it is available? ______________________

____

____

14–12 Describe a debit card. ______________________

____

14–13 Can payment plans be set up over the telephone? Explain. yes.

14–14 To collect on an account, important factors are the insurance billing specialist's ability to ______ and ______ with the patient and the patient's ______ to pay.

14–15 When making a telephone collection call and the patient gets angry and raises his or her voice, how should you respond? ______

14–16 When organizing accounts to make collection calls, which account should be targeted? ______

14–17 Where should the telephone be located that is used to make collection calls? ______

14–18 What staff member in the physician's office usually composes collection letters and devises a plan for follow-up? ______

14–19 Generally speaking, when should a patient's account be turned over to a collection agency? ______

14–20 Name several advantages of using the small claims court system.

(a) ______
(b) ______
(c) ______
(d) ______

14–21 According to the Fair Debt Collection Practices Act, how should the following situations be handled?

(a) Hours to place telephone calls After 8am + Before 9pm
(b) Leaving messages for debtors ______
(c) Postcards NO
(d) Number of times a debtor can be contacted Once daily
(e) Contacting the debtor at work ______

14–22 If a patient declares bankruptcy, what should the physician's office do and not do?

______

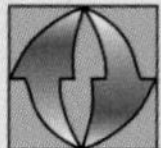

Exercise Exchange

14–1 Calculate the Accounts Receivable Ratio for College Clinic.

Directions

1. Refer to the formula used to determine the A/R ratio in the example presented in the section Age Analysis.

2. Refer to the formula presented in Example 14–1 for the range of a normal A/R ratio.
3. Calculate the A/R ratio for the following scenario.

Scenario: The month-end A/R balance for College Clinic as of March 2002 is $46,000. Following are the total monthly charges for the 12-month period preceding this. Find the monthly average charges by adding all monthly totals and dividing this amount by the number of months (12). Now divide the month-end A/R balance by the average monthly charges.

February	$18,000
January	$20,000
December	$16,000
November	$18,200
October	$19,990
September	$26,000
August	$36,000
July	$33,000
June	$32,000
May	$25,550
April	$26,000
March	$30,000

a. Total charges for 12 months $____________
b. Average monthly total charges $____________
c. A/R ratio ____________%
d. Does the College Clinic A/R ratio fall within the range mentioned? ____________

14–2 **Determine How Much of College Clinic's A/R Is over 90 Days.**

Directions

1. Refer to the formula used to determine the A/R ratio in the section Age Analysis and Example 14–3.
2. Calculate the percentage of accounts over 90 days in the following scenario.

Scenario: The month-end A/R balance for College Clinic as of March 2002 is $46,000. The amount of money that is over 90 days is $9,000. What percentage of the A/R is over 90 days? ______________

14–3 **Calculate the Collection Rate for College Clinic for the Month of March 2002.**

Directions

1. Refer to the formula used to determine the collection ratio in the section Age Analysis and in Example 14–4.
2. Calculate the collection rate for the following scenario.

Scenario: The month-end A/R balance for College Clinic as of March 2002 is $46,000. The amount of monies collected during March is $43,000. What is the collection rate? ________%

14–4 **Prepare a Credit Card Voucher.**

Directions

1. Read the case scenario and abstract information to fill in a credit card voucher on page 454.

Scenario: You are performing collection calls on October 24 (current year) and are speaking to Susie Willey. She owes an unpaid balance of $272.83 for a diagnostic D & C to Dr. Caesar of College Clinic. After discussion, it is decided that Ms. Willey will pay the entire unpaid balance by using her Visa credit card. She gives you her verbal authorization, account number (6765 2431 7345 5543), expiration date (3/31/XX), and indicates that the card is listed under the name "Susan Joy Willey." You call the bank and receive an authorization number (988435).

14–5 **Complete a Financial Agreement.**

Directions

1. Read the case scenario and abstract information to fill out the financial agreement.

BANKCARD SALES SLIP 3PT.

MOORE© SPEEDISET© MOORESCAN© PATENTED 205 PRINTED IN USA FORM 50983C (12-08) P689

DO NOT WRITE ABOVE THIS LINE

A555A

↑ PLEASE DO NOT WRITE ABOVE THIS LINE ↑

EXPIRATION DATE CHECKED

QTY.	CLASS	DESCRIPTION	PRICE	AMOUNT
DATE	AUTHORIZATION		SUB TOTAL	
	REG./DEPT.	CLERK	TAX	
			TIPS / MISC.	
VISA	MC	5882352	TOTAL	

SALES SLIP CUSTOMER COPY

SIGN HERE

X

The issuer of the card identified on this item is authorized to pay the amount shown as TOTAL upon proper presentation. I promise to pay such TOTAL (together with any other charges due thereon) subject to and in accordance with the agreement governing the use of such card.

CUSTOMER: RETAIN THIS COPY FOR YOUR RECORDS

Scenario: You are making telephone collection calls on October 24 (current year) and have called Jason Craiglow at (555) 486-3092. He is a patient of Dr. Ulibarri and has a large balance due ($1,450) with no medical insurance. You discuss a payment plan and Mr. Craiglow agrees to pay $250 as a cash down payment. The balance is to be divided into six equal payments due on the 15th of each month starting November 15 (current year). There will be no finance charge. An itemization of the agreement will be supplied to Mr. Craiglow when he comes into the office tomorrow and signs the agreement.

FINANCIAL AGREEMENT

For PROFESSIONAL SERVICES rendered or to be rendered to:

Patient ____________________ Daytime phone____________________

Parent if patient is a minor ____________________

1. Cash price for services...$ ________
2. Cash down payment...$ ________
3. Charges covered by insurance service plan.............................$ ________
4. Unpaid balance of cash price...$ ________
5. Amount financed (the amount of credit provided to you)...........$ ________
6. **FINANCE CHARGE** (the dollar amount the credit will cost you).$ ________
7. **ANNUAL PERCENTAGE RATE** (the cost of credit as a yearly rate)...________ %
8. Total of payments (5 + 6 above – the amount you will have paid when you have made all scheduled payments)..........................$ ________
9. Total sales price (1 + 6 above – sum of cash price, financing charge and any other amounts financed by the creditor, not part of the finance charge)...$ ________

You have the right at any time to pay the unpaid balance due under this agreement without penalty. You have the right at this time to receive an itemization of the amount financed.

☐ I want an itemization ☐ I do not want an itemization

Total of payments (#8 above) is payable to Dr.____________________ in________ monthly installments of $____________ each and __________ installments of $____________ each. The first installment being payable on ______________ 20 ____ and subsequent installments on the same day of each consecutive month until paid in full.

NOTICE TO PATIENT

Do not sign this agreement if it contains any blank spaces. You are entitled to an exact copy of any agreement you sign. You have the right at any time to pay the unpaid balance due under this agreement.

The patient (parent or guardian) agrees to be and is fully responsible for total payment of services performed in this office including any amounts not covered by any health insurance or prepayment program the responsible party may have. See your contract documents for any additional information about nonpayment, default, any required prepayment in full before the scheduled date and prepayment refunds and penalties.

Signature of patient or one parent if patient is a minor:

X ____

Doctor's Signature ____

Form 1826 • 1882

SCHEDULE OF PAYMENT

No.	Date due	Amount of installment	Date paid	Amount paid	Balance owed
		Total amount			
D.P.			Ck#		
1					
2					
3					
4					
5					
6					
7					
8					
9					
10					
11					
12					
13					
14					
15					
16					
17					
18					
19					
20					
21					
22					
23					

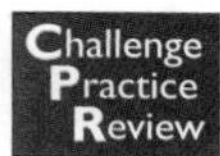

CPR Session: Answers

REVIEW SESSIONS 14–1 AND 14–2

14–1 (a) dates of service
(b) detailed charges
(c) payments
(d) date insurance claim was submitted
(e) adjustments
(f) account balance

14–2 within the first 30 days after the service is rendered

PRACTICE SESSIONS 14–3 THROUGH 14–6

14–3 Two

14–4 9/17/XX and 10/24/XX

14–5 Four (NP OV, CXR, spirometry on 9/17/XX, and Est Pt OV on 10/24/XX)

14–6 Because services were performed on 9/17/XX and the statement is dated 10/27/XX; therefore 40 days have lapsed without payment.

REVIEW SESSIONS 14–7 THROUGH 14–11

14–7 (a) typed statement on continuous form paper
(b) photocopy of patient's ledger

14–8 install software that controls the A/R

14–9 (a) types of account
(b) dates of service
(c) insurance types

14–10 (a) specialty of the practice
(b) number of accounts
(c) number of staff members assigned to the collection process

14–11 monthly billing and cycle billing

REVIEW SESSIONS 14–12 THROUGH 14–14

14–12 (a) display a credit card acceptance sign
(b) include an insignia or message on the statement
(c) include the credit card policy in the new patient brochure
(d) have staff members tell patients that this option is available

14–13 four or more installments, excluding a down payment

14–14 A medical practice cannot refuse an immediate appointment of an established patient because of a debt. The patient should be asked for payment when he or she is in the office and the physician must ultimately determine whether to continue treating the patient or terminate care.

REVIEW SESSIONS 14–15 THROUGH 14–19

14–15 medical insurance billing specialist

14–16 confidence

14–17 Follow up the telephone call with a letter verifying the amount of payment and the date that was agreed on.

14–18 (a) individual letter—can be personalized to the patient's situation
(b) form letter—saves time and goes out automatically at specific times
(c) letters with checklists—makes it easy for the patient to choose a payment option

14–19 A letter of withdrawal should be sent by certified mail and a note indicating the account was assigned to a collection agency should be attached to the patient's ledger/account so no further statements are sent.

REVIEW SESSIONS 14–20 THROUGH 14–23

14–20 Federal Truth in Lending Act

14–21 Fair Debt Collection Practices Act

14–22 as a continuation of care and an extension of credit

14–23 skip

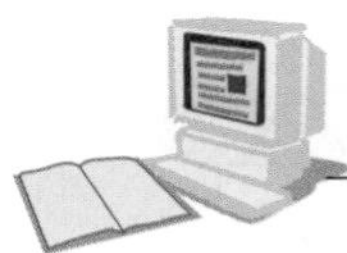

Resources

It is important to keep up-to-date on credit and collection issues so that collecting on accounts is successful and following up on delinquent accounts is done lawfully. There are several resources listed that may be obtained to receive the latest information.

Today, since our society is more transient than ever, another important function is learning how to trace a skip so that income is not lost to the medical practice. Refer to "skip tracing" for resources on the Internet that may be utilized.

Internet

Skip tracing

- Bigfoot
  Web site: http://www.bigfoot.com
- InfoUSA
  Web site: http://www.infousa.com
- Reverse Directories
  Web site: http://www.anywho.com
  http://www.infospace.com
- Search-It-All
  Web site: http://www.searchbug.com
- Switchboard
  Web site: http://www.switchboard.com
- WhoWhere?
  Web site: http://www.whowhere.com
- Yahoo
  Web site: http://www.yahoo.com
  (key term "people search")

Newsletters

- *Health Care Collector* (monthly), Aspen Publishers, Inc., P. O. Box 990, Frederick, MD 21705-9727, (800) 638-8437
- *How To Get Paid,* Opus Communications, P.O. Box 1168, Marblehead, MA 01945, (800) 650-6787

Reference Books

- *Health Care Billing and Collections: Forms, Checklists, and Guidelines,* Aspen Health and Administration Development Group, Aspen Publishers, Inc., P. O. Box 990, Frederick, MD 21705-9727, (800) 638-8437
- *Small Claims Court: Making Your Way Through the System: A Step-by-Step Guide,* Theresa Meehan Rudy in association with HALT, 1990, published by Random House, New York, NY; order from HALT, 1612 K Street, NW, Suite 510, Washington, DC 20006, (888) 367-4258
- *State-by-State Health Care Collection Laws and Regulations,* Sarah O. Rollman, 2000, Aspen Publishers, Inc., 200 Orchard Ridge Drive, Suite 200, Gaithersburg, MD, (800) 638-8437
- *Successful Billing and Collection Handbook,* Conomikes Reports, Inc., Conomikes Association, Inc., 151 Kalmus Drive, Suite B150, Costa Mesa, CA 92626-9627, (800) 421-6512

NOTES

Objectives

After reading this chapter and completing the exercise sessions, you should be able to:

Learning Objectives:

✔ List components of an explanation of benefits.

✔ Name three claim management techniques.

✔ State time limits for receiving payments for manual and electronic claims.

✔ Describe situations for filing an appeal.

✔ List possible solutions to insurance carrier collection problems.

Performance Objectives:

✔ Interpret an explanation of benefits, abstract information, and post payments and adjustments to a patient's ledger/account.

✔ Complete an insurance claim tracer.

✔ Type a letter of appeal for a rejected claim.

Key Terms

appeal
delinquent claim
denied claim
explanation of benefits (EOB)
inquiry
lost claim
overpayment
peer review
prompt payment laws
rebill
suspended claim
tracer

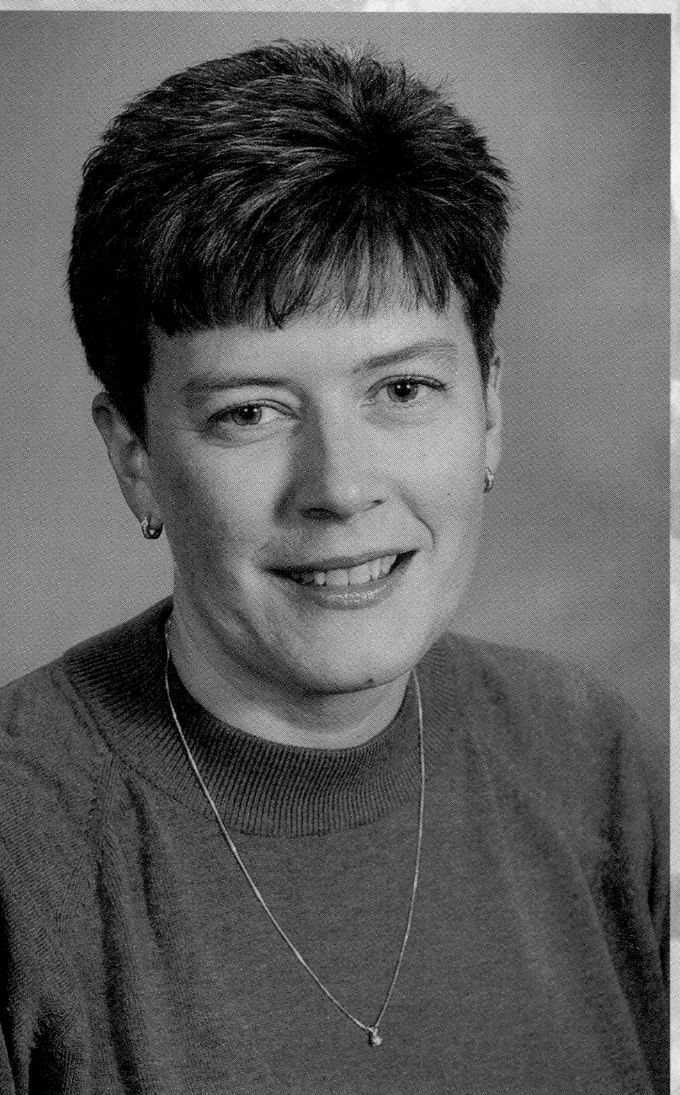

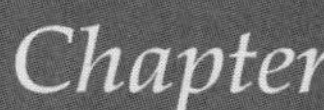

Over the course of 17 years in medical offices I have occupied every front office position. I am currently responsible for billing all insurance carriers, following up on problem claims, posting insurance payments, and making contract adjustments for a pediatric office that has over 6,000 patients.

I once worked for a physician who believed that there was no job too small for any of his staff. When hired, we were expected to do everything from assembling chairs and painting walls, to computerizing the office and enforcing Medicare guidelines. This quickly spread a sense of teamwork between all staff members and the physician. Often our conversations (over a paint brush) were about how we could maximize the then sparse medical software selections available to make our office on the cutting edge of the electronic world. These experiences have made me a more versatile employee.

Cathy Petersen
Billing Specialist
Pediatrics

Tracking Reimbursement

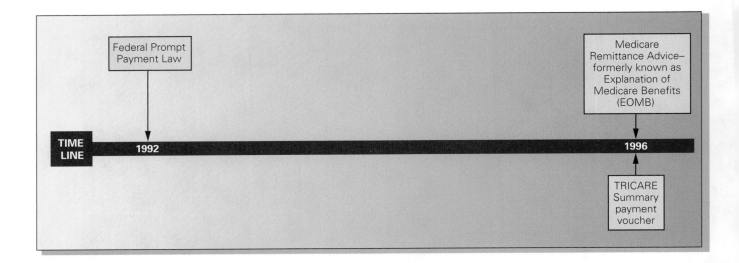

TRACKING REIMBURSEMENT

Now that you have learned how to fill out and process claim forms for private insurance carriers, Medicare, Medicaid, TRICARE, and workers' compensation cases, the next step is to learn what happens after claim submission. Once an insurance claim has been sent to the proper carrier, there are three major functions that need to regularly take place: (1) sending statements to patients and collecting on accounts, (2) posting payments received from patients and insurance companies, and (3) following up on claims that have been submitted to insurance carriers. The first function, billing patients and the collection process, was covered in the preceding chapter. Posting payments and following up on claims will be presented in this chapter. You will learn how to be a detective—how to investigate, look for clues, and follow through on claims that have been submitted in order to gain maximum reimbursement for the physician's practice.

GETTING PAID

Building a constructive relationship with insurers before conflicts arise is the best way to keep your practice's cash flow healthy. Having ongoing communication with provider representatives helps establish a professional understanding and a cooperative relationship.

It is currency that keeps a practice alive, and as stated before, the medical insurance billing specialist is the life support of the medical office, for it is he or she who obtains reimbursement for services rendered. Arrival of an insurance check or maximum reimbursement received on a delinquent account is the reward for a job well done. It motivates an insurance specialist to do an even better job.

Explanation of Benefits

Accompanying the insurance check is an **explanation of benefits (EOB)** notice which itemizes the payment received. This document should be reviewed carefully to determine if reimbursement has been made according to the insurance contract. If benefits have been assigned, the physician receives a copy of the EOB along with a payment check, also called a *voucher.*

Insurance Check Sent to Patient

Payment with Assignment of Benefits

If you suspect that the insurance check is sent to the patient after an assignment of benefits has been obtained, call the insurance company to verify that a payment was made and to whom. Ask for a copy of the endorsed check or EOB statement that indicates where payment was sent. There are then two courses of action to take:

1. Call or send a letter by certified mail to notify the patient that the insurance company sent payment to him or her in error. State that the account is due and payable within 10 days and ask when you can expect full payment. Document a promise of payment in the patient's financial record. Do not send continual monthly statements. If the patient refuses to pay and the physician does not want the patient to return, send a 10-day notification advising the pa-

Expressions from Experience

By computerizing most of our claims filing process, our turnaround time on claims can be as low as three days and averages less than two weeks. This has provided the physicians with a much clearer and more consistent financial picture and has allowed us to better budget for the long run.

Cathy Petersen
Billing Specialist
Pediatrics

tient that the account will be turned over to a collection agency. In order to follow this policy, the patient *must* be billed consistently from the date of service and all bills must state that the "account is due and payable."

2. Send a letter to the insurance company and include a copy of the claim and assignment of benefits along with the EOB indicating payment was made to the patient. It is the insurance carrier's responsibility to recover payment from the patient. If after pursuing reimbursement from the insurance company you run into a dead end, file a complaint with the state insurance commissioner. The insurance commissioner will request a review of the claim. When the assignment of benefits is discovered and it is realized that payment was sent to the patient inadvertently, the insurance company will be directed to honor the assignment of benefits, pay the physician directly, and recover money from the patient.

Payment without Assignment of Benefits

If benefits have not been assigned, payment goes to the patient and the physician may have a difficult time collecting payment and obtaining a copy of the EOB. It is wise to collect all fees at the time of service for unassigned claims.

Overpayment

An **overpayment** is a sum of money paid to the provider of service by the insurance carrier that is more than the allowed amount, or money paid by the patient that is more than the bill. Overpayment may be discovered immediately, called to your attention by the patient or insurance carrier, or not discovered for several months or years. First, examine all documents (ledger/account, day sheet, deposit, EOB) and verify that an overpayment has been made.

In any type of overpayment situation, always cash the third party payer's check and make out a provider's refund check—never refund in cash. In case of an audit, this establishes documentation proving a refund was made to reconcile the problem. Refund checks are usually written once a month by the bookkeeper or accounts payable manager. Make sure this policy is written and adhered to in all cases. If the patient paid by credit card, wait until the charges have cleared to draft a check.

Overpayments from private insurance carriers may be refunded if found immediately, or kept as a negative balance on the books. If 6 months have passed before the provider is notified of an overpayment and asked to refund money, wait until the patient is notified and proceed cautiously before refunding money. Refund all payments to Medicare immediately. If not paid back, future claims may be held up and past claims reviewed.

Components of an EOB

At first glance, the EOB document may seem difficult to understand. Unfortunately, there is no standardized format for an EOB from one carrier to the next, but categories of information contained in each one are similar (Fig. 15–1).

Interpretation of an EOB

If you read one line at a time, you can easily understand the description and calculations for each line of service. However, the EOB received from one insurance carrier may reflect more than one patient who has received services for more than one date of service. The insurance company processes all claims from a physician (or practice), issues one payment check, and submits a combined EOB reflecting the status of all charges (line by line). In addition, if more than one physician is in the medical practice and the practice is submitting claims using one group tax identification number, more than one physician's patient claims may appear on a single EOB. Read the explanation of benefits shown in Figure 15–1 line by line to see if you can interpret the meanings under each category or column. Examine the entire form carefully and refer to the numbered explanations when needed.

Posting an EOB

On receipt of an EOB, pull a copy of all claims listed according to dates of service. If the EOB contains information on more than one patient, copies may be made with the patient's name highlighted to accompany each file. If the office is computerized, refer to the patient's computerized account. Check every payment against the applicable insurance contract to find out whether the amount paid is correct. Post contractual adjustments at the time you post the insurance payment. If the EOB does not explain the breakdown of payment, call the insurance carrier for clarification. The entire EOB must be reconciled prior to depositing the check to make sure that all transactions are correct. Refer, if necessary, to the step-by-step directions for posting to a patient's ledger presented in Table 3–1 and an example of a ledger card in Figure 3–7 of Chapter 3.

Expressions from Experience

The health care industry changes daily and it is a challenge to keep abreast of those changes. Where I live, good continuing educational opportunities specific to my job are hard to find. I have found that books teach good basics on which you can expand in the medical setting.

Cathy Petersen
Billing Specialist
Pediatrics

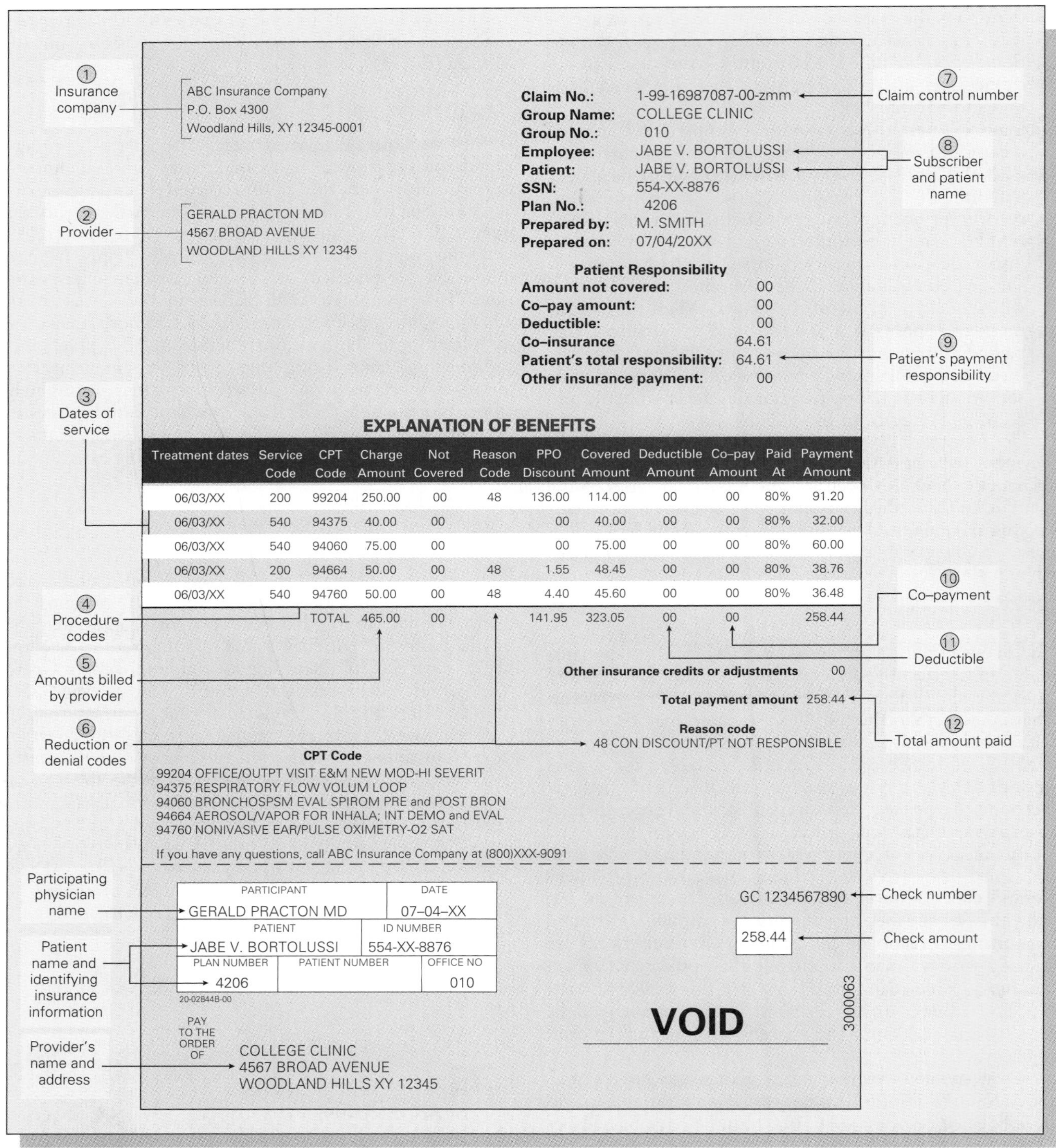

ABC Insurance Company
P.O. Box 4300
Woodland Hills, XY 12345-0001

GERALD PRACTON MD
4567 BROAD AVENUE
WOODLAND HILLS XY 12345

Claim No.: 1-99-16987087-00-zmm
Group Name: COLLEGE CLINIC
Group No.: 010
Employee: JABE V. BORTOLUSSI
Patient: JABE V. BORTOLUSSI
SSN: 554-XX-8876
Plan No.: 4206
Prepared by: M. SMITH
Prepared on: 07/04/20XX

Patient Responsibility

Amount not covered:	00
Co-pay amount:	00
Deductible:	00
Co-insurance	64.61
Patient's total responsibility:	64.61
Other insurance payment:	00

EXPLANATION OF BENEFITS

Treatment dates	Service Code	CPT Code	Charge Amount	Not Covered	Reason Code	PPO Discount	Covered Amount	Deductible Amount	Co-pay Amount	Paid At	Payment Amount
06/03/XX	200	99204	250.00	00	48	136.00	114.00	00	00	80%	91.20
06/03/XX	540	94375	40.00	00		00	40.00	00	00	80%	32.00
06/03/XX	540	94060	75.00	00		00	75.00	00	00	80%	60.00
06/03/XX	200	94664	50.00	00	48	1.55	48.45	00	00	80%	38.76
06/03/XX	540	94760	50.00	00	48	4.40	45.60	00	00	80%	36.48
		TOTAL	465.00	00		141.95	323.05	00	00		258.44

Other insurance credits or adjustments 00

Total payment amount 258.44

Reason code
48 CON DISCOUNT/PT NOT RESPONSIBLE

CPT Code
99204 OFFICE/OUTPT VISIT E&M NEW MOD-HI SEVERIT
94375 RESPIRATORY FLOW VOLUM LOOP
94060 BRONCHOSPSM EVAL SPIROM PRE and POST BRON
94664 AEROSOL/VAPOR FOR INHALA; INT DEMO and EVAL
94760 NONIVASIVE EAR/PULSE OXIMETRY-O2 SAT

If you have any questions, call ABC Insurance Company at (800)XXX-9091

PARTICIPANT		DATE
GERALD PRACTON MD		07–04–XX
PATIENT		ID NUMBER
JABE V. BORTOLUSSI		554-XX-8876
PLAN NUMBER	PATIENT NUMBER	OFFICE NO
4206		010

20-02844B-00

GC 1234567890

258.44

PAY TO THE ORDER OF
COLLEGE CLINIC
4567 BROAD AVENUE
WOODLAND HILLS XY 12345

VOID

3000063

Figure 15–1. Example of an explanation of benefits document with accompanying payment check that provider received from a private insurance company.

Claims paid according to the insurance contract are put into a file designated "closed claims." Each copy of the EOB may then be stapled to each claim form and filed with the closed claim according to the date payment was posted. If needed for future reference, check the payment date on the patient's account and look in the closed claim date file accordingly. The office manager should periodically do a review of random EOBs to assure accurate posting.

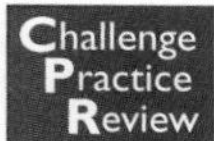

Pause and Practice CPR

REVIEW SESSIONS 15–1 THROUGH 15–3

Directions: *Complete the following questions as a review of information you have just read.*

15–1 What is the reward that a medical insurance billing specialist strives for?

____

15–2 What accompanies an insurance check? ______________________________

15–3 On receipt of an EOB, what should be done? ______________________________

____

____

CHECK YOUR HEARTBEAT! Turn to the end of the chapter for answers to these review sessions.

FOLLOW-UP AFTER CLAIM SUBMISSION

For specific knowledge of where and when insurance claim problems occur after submission, you must study all aspects of the insurance process from beginning to end. This section begins with tracking insurance claims. Next, you learn how to analyze claim problems, and last you learn how to make claim inquiries and handle suspended and denied claims. With the development of proficient skills and experience in following up on claims, you will become an invaluable asset to your employer and will consistently bring in revenue that might otherwise be lost to the business.

Tracking Insurance Claims

In Chapter 3 you learned to establish a follow-up procedure for insurance claims by either (1) logging the completed claims onto an insurance claims register (Fig. 15–2), (2) using a tickler file, or (3) generating a practice management report that can be used to track insurance payments. The ease of tracking unpaid insurance claims quickly and accurately should be the goal in choosing and setting up a system.

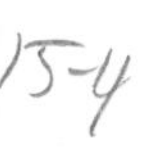

When using a manual system (log or tickler file) a copy of the insurance claim is filed chronologically in a pending file according to the date of service. Claims may be further divided by insurance carrier type so

INSURANCE CLAIMS REGISTER Page No. ________

Patient's Name Group/policy No.	Name of Insurance Company	Claim Submitted Date	Claim Submitted Amount	Follow-Up Date	Follow-Up Date	Claim Paid Date	Claim Paid Amt	Difference
Davis, Bob	BC/BS	1-7-00	319.37			2/28/00	294.82	24.55
Cash, David	BC	1-8-00	268.08	2-10-00	3-10-00			
Smythe, Jan	Medicaid	1-9-00	146.15	2-10-00				
Phillips, Emma	Medicare	1-10-00	96.28	2-10-00				
Perez, Jose	Medi-Medi	1-10-00	647.09	2-10-00				
Amato, Joe	TRICARE	2-1-00	134.78	3-10-00				
Rubin, Billy	Aetna	2-4-00	607.67	3-10-00				
Pfeifer, Renee	Travelers	2-10-00	564.55	3-10-00				
Tam, Chang	Prudential	2-15-00	1515.79					
Brown, Harry	Allstate	2-21-00	121.21					
Park, James	BC	2-24-00	124.99					

Figure 15–2. Insurance Claims Register used to track claims and follow-up activity.

that multiple outstanding claims can be addressed in one telephone call, letter, or tracer.

When payment is received from the insurance company, pull the copy of the claim and attach it to the EOB. Post payment to the patient's ledger/account and day sheet, post the contractual adjustment, then file the claim. A line may be drawn through the information in the insurance claim register without obscuring data, thus alerting the insurance specialist that no more follow-up is needed. On a regular basis (daily or weekly) check the log or file under "today's date" and follow up on all unpaid claims remaining in the tickler file that exceed the contract time limit.

When referring to a report generated by the medical software program, claims will be aged according to date submitted. Paid claims will not appear in the report that is being reviewed for follow-up.

Table 15–1 **Time Limit for Receiving Insurance Reimbursement**

Program	From Date Claim Was Manually Submitted (by mail)	From Date Claim Was Electronically Submitted
Private insurance companies	4–6 wks	2 wks or less
TRICARE Standard	8–12 wks	2 wks or less
Medicare	4–6 wks	2½ wks for participating physicians 3½ wks for nonparticipating physicians
Workers' compensation	4–8 wks	2 wks or less

Analyzing Claim Problems

Always identify why payment has not been received and pinpoint the source of the error that occurs within the medical office. A claim may be suspended or denied because of an error that occurred when collecting registration information at the front desk, when posting charges to an account, during the coding process, when assigning provider identification numbers, and so forth. A large number of claims are denied for wrong sex and wrong year of birth. The more unusual or foreign-sounding a name is, the more denials occur based on gender. Identified errors should be brought to the attention of the individual(s) responsible to improve accuracy of outgoing claims and avoid future problems.

Determine which insurance carriers are presenting the most problems. Use your payment records and document those that consistently fail to pay within 90 days. Note how many times claims have to be resubmitted, what proportion of claims are rejected, the dollar amount of claims submitted versus monies received, and the lag time between claim submission and payment. These statistics will help persuade carriers to improve the promptness of reimbursement. If a particular insurance company pays significantly slower than others, draw up a plan of action to approach the company. It is wise to select cases of slow or inadequate reimbursement problems rather than individual claim disputes. While making your case, you can have individual examples at hand to refer to when necessary.

Contract Payment Time Limits

When following up after claim submission the first thing to determine is the payment time limit stated in the insurance contract. The health insurance policy has a provision regarding the insurance company's obligation to pay benefits promptly when a claim is submitted. It is reasonable to expect payment as shown in Table 15–1. A claim awaiting overdue payment from a nonpayer is referred to as a **delinquent claim.**

If the claim was filed in a timely manner, submit proof to substantiate the original filing date. A demand letter may be attached to encourage payment, stating the contracted time limit and asking why the claim has not been paid; retain a copy for the physician's file. Obtain a Certificate of Mailing or send all high-dollar claims by certified mail to alleviate the problem of the insurance company saying that "it was never received." If the claim was submitted late, provide an explanation for the late filing.

Prompt payment laws are emerging in many states which are designed to govern the actions of insurers and other third party payers, while outlining actions collectors can take against the companies. Go to the web site (http://www.wbsaunders.com/MERLIN/Fordney/insurance/) for a list of prompt payment laws for each state, which includes a brief statute of the law and specifies a state agency contact.

Managed Care Contract Time Limits

Managed care plans usually process claims on a daily basis and issue capitated payment monthly; however, some plans release payments quarterly. There are plans that withhold a percentage of the reimbursement that is reserved in a pool and distributed at the end of the fiscal year. Usually state laws dictate the time limit within which a managed care plan must pay. In some states, an agency other than the state insurance commissioner has jurisdiction over managed care plans. Contact your state medical society to find out who the responsible entity is.

The contract should state the terms of payment, time limits, and late payment penalties, all of which can vary from one plan to another. To diminish late payment of claims, a contract can specify that late claims accrue interest (e.g., 15% of the reimbursement amount for claims paid after the payment time limit has elapsed).

If claims are not being paid in a timely manner (e.g., 30 to 45 days), take the following steps.

1. Write to the plan representative and list all unpaid claims, claims paid after the payment time limit, and claims paid in error.
2. Send a statement of all unpaid claims to the director of the managed care plan notifying him or her that

if the bill is not paid you will contact the employer's benefits manager (or patient) and alert that person to the outstanding, slow-paying accounts. State that this will prevent the physician from renewing the plan's contract. Ask the patient to also contact the plan's representative.

3. Take examples and statistics to the next renegotiating session when the physician's contract is expiring.

Before a medical practice participates in a managed care plan, a time limit payment provision is an important factor to consider when reviewing the contract.

Claim Inquiries

Once payment is delayed, recheck the insurance claim and affirm that a clean claim was sent with all necessary precertification, preauthorization, and documentation for services. If it is discovered that an error has been made in billing a case, send a *corrected* claim indicating this in Block 19. Do not **rebill** the insurance carrier by sending a duplicate claim; the practice could be accused of trying to collect double payment. Instead, send an insurance **tracer** (Fig. 15–3).

An **inquiry**, sometimes called a tracer or follow-up, is made to an insurance company to locate the status of

College Clinic

Telephone (555) 486-9002 | 4567 Broad Avenue, Woodland Hills, XY 12345-0001 | Fax (555) 487-8976

INSURANCE CLAIM TRACER

INSURANCE COMPANY NAME American Insurance DATE 09/14/XX

ADDRESS P.O. Box 5300, New York, New York 12345

Patient: Marcella Austin

Insured: Marcella Austin

Employer: T C Corporation

Policy/certificate no. 9635 402-A

Group name/no. B0105

Date of initial claim submission: 08/02/XX

Amount of claim: $536.24

An inordinate amount of time has passed since the submission of our original claim. We have not received a request for additional information and still await payment of this assigned claim. Please review the attached duplicate and process for payment within 7 days.

If there is any difficulty with this claim, please check the reason below and return this letter to our office. Thank you.

- ☐ No record of claim.
- ☐ Claim received and payment is in process.
- ☐ Claim is in suspense (comment please).
- ☐ Claim is in review (comment please).
- ☐ Additional information needed (comment please)
- ☐ Claim paid. Date:______ Amount:$______ To whom:______
- ☐ Claim denied (comment please).

Comments:______

Thank you for your assistance in this important matter. Please contact the insurance specialist named below if you have any questions regarding this claim.

Katelyn Chang — Insurance Specialist (555) 486-9002 Ext. 236

Gene Ullibarri, MD — Treating Physician

Figure 15–3. Example of an Insurance Claim Tracer used to follow up on delinquent insurance claims.

an insurance claim or to inquire about payment determination shown on the EOB. With some insurance companies, claim status can be easily accessed by means of computer or teledigital response systems, thus speeding up inquiry/response time. It may also be accessed by telephone or mail. Following are some reasons for making inquiries.

- No response or payment received on submitted claim
- Payment received, amount incorrect
- Payment received, amount allowed, and patient's responsibility not defined
- Payment received for individual/patient not seen by physician
- Change in procedure or diagnostic code from code submitted
- Error on EOB
- Insurance check made out to wrong physician or party

If the inquiry is submitted in writing, a form used by the insurance carrier may be required with the claim attached. If there is no response from the insurance carrier within 2 to 4 weeks, call the carrier and/or patient to find out the reason for the delay. Direct your call to the claims representative.

Insurance Carrier Telephone Inquiries

When calling a third party payer, get the names and direct-dial numbers of all the employees who can answer questions about precertification, coverage and limitation, reason for denials, and so forth. Be ready to give the following facts relating to the case.

- Physician's PIN, UPIN, or NPI; tax I.D.; and provider number
- Patient's name and date of birth
- Patient's insurance I.D.; contract, employer, or group number
- Date of service and dollar amount of claim
- All relevant procedure/service codes and diagnostic codes
- Brief but complete recap of complaint

Be calm and factual as you present your case. Invite the insurance adjuster to call you back if he or she cannot come up with the answers you need right away.

Lost Claims

When an insurance claim is received by the insurance carrier it is date-stamped (usually within 24 hours), assigned a number, and logged into the payer system. If there is a backlog of claims it may take 7 to 15 days (or longer) to be recorded. If you call to find out the status of a claim during that time, you may be told it was not received, or it may be considered a **lost claim.**

To determine if this is the situation, ask if there is a backlog of claims, and if so, ask for the expected turnaround time. At this point you need to either wait until the carrier processes the claim or gather documentation on claims that have been "lost" or paid late by the same carrier and file a complaint with the state insurance commissioner. If the carrier does not admit to having a backlog of claims and it is determined to be lost, submit a copy of the original claim, referencing it in Block 19, "copy of original claim submitted on [date]."

History of Account

If you cannot get a satisfactory answer over the telephone as to why the claim has not been paid, or if the insurance company seems to be ignoring all efforts to trace the claim, an exact history of the account may be the best weapon with which to proceed. A *history of the account* is a chronologic record of all events that have occurred. Keep all communications received from the insurance company, note all telephone calls, and keep copies of all documents sent. Send a copy of the history of the account directly to the insurance company and demand a reply. If payment or reason for delay is not received, notify the patient and file a complaint with the regulatory agency.

Suspended and Denied Claims

Claims that are listed on the EOB as a **suspended claim** or **denied claim** must be analyzed to determine the problem causing delay or nonpayment. First, look at the reason/denial code on the EOB to determine the cause. Example 15–1 lists some denial codes used by insurance companies. Next, look at the problem claim and categorize it in one of the five compliance risk areas: (1) insurance policy requirements, (2) correct coding, (3) appropriate billing guidelines, (4) reasonable and necessary services, and (5) proper documentation. Once it has been categorized, follow the necessary steps to correct the problem. Various claim problems and solutions may be found by going to the worktext web site http://www.wbsaunders.com/MERLIN/Fordney/insurance/.

Example 15–1

Denial Codes

D11 Denied	Claim is not eligible for payment based on medical information received.
D12 Denied	Office procedure is not payable in connection with surgery.
D13 Denied	Member ineligible on the date of service.
D14 Denied	These charges were incurred after the member's coverage terminated.
D23 Denied	This member has maternity benefits only.
D29 Denied	Duplicate; these charges have been previously considered.
D43 Denied	Claim was received past the plan's filing limit.

State Insurance Commission

If a complaint arises about an insurance policy, medical claim, or insurance agent/broker, contact the insurance department of the state you reside in or the state

Example 15–2

Communication Involving the Insurance Commissioner

Problem: XYZ Insurance Company is historically a slow payer.

Letter to Insurance Company: Unless this claim is paid or denied within 30 days, a formal written complaint will be filed with the state insurance commissioner.

Problem Unresolved: No response from XYZ Insurance Company.

Letter to Insurance Commissioner: The attached claim has been submitted to the XYZ Insurance Company. It has not been paid or denied (see enclosed history of the account). Please accept this letter as a formal written complaint against the XYZ Insurance Company.

where the insurance company's corporate office is headquartered. Sometimes this department is referred to as the insurance commission of the state. State insurance departments usually have various objectives, including the following:

- Verifying insurance company solvency
- Protecting policyholders' interests
- Ensuring contract provisions are carried out in good faith
- Monitoring compliance of insurance laws by organizations authorized to transact insurance (e.g., agents and brokers)
- Tracking and release of complaint information
- Explaining correspondence related to insurance company bankruptcies and other financial difficulties
- Assisting companies that fund their own insurance plan
- Helping resolve insurance conflicts

The insurance commissioner does not have the authority vested in a court of law to order an insurance company to make payment on a specific claim. The commissioner will review an insurance policy to see whether the denial of a claim by the insurance company was based on legal provisions of the insurance contract and will advise the patient if there is an infraction of the law. If there is an infraction, the patient should consult an attorney to determine whether the claim should be submitted to a court of law.

The types of problems that should be submitted to the insurance commissioner are as follows:

1. Improper denial of a claim or a settlement of an amount less than that indicated by the policy, after proper appeal has been made
2. Delay in settlement of a claim, after proper appeal has been made
3. Illegal cancellation or termination of an insurance policy
4. Misrepresentation by an insurance agent or broker
5. Misappropriation of premiums paid to an insurance agent or broker
6. Problems about insurance premium rates
7. Dispute of coordination of benefits

Commission Inquiries

Requests to the insurance commissioner must be submitted in writing. In some states, the insurance commissioner requires that the complaint come from the patient even if the patient has assigned benefits to the physician. In such cases, prepare a letter for the patient and submit with the patient's signature. Copies may be sent to the state medical association and/or attorney. Mail may be sent certified, return receipt requested. Insurance companies are rated according to the number of complaints received about them, so they do not want the insurance commissioner to be alerted to any problems.

Example 15–2 illustrates a scenario where an insurance carrier has been categorized by the physician's office as a slow payer. The insurance company ignores a demand for payment and a letter is sent to the insurance commissioner.

Contact your state insurance commission and obtain copies of your state laws. Become familiar with the laws and use them in communication with the insurance carrier when necessary (see Example 15–3).

Example 15–3

Complaints to Insurance Commissioner

- This claim is being monitored pursuant to [_______ Insurance Code §_______] which requires all claims to be paid not later than [_______] days.
- This claim is NOW DELINQUENT pursuant to [_______ Insurance Code §_______] which requires all claims to be paid not later than [_______] days, or interest/penalties will be assessed.

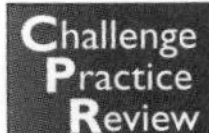

Pause and Practice CPR

REVIEW SESSIONS 15–4 THROUGH 15–9

Directions: *Complete the following questions as a review of information you have just read.*

15–4 When using a manual system to track insurance claims, how should they be filed?

____

15–5 When referring to a computer-generated report, claims are aged according to ____________ ______________________________.

15–6 When following up after claim submission, what is the first thing that needs to be determined? ______________________________

15–7 A claim awaiting overdue payment from a nonpayer is called a ______________________________.

15–8 A follow-up made to an insurance carrier is also called a/an ______________________________ or ______________________________.

15–9 If claims are being denied because of noncovered services, what should be done to prevent this from happening in the future? ______________________________
____
____
____

CHECK YOUR HEARTBEAT! Turn to the end of the chapter for answers to these review sessions.

REVIEW AND APPEAL PROCESS

It is worth investing money and staff resources to identify the cause of claim denials. When efforts to resolve denials or underpayment issues have not been satisfied, the next step is to appeal the claim.

Appeal

An **appeal** is a request for payment by asking for a review of an insurance claim for one of the following reasons:

- Payment is denied for unknown reason.
- Payment is received but the amount is incorrect (e.g., excessive reduction in allowed payment or usual and customary fee).
- Physician disagrees with insurance carrier's decision about a preexisting condition.
- Medical treatment rendered due to unusual circumstances is not adequately reimbursed.
- Precertification/preauthorization not obtained prior to service due to extenuating circumstances; claim denied.
- Inadequate payment received for complicated procedure.
- Physician disagrees with decision for denial of claim, "not medically necessary."

Usually, there is a time limit for appealing a claim. To determine whether payment has been issued correctly, read the EOB document or refer to provider manuals for the various programs.

You should base appealing a claim on billing guidelines and on state and federal insurance laws and regulations. A bimonthly newsletter is available online that links to regulatory information (see Resources at the end of this chapter).

The decision to appeal a claim should be decided after asking three questions: (1) Is there sufficient information and documentation to back up the claim? (2) Is the amount of money in question sufficient (in the physician's opinion)? (3) How much time and energy do you want to expend to appeal a claim?

Studies indicate that in over 50% of claims that are initially denied, the decision is reversed and the claims are reimbursed. Ultimately, the decision to appeal often rests in the physician's hands, not with the insurance billing specialist. It takes a team effort to successfully appeal a claim. Following are basic guidelines for filing an appeal:

1. Assemble all documents needed (i.e., patient's medical record, copy of the insurance claim form, EOB, and any communication that has taken place with the insurance carrier).
2. Complete an appeal form or compose a letter explaining the reason why the provider does not agree with the claim denial (or insufficient payment) listed on the EOB.
3. Send documentation that supports your view. Photocopy sections from the coding manual, or abstract and photocopy excerpts from a coding resource book or newsletter and include the name and date of the publication and the title of the article (if applicable).
4. Send copies of similar cases with increased reimbursement from the same insurance carrier, if available.

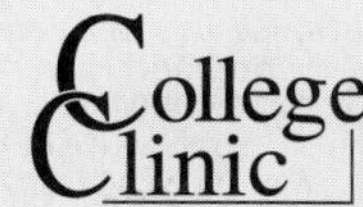

4567 Broad Avenue
Woodland Hills, XY
12345-0001
Telephone (555) 486-9002
Fax (555) 487-8976

September 12, 20XX

Ms. Jane Hatfield
Appeals Division
XYZ Managed Care Plan
100 South H Street
Anytown, XY 12345-0001

Dear Ms. Hatfield:

Re: Claim number: A0958
Patient: Carolyn B. Little
Dates of service: August 2–10, 20XX

Recently I received a denied claim from your office (see enclosure). A review of the contract I have with your managed care plan shows that these hospital services should have been approved and paid according to your fee schedule.

Enclosed is a photocopy of the history and physical, progress notes, and discharge summary for these dates of service. All services were medically necessary. Please review the laboratory results and abdominal ultrasound enclosed which substantiate the patient's complaint.

If after review of this claim you still feel reimbursement is not appropriate, please forward this request to the Peer Review Committee for a final determination.

If you need additional information, please telephone, fax, or write my office.

Sincerely,

Gerald Practon, MD

mtf
Enclosures

Figure 15–4. Example of a letter asking for a review of a claim submitted and denied by a managed care plan.

5. Call the insurance company and speak to the individual responsible for appeals, explaining what you are trying to accomplish with the appeal. Direct the correspondence to this person.
6. Retain copies of all data sent for the physician's files.

Figure 15–4 is an example of a letter that was submitted to a managed care plan when appealing a denied claim. Track the appeal until the case is resolved. If an appeal is not successful, the physician may want to proceed to the next step, which is a peer review.

Peer Review

A **peer review** is an examination done by a group of unbiased practicing physicians who judge the effectiveness and efficiency of the professional care rendered. This group determines the medical necessity and subsequent payment for the case in question. Some insurance carriers send a claim for review routinely for certain procedures that have been done for certain diagnoses. If you need to have a claim reviewed after payment has been rendered, send in the letter as shown in Figure 15–5.

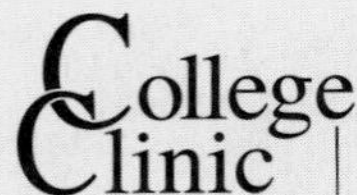

4567 Broad Avenue
Woodland Hills, XY
12345-0001
Telephone (555) 486-9002
Fax (555) 487-8976

Committee on Physician's Services

Re: Underpayment
Identification No.: M18876782
Patient: Peaches Melba
Type of Service: Plastic & Reconstructive Surgery
Date of Service: 1 - 3 - XX
Amount Paid: $ 75.00
My Fees: $ 180.00

Dear Sirs:

Herewith a request for a committee review of the above-named case, since I consider the allowance paid very low having in mind the location, the extent, the type and the necessary surgical procedure performed:
The skin graft, one inch in diameter included the lateral third of eyebrow and was full thickness to preserve hair follicles.

Operative report for the surgery has been sent to you with the claim.

Considering these facts I hope that you will authorize additional payment in order to bring the total fee to within reasonable and customary charges.

Sincerely,

Cosmo Graff, M.D.

mf
enclosure

Figure 15–5. Example of a letter appealing a fee reduction. This letter itemizes important data and is submitted to the insurance carrier after payment has been received that the physician believes is below standard.

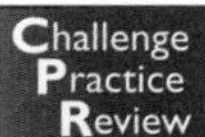

Pause and Practice CPR

REVIEW SESSIONS 15–10 AND 15–11

Directions: *Complete the following questions as a review of information you have just read.*

15–10 What questions should be asked to help determine if a claim should be appealed?

(a) __________

(b) __________

(c) __________

15–11 An examination done by a group of unbiased practicing physicians who judge the effectiveness and efficiency of professional care rendered is called a/an ______________________.

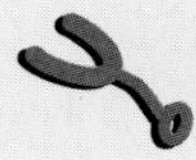

CHECK YOUR HEARTBEAT! Turn to the end of the chapter for answers to these review sessions.

FOLLOW-UP ON SPECIFIC CLAIM TYPES

For follow-up information on specific claim types (e.g., Medicaid, Medicare, TRICARE, and so forth), including visual examples and an exercise session, go to the worktext web site http://www.wbsaunders.com/MERLIN/Fordney/insurance/.

SUMMATION AND PREVIEW

All reimbursement activity begins with the gathering of information, which is the underpinning of an effective practice. The information flow, documentation, coding, statements, and insurance forms can all affect reimbursement. When payment is not received, the insurance billing specialist needs to be able to turn obstacles into challenges as he or she analyzes problems in the reimbursement cycle.

Techniques used to follow up on delinquent claims are the final skills needed to assure financial success for the physician's practice. You will now have an opportunity to practice these skills. As you add these skills to the solid foundation and structure you have meticulously built, you will be securing the protective roof to ensure that all of your hard efforts of claim filing will be successful. Without good follow-up techniques, many claims go unpaid and medical practices lose large amounts of money. Secure your employer's medical practice against loss, and ensure maximum reimbursement by learning how to post payments, adjustments, and follow-up on unpaid claims.

You may want to return to Chapter 1 and reread sections on certifications and various forms of job search found in the Resources section.

GOLDEN RULE

Be a detective; look for a clue and follow through.

NOTES

Chapter 15 Review and Practice

Study Session

Directions: *Review the objectives, key terms, and chapter information before completing the following study questions.*

460 15–1 What is another name for the insurance payment check? voucher

15–2 What should you do if an EOB does not explain the breakdown of the payment?

____

15–3 What do you do with claims that are paid according to the insurance contract? ______________________________

____

15–4 Name three methods used to track and follow up on insurance claims.

463 (a) logging completed claims onto an insurance claims register

(b) using a tickler file

(c) generating a practice

15–5 What statistics should be gathered to present to a slow-paying insurance carrier?

(a) ______________________________

(b) ______________________________

(c) ______________________________

(d) ______________________________

15–6 If a claim is submitted late, what should be done? ______________________________

____

15–7 What types of laws are emerging in states that are designed to govern the actions of insurers and other third party payers, while outlining actions collectors can take against insurance companies? ______________________________

15–8 List the time limits for receiving insurance reimbursement from the following insurance plans.

(a) Medicare ______________________________

(b) TRICARE Standard ______________________________

(c) Private carriers ______________________________

(d) Workers' compensation ______________________________

15–9 Once payment is delayed, recheck the insurance claim for ______________________________

______________________________.

15–10 Claim status can be obtained by:

(a) ______________________________

(b) ______________________________

(c) ______________________________

(d) ______________________________

15–11 To analyze a suspended or denied claim, what should you look at? ______________________

____

15–12 If claims are being denied stating services are "unbundled," what can be done to determine what services are bundled? ______________________________

____

15–13 *Most* billing problems originate from ______________________________,
and ______________________________ is one of the top causes.

15–14 If services are declared "not medically necessary" and denied, what is the *first* step that should be taken? ______________________________

____

15–15 Describe what an appeal is. ______________________________

____

15–16 What is the approximate percentage of claims originally denied where the decision is reversed after appeal? ______________%

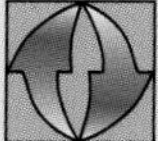

Exercise Exchange

15–1 **Trace a Delinquent Claim.**

Scenario: You are following up on insurance claims using an insurance claims register and notice that a private insurance claim for Sondra Still has not been paid.

Directions

1. Refer to the patient ledger for Sondra Still and complete a claim tracer found in Appendix F (Form F–16).
2. The patient is employed by Giraffe Graphics.
3. List today's date as 12/15/XX.
4. Your telephone extension is 236.
5. The patient is the insured and the claim was originally filed the day the patient was discharged from the hospital.
6. Note: On the insurance claims register you would indicate that the claim has had an insurance claim tracer sent.

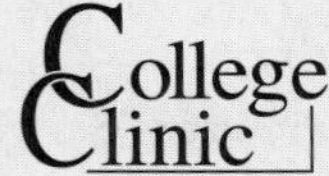

4567 Broad Avenue
Woodland Hills, XY
12345-0001
Tel (555) 486-9002
Fax (555) 487-8976

Sondra T. Still
1515 Grand Street Apt. 5
Orange Grove, XY 12345-0001

Phone No. (H) 555/967-8021 (W) 555/967-7772 Birthdate 03/30/57
Insurance Co. Highmark Ins. Co. PO Box 43, NY, NY 12345-0001 Policy No. 486-60973 Group A77

DATE	REFERENCE	PROFESSIONAL SERVICE DESCRIPTION	CHARGE	CREDITS		CURRENT BALANCE
				PAYMENTS	ADJUSTMENTS	
10/25/20XX	99253	Inpatient Consult Level 3	106 10			106 10
10/26/20XX	43820	Gastrojejunostomy (Cutler)	971 86			1077 96
10/27/20XX	99253	HV Level 3	N C			1077 96
10/28/20XX	99252	HV Level 2	N C			1077 96
10/29/20XX	99251	HV Level 1	N C			1077 96
10/30/20XX	99238	Discharge (30 min)	N C			1077 96
10/30/20XX	10/25–10/26/XX	Billed Highmark Insurance Company				1077 96

Due and payable within 10 days **Pay last amount in balance column** ⇧

Key: PF: Problem-focused
EPF: Expanded problem-focused
D: Detailed
SF: Straightforward
L: Low complexity
M: Moderate complexity
CON: Consultation
HX: History
PX: Phys Exam
ED: Emergency Dept.
HC: House Call
HV: Hospital visit

15–2 **Compose a Letter of Appeal.**

Scenario: It is 12/30/XX and you receive check number 20190 from Highmark Insurance Company payable to Dr. Cutler in the amount of $777.49 for services provided to patient Sondra Still on 10/26/20XX. This payment is 80% of the submitted charge, which is in agreement with the insurance contract. The consult, however, on 10/25/20XX, which was requested by Dr. Practon, is denied stating it is bundled with the surgery. Dr. Cutler does not agree with this denial because an extensive workup was done on the patient on 10/25/20XX (diagnostic and radiology testing) which resulted in a decision for surgery. The consultation report from the hospital as well as the history and physical and laboratory and radiology reports substantiate this and Dr. Cutler would like you to appeal the claim.

Directions

1. Post the insurance payment to the patient's ledger card using the ledger from Exercise Exchange 15–1.
2. Use the College Clinic letterhead (Form 01 found in Appendix F) and compose a letter of appeal addressed to Mr. William Robinson in the Appeals Division of Highmark Insurance.
3. Enclose the above documents and list the claim number as B55689.
4. Refer to Figure 15–4 for guidance but individualize the letter according to the case at hand.

15–3 **Interpret an Explanation of Benefits, Abstract Data. Calculate and Post Payments and Adjustments to Three Patient's Ledger Cards.**

Directions

1. Remove the ledgers found in Appendix F for Kenneth Kozak (Form 17), Larry Slomkowski (Form 18), and Julie Vale (Form 19). They all are insured by Temple Insurance Company and received services during the month of September 20XX from Dr. Practon.
2. Refer to the Explanation of Benefits from Temple Insurance listing these patients' services.
3. Today is October 17, 20XX. Verify all figures on the EOB, paying close attention to the services that are being paid at an amount less than the charged amount.
4. Post the insurance payment for each of these patients. Refer, if necessary, to instructions on how to post to a patient ledger found in Chapter 3, Table 3–1 and Figure 3–7.
5. Determine if there is a contractual insurance adjustment, and if so, post it to the ledger.
6. Bill the patient for the balance.

Gerald Practon MD
College Clinic
4500 Broad Avenue
Woodland Hills, XY
12345-0001

Temple Insurance Company

10/15/20XX

EXPLANATION OF BENEFITS

PATIENT NAME	TREATMENT DATES	CPT CODE	CHARGE AMOUNT	REASON CODE	COVERED AMOUNT	DEDUCTIBLE AMOUNT	CO-PAY AMOUNT	PAID AT	PAYMENT AMOUNT
KOZAK, KENNETH	09/02/20XX	99205	132.28	03	125.00	00	00	80%	100.00
	09/02/20XX	82947	15.00		15.00	00	00	80%	12.00
	09/02/20XX	86580	11.34		11.34	00	00	80%	9.07
	TOTALS		158.62		151.34		PAYMENT TOTAL		121.07
SLOMKOWSKI, LARRY	09/05/20XX	99212	28.55		28.55	00	00	80%	22.84
	TOTALS		28.55		28.55		PAYMENT TOTAL		22.84
VALE, JULIE	09/03/20XX	99203	70.92	03	69.23	00	00	80%	55.38
	09/03/20XX	71020	40.97	03	34.95	00	00	80%	27.96
	TOTALS		111.89		104.18		PAYMENT TOTAL		83.34

Reason Code: 03 Allowed amount per insurance contract **Check No. 56390** **$227.25**

NOTES

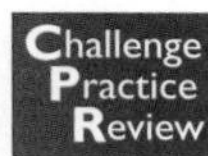

CPR Session: Answers

REVIEW SESSIONS 15–1 THROUGH 15–3

15–1 the arrival of an insurance check or maximum reimbursement on a delinquent account

15–2 explanation of benefit (EOB)

15–3 Pull copies of all claims listed according to dates of service, make copies of the EOB if it contains more than one patient, refer to the patient's ledger or computerized account, check every payment against the insurance contract to assure that it was paid correctly, post adjustments and payments.

REVIEW SESSIONS 15–4 THROUGH 15–9

15–4 chronologically according to DOS and insurance type

15–5 date submitted

15–6 payment time limit stated in the insurance contract

15–7 delinquent claim

15–8 tracer or inquiry

15–9 Call the insurance carrier and keep a list of all noncovered services that the physician does routinely. Have the patient sign a waiver of liability agreement prior to these services being rendered.

REVIEW SESSIONS 15–10 AND 15–11

15–10 (a) Is there sufficient information and documentation to back up the claim?
(b) Is the amount of money in question sufficient?
(c) How much time and energy do you want to expend to appeal a claim?

15–11 peer review

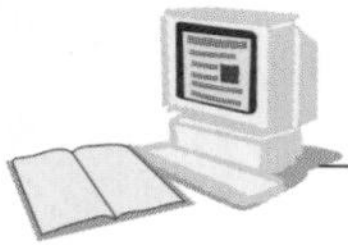

Resources

Reading documentation, gathering facts, and composing letters that justify services performed are skills that are learned over time. One must first determine that a claim is worthy of entering the appeals process. Resources listed under "appeals" may help with this task.

Internet

Appeals

- Bimonthly newsletter for regulatory information on appeals
  Web site: www.appealsolutions.com

Publications

- *CHAMPVA Handbook* (booklet featuring data on review and appeals), CHAMPVA, P. O. Box 65023, Denver, CO 80206-9023, (800) 733-8387
  Web site: www.va.gov/hac/champva
- *Medicare Appeals and Grievances (Complaints)* booklet—CMS Publication no. 10119, (800) 633-4227
  Web site: www.medicare.gov
- *TRICARE Network Provider Manual, Medical and Surgical,* HealthNet Federal Services, 2025 Aerojet Road, Rancho Cordova, CA 95742, (800) 977-1255
  Web site: www.tricare.osd.mil

Software

- *Appeal Solutions* (450 appeal letters), Appeal Solutions, 703 Blue Oak, Lewisville, TX, (888) 399-4925
  Web site: www.appealsolutions.com

Appendix

A

College Clinic—Medical Practice Simulation

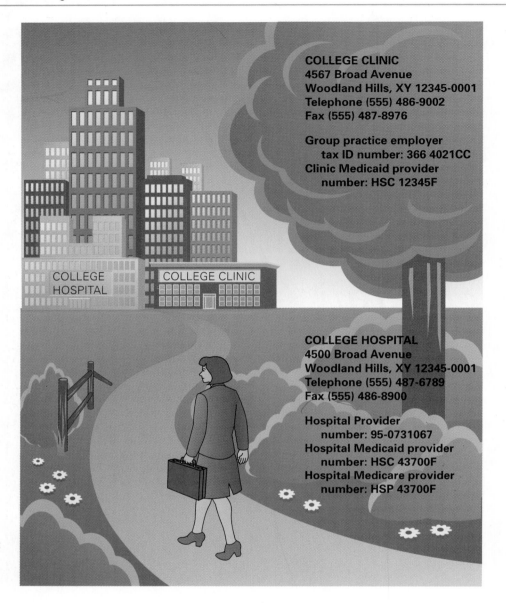
COLLEGE CLINIC
4567 Broad Avenue
Woodland Hills, XY 12345-0001
Telephone (555) 486-9002
Fax (555) 487-8976
Group practice employer tax ID number: 366 4021CC
Clinic Medicaid provider number: HSC 12345F
COLLEGE HOSPITAL
COLLEGE CLINIC
COLLEGE HOSPITAL
4500 Broad Avenue
Woodland Hills, XY 12345-0001
Telephone (555) 487-6789
Fax (555) 486-8900
Hospital Provider number: 95-0731067
Hospital Medicaid provider number: HSC 43700F
Hospital Medicare provider number: HSP 43700F

College Clinic

4567 Broad Avenue
Woodland Hills,
XY 12345-0001
Telephone (555) 486-9002
Fax (555) 487-8976

Student-Employee

To gain practical experience and put theory to work, assume that you have been hired to work as a medical insurance billing specialist for College Clinic.

You will be filing insurance claims and asked to perform a number of tasks in the exercises presented in this Worktext as if you were on the job.

Various reference materials that you will be using are listed in Appendices described in sections on this page.

Staff Physicians

College Clinic has ten staff physicians in various specialties to serve patient needs. A complete listing with provider and reference numbers is on the following page.

All physicians are on staff at College Hospital.

Physicians have signed contracts with Medicaid, Medicare, CHAMPVA, TRICARE, workers' compensation carriers, as well as many private insurance plans and will be accepting assignment of medical benefits.

Fee Schedule
Appendix B

A Mock Fee Schedule is listed in Appendix B.
All physicians accept assignment unless otherwise specified.

The figures in the first column (mock fees) are the physicians' standard fees and should be used when billing private insurance plans, Medicaid, CHAMPVA, TRICARE, and workers' compensation carriers.

Use the Medicare Participating Provider column for Medicare Claims.

Claim Submission
Appendices D and F

Copy the HCFA-1500 claim form (Form 09) in Appendix F and submit all claims using OCR guidelines.

Refer to "Block by Block Instructions" and "Insurance Templates" in Appendix D for guidelines and visual examples when completing the claim form.

Other forms will also be found in Appendix F for your use.

Student Worksheets found in Appendix F may be used for coding assignments and to keep track of your progress.

HCPCS Level II Codes
Appendix C

A selected listing of HCPCS Level II Codes including some modifiers is found in Appendix C.

Glossary
Appendix E

Refer to Appendix E for definitions of key terms.

Concha Antrum, MD Dr. #1
Otolaryngologist
Social Security
082-XX-1707
State License
C01602X
Federal Tax ID (EIN)
74-10640XX
UPIN/PIN/NPI
12458977XX

Pedro Atrics, MD Dr. #2
Pediatrician
Social Security
134-XX-7600
State License
D06012X
Federal Tax ID (EIN)
71-32061XX
UPIN/PIN/NPI
37640017XX

Bertha Caesar, MD Dr. #3
Obstetrician/Gynecologist
Social Security
230-XX-6700
State License
A01817X
Federal Tax ID (EIN)
72-57130XX
UPIN/PIN/NPI
43056757XX

Perry Cardi, MD Dr. #4
Internist/Cardiologist
Social Security
557-XX-9980
State License
C02140X
Federal Tax ID (EIN)
70-64217XX
UPIN/PIN/NPI
67805027XX

Brady Coccidioides, MD Dr. #5
Internist/Pulmonologist
Social Security
670-XX-0874
State License
C04821X
Federal Tax ID (EIN)
75-67321XX
UPIN/PIN/NPI
64211067XX

Waiting Room

Receptionist Area

Rest Room

Minor Surgery/Treatment Room

Laboratory

Storage

COLLEGE CLINIC
4567 Broad Avenue
Woodland Hills, XY 12345-0001
Telephone (555) 486-9002
Fax (555) 487-8976
Group Practice Employer Tax ID Number 366 4021CC

Office Manager

Doctor's Office

Doctor's Office

Doctor's Office

Doctor's Office

Medical Insurance Billing Office

Vera Cutis, MD Dr. #6
Dermatologist
Social Security
409-XX-8620
State License
C06002X
Federal Tax ID (EIN)
71-80561XX
UPIN/PIN/NPI
70568717XX

Clarence Cutler, MD Dr. #7
General Surgeon
Social Security
410-XX-5630
State License
B07600X
Federal Tax ID (EIN)
71-57372XX
UPIN/PIN/NPI
43050047XX

Gerald Practon, MD Dr. #8
General Practitioner
Social Security
123-XX-6789
State License
C01402X
Federal Tax ID (EIN)
70-34597XX
UPIN/PIN/NPI
46278897XX

Raymond Skeleton, MD Dr. #9
Orthopedist
Social Security
432-XX-4589
State License
C04561X
Federal Tax ID (EIN)
74-65412XX
UPIN/PIN/NPI
12678547XX

Gene Ulibarri, MD Dr. #10
Urologist
Social Security
990-XX-3245
State License
C06430X
Federal Tax ID (EIN)
77-86531XX
UPIN/PIN/NPI
25678831XX

Appendix

B

College Clinic—Mock Fee Schedule

The mock fee schedule is provided to use while completing ledger cards and claim forms with Billing Break exercises. It offers a realistic approach in locating fees after services and procedures have been coded. The fees listed are hypothetical and are intended only for use in completing the exercises. The mock fee schedule is arranged in the same sequence as the CPT code book sections (i.e., Evaluation and Management, Anesthesia, Surgery, Radiology, Pathology/Laboratory, and Medicine). If you do not have access to the latest edition of CPT, you may use the code numbers provided in the mock fee schedule; however, do so with the understanding that the code numbers provided in this schedule are not comprehensive and descriptions are not complete. A complete list of modifiers may be found in Appendix C. A comprehensive list of modifiers may be found on the worktext web site at http://www.wbsaunders.com/MERLIN/Fordney/Insurance/

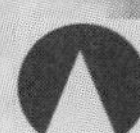
Private Payers—Use the mock fee column.

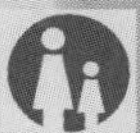
Medicaid—Use the mock fee column.

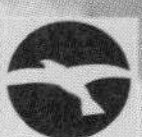
Medicare—Refer to the three columns pertaining to Medicare and use the Participating column unless otherwise specified.

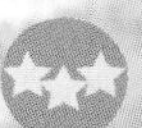
TRICARE—Use the mock fee column.

CHAMPVA—Use the mock fee column.

Workers' Compensation—use the mock fee column.

Table B–1 **College Clinic—Mock Fee Schedule**

Code No. and Description		Mock Fee	Medicare		
			Participating	Non-participating	Limiting Charge
EVALUATION AND MANAGEMENT					
OFFICE					
New Patient					
99201	PF hx/exam SF DM	33.25	30.43	28.91	33.25
99202	EPF hx/exam SF DM	51.91	47.52	45.14	51.91
99203	D hx/exam LC DM	70.92	64.92	61.67	70.92
99204	C hx/exam MC DM	106.11	97.13	92.27	106.11
99205	C hx/exam HC DM	132.28	121.08	115.03	132.38
Established Patient					
99211	May not require presence of physician (5 min)	16.07	14.70	13.97	16.07
99212	PF hx/exam SF DM	28.55	26.14	24.83	28.55
99213	EPF hx/exam LC DM	40.20	36.80	34.96	40.20
99214	D hx/exam MC DM	61.51	56.31	53.49	61.51
99215	C hx/exam HC DM	96.97	88.76	84.32	96.97
HOSPITAL					
Observation Services (new/est pt)					
99217	Discharge	66.88	61.22	58.16	66.88
99218	D/C hx/exam SF/LC DM	74.22	67.94	64.54	74.22
99219	C hx/exam MC DM	117.75	107.78	102.39	117.75
99220	C hx/exam HC DM	147.48	134.99	128.24	147.48
Inpatient Services (new/est pt)					
99221	D/C hx/exam SF/LC DM	73.00	66.82	63.48	73.00
99222	C hx/exam MC DM	120.80	110.57	105.04	120.80
99223	C hx/exam HC DM	152.98	140.03	133.03	152.98
Subsequent Hospital Care					
99231	PF hx/exam SF/LC DM	37.74	34.55	32.82	37.74
99232	EPF hx/exam MC DM	55.56	50.85	48.31	55.56
99233	D hx/exam HC DM	76.97	70.45	66.93	76.97
99238	Discharge 30 min	65.26	59.74	56.75	65.26
CONSULTATIONS					
Office (new/est pt)					
99241	PF hx/exam SF DM	51.93	47.54	45.16	51.93
99242	EPF hx/exam SF DM	80.24	73.44	69.77	80.24
99243	D hx/exam LC DM	103.51	94.75	90.01	103.51
99244	C hx/exam MC DM	145.05	132.77	126.13	145.05
99245	C hx/exam HC DM	195.48	178.93	169.98	195.48
Inpatient (new/est pt)					
99251	PF hx/exam SF DM	53.29	48.78	46.34	53.29
99252	EPF hx/exam SF DM	80.56	73.74	70.05	80.56
99253	D hx/exam LC DM	106.10	97.12	92.26	106.10
99254	C hx/exam MC DM	145.26	132.96	126.31	145.26
99255	C hx/exam HC DM	196.55	179.91	170.91	196.55
Follow-up Inpatient (new/est pt)					
99261	PF hx/exam SF/LC DM	29.66	27.15	25.79	29.66
99262	EPF hx/exam MC DM	50.57	46.28	43.97	50.57
99263	D hx/exam HC DM	76.36	69.90	66.40	76.36
Confirmatory 2nd-3rd opinion (new/est pt)					
99271	PF hx/exam SF DM	45.47	41.62	39.54	45.47
99272	EPF hx/exam SF DM	67.02	61.35	58.28	67.02
99273	D hx/exam LC DM	95.14	87.08	82.73	95.14
99274	C hx/exam MC DM	125.15	114.56	108.83	125.15
99275	C hx/exam HC DM	172.73	158.10	150.20	172.73

Table B–1 College Clinic—Mock Fee Schedule *(Continued)*

Code No. and Description		Mock Fee	Medicare* Participating	Medicare* Non-participating	Medicare* Limiting Charge
EMERGENCY DEPARTMENT (new/est pt)					
99281	PF hs/exam SF DM	24.32	22.26	21.15	24.32
99282	EPF hx/exam LC DM	37.02	33.88	32.19	37.02
99283	EPF hx/exam MC DM	66.23	60.62	57.59	66.23
99284	D hx/exam MC DM	100.71	92.18	87.57	100.71
99285	C hx/exam HC DM	158.86	145.41	138.14	158.86
CRITICAL CARE SERVICES					
99291	First 30–74 min	208.91	191.22	181.66	208.91
99292	Each additional 30 min	102.02	92.46	87.84	102.02
NEONATAL INTENSIVE CARE					
99295	Initial/day	892.74	817.16	776.30	892.74
99296	Subsequent unstable case	418.73	383.27	364.11	418.73
99297	Subsequent stable case	214.68	196.50	186.68	214.68
NURSING FACILITY					
99301	D hx/exam SF/LC DM	64.11	58.68	55.75	64.11
99302	D hx C exam MC/HC DM	90.55	82.88	78.74	90.55
99303	C hx/exam MC/HC DM	136.76	125.18	118.92	136.76
Subsequent (new/est pt)					
99311	PF hx/exam SF/LC DM	37.95	34.74	33.00	37.95
99312	EPF hx/exam MC DM	55.11	50.44	47.92	55.11
99313	D hx/exam MC/HC DM	69.61	63.72	60.53	69.61
DOMICILIARY, REST HOME, CUSTODIAL CARE					
New Patient					
99321	PF hx/exam SF/LC DM	46.10	42.20	40.09	46.10
99322	EPF hx/exam MC DM	65.02	59.52	56.54	65.02
99323	D hx/exam HC DM	86.18	78.88	74.94	86.18
Established Patient					
99331	PF hx/exam SF/LC DM	37.31	34.15	32.44	37.31
99332	EPF hx/exam MC DM	49.22	45.05	42.80	49.22
99333	D hx/exam HC DM	60.61	55.47	52.70	60.61
HOME SERVICES					
New Patient					
99341	PF hx/exam SF DM	70.32	64.37	61.15	70.32
99342	EPF hx/exam LC DM	91.85	84.07	79.87	91.85
99343	D hx/exam MC DM	120.24	110.06	104.56	120.24
Established Patient					
99347	PF hx/exam SF DM	54.83	50.19	47.68	54.83
99348	EPF hx/exam LC DM	70.06	64.13	60.92	70.06
99349	D hx/exam MC DM	88.33	80.85	76.81	88.33
PROLONGED SERVICES WITH CONTACT					
Outpatient					
99354	First 30–74 minutes	96.97	88.76	84.32	96.97
99355	Each additional 30 minutes	96.97	88.76	84.32	96.97
Inpatient					
99356	First hour	96.42	88.25	83.84	96.42
99357	Each additional 30 minutes	96.42	88.25	83.84	96.42
PROLONGED SERVICES WITHOUT DIRECT CONTACT					
99358	First hour	90.00			
99359	Each additional 30 minutes	90.00			

*Some services and procedures may not be considered a benefit under the Medicare program, and when listed on a claim form, no reimbursement may be received. For this reason, some of the services shown in this mock fee schedule do not have any amounts listed under the three Medicare columns.

Table continued on following page

Table B–1 College Clinic—Mock Fee Schedule *(Continued)*

Code No. and Description		Mock Fee	Medicare*		
			Participating	Non-participating	Limiting Charge
PHYSICIAN STANDBY SERVICE					
99360	Each 30 min	95.00			
CASE MANAGEMENT SERVICES					
Team Conferences					
99361	30 min	85.00			
99362	60 min	105.00			
Telephone Calls					
99371	Simple or brief	30.00			
99372	Intermediate	40.00			
99373	Complex or lengthy	60.00			
CARE PLAN OVERSIGHT SERVICES					
99375	30 min or more	93.40	85.49	81.22	93.40
PREVENTIVE MEDICINE					
New Patient					
99381	Infant under age 1 year	50.00			
99382	1–4 years	50.00			
99383	5–11 years	45.00			
99384	12–17 years	45.00			
99385	18–39 years	50.00			
99386	40–64 years	50.00			
99387	65 years and over	55.00			
Established Patient					
99391	Infant under age 1 year	35.00			
99392	1–4 years	35.00			
99393	5–11 years	30.00			
99394	12–17 years	30.00			
99395	18–39 years	35.00			
99396	40–64 years	35.00			
99397	65 years and over	40.00			
COUNSELING (new/est pt)					
Individual					
99401	15 min	35.00			
99402	30 min	50.00			
99403	45 min	65.00			
99404	60 min	80.00			
Group					
99411	30 min	30.00			
99412	60 min	50.00			
Other Preventive Medicine Services					
99420	Health hazard appraisal	50.00			
99429	Unlisted preventive med serv	variable			
NEWBORN CARE					
99431	Birthing room delivery hx/exam	102.15	93.50	88.83	102.15
99432	Other than birthing room exam	110.16	100.83	95.79	110.16
99433	Subsequent hospital care	54.02	49.44	46.97	54.02
99440	Newborn resuscitation	255.98	234.30	222.59	255.98

*Some services and procedures may not be considered a benefit under the Medicare program, and when listed on a claim form, no reimbursement may be received. For this reason, some of the services shown in this mock fee schedule do not have any amounts listed under the three Medicare columns.

Table B–1 **College Clinic—Mock Fee Schedule *(Continued)***

Code No. and Description		Mock Fee	Medicare* Participating	Medicare* Non-participating	Medicare* Limiting Charge
ANESTHESIOLOGY					
Anesthesiology fees are presented here for CPT codes. However, each case would require a fee for time, e.g., every 15 minutes would be worth $55. This fee is determined according to the relative value system, calculated, and added into the anesthesia (CPT) fee. Some anesthesiologists may list a surgical code using an anesthesia modifier on a subsequent line for carriers that do not acknowledge anesthesia codes.					
99100	Anes for pt under 1 year/over 70	55.00			
99116	Anes complicated-total hypothermia	275.00			
99135	Anes complicated-hypotension	275.00			
99140	Anes complicated emerg cond	110.00			
Physician Status Modifier Codes					
P-1	Normal healthy patient	00.00			
P-2	Patient with mild systemic disease	00.00			
P-3	Patient with severe systemic disease	55.00			
P-4	Patient with severe systemic disease (constant threat to life)	110.00			
P-5	Moribund pt not expected to survive for 24 hr with or without operation	165.00			
P-6	Declared brain-dead pt, organs being removed for donor	00.00			
Head					
00160	Anes for proc nose & accessory sinuses: NOS	275.00			
00172	Anes; repair cleft palate	165.00			
Thorax					
00400	Anes for proc integumentary system/ extremities, anterior trunk	165.00			
00402	Anes breast reconstruction	275.00			
00546	Anes; pulmonary resection with thoracoplasty	275.00			
00600	Anes cervical spine and cord	550.00			
Lower Abdomen					
00800	Anes for proc lower ant abdominal wall	165.00			
00840	Anes intraperitoneal proc lower abdomen: NOS	330.00			
00842	Amniocentesis	220.00			
00914	Anes; TURP	275.00			
00942	Anes; colporrhaphy, colpotomy/vaginectomy	220.00			
Upper Leg					
01210	Anes open proc hip joint; NOS	330.00			
01214	Total hip replacement	440.00			
Upper Arm and Elbow					
01740	Anes open proc humerus/elbow; NOS	220.00			
01758	Exc cyst/tumor humerus	275.00			
Radiologic Procedures					
01922	Anes CAT scan/radiation therapy	385.00			
Miscellaneous Procedure(s)					
01999	Unlisted anes proc	variable			

*Some services and procedures may not be considered a benefit under the Medicare program, and when listed on a claim form, no reimbursement may be received. For this reason, some of the services shown in this mock fee schedule do not have any amounts listed under the three Medicare columns.

Table continued on following page

Table B–1 **College Clinic—Mock Fee Schedule *(Continued)***

Code No. and Description		Mock Fee	Medicare Participating	Medicare Non-participating	Medicare Limiting Charge	Follow-up Days†
SURGERY SECTION						
10060*	I & D abscess furuncle, paronychia; single	75.92	69.49	66.02	75.92	10
11040*	Debridement; skin, partial thickness	79.32	75.60	68.97	79.32	10
11044	Debridement; skin, subcu, muscle, bone	269.28	246.48	234.16	269.28	10
11100	Biopsy of skin, SC tissue &/or mucous membrane; 1 lesion	65.43	59.89	56.90	65.43	10
11200*	Removal skin tags; up to 15	55.68	50.97	48.42	55.68	10
11401	Exc, benign lesion, 0.6–1.0 cm trunk, arms, legs	95.62	87.53	83.15	96.62	10
11402	1.1–2.0 cm	121.52	111.23	105.67	121.52	10
11403	2.1–3.0 cm	151.82	138.97	132.02	151.82	10
11420	Exc, benign lesion, 0.5 cm or less scalp, neck, hands, feet, genitalia	75.44	69.05	65.60	75.44	10
11422	1.1–2.0 cm	131.35	120.23	114.22	131.35	10
11441	Exc, benign lesion face, ears, eyelids, nose, lips, or mucous membrane; 0.6–1.0 cm dia or less	119.08	109.00	103.55	119.08	10
11602	Exc, malignant lesion, trunk, arms, or legs; 1.1–2.0 cm dia	195.06	178.55	169.62	195.06	10
11719	Trimming of nondystrophic nails, any number	30.58	27.82	26.33	30.58	0
11720	Debridement of nails, any method, 1–5	32.58	29.82	28.33	32.58	0
11721	6 or more	32.58	29.82	28.33	32.58	0
11730*	Avulsion nail plate, partial or complete, simple repair; single	76.91	70.40	66.88	76.91	0
11750	Exc, nail or nail matrix, partial or complete	193.45	177.07	168.22	193.45	10
11765	Wedge excision of nail fold	57.95	53.04	50.39	57.95	10
12001*	Simple repair (scalp, neck, axillae, ext genitalia, trunk, or extremities incl hands & feet); 2.5 cm or less	91.17	83.45	79.28	91.17	10
12011*	Simple repair (face, ears, eyelids, nose, lips, or mucous membranes); 2.5 cm or less	101.44	92.85	88.21	101.44	10
12013*	2.6–5.0 cm	123.98	113.48	107.81	123.98	10
12032*	Repair, scalp, axillae, trunk (intermediate)	169.73	155.36	147.59	169.73	10
12034	7.6–12.5 cm	214.20	196.06	186.26	214.20	10
12051*	Layer closure of wounds (face, ears, eyelids, nose, lips, or mucous membranes); 2.5 cm	167.60	153.41	145.74	167.60	10
17000*	Destruction, any method, 1 lesion	52.56	48.11	45.70	52.56	10
17003	Second through fourteen lesions, each	15.21	17.77	16.88	15.21	10
17110*	Destruction flat warts, molluscum contagiosum, up to 14	47.37	43.36	41.19	47.37	10
19020	Mastotomy, drainage/exploration deep abscess	237.36	217.26	206.40	237.36	90
19100*	Biopsy, breast, needle	96.17	88.03	83.63	96.17	0
19101	Open, incisional	281.51	257.67	244.79	281.51	10
20610*	Arthrocentesis, aspiration or injection joint (should, hip, knee) or bursa	52.33	47.89	45.50	52.33	0
21330	Nasal fracture, open treatment complicated	599.46	548.71	521.27	599.46	90
21555	Excision tumor, soft tissue (neck/thorax); subcutaneous	280.06	256.35	243.53	280.06	90
21556	deep, subfascial, intramuscular	463.39	424.16	402.95	463.39	90
24066	Biopsy, deep, soft tissue, upper arm, elbow	383.34	350.88	333.34	383.34	90
26720	Closed treatment prolonged shaft fx, proximal/midphalanx, finger/thumb without manipulation	134.50	123.12	116.96	134.50	90
27130	Arthroplasty (total hip replacement)	2266.32	2074.43	1970.71	2266.32	90
27455	Osteotomy, proximal tibia	1248.03	1142.36	1085.24	1248.03	90
27500	Closed treatment femoral shaft fracture without manipulation	554.90	507.92	482.52	554.90	90

†Data for the surgical follow-up days from *St. Anthony's Medicare Correct Coding and Payment Manual for Procedures and Services*, Reston, VA, 2001.

Table B–1 **College Clinic—Mock Fee Schedule *(Continued)***

Code No. and Description		Mock Fee	Medicare Participating	Medicare Non-participating	Medicare Limiting Charge	Medicare Follow-up Days†
27530	Closed treatment tibial fracture, proximal, without manipulation	344.24	315.09	299.34	344.24	90
27750	Closed treatment tibial shaft fracture without manipulation	400.94	366.99	348.64	400.94	90
27752	With manipulation	531.63	486.62	462.29	531.63	90
29280	Strapping of hand/finger	35.13	31.36	29.79	35.13	0
29345	Appl long leg cast (thigh to toes)	123.23	112.80	107.16	123.23	0
29355	Walker or ambulatory type	133.75	122.42	116.30	133.75	0
29425	Appl short leg walking cast	102.10	93.45	88.78	102.10	0
30110	Excision, simple nasal polyp	145.21	132.92	126.27	145.21	10
30520	Septoplasty	660.88	604.93	574.68	660.88	90
30903*	Control nasal hemorrhage; anterior, complex	118.17	108.17	102.76	118.17	0
30905*	Control nasal hemorrhage, posterior with posterior nasal packs; initial	190.57	174.43	165.71	190.57	0
30906*	Subsequent	173.01	158.36	150.44	173.01	0
31540	Laryngoscopy with excision of tumor and/or stripping of vocal cords	488.95	447.55	425.17	488.95	0
31541	With operating microscope	428.33	392.06	372.46	428.33	0
31575	Laryngoscopy, flexible fiberoptic; diagnostic	138.48	126.76	120.42	138.48	0
31625	Bronchoscopy; with biopsy	312.87	286.38	272.06	312.87	0
32310	Pleurectomy, parietal	1234.79	1130.24	1073.73	1234.79	90
32440	Pneumonectomy, total	1972.10	1805.13	1714.87	1972.10	90
33020	Pericardiotomy	1289.25	1180.09	1121.09	1289.25	90
33206	Insertion (or replacement) of pacemaker; atrial	728.42	666.75	633.41	728.42	90
33208	atrial and ventricular	751.57	687.89	653.50	751.57	90
35301	Thromboendarterectomy, with or without patch graft; carotid, vertebral, subclavian, by neck incision	1585.02	1450.82	1378.28	1585.02	90
36005	Intravenous injection for extremity venography	59.18	54.17	51.46	59.18	0
36248	Catheter placement (selective) arterial system, 2nd, 3rd and beyond	68.54	62.74	59.60	68.54	0
36415*	Routine venipuncture for collection of specimen(s)	10.00	—	—	—	XXX
38101	Splenectomy, partial	994.44	910.24	864.73	994.44	90
38510	Biopsy/excision deep cervical node/s	327.42	299.69	284.71	327.42	90
39520	Repair, diaphragmatic hernia; transthoracic	1436.50	1314.87	1249.13	1436.50	90
42820	T & A under age 12 years	341.63	312.71	297.07	341.63	90
42821	over age 12 years	410.73	375.96	357.16	410.73	90
43234	Upper GI endoscopy, simple primary exam	201.86	184.77	175.53	201.86	0
43235	Upper GI endoscopy incl esophagus, stomach, duodenum, or jejunum; diagnostic	238.92	218.69	207.76	238.92	0
43456	Dilation esophagus (balloon/dilator) retrograde	254.52	232.97	221.32	254.52	0
43820	Gastrojejunostomy	971.86	889.58	845.10	971.86	90
44150	Colectomy, total, abdominal	1757.81	1608.98	1528.53	1757.81	90
44320	Colostomy or skin level cecostomy	966.25	884.44	840.22	966.25	90
44950	Appendectomy	568.36	520.24	494.23	568.36	90
45308	Proctosigmoidoscopy for removal of polyp	135.34	123.88	117.69	135.34	0
45315	Multiple polyps	185.12	169.44	160.97	185.12	0
45330	Sigmoidoscopy, diagnostic (for biopsy or collection of specimen by brushing or washing)	95.92	87.80	83.41	95.92	0
45380	Colonoscopy with biopsy (single/multiple)	382.35	349.98	332.48	382.35	0

†Data for the surgical follow-up days from *St. Anthony's Medicare Correct Coding and Payment Manual for Procedures and Services*, Reston, VA, 2001.

Table continued on following page

Table B–1 **College Clinic—Mock Fee Schedule *(Continued)***

Code No. and Description		Mock Fee	Medicare			
			Participating	Non-participating	Limiting Charge	Follow-up Days†
46255	Hemorrhoidectomy int & ext, simple	503.57	460.94	437.89	503.57	90
46258	Hemorrhoidectomy with fistulectomy	636.02	582.17	553.06	636.02	90
46600	Anoscopy; diagnostic	32.86	30.07	28.57	32.86	0
46614	With control of hemorrhage	182.10	166.68	158.35	182.10	0
46700	Anoplastic, for stricture, adult	657.39	601.73	571.64	657.39	90
47600	Cholecystectomy	937.74	858.35	815.43	937.74	90
49505	Inguinal hernia repair, age 5 or over	551.07	504.41	479.19	551.07	90
49520	Repair, inguinal hernia, any age; recurrent	671.89	615.00	584.25	671.89	90
50080	Nephrostolithotomy, percutaneous	1323.93	1211.83	1151.24	1323.93	90
50780	Ureteroneocystostomy	1561.23	1429.84	1357.59	1561.23	90
51900	Closure of vesicovaginal fistula, abdominal approach	1196.82	1095.48	1040.71	1196.82	90
52000	Cystourethroscopy	167.05	152.90	145.26	167.05	0
52601	Transurethral resection of prostate	1193.53	1092.47	1037.85	1193.53	90
53040	Drainage of deep periurethral abscess	379.48	347.35	329.98	379.48	90
53230	Excision, female diverticulum (urethral)	859.69	786.91	747.56	859.69	90
53240	Marsupialization of urethral diverticulum, M or F	520.11	476.07	452.27	520.11	90
53620*	Dilation, urethra, male	100.73	92.20	87.59	100.73	0
53660*	Dilation urethra, female	48.32	44.23	42.02	48.32	0
54150	Circumcision-newborn (clamp/other device)	111.78	102.32	97.20	111.78	10
54520	Orchiectomy, simple	523.92	479.56	455.58	523.92	90
55700	Biopsy of prostate, needle or punch	156.22	142.99	135.84	156.22	0
55801	Prostatectomy, perineal subtotal	1466.56	1342.39	1275.27	1466.56	90
57250	Posterior colporrhaphy, repair of rectocele	616.86	564.63	536.40	616.86	90
57260	Combined anteroposterior colporrhaphy	864.85	791.62	752.04	864.85	90
57265	With enterocele repair	902.24	825.85	784.56	902.24	90
57452*	Colposcopy	84.18	77.05	73.20	84.18	0
57510	Cauterization of cervix, electro or thermal	115.15	105.40	100.13	115.15	10
57520	Conization of cervix with or without D & C, with or without fulguration; cold knife/laser	387.08	354.30	336.59	387.08	90
58100*	Endometrial biopsy	71.88	65.79	62.50	71.88	0
58120	D & C, diagnostic and/or therapeutic (nonOB)	272.83	249.73	237.24	272.83	10
58150	TAH w/without salpingo-oophorectomy	1167.72	1068.85	1015.41	1167.72	90
58200	Total hysterectomy, including partial vaginectomy, lymph node sampling	1707.24	1562.69	1484.56	1707.24	90
58210	Radical abdominal hysterectomy with bilateral pelvic lymphadenectomy	2160.78	1977.83	1878.94	2160.78	90
58300*	Insertion of intrauterine device	100.00				0
58340*	Hysterosalpingography, inj procedure	73.06	66.87	63.53	73.06	0
58400	Uterine suspension	594.47	544.14	516.93	594.47	90
58720	Salpingo-oophorectomy, complete or partial, unilateral or bilateral	732.40	670.39	636.87	732.40	90
	Surgical treatment of ectopic pregnancy					
59120	Salpingectomy and/or oophorectomy for ectopic pregnancy (abdominal/vaginal)	789.26	722.43	686.31	789.26	90
59121	Without salpingectomy and/or oophorectomy	638.84	584.75	555.51	638.84	90
59130	Abdominal pregnancy	699.12	639.93	607.93	699.12	90
59135	Interstitial, uterine pregnancy	1154.16	1056.44	1003.62	1154.16	90
59136	Partial uterine resection, interstitial uterine pregnancy	772.69	707.26	671.90	772.69	90
59140	Cervical, with evacuation	489.68	448.22	425.81	489.68	90

†Data for the surgical follow-up days from *St. Anthony's Medicare Correct Coding and Payment Manual for Procedures and Services,* Reston, VA, 2001.

Table B–1 **College Clinic—Mock Fee Schedule *(Continued)***

Code No.	Description	Mock Fee	Medicare Participating	Medicare Non-participating	Medicare Limiting Charge	Medicare Follow-up Days†
59160	Curettage postpartum	293.46	268.61	255.18	293.46	10
59400	OB care—routine, incl antepartum/vag delvy postpartum care	1864.30	1706.45	1621.13	1864.30	N/A
59510	C-section including antepartum and postpartum care	2102.33	1924.33	1828.11	2102.33	N/A
59515	C-section incl postpartum care	1469.80	1345.36	1278.09	1469.80	N/A
59812	Treatment of incompl abortion, any trimester; completed surgically	357.39	327.13	310.77	357.39	90
61314	Craniotomy; extradural/subdural	2548.09	2332.35	2215.73	2548.09	90
62270*	Spinal puncture, lumbar; diagnostic	77.52	70.96	67.41	77.52	0
65091	Excision of eye, without implant	708.22	648.25	615.84	708.22	90
65205*	Removal of foreign body, ext eye	56.02	51.27	48.71	56.02	0
65222*	Corneal, with slit lamp	73.81	67.56	64.18	73.81	0
69420*	Myringotomy	97.76	89.48	85.01	97.76	10
RADIOLOGY, NUCLEAR MEDICINE, AND DIAGNOSTIC ULTRASOUND						
70120	X-ray mastoids, 1–2 views per side	38.96	35.66	33.88	38.96	
70130	X-ray mastoids, 3 views per side	56.07	51.33	48.76	56.07	
71010	X-ray chest, 1 view	31.95	29.24	27.78	31.95	
71020	Chest x-ray, 2 views	40.97	37.50	35.63	40.97	
71030	Chest x-ray, compl, 4 views	54.02	49.44	46.97	54.02	
71060	Bronchogram, bilateral	143.75	131.58	125.00	143.75	
72100	X-ray spine, LS; 2–3 views	43.23	39.57	37.59	43.23	
72114	Complete, incl bending views	74.97	68.62	65.19	74.97	
73070	X-ray elbow, 2 views	32.58	29.82	28.33	32.58	
73080	Complete, min 3 views	35.87	32.83	31.19	35.87	
73100	X-ray wrist, 2 views	31.61	28.94	27.49	31.61	
73110	Complete, min 3 views	34.26	31.36	27.79	34.26	
73500	X-ray hip, 1 view (unilateral)	31.56	28.88	27.44	31.56	
73510	Complete, min 2 views	38.33	35.08	33.33	38.33	
73540	X-ray pelvis & hips, infant or child, 2 views	37.94	34.73	32.99	37.94	
73590	X-ray tibia & fibula, 2 views	33.35	30.53	29.00	33.35	
73620	Radiologic exam, foot; 2 views	31.61	28.94	27.49	31.61	
73650	X-ray calcaneus, 2 views	30.71	28.11	26.70	30.71	
74241	Radiologic exam, upper gastrointestinal tract, with/without delayed films with KUB	108.93	99.71	94.72	108.93	
74245	Small intestine	161.70	148.01	140.61	161.70	
74270	Barium enema	118.47	108.44	103.02	118.47	
74290	Cholecystography, contrast, oral	52.59	48.14	45.73	52.59	
74400	Urography (pyelography), intravenous, with or without KUB	104.78	95.90	91.11	104.78	
74410	Urography, infusion	116.76	106.87	101.53	116.76	
74420	Urography, retrograde	138.89	127.13	120.77	138.89	
75982	Percutaneous placement of drainage catheter	359.08	328.67	312.24	359.08	
76090	Mammography, unilateral	62.57	57.27	54.41	62.57	
76091	Bilateral	82.83	75.82	72.03	82.83	
76805	Ultrasound, pregnant uterus, B-scan or real time; complete fetal/maternal eval.	154.18	141.13	134.07	154.18	
76810	Ultrasound, pregnant uterus, complete: multiple gestation, after first trimester	306.54	280.59	266.56	306.54	
76946	Ultrasonic guidance for amniocentesis	91.22	83.49	79.32	91.22	

†Data for the surgical follow-up days from *St. Anthony's Medicare Correct Coding and Payment Manual for Procedures and Services,* Reston, VA, 2001.

Table continued on following page

Table C–1 College Clinic—Mock Fee Schedule *(Continued)*

Code No. and Description		Mock Fee	Medicare		
			Participating	Non-participating	Limiting Charge
77300	Radiation dosimetry calculation	97.58	89.32	84.85	97.58
78104	Bone marrow imaging; whole body	230.56	211.04	200.49	230.56
78215	Liver and spleen imaging	160.44	146.85	139.51	160.44
78800	Tumor localization, limited area	191.53	175.32	166.55	191.53
PATHOLOGY AND LABORATORY‡					
Organ or Disease-Oriented Panels					
80048	Basic metabolic panel	15.00	14.60	13.87	16.64
80050	General health panel	20.00	19.20	15.99	21.87
80051	Electrolyte panel	20.00	19.20	15.99	21.87
80053	Comprehensive metabolic panel	25.00	20.99	19.94	23.93
80055	Obstetric panel	25.00	20.99	19.94	23.93
80069	Renal function panel	30.00	28.60	25.97	32.16
80074	Acute hepatitis panel	30.00	28.60	25.97	32.16
80076	Hepatic function panel	30.00	28.60	25.97	32.16
80090	TORCH antibody panel	32.00	30.70	27.54	34.15
Urinalysis					
81000	Urinalysis, nonautomated, with microscopy	8.00	7.44	5.98	8.84
81001	Urinalysis, automated, with microscopy	8.00	7.44	5.98	8.84
81002	Urinalysis, nonautomated without microscopy	8.00	7.44	5.98	8.84
81015	Urinalysis, microscopy only	8.00	7.44	5.98	8.84
Chemistry					
82270	Blood, occult; feces screening 1–3	4.05	3.56	3.31	4.05
82565	Creatinine; blood	10.00	9.80	8.88	12.03
82947	Glucose; quantitative	15.00			
82951	Glucose tol test (GTT) 3 spec	40.00	41.00	36.80	45.16
82952	Each add spec beyond 3	30.00	28.60	25.97	32.16
83020	Hemoglobin, electrophoresis	25.00	20.00	19.94	23.93
83715	Lipoprotein, blood; electrophoretic separation	25.00	20.00	19.94	23.93
84478	Triglycerides, blood	20.00	19.20	15.99	21.87
84479	Thyroid hormone (T-3/T-4)	20.00	19.20	15.99	21.87
84520	Urea nitrogen, blood (BUN); quantitative	25.00	20.99	19.94	23.93
84550	Uric acid, blood	20.00	19.20	15.99	21.87
84702	Gonadotropin, chorionic; quantitative	20.00	19.20	15.99	21.87
84703	Qualitative	20.00	19.20	15.99	21.87
Hematology					
85022	Hemogram, automated manual differential WBC count (CBC)	20.00	19.20	15.99	21.87
85025	Hemogram, platelet count, automated, differential WBC count (CBC)	25.00	20.00	19.94	23.93
85031	Complete blood count, manual (hemogram)	25.00	20.00	19.94	23.93
85097	Bone marrow, smear interpretation	73.52	67.29	63.93	73.52
85345	Coagulation time; Lee & White	20.00	19.20	15.99	21.87
85590	Platelet count; manual count	20.00	19.20	15.99	21.87
Immunology					
86038	Antinuclear antibodies (ANA)	25.00	20.00	19.94	23.93
86490	Skin test; coccidioidomycosis	13.14	12.03	11.43	13.14
86580	TB, intradermal	11.34	10.38	9.86	11.34
Microbiology					
87081	Culture, screening only	25.00	20.00	19.94	23.93

‡Mock fees for laboratory tests presented in this schedule may not be representative of fees in your region due to the variety of capitation and managed care contracts as well as discount policies made by laboratories.

Table C–1 College Clinic—Mock Fee Schedule *(Continued)*

Code No.	Description	Mock Fee	Medicare Participating	Medicare Non-participating	Medicare Limiting Charge
87181	Sensitivity studies, antiobiotic; per (antibiotic) agent	20.00	19.20	15.99	21.87
87184	Disk method, per plate (12 disks or less)	20.00	19.20	15.99	21.87
87210	Smear, primary source; wet mount with simple stain, for bacteria, fungi, ova, and/or parasites	35.00	48.35	45.93	55.12
Cytopathology					
88150	Papanicolaou cytopath	35.00	48.35	45.93	55.12
Surgical Pathology					
88302	Surgical pathology, Level II gross & micro exam (skin, fingers, nerve, testis)	24.14	22.09	20.99	24.14
88305	Surgical pathology Level IV (bone marrow)	77.69	71.12	67.56	77.69
MEDICINE					
Immunization Injections					
90701	Diphtheria, tetanus, pertussis	34.00			
90703	Tetanus toxoid	28.00			
90712	Poliovirus vaccine, oral	28.00			
Therapeutic Injections					
90782	IM or SC medication, therapeutic, prophylactic, diagnostic	4.77	4.37	4.15	4.77
90784	IV	21.33	19.53	18.55	21.33
90788	IM antibiotic	5.22	4.78	4.54	5.22
Psychiatry					
90816	Individual psychotherapy 20–30 min	60.25	55.15	52.39	60.25
90853	Group therapy	29.22	26.75	25.41	29.22
Hemodialysis					
90935	Single phys evaluation	117.23	107.31	101.94	117.23
90937	Repeat evaluation	206.24	188.78	179.34	206.24
Gastroenterology					
91000	Esophageal intubation	69.82	63.91	60.71	69.82
91055	Gastric intubation	87.41	80.01	76.01	87.41
Ophthalmologic Services					
92004	Comprehensive eye exam	90.86	83.17	79.01	90.86
92100	Tonometry	47.31	43.31	41.14	47.31
92230	Fluorescein angioscopy	55.49	50.79	48.25	55.49
92275	Electroretinography	81.17	74.29	70.58	81.17
92531	Spontaneous nystagmus	26.00			
Audiologic Function Tests					
92557	Basic comprehensive audiometry	54.33	49.73	47.24	54.33
92596	Ear measurements	26.81	24.54	23.31	26.81
Cardiovascular Therapeutic Services					
93000	Electrocardiogram (ECG)	34.26	31.36	29.79	34.26
93015	Treadmill ECG	140.71	128.80	122.36	140.71
93040	Rhythm ECG, 1–3 leads	18.47	16.90	16.06	18.47
93230	ECG monitoring 24 hr	217.99	199.54	189.56	217.99
Pulmonary					
94010	Spirometry	38.57	35.31	33.54	38.57
94060	Spirometry before and after bronchodilator	71.67	65.60	62.32	71.67
94150	Vital capacity, total	13.82	12.65	12.02	13.82
Allergy and Clinical Immunology					
95004	Percutaneous tests with allergy extracts	4.31	3.95	3.75	4.31
95024	Intradermal tests	6.58	6.02	5.72	6.58
95044	Patch/application tests	8.83	8.08	7.68	8.83

Table continued on following page

Table C–1 College Clinic—Mock Fee Schedule *(Continued)*

Code No. and Description		Mock Fee	Medicare Participating	Medicare Non-participating	Medicare Limiting Charge
95115	Treatment for allergy, corticosteroids, single inj	17.20	15.75	14.96	17.20
95117	Two or more inj	22.17	20.29	19.28	22.17
95165	Allergen immunotherapy, single or multiple antigens (specify no. of doses)	7.11	6.50	6.18	7.11
Neurology					
95812	Electroencephalogram up to 1 hr	129.32	118.37	112.45	129.32
95819	Electroencephalogram—awake and asleep	126.81	116.07	110.27	126.81
95860	Electromyography, 1 extremity	88.83	81.31	77.24	88.83
95864	Electromyography, 4 extremities	239.99	219.67	208.69	239.99
Physical Medicine					
97024	Diathermy	14.27	13.06	12.41	14.27
97036	Hubbard tank, each 15 min	24.77	22.67	21.54	24.77
97110	Physical therapy, initial 30 min	23.89	21.86	20.77	23.89
Special Services and Reports					
99000	Handling of specimen (transfer from Dr.'s office to lab)	5.00			
99025	Initial surg eval (new pt) with starred procedure	50.00			
99050	Services requested after office hours in addition to basic service	25.00			
99052	Services between 10 p.m. and 8 a.m. in addition to basic service	35.00			
99054	Services on Sundays and holidays in addition to basic service	35.00			
99058	Office services provided on an emergency basis	65.00			
99070	Supplies and materials (itemize drugs and materials provided)	25.00			
99080	Special reports:				
	Insurance forms	10.00			
	Review of data to clarify pt's status	20.00			
	WC reports	50.00			
	WC extensive review report	250.00			

Appendix

C

CPT Modifiers, Medicare's National HCPCS Level II Modifiers and Codes

Fee Schedule—For simplicity, the mock fee of $15 is assigned to all HCPCS Level II codes and should be used when completing Billing Break exercises that require the use of these codes.

Following is a complete list of CPT modifiers and a partial alpha/numeric list of the Health Care Financing Administration's Common Procedure Coding System national Level II Modifiers and codes referred to as HCPCS (pronounced hick-picks). This system was developed by Medicare to code services/procedures not listed in the American Medical Association's *Current Procedure Terminology (CPT)* code book and is used in some states by Medicaid, TRICARE, and many private carriers.

Table C–1 **CPT Modifiers**

Modifier	Description
-21	Prolonged Evaluation and Management Services—greater than usually required for highest level E/M
-22	Unusual Procedures—greater than usually required
-23	Unusual Anesthesia—requiring general anesthesia when usually not necessary
-24	Unrelated E/M Service during Post Operative Period by Same Physician
-25	Significant, Separately Identifiable E/M Service by (1) Same Physician, on (2) Same Day of the Procedure/Service—above and beyond other service requiring unrelated diagnostic statement
-26	Professional Component—when physician portion reported separately
-32	Mandated Services—e.g., by third party payer
-47	Anesthesia by Surgeon—regional or general
-50	Bilateral Procedure—unless described by CPT code description
-51	Multiple Procedure—other than E/M service (same day, same provider—except "add on" codes)
-52	Reduced Services
-53	Discontinued Procedure—because of a threat to the well being of the patient (after administration of anesthesia)
-54	Surgical Care Only—no preoperative and/or postoperative care given
-55	Postoperative Management Only—another surgeon performs surgery
-56	Preoperative Management Only—another surgeon performs surgery
-57	Decision for Surgery—append to E/M service for *initial* decision
-58	Stage/Related Procedure/Service by Same Physician during Postoperative Period—either (1) planned at the time of the original procedure/service, (2) more extensive than the original procedure/service, or (3) for therapy following diagnostic surgical procedure
-59	Distinct Procedure/Service—or independent from other procedure/service and not normally reported together, such as (1) different session/encounter, (2) different procedure/surgery, (3) different site/organ system, (4) separate lesion, (5) separate injury
-62	Two Surgeons—work together as primary surgeons
-66	Surgical Team—for highly complex procedures
-76	Repeat Procedure by Same Physician
-77	Repeat Procedure by Another Physician
-78	Return to Operating Room for Related Procedure during Postoperative Period
-79	Unrelated Service/Procedure by Same Physician during Postoperative Period
-80	Assistant Surgeon
-81	Minimum Assistant Surgeon
-82	Assistant Surgeon—when qualified resident surgeon not available—use in teaching institution
-90	Reference Laboratory—laboratory service provided *outside* of the physician's office, performed by party other than treating physician, and billed by treating physician
-91	Repeat Clinical Diagnostic Laboratory Test—on same day
-99	Multiple Modifiers—use when two or more modifiers apply to one code

Table C–2 HCPCS Level II Modifiers

Modifier	Description
-AA	Anesthesia service personally furnished by anesthesiologists*
-AD	Medical supervision by a physician; more than four concurrent anesthesia procedures*
-AH	Clinical psychologist
-AJ	Clinical social worker
-AM	Physician, team member service
-AS	Physician assistant, nurse practitioner, or clinical nurse specialist services for assistant at surgery
-AT	Acute treatment (this modifier should be used when reporting chiropractic service 98940, 98941, 98942)
-BP	The beneficiary has been informed of the purchase and rental options and has elected to purchase the item
-BR	The beneficiary has been informed of the purchase and rental options and has elected to rent the item
-BU	The beneficiary has been informed of the purchase and rental options and after 30 days has not informed the supplier of his/her decision
-CC	Procedure code change. Use modifier when the procedure code submitted was changed either for administrative reasons or when an incorrect code was filed
-EP	Service provided as part of Medicaid Early Periodic Screening Diagnosis and Treatment (EPSDT) program
-E1	Upper left, eyelid
-E2	Lower left, eyelid
-E3	Upper right, eyelid
-E4	Lower right, eyelid
-FA	Left hand, thumb
-FP	Service provided as part of Medicaid family planning program
-F1	Left hand, second digit
-F2	Left hand, third digit
-F3	Left hand, fourth digit
-F4	Left hand, fifth digit
-F5	Right hand, thumb
-F6	Right hand, second digit
-F7	Right hand, third digit
-F8	Right hand, fourth digit
-F9	Right hand, fifth digit
-GA	Waiver of liability statement on file
-GY	Item or service excluded or does not meet the definition of any Medicare benefit
-GZ	Item or service expected to be denied as not reasonable and necessary
-LC	Left circumflex coronary artery
-LD	Left anterior descending coronary artery
-LT	Left side. Used to identify procedures performed on the left side of the body. This modifier has no direct effect on payment
-NU	New equipment
-QB	Physician providing service in a rural HPSA. The -QB and -QU modifiers describe covered Medicare services performed by a physician within the geographic boundaries of a rural or urban health professional shortage area (HPSA)
-QK	Medical direction of two, three, or four concurrent anesthesia procedures involving qualified individuals
-QL	Patient pronounced dead after ambulance called
-QM	Ambulance service provided under arrangement by hospital
-QN	Ambulance service furnished directly by a provider of services
-QR	Repeat laboratory test performed on the same day
-QS	Monitored anesthesia care service
-QT	Recording and storage on tape by an analog tape recorder
-QX	CRNA service: With medical direction by a physician
-QY	Medical direction of one certified registered nurse anesthetist (CRNA) by an anesthesiologist
-QZ	CRNA service: Without medical direction by a physician
-Q5	Service furnished by a substitute physician under a reciprocal billing arrangement
-Q6	Service furnished by a locum tenens physician
-RC	Right coronary artery

*This modifier affects the fee schedule amount received.

Table continued on following page

Table C–2 HCPCS Level II Modifiers *(Continued)*

Modifier	Description
-RR	Rental. Use this modifier when durable medical equipment is to be rented
-RT	Right side. Used to identify procedures performed on the right side of the body. This modifier has no direct effect on payment
-SF	Second opinion ordered by a professional review organization (PRO). 100% reimbursement; no Medicare deductible or coinsurance
-SG	Ambulatory surgical center facility service
-TA	Left foot, great toe
-TC	Technical component: Under certain circumstances a charge may be made for the technical component alone. Under those circumstances the technical component charge is identified by adding modifier -TC to the usual procedure number. Technical component charges are institutional charges and not billed separately by physicians. However, portable x-ray suppliers only bill for the technical component and should use modifier -TC. The charge data from portable x-ray suppliers will then be used to build customary and prevailing profiles
-T1	Left foot, second digit
-T2	Left foot, third digit
-T3	Left foot, fourth digit
-T4	Left foot, fifth digit
-T5	Right foot, great toe
-T6	Right foot, second digit
-T7	Right foot, third digit
-T8	Right foot, fourth digit
-T9	Right foot, fifth digit
-UE	Used durable medical equipment.

Table C–3 **HCPCS Level II Codes Alpha Index**

Description	Code
A	
acetazolamide sodium (Diamox sodium), injection	J1120
adrenaline, injection	J0170
Adriamycin, injection (doxorubicin HCl)	J9000
air ambulance	A0030
air bubble detector, dialysis	E1530
air travel and nonemergency transport	A0140
alarm, pressure dialysis	E1540
alcohol	A4244
alcohol wipes	A4245
alternating pressure pad/mattress	E0180
amitriptyline HCl (Elavil)	J1320
ammonia test paper	A4774
ampicillin sodium injection	J0290
amputee wheelchair, detachable elevating leg rests	E1170
amygdalin, injection	J3570
anesthetics for dialysis	A4735
apnea monitor	E0608
appliance, pneumatic	E0655
arms, adjustable, wheelchair	E0973
atropine sulfate, injection	J0460
B	
bacterial sensitivity study	P7001
bandage, elastic	A4460
battery, wheelchair,	A4631
bed rail; full length	E0315
bed pan	E0276
belt, extremity	E0945
belt, ostomy	A4367
belt, pelvic	E0944
bench, bathtub	E0245
benztropine, injection	J0515
bicarbonate dialysate	A4705
bilirubin (phototherapy) light	E0202
blood pressure monitor	A4670
blood pump, dialysis	E1620
blood strips	A4253
blood testing supplies	A4770
bond or cement, ostomy skin	A4364
C	
cane	E0100
catheter caps, disposable (dialysis)	A4860
catheter insertion tray	A4354
catheter irrigation set	A4355
cellular therapy	M0075
cement, ostomy	A4364
cephalin flocculation, blood	P2028
cervical head harness/halter	E0942
cervical pillow	E0943
chair, adjustable, dialysis	E1570
chelation therapy, IV (chemical endarterectomy)	M0300
chin cup, cervical	L0150
chorionic gonadotropin, injection	J0725
commode seat, wheelchair	E0968
compressor, pneumatic	E0650
conductive paste or gel	A4558
Congo red blood	P2029
contraceptive; cervical cap	A4261
crutches, underarm, wood, pair	E0112
culture sensitivity study	P7001
D	
decubitus care, protector, heel/elbow	E0191
deionizer, water purification system	E1615
Depo-Estradiol, injection	1000
Dextran	J7100
dextrose/normal saline, solution	J7042
Dextrostix	A4772
dialyzers	A4690
diazepam (Valium), injection	J3360
digoxin, injection	J1160
dimenhydrinate (Dramamine), injection	J1240
diphenhydramine HCl (Benadryl), injection	J1200
disarticulation, elbow, prostheses	L6200
drainage bag	A4358
drainage board	E0606
E	
elbow protector	E0191
electrodes, per pair	A4556
elevating leg rest, wheelchair	K0195
endarterectomy, chemical	M0300
epinephrine, injection	J0170
estrone, injection	J1435
etoposide, 50 mg, injection	J9181
external ambulatory infusion pump with adm equip	E0781
extremity belt-harness	E0945
F	
faceplate, ostomy	A4361
fentanyl citrate, injection	J3010
fern test	Q0114
fistula cannulation set	A4730
floxuridine, 500 mg, injection	J9200
fluid barriers, dialysis	E1575
fluorouracil, injection	J9190
foam pad adhesive	A5126
forearm crutches	E0110
furosemide (Lasix), injection	J1940
G	
Garamycin, injection	J1580
gauze bandages (gauze elastic)	A6263
gel, conductive	A4558
gel pressure pad for mattress	E0185
gentamicin, injection	J1580

Table continued on following page

Table C–2 **HCPCS Level II Codes Alpha Index *(Continued)***

Description	Code
gloves, dialysis	A4927
glucose test strips	A4772
Gomco drain bottle	A4912
Grade-Aid, wheelchair	E0974
gravity traction device	E0941
Gravlee jet washer	A4470
H	
hair analysis	P2031
hallux-valgus dynamic splint	L3100
haloperidol (Haldol), injection	J1630
halter, cervical head	E0942
harness, extremity	E0945
harness, pelvic	E0944
harness/halter, cervical head	E0942
heater for nebulizer	E1372
heel or elbow protector	E0191
heel stabilizer	L3170
helicopter ambulance	A0431
hemipelvectomy prostheses	L5280
hemodialysis kit	A4820
hemostats	A4850
Hemostix	A4773
heparin infusion pump, dialysis	E1520
Hexcelite, cast material	A4590
hot water bottle	E0220
hydrocortisone acetate, up to 25 mg, injection	J1700
hydrocortisone phosphate, injection	J1710
I	
ice cap or collar	E0230
infusion pump, external ambulatory with adm equip	E0781
infusion pump, heparin, dialysis	E1520
insulin, injection	J1820
intercapsular thoracic endoskeletal prostheses	L6570
intraocular lenses, anterior chamber	V2630
intraocular lenses, iris supported	V2631
intraocular lenses, posterior chamber	V2632
iodine swabs/wipes	A4247
iron dextran (Imferon), injection	J1750
IV pole	E0776
J	
jacket, body	L0500
Jewett, spinal orthosis (hyperextension)	L0370
K	
Kartop patient list, toilet or bathroom	E0625
kit, CAPD supply	A4900
kit, CCPD supply	A4901
kit, surgical dressing (tray)	A4550
Knee-O-Prene™ Hinged Kneesleve (orthosis)	L1810
L	
Laetrile, amygdalin (vitamin B_{17}), injection	J3570
lancets	A4259
lead wires	A4557
leg extension, walker	E1058
leg rest, wheelchair, elevating	E0990
leukocyte-poor blood, each unit	P9016
lidocaine (Xylocaine), injection	J2000
lubricant, ostomy	A4402
lumbar flexion	L0540
M	
measuring cylinder, dialysis	A4921
medroxyprogesterone acetate (Depo-Provera), injection	J1050
meter, bath conductivity, dialysis	E1550
methadone HCl, injection	J1230
microbiology tests	P7001
mini-bus, nonemergency transportation	A0120
monitor, apnea	E0608
monitor, blood pressure	A4670
mucoprotein, blood	P2038
N	
narrowing device, wheelchair	E0969
nasal vaccine inhalation	J3530
nebulizer, portable	E0570
needle with syringe	A4206
neonatal transport, ambulance, base rate	A0225
neuromuscular stimulator	E0745
nonprescription drugs	A9150
O	
occipital/mandibular support, cervical	L0160
occupational therapy (hospital)	G0129
occupational therapy (home)	S9129
orthotic additions (halo)	L0860
orthotic device, thoracic	L0210
P	
pacemaker monitor, includes audible/visible check systems	E0610
pacemaker monitor, includes digital/visible check systems	E0615
pad for water circulating heat unit	E0249
pail or pan for use with commode chair	E0167
paste, conductive	A4558
pelvic belt/harness/boot	E0944
penicillin G banzathine (Bicillin), injection	J0540
penicillin G potassium (Pfizerpen), injection	J2540
penicillin procaine, aqueous, injection	J2510
peroxide	A4244
personal comfort items	A9190
pessary; rubber	A4561
pHisoHex solution	A4246

Table C–2 HCPCS Level II Codes Alpha Index *(Continued)*

Description	Code
phototherapy, light	E0202
pillow, cervical	E0943
plasma, protein fraction, each unit	P9018
plasma, single donor, fresh frozen, each unit	P9017
platelet-rich plasma, each unit	P9020
platform attachment; wheelchair	E0154
portable hemodialyzer system	E1635
portable nebulizer	E1375
prolotherapy	M0076
prosthesis, breast, silicone	L8030
prosthesis, eye (ocular)	L8610
prosthesis, hemifacial (maxillofacial)	K0444
prosthesis, larynx	L8500
prosthesis, nasal (maxillofacial)	K0440
prosthesis, upper facial (maxillofacial)	K0443
protector, heel or elbow	E0191
Q	
Quad cane	E0105
R	
rack/stand, oxygen	E1355
reciprocating peritoneal dialysis system	E1630
red blood cells, each unit	P9021
regulator, oxygen	E1353
replacement tanks, dialysis	A4880
restraints, any type	E0710
rib belt, elastic	A4572
Ringer's, lactate infusion	J7120
rings, ostomy	A4404
S	
safety equipment	E0700
scale or scissors, dialysis	A4910
seat attachment, walker	E0156
seat insert, wheelchair	E0992
sensitivity study	P7001
serum clotting time tube	A4771
shunt accessories, for dialysis	A4740
sitz bath, portable	E0160
skin barrier, ostomy	A4362
skind bond or cement, ostomy	A4364
sling, patient lift	E0621
slings	A4565
splint	A4570
splint; foot drop	L4398
surgical stockings, above-knee length	A4490
surgical supplies, miscellaneous	A4649
surgical trays	A4550
swabs, Betadine or iodine	A4247
syringe	A4213
syringes, dialysis	A4655
T	
tape, all types, all sizes	A4454
taxi, nonemergency transportation	A0100
tent, oxygen	E0455
tetanus immune globulin (Homo-Tet), injection	J1670
tetracycline, injection	J0120
toilet seat, raised	E0244
tool kit, dialysis	A4910
tourniquet, dialysis	A4910
tracheotomy collar or mask	A4621
traction equipment, overdoor	E0860
trays, surgical	A4550
U	
ultraviolet cabinet	E0690
unclassified drugs (contraceptives)	J3490
urinary leg bag, latex (incontinence supply)	A5112
urine sensitivity study	P7001
V	
vaporizer	E0605
vascular catheters	A4300
venous pressure clamps, dialysis	A4918
venipuncture, routine	G0001
ventilator, volume	E0450
vest, safety, wheelchair	E0980
vitamin B_{12}, injection, cyanocobalamin	J3420
vitamin K, injection	J3430
W	
walker, wheeled, without seat	E0141
water, distilled (for nebulizer)	A7018
water softening system, ESRD	E1625
water tanks, dialysis	A4880
wrist disarticulation prosthesis	L6050
X	
X caliber power wheelchair	K0014

Appendix D

HCFA-1500* Claim Form Block by Block Instructions and Insurance Templates

The following instructions are straightforward and contain all pertinent information needed to complete the HCFA-1500 claim form using Optical Character Recognition (OCR) guidelines for private carriers, Medicaid, Medicare (Medicare/Medicaid, Medicare/Medigap, Medicare Secondary Payer), TRICARE, CHAMPVA, and workers' compensation programs. However, much information on specific coverage guidelines, program policies, and practice specialties could not be included here. Because claim form completion guidelines vary at the state and local levels, consult your local intermediary or private carrier for detailed instruction.

Block numbers match those on the Health Insurance Claim Form. First, locate the block number you would like instruction for. Second, use the insurance icon and color-coded section to quickly locate the type of insurance program you are billing for. Last, read the specific guidelines for block requirements. Italicized sections refer students to guidelines in completing Billing Break assignments when there are optional ways of completing a block.

When generating paper claims via computer, many software programs insert the insurance carrier's name and address in the top right corner of the HCFA-1500 claim form. When typing a claim form or producing one using the Student Software Challenge on the enclosed CD-ROM, it is suggested that this same procedure be followed. All Billing Break exercises may be completed using the Student Software Challenge. Just click on *"Other Patients"* in the file folder, make up a file for the Billing Break exercise using the patient's name, complete the form, and print the completed assignment.

Following is a list of the most common insurance programs encountered in a medical practice illustrated in claim form templates, each identified by an icon. Screened areas on each form do not apply to the insurance program example illustrated and should be left blank.

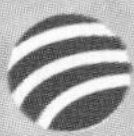
All Payers: All payer guidelines include all private insurance companies and all federal and state programs.

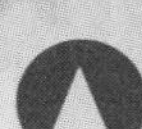
All Private Payers: All private insurance companies (see Fig. D–3).

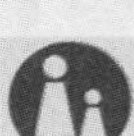
Medicaid: State Medicaid programs (see Fig. D–5).

Medicare: Federal Medicare programs, Medicare/Medicaid, Medicare/Medigap, and Medicare Secondary Payer (MSP) (see Figs. D–6 to D–9).

TRICARE: TRICARE Standard (formerly CHAMPUS), TRICARE Prime, TRICARE Extra (see Fig. D–10).

CHAMPVA: Civilian Health and Medical Program of the Department of Veterans' Affairs (see Fig. D–11).

Workers' Compensation: State workers' compensation programs (see Fig. D–12).

*Now known as CMS-1500.

Top of Form

Enter name and address of insurance company in the top right corner of the insurance form using all capital letters and no punctuation. This format is being used to demonstrate that the student knows where to direct the claim even though some carriers (e.g., Medicare) do not follow this guideline.

APPROVED OMB-0938-008

PLEASE DO NOT STAPLE IN THIS AREA

PRUDENTIAL INSURANCE COMPANY
5540 WILSHIRE BOULEVARD
WOODLAND HILLS XY 12345 0000

CARRIER

PICA — HEALTH INSURANCE CLAIM FORM — PICA

1. MEDICARE	MEDICAID	CHAMPUS	CHAMPVA	GROUP Health Plan	FECA BLK LUNG	OTHER	1a. INSURED I.D. NUMBER	(FOR PROGRAM IN ITEM 1)
☐ (Medicare #)	☐ (Medicaid #)	☐ (Sponsor's SSN)	☐ (VA File #)	X (SSN or ID)	☐ (SSN)	☐ (ID)	111704521	A482

2. PATIENT'S NAME (Last Name, First Name, Middle Initial)	3. PATIENT'S BIRTH DATE MM DD YYYY	SEX	4. INSURED'S NAME (LAST NAME, FIRST NAME, MIDDLE INITIAL)
FOREHAND HARRY N	01 06 1946	M X F ☐	SAME

Block 1

APPROVED OMB-0938-008

PLEASE DO NOT STAPLE IN THIS AREA

PRUDENTIAL INSURANCE COMPANY
5540 WILSHIRE BOULEVARD
WOODLAND HILLS XY 12345 0000

CARRIER

PICA — HEALTH INSURANCE CLAIM FORM — PICA

1. MEDICARE	MEDICAID	CHAMPUS	CHAMPVA	GROUP Health Plan	FECA BLK LUNG	OTHER	1a. INSURED I.D. NUMBER	(FOR PROGRAM IN ITEM 1)
☐ (Medicare #)	☐ (Medicaid #)	☐ (Sponsor's SSN)	☐ (VA File #)	X (SSN or ID)	☐ (SSN)	☐ (ID)	111704521	A482

2. PATIENT'S NAME (Last Name, First Name, Middle Initial)	3. PATIENT'S BIRTH DATE MM DD YYYY	SEX	4. INSURED'S NAME (LAST NAME, FIRST NAME, MIDDLE INITIAL)
FOREHAND HARRY N	01 06 1946	M X F ☐	SAME

All Private Payers:
Individual Health Plan: Check "Other" for an individual who is covered under an individual policy.
Group Health Plan: Check this box for those covered under any group contract insurance (e.g., insurance obtained through employment); also for patients who receive services paid by managed care programs (e.g., HMOs, PPOs, IPAs).

- *When completing Billing Break assignments, if the insured is employed, assume the insurance is through the employer and is "group" insurance; otherwise, assume it is an individual policy and enter "other."*

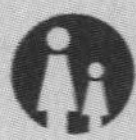

Medicaid: Check for person receiving Medicaid benefits.

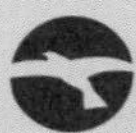

Medicare: Check for patient who receives Medicare benefits.

Medicare/Medicaid: Check "Medicare" and "Medicaid" if the patient is covered under Medicare and Medicaid programs.

Medicare/Medigap: Check "Medicare" and, if the patient has group or individual Medigap coverage, check "Group" or "Other," depending on health plan.

- *When completing Billing Break assignments, if the insured is employed, assume the insurance is through the employer and is "group" insurance; otherwise, assume it is an individual policy and enter "other."*

MSP: Check "Group" or "Other" (depending on health plan) and "Medicare" when a Medicare patient has insurance primary to Medicare coverage.

TRICARE: Check "CHAMPUS" for individual receiving TRICARE benefits.

CHAMPVA: Check "CHAMPVA" for individual receiving CHAMPVA benefits.

Workers' Compensation: Check "Other" for all workers' compensation claims except FECA Black Lung. Check "FECA Black Lung" for patients who receive black lung benefits under the Federal Employee Compensation Act.

Block 1a

APPROVED OMB-0938-008

PLEASE DO NOT STAPLE IN THIS AREA

PRUDENTIAL INSURANCE COMPANY
5540 WILSHIRE BOULEVARD
WOODLAND HILLS XY 12345 0000

CARRIER

PICA **HEALTH INSURANCE CLAIM FORM** PICA

1. MEDICARE	MEDICAID	CHAMPUS	CHAMPVA	GROUP Health Plan	FECA BLK LUNG	OTHER	1a. INSURED I.D. NUMBER	(FOR PROGRAM IN ITEM 1)
☐ (Medicare #)	☐ (Medicaid #)	☐ (Sponsor's SSN)	☐ (VA File #)	☒ (SSN or ID)	☐ (SSN)	☐ (ID)	111704521	A482

2. PATIENT'S NAME (Last Name, First Name, Middle Initial)	3. PATIENT'S BIRTH DATE MM DD YYYY	SEX	4. INSURED'S NAME (LAST NAME, FIRST NAME, MIDDLE INITIAL)
FOREHAND HARRY N	01 06 1946	M ☒ F ☐	SAME

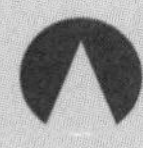

All Private Payers: Enter the patient's policy (identification or certificate) number in the left portion of the block and the group number, if applicable, in the right portion of the block as it appears on the insurance card, without punctuation.

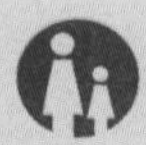

Medicaid: Enter the Medicaid number in the left portion of the block. Do not enter dashes or other special characters in this block.

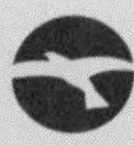

Medicare: Enter the patient's Medicare Health Insurance Claim (HIC) number from the patient's Medicare card in the left portion of this block, regardless of whether Medicare is the primary or secondary payer.
Medicare/Medicaid: Enter the patient's Medicare number in the left portion of this block.
Medicare/Medigap: Enter the patient's Medicare number in the left portion of this block.
MSP: Enter the patient's Medicare number in the left portion of this block. Refer to Block 11 for primary insurance.

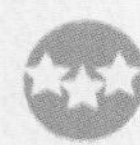

TRICARE: First enter sponsor's Social Security number (SSN) in the left portion of this block. Then, if the patient is a NATO beneficiary, add "NATO" or, if sponsor is a security agent, add "SECURITY." Do not provide the patient's SSN unless the patient and sponsor are the same.

CHAMPVA: Enter the Veterans Affairs file number (omit prefix or suffix) or sponsor's Social Security number in the left portion of this block. Do not use any other former service numbers.

Workers' Compensation: Enter the claim number. If none is assigned, enter the employer's policy number or patient's Social Security number.

Block 2

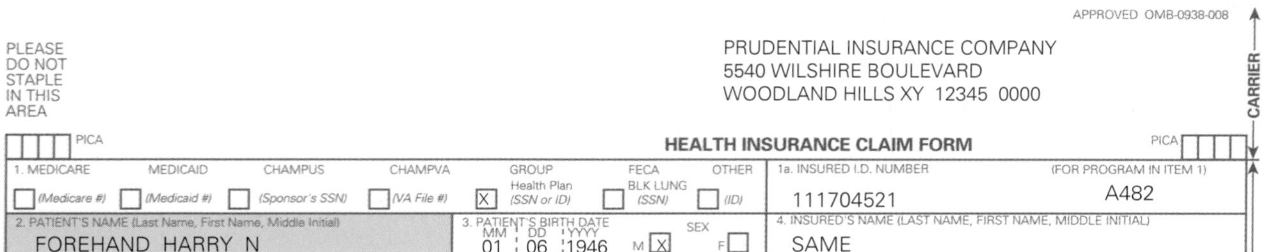
APPROVED OMB-0938-008

PLEASE DO NOT STAPLE IN THIS AREA

PRUDENTIAL INSURANCE COMPANY
5540 WILSHIRE BOULEVARD
WOODLAND HILLS XY 12345 0000

CARRIER

PICA HEALTH INSURANCE CLAIM FORM PICA

1. MEDICARE	MEDICAID	CHAMPUS	CHAMPVA	GROUP Health Plan	FECA BLK LUNG	OTHER	1a. INSURED I.D. NUMBER	(FOR PROGRAM IN ITEM 1)
☐ (Medicare #)	☐ (Medicaid #)	☐ (Sponsor's SSN)	☐ (VA File #)	☒ (SSN or ID)	☐ (SSN)	☐ (ID)	111704521	A482

2. PATIENT'S NAME (Last Name, First Name, Middle Initial)	3. PATIENT'S BIRTH DATE MM DD YYYY	SEX	4. INSURED'S NAME (LAST NAME, FIRST NAME, MIDDLE INITIAL)
FOREHAND HARRY N	01 06 1946	M ☒ F ☐	SAME

All Payers: Enter the last name, first name, and middle initial of the patient—in that order—as shown on the patient's identification card, even if it is misspelled. Do not use nicknames or abbreviations. Do not use commas. If a name is hyphenated, a hyphen may be used (see Example D–1).

Example D–1

Hyphenated name: Smith-White = SMITH-WHITE
Prefixed name: MacIverson = MACIVERSON
Seniority name with numeric suffix: John R. Ellis, III = ELLIS III JOHN R

Block 3

APPROVED OMB-0938-008

PLEASE DO NOT STAPLE IN THIS AREA

PRUDENTIAL INSURANCE COMPANY
5540 WILSHIRE BOULEVARD
WOODLAND HILLS XY 12345 0000

CARRIER

PICA HEALTH INSURANCE CLAIM FORM PICA

1. MEDICARE	MEDICAID	CHAMPUS	CHAMPVA	GROUP Health Plan	FECA BLK LUNG	OTHER	1a. INSURED I.D. NUMBER	(FOR PROGRAM IN ITEM 1)
☐ (Medicare #)	☐ (Medicaid #)	☐ (Sponsor's SSN)	☐ (VA File #)	☒ (SSN or ID)	☐ (SSN)	☐ (ID)	111704521	A482

2. PATIENT'S NAME (Last Name, First Name, Middle Initial)	3. PATIENT'S BIRTH DATE MM DD YYYY	SEX	4. INSURED'S NAME (LAST NAME, FIRST NAME, MIDDLE INITIAL)
FOREHAND HARRY N	01 06 1946	M ☒ F ☐	SAME

All Payers: Enter the patient's birth date using eight digits (01272000). The patient's age must be as follows to correlate with the diagnosis in Block 21:

- Birth: Newborn diagnosis
- Birth to 17 years: Pediatric diagnosis
- 12 to 55 years: Maternity diagnosis
- 15 to 124 years: Adult diagnosis

Check the appropriate box for the patient's sex. If left blank, gender block defaults to "female."

Block 4

APPROVED OMB-0938-008

PLEASE DO NOT STAPLE IN THIS AREA

PRUDENTIAL INSURANCE COMPANY
5540 WILSHIRE BOULEVARD
WOODLAND HILLS XY 12345 0000

CARRIER

PICA — HEALTH INSURANCE CLAIM FORM — PICA

1. MEDICARE / MEDICAID / CHAMPUS / CHAMPVA / GROUP / FECA / OTHER	1a. INSURED I.D. NUMBER (FOR PROGRAM IN ITEM 1)
☐ (Medicare #) ☐ (Medicaid #) ☐ (Sponsor's SSN) ☐ (VA File #) ☒ GROUP Health Plan (SSN or ID) ☐ FECA BLK LUNG (SSN) ☐ (ID)	111704521 A482
2. PATIENT'S NAME (Last Name, First Name, Middle Initial): FOREHAND HARRY N	3. PATIENT'S BIRTH DATE MM DD YYYY: 01 06 1946; SEX M ☒ F ☐
4. INSURED'S NAME (LAST NAME, FIRST NAME, MIDDLE INITIAL): SAME	

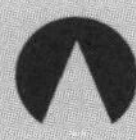

All Private Payers: Enter "SAME" when the insured is also the patient. If the insured is not the patient, enter the name of the insured (last name first).

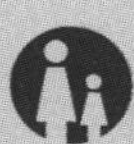

Medicaid: Refer to Medicare guidelines.

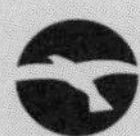

Medicare: Leave blank if the insured is also the patient. Enter the insured's name, if different from the patient's.
Medicare/Medicaid: Refer to Medicare guidelines.
Medicare/Medigap: Refer to Medicare guidelines.
MSP: Enter the name of the insured (last name first).

TRICARE: Enter the sponsor's last name, first name, and middle initial, not a nickname or abbreviation. Do not complete if "self" is checked in Block 6.

CHAMPVA: Enter the veteran's name, last name first.

Workers' Compensation: Enter the employer's name. If the employer is a large corporation, enter the name of the insured corporation in Block 4 and the local employer in Block 11b (e.g., Elsevier Science is the insured corporation [4] and W. B. Saunders is the employer and would be typed in Block 11b).

Block 5

5. PATIENT'S ADDRESS (No., Street)		6. PATIENT RELATIONSHIP TO INSURED	7. INSURED'S ADDRESS (No, Street)	
1456 MAIN STREET		Self ☒ Spouse ☐ Child ☐ Other ☐		
CITY: WOODLAND HILLS	STATE: XY	8. PATIENT STATUS: Single ☐ Married ☒ Other ☐	CITY	STATE
ZIP CODE: 12345 0000	TELEPHONE (Include Area Code): (555) 490 9876	Employed ☒ Full-Time Student ☐ Part-Time Student ☐	ZIP CODE	TELEPHONE (INCLUDE AREA CODE) ( )

FORMATION

All Private Payers: Enter the patient's mailing address and residential telephone number.

Medicaid: Enter the patient's mailing address and residential telephone number.

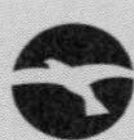

Medicare: Enter the patient's mailing address and residential telephone number. On the first line, enter the street address; on the second line, the city and two-character state code (e.g., AZ = Arizona); on the third line, enter the ZIP code and residential telephone number. Punctuation is not necessary (e.g., ST LOUIS, no period after ST).
Medicare/Medicaid: Enter the patient's mailing address and residential telephone number.
Medicare/Medigap: Enter the patient's mailing address and residential telephone number.
MSP: Enter the patient's mailing address and residential telephone number.

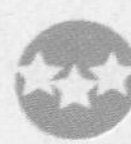

TRICARE: Enter the patient's mailing address and residential telephone number. Do not enter a post office box number; provide the actual place of residence. If a rural address, the address must contain the route and box number. An APO/FPO address should not be used unless that person is residing overseas.

CHAMPVA: Enter the patient's mailing address and residential telephone number. Do not enter a post office box number; provide the actual place of residence. If a rural address, the address must contain the route and box number. An APO/FPO address should not be used unless that person is residing overseas.

Workers' Compensation: Enter the patient's mailing address and residential telephone number.

Block 6

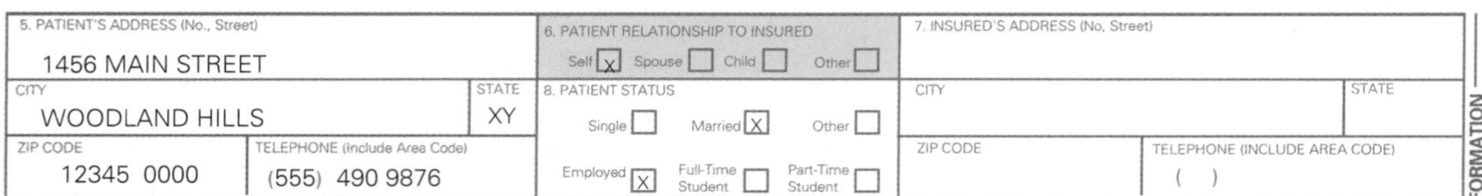

5. PATIENT'S ADDRESS (No., Street)
1456 MAIN STREET
CITY: WOODLAND HILLS — STATE: XY
ZIP CODE: 12345 0000 — TELEPHONE (Include Area Code): (555) 490 9876

6. PATIENT RELATIONSHIP TO INSURED
Self [X] Spouse [ ] Child [ ] Other [ ]

8. PATIENT STATUS
Single [ ] Married [X] Other [ ]
Employed [X] Full-Time Student [ ] Part-Time Student [ ]

7. INSURED'S ADDRESS (No. Street)
CITY — STATE
ZIP CODE — TELEPHONE (INCLUDE AREA CODE) ( )

FORMATION

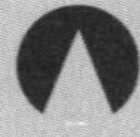

All Private Payers: Check the patient's relationship to the insured. If the patient is an unmarried "domestic partner," check "Other."

Medicaid: Leave blank. Check appropriate box only if there is third party coverage.

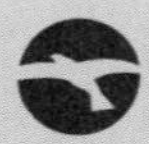

Medicare: Indicate relationship to insured when Block 4 is completed; otherwise, leave blank.
Medicare/Medicaid: Refer to Medicare guidelines.
Medicare/Medigap: Refer to Medicare guidelines.
MSP: Indicate relationship to insured.

TRICARE: Check the patient's relationship to the sponsor. If patient is the sponsor, check "self" (e.g., retiree). If the patient is a child or stepchild, check the box for child. If "other" is checked, indicate how the patient is related to the sponsor in Block 19 or on an attachment (e.g., former spouse).

CHAMPVA: Indicate the patient's relationship to the sponsor. If patient is the sponsor, check "self." If the patient is a child or stepchild, check the box for child. If "other" is checked, indicate how the patient is related to the sponsor in Block 19 or on an attachment (e.g., former spouse).

Workers' Compensation: Check "Other."

Block 7

5. PATIENT'S ADDRESS (No., Street)		6. PATIENT RELATIONSHIP TO INSURED	7. INSURED'S ADDRESS (No, Street)	
1456 MAIN STREET		Self [X] Spouse [ ] Child [ ] Other [ ]		
CITY WOODLAND HILLS	STATE XY	8. PATIENT STATUS Single [ ] Married [X] Other [ ]	CITY	STATE
ZIP CODE 12345 0000	TELEPHONE (Include Area Code) (555) 490 9876	Employed [X] Full-Time Student [ ] Part-Time Student [ ]	ZIP CODE	TELEPHONE (INCLUDE AREA CODE) ( )

FORMATION

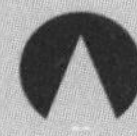

All Private Payers: Leave blank if Block 4 indicates "same." Enter "SAME" if Block 4 is completed and the address is identical to that listed in Block 5. Enter address if different from that listed in Block 5.

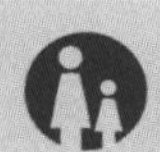

Medicaid: Refer to Medicare guidelines.

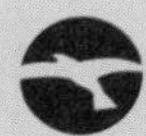

Medicare: Leave blank if Block 4 is blank. Enter "SAME" if Block 4 is completed and the address is identical to that listed in Block 5. Enter address if different from that listed in Block 5.
Medicare/Medicaid: Refer to Medicare guidelines.
Medicare/Medigap: Refer to Medicare guidelines.
MSP: Complete only when Block 4 is completed. If insured is other than the patient, list insured's address and if the address is the same as in Block 5, enter "SAME."

TRICARE: Enter "SAME" if address is the same as that of the patient listed in Block 5. Enter the sponsor's address (e.g., an APO/FPO address or active duty sponsor's duty station or the retiree's mailing address) if different from the patient's address.

CHAMPVA: Enter "SAME" if address is the same as that of the patient. Enter the sponsor's address if different from the patient's address.

Workers' Compensation: Enter the employer's address.

Block 8

5. PATIENT'S ADDRESS (No., Street)		6. PATIENT RELATIONSHIP TO INSURED	7. INSURED'S ADDRESS (No, Street)	
1456 MAIN STREET		Self [X] Spouse [ ] Child [ ] Other [ ]		
CITY	STATE	8. PATIENT STATUS	CITY	STATE
WOODLAND HILLS	XY	Single [ ] Married [X] Other [ ]		
ZIP CODE	TELEPHONE (Include Area Code)		ZIP CODE	TELEPHONE (INCLUDE AREA CODE)
12345 0000	(555) 490 9876	Employed [X] Full-Time Student [ ] Part-Time Student [ ]		( )

FORMATION

All Private Payers: Check the appropriate box for the patient's marital status and whether employed or a student. The "other" box should be checked when a patient is covered under his or her children's health insurance plan or for a domestic partner. For individuals between the ages of 19 and 23, some insurance carriers require documentation from the school verifying full-time student status. This may be obtained as a signed letter from the school or by using a special form supplied by the insurance company.

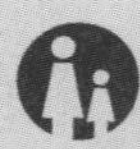

Medicaid: Leave blank.

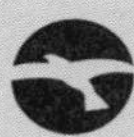

Medicare: Check the appropriate box or boxes for the patient's marital status and whether employed or a student (e.g., a beneficiary may be employed, a student, and married). Check "single" if widowed or divorced. In some locales, this block is not required by Medicare.
Medicare/Medicaid: Check appropriate box for the patient's marital status and whether employed or a student. Check "single" if widowed or divorced.
Medicare/Medigap: Check appropriate box for the patient's marital status and whether employed or a student. Check "single" if widowed or divorced.
MSP: Check appropriate box for the patient's marital status and whether employed or a student. Check "single" if widowed or divorced.

TRICARE: Check the appropriate box for the patient's marital status and whether employed or a student.

CHAMPVA: Check the appropriate box for the patient's marital status and whether employed or a student.

Workers' Compensation: Check "Employed." Some workers' compensation carriers may have requirements for marital status; otherwise, leave blank.

- *When completing the Billing Break assignments, leave marital status blank.*

Block 9

9. OTHER INSURED'S NAME (Last Name, First Name, Middle Initial)	10. IS PATIENT'S CONITION RELATED TO:	11. INSURED'S POLICY GROUP OR FECA NUMBER
a. OTHER INSURED'S POLICY OR GROUP NUMBER	a. EMPLOYMENT? (CURRENT OR PREVIOUS) ☐ YES ☒ NO	a. INSURED'S DATE OF BIRTH MM DD YYYY SEX M☐ F☐
b. OTHER INSURED'S DATE OF BIRTH MM DD YY SEX M☐ F☐	b. AUTO ACCIDENT? ☐ YES ☒ NO PLACE (State)	b. EMPLOYER'S NAME OR SCHOOL NAME
c. EMPLOYER'S NAME OR SCHOOL NAME	c. OTHER ACCIDENT? ☐ YES ☒ NO	c. INSURANCE PLAN NAME OR PROGRAM NAME
d. INSURANCE PLAN NAME OR PROGRAM NAME	10d. RESERVED FOR LOCAL USE	d. IS THERE ANOTHER HEALTH BENEFIT PLAN? ☐ YES ☒ NO *If yes*, return to and complete item 9 a-d

All Private Payers: For submission to primary insurance, leave blank. If patient has secondary insurance, enter patient's full name in last name, first name, and middle initial order.

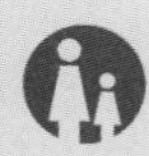

Medicaid: For primary insurance, leave blank. For secondary insurance, enter patient's full name in last name, first name, and middle initial order.

Medicare: For primary insurance, leave blank. Do not list Medicare supplemental coverage (private, not Medigap) on the primary Medicare claim. Beneficiaries are responsible for filing a supplemental claim if the private insurer does not contract with Medicare to send claim information electronically.
Medicare/Medicaid: Enter Medicaid patient's full name in last name, first name, and middle initial order.
Medicare/Medigap: Enter the last name, first name, and middle initial of the Medigap enrollee if it differs from that in Block 2; otherwise, enter "SAME." Only Medicare participating physicians and suppliers should complete Block 9 and its subdivisions, and only when the beneficiary wishes to assign his/her benefits under a Medigap policy to the participating physician or supplier. If no Medigap benefits are assigned, leave blank.
MSP: Leave blank.

TRICARE: For primary insurance, leave blank. For secondary insurance held by someone other than the patient, enter the name of the insured. Blocks 11a–d should be used to report other health insurance held by the patient.

CHAMPVA: For primary insurance, leave blank. For secondary insurance held by someone other than the patient, enter the name of the insured. Blocks 11a–d should be used to report other health insurance held by the patient.

Workers' Compensation: Leave blank. If case is pending and not yet declared workers' compensation, insert other insurance.

Block 9a

All Private Payers: Enter the policy and/or group number of the other (secondary) insured's insurance coverage.

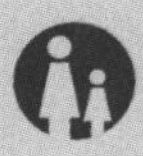

Medicaid: Leave blank.

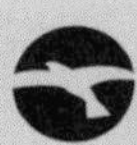

Medicare: Refer to appropriate secondary coverage guidelines.
Medicare/Medicaid: Enter Medicaid policy number here or in Block 10d. However, some states may have different guidelines, so, if in doubt, check with your local fiscal intermediary.
- *When completing Billing Break assignments, enter the Medicaid policy number in Block 10d.*

Medicare/Medigap: Enter the policy and/or group number of the Medigap enrollee preceded by the word "MEDIGAP," "MG," or "MGAP." In addition to Medicare/Medigap, if a patient has a third insurance (i.e., employer-supplemental), all information for the third insurance should be submitted on an attachment.
- *When completing Billing Break assignments, enter the word "MEDIGAP."*

MSP: Leave blank.

TRICARE: Enter the policy or group number of the other (secondary) insurance policy.

CHAMPVA: Enter the policy or group number of the other (secondary) insurance policy.

Workers' Compensation: Leave blank.

Block 9b

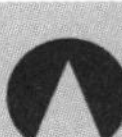

All Private Payers: Enter the other insured's date of birth and gender.

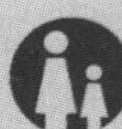

Medicaid: Leave blank.

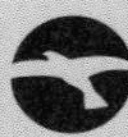

Medicare: Refer to appropriate secondary coverage guidelines.
Medicare/Medicaid: Enter the Medicaid enrollee's birth date, using eight digits (e.g., 03062000), and gender. If same as patient's, leave blank.
Medicare/Medigap: Enter the Medigap enrollee's birth date, using eight digits (e.g., 03062000), and gender. If same as patient's, leave blank.
MSP: Leave blank.

TRICARE: For secondary coverage held by someone other than the patient, enter the other insured's date of birth and check the appropriate box for gender.

CHAMPVA: For secondary coverage held by someone other than the patient, enter the other insured's date of birth and check the appropriate box for gender.

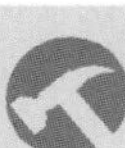

Workers' Compensation: Leave blank.

Block 9c

All Private Payers: For secondary coverage, enter employer's name, if applicable.

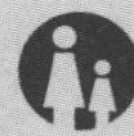

Medicaid: Leave blank.

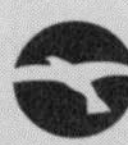

Medicare: Refer to appropriate secondary coverage guidelines.
Medicare/Medicaid: Leave blank.
Medicare/Medigap: Enter the Medigap insurer's claims processing address. Ignore "employer's name or school name." Abbreviate the street address to fit in this block by deleting the city, and using the two-letter state postal code and ZIP code. For example, 1234 Wren Drive, Any City, Pennsylvania 19106 would be typed "1234 WREN DR PA 19106." *Note: If a carrier-assigned unique identifier (sometimes called "Other Carrier Name and Address," or OCNA) for a Medigap insurer appears in Block 9d, then Block 9c may be left blank.*
MSP: Leave blank.

TRICARE: For secondary coverage held by someone other than the patient, enter the name of the other insured's employer or name of school.

CHAMPVA: For secondary coverage held by someone other than the patient, enter the name of the other insured's employer or name of school.

Workers' Compensation: Leave blank.

Block 9d

All Private Payers: Enter name of secondary insurance plan or program.

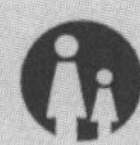

Medicaid: Leave blank.

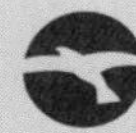

Medicare: Refer to appropriate secondary coverage guidelines.
Medicare/Medicaid: Leave blank.
Medicare/Medigap: Enter the Medigap insurer's nine-digit alphanumeric PAYERID number if known (often called the OCNA key), and Block 9c may be left blank. If not known, enter the name of the Medigap enrollee's insurance company. If you are a participating provider, all of the information in Blocks 9 through 9d must be complete and correct or the Medicare carrier cannot electronically forward the claim information to the Medigap insurer. For multiple insurance information, enter "ATTACHMENT" in Block 10d and provide information on an attached sheet.
MSP: Leave blank.

TRICARE: For secondary coverage held by someone other than the patient, insert name of insured's other health insurance program. On an attached sheet, provide a complete mailing address for all other insurance information and enter the word "ATTACHMENT" in Block 10d. If the patient is covered by a Health Maintenance Organization, attach a copy of the brochure showing that the service is not covered by the HMO.

CHAMPVA: For secondary coverage held by someone other than the patient, insert name of insured's other health insurance program. On an attached sheet, provide a complete mailing address for all other insurance information and enter the word "ATTACHMENT" in Block 10d. If the patient is covered by a Health Maintenance Organization, attach a copy of the brochure showing that the service is not covered by the HMO.

Workers' Compensation: Leave blank.

Block 10a

9. OTHER INSURED'S NAME (Last Name, First Name, Middle Initial)	10. IS PATIENT'S CONITION RELATED TO:	11. INSURED'S POLICY GROUP OR FECA NUMBER
a. OTHER INSURED'S POLICY OR GROUP NUMBER	a. EMPLOYMENT? (CURRENT OR PREVIOUS) ☐ YES ☒ NO	a. INSURED'S DATE OF BIRTH MM | DD | YYYY SEX M ☐ F ☐
b. OTHER INSURED'S DATE OF BIRTH MM | DD | YY SEX M ☐ F ☐	b. AUTO ACCIDENT? PLACE (State) ☐ YES ☒ NO	b. EMPLOYER'S NAME OR SCHOOL NAME
c. EMPLOYER'S NAME OR SCHOOL NAME	c. OTHER ACCIDENT? ☐ YES ☒ NO	c. INSURANCE PLAN NAME OR PROGRAM NAME
d. INSURANCE PLAN NAME OR PROGRAM NAME	10d. RESERVED FOR LOCAL USE	d. IS THERE ANOTHER HEALTH BENEFIT PLAN? ☐ YES ☒ NO *If yes*, return to and complete item 9 a-d

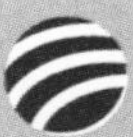

All Payers: Check "yes" or "no" to indicate whether patient's diagnosis described in Block 21 is the result of an accident or injury that occurred on the job or an industrial illness.

Block 10b

All Private Payers: A "yes" checked in Block 10b indicates a third party liability case; file the claim with the other liability insurance or automobile insurance company. List the abbreviation of the state in which the accident took place (e.g., CA for California).

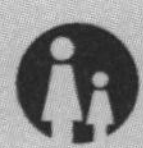

Medicaid: Check appropriate box.

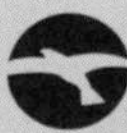

Medicare: Check "no." If "yes," bill the liability insurance as primary insurance and Medicare as secondary insurance.
Medicare/Medicaid: Refer to Medicare guidelines.
Medicare/Medigap: Refer to Medicare guidelines.
MSP: Refer to Medicare guidelines.

TRICARE: Check "yes" or "no" to indicate whether automobile liability applies to one or more of the services described in Block 24. If "yes," provide information concerning potential third party liability. If a third party is involved in the accident, the beneficiary must complete Form DD 2527 (Statement of Personal Injury—Possible Third-Party Liability) and attach it to the claim.

CHAMPVA: Check "yes" or "no" to indicate whether automobile liability applies to one or more of the services described in Block 24. If "yes," provide information concerning potential third party liability.

Workers' Compensation: Check "yes" to indicate an automobile accident that occurred while the patient was on the job.

Block 10c

All Private Payers: Check "yes" or "no" to indicate whether the patient's condition is related to an accident other than automobile or employment. Verify primary insurance.

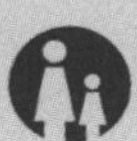

Medicaid: Check if applicable.

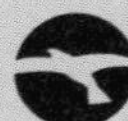

Medicare: Check "yes" or "no" to indicate whether the patient's condition is related to an accident other than automobile or employment. Verify primary insurance.
Medicare/Medicaid: Refer to Medicare guidelines.
Medicare/Medigap: Refer to Medicare guidelines.
MSP: Refer to Medicare guidelines.

TRICARE: Check "yes" or "no" to indicate whether another accident (not work related or automobile) applies to one or more of the services described in Block 24. If so, provide information concerning potential third party liability. If third party is involved in the accident, the beneficiary must complete Form DD 2527 (Statement of Personal Injury—Possible Third-Party Liability) and attach it to the claim.

CHAMPVA: Refer to TRICARE guidelines.

Workers' Compensation: Check "no."

Block 10d

All Private Payers: Leave blank.

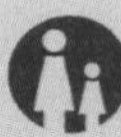

Medicaid: Leave blank. Generally, this block is used exclusively for Medicaid as a secondary payer. In some states the share of cost may be entered (e.g., SOC 5000).

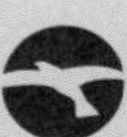

Medicare: Leave blank.
Medicare/Medicaid: Enter the patient's Medicaid (MCD) number preceded by "MCD."
Medicare/Medigap: Leave blank.
MSP: Leave blank.

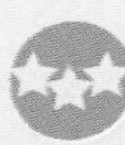

TRICARE: Generally, leave blank unless regional fiscal intermediary gives special guidelines. However, if Block 11d is checked "yes," the mailing address of the insurance carrier must be attached to the claim form, and in this block enter "ATTACHMENT."

- *When completing Billing Break assignments, leave blank.*

CHAMPVA: Generally, leave blank unless regional fiscal intermediary gives special guidelines. If Block 11d is checked "yes," the mailing address of the insurance carrier must be attached to the claim form, and in this block enter "ATTACHMENT."

- *When completing Billing Break assignments, leave blank.*

Workers' Compensation: Leave blank.

Block 11

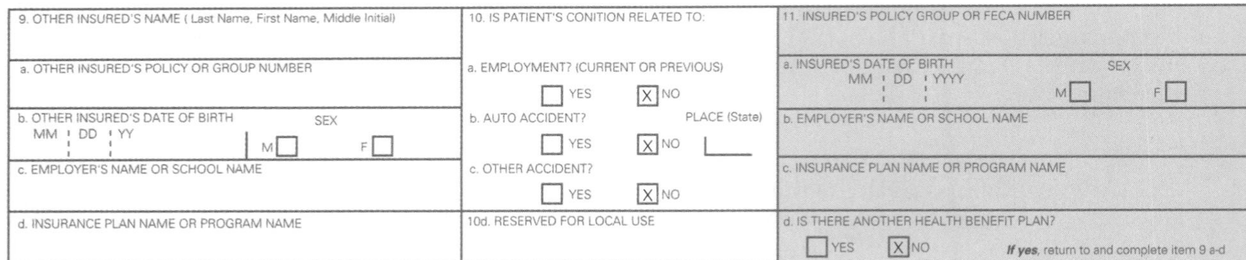

9. OTHER INSURED'S NAME (Last Name, First Name, Middle Initial)	10. IS PATIENT'S CONITION RELATED TO:	11. INSURED'S POLICY GROUP OR FECA NUMBER
a. OTHER INSURED'S POLICY OR GROUP NUMBER	a. EMPLOYMENT? (CURRENT OR PREVIOUS) ☐ YES ☒ NO	a. INSURED'S DATE OF BIRTH MM DD YYYY SEX M ☐ F ☐
b. OTHER INSURED'S DATE OF BIRTH MM DD YY SEX M ☐ F ☐	b. AUTO ACCIDENT? PLACE (State) ☐ YES ☒ NO	b. EMPLOYER'S NAME OR SCHOOL NAME
c. EMPLOYER'S NAME OR SCHOOL NAME	c. OTHER ACCIDENT? ☐ YES ☒ NO	c. INSURANCE PLAN NAME OR PROGRAM NAME
d. INSURANCE PLAN NAME OR PROGRAM NAME	10d. RESERVED FOR LOCAL USE	d. IS THERE ANOTHER HEALTH BENEFIT PLAN? ☐ YES ☒ NO *If yes*, return to and complete item 9 a-d

All Private Payers: Leave Blocks 11 through 11c blank if no private secondary coverage. If (private) secondary insurance, see Blocks 9–9d.

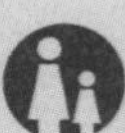

Medicaid: Generally, leave blank. Enter a rejection code if the patient has other third party insurance coverage and the claim was rejected.

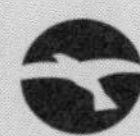

Medicare: If other insurance is not primary to Medicare, enter "NONE" and go to Block 12. Block 11 must be completed. By completing this block, the physician/supplier acknowledges having made a good faith effort to determine whether Medicare is the primary or secondary payer.
Medicare/Medicaid: Refer to Medicare guidelines.
Medicare/Medigap: Refer to Medicare guidelines.
MSP: When insurance is primary to Medicare, enter the insured's policy and/or group number and complete Blocks 11a through 11c.

TRICARE: Leave blank.

CHAMPVA: Enter the three-digit number of the VA station that issued the identification card.

Workers' Compensation: Leave blank.

Block 11a

All Private Payers: Leave blank.

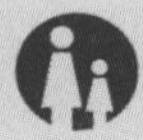

Medicaid: Leave blank.

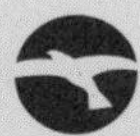

Medicare: Leave blank.
Medicare/Medicaid: Leave blank.
Medicare/Medigap: Leave blank.
MSP: Enter the insured's eight-digit date of birth (06122000) and gender if different from that listed in Block 3; otherwise leave blank.

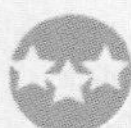

TRICARE: Enter sponsor's date of birth and gender, if different from that listed in Block 3; otherwise leave blank.

CHAMPVA: Enter sponsor's date of birth and gender, if different from that listed in Block 3; otherwise leave blank.

Worker's Compensation: Leave blank.

Block 11b

All Private Payers: When submitting to secondary insurance, enter the name of the employer, school, or organization if primary policy is a group plan; otherwise, leave blank.

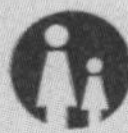

Medicaid: Leave blank.

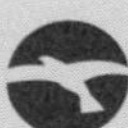

Medicare: Leave blank.
Medicare/Medicaid: Leave blank.
Medicare/Medigap: Leave blank.
MSP: Enter the employer's name of primary insurance. Also use this block to indicate a change in the insured's insurance status (e.g., "RETIRED" and the eight-digit retirement date). Submit paper claims with a copy of the primary payer's Remittance Advice (RA) document to be considered for Medicare Secondary Payer benefits. Instances when Medicare may be secondary include the following:

1. Group health plan coverage
   a. Working aged
   b. Disability (large group health plan)
   c. End-stage renal disease
2. No fault and/or other liability
   a. Automobile
   b. Homeowner
   c. Commercial
3. Work-related illness/injury
   a. Workers' compensation
   b. Black lung
   c. Veterans' benefits

TRICARE: Indicate sponsor's branch of service, using abbreviations (e.g., United States Navy = USN).

CHAMPVA: Indicate sponsor's branch of service, using abbreviations (e.g., United States Army = USA).

Workers' Compensation: If a large corporation's name is listed in Block 4, enter the name of the patient's local employer; otherwise, leave this block blank.

Block 11c

All Private Payers: When submitting to secondary insurance, enter the name of the primary insurance plan; otherwise, leave this block blank.

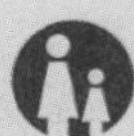

Medicaid: Leave blank.

Medicare: Leave blank.
Medicare/Medicaid: Leave blank.
Medicare/Medigap: Leave blank.
MSP: Enter the complete name of the insurance plan or program that is primary to Medicare. Include the primary payer's claim processing address directly on the EOB.

TRICARE: Enter TRICARE/CHAMPUS.

CHAMPVA: Indicate name of the secondary coverage held by the patient, if applicable; otherwise, leave blank.

Workers' Compensation: Leave blank.

Block 11d

All Private Payers: Check "yes" or "no" to indicate if there is another health plan. If "yes," Blocks 9a through 9d must be completed.

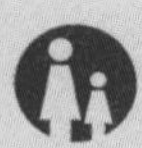

Medicaid: Leave blank.

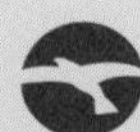

Medicare: Generally leave blank; some regions require "yes" or "no" checked, so verify this requirement with your local fiscal intermediary.
- *When completing Billing Break assignments, leave blank.*

Medicare/Medicaid: Refer to guidelines for Medicare.
Medicare/Medigap: Refer to guidelines for Medicare.
MSP: Leave blank.

TRICARE: Check "yes" or "no" to indicate if there is another health plan. If "yes," Blocks 9a through 9d must be completed.

CHAMPVA: Check "yes" or "no" to indicate if there is another health plan. If "yes," Blocks 9a through 9d must be completed.

Workers' Compensation: Leave blank.

Block 12

READ BACK OF FORM BEFORE COMPLETING & SIGNING THIS FORM.
12. PATIENT'S OR AUTHORIZED PERSON'S SIGNATURE. I authorize the release of any medical or other information necessary to process this claim. I also request payment of government benefits either to myself or to the party who accepts assignment below.
SIGNED ______ March 3 20xx

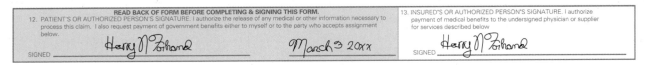

13. INSURED'S OR AUTHORIZED PERSON'S SIGNATURE. I authorize payment of medical benefits to the undersigned physician or supplier for services described below
SIGNED ______

or

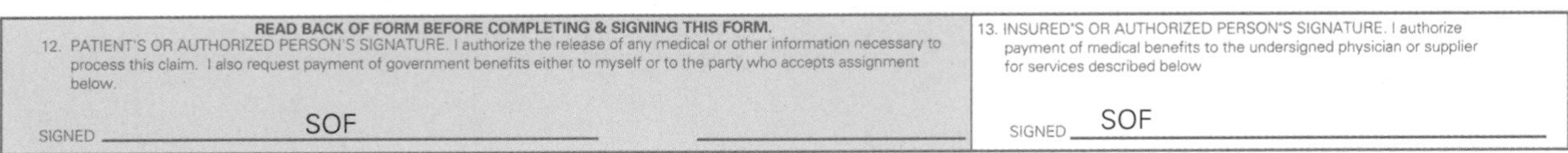
READ BACK OF FORM BEFORE COMPLETING & SIGNING THIS FORM.
12. PATIENT'S OR AUTHORIZED PERSON'S SIGNATURE. I authorize the release of any medical or other information necessary to process this claim. I also request payment of government benefits either to myself or to the party who accepts assignment below.
SIGNED SOF

13. INSURED'S OR AUTHORIZED PERSON'S SIGNATURE. I authorize payment of medical benefits to the undersigned physician or supplier for services described below
SIGNED SOF

All Private Payers: A signature here authorizes the release of medical information for claims processing. Have the patient or the authorized representative sign and date this block. If the patient has signed a consent form, "Signature on File" or "SOF" can be entered here. The consent form must be current, may be lifetime, and must be in the physician's file. When the patient's representative signs, the relationship to the patient must be indicated. If the signature is indicated by a mark (X), a witness must sign his or her name and enter the address next to the mark.
- *When completing Billing Break assignments, enter "SOF" in this block.*

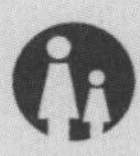

Medicaid: Leave blank.

Medicare: A signature here authorizes payment of benefits to the physician (if the physician accepts assignment) *and* release of medical information for claims processing. Have the patient or the authorized representative sign and date this block. If the patient has signed a consent form, "Signature on File" or "SOF" can be typed here. Be sure the form includes both authorizations just mentioned. The form must be current, may be lifetime, and must be in the physician's file. When the patient's representative signs, the relationship to the patient **must** be indicated. If the signature is by mark (X), a witness must sign his or her name and enter the address next to the mark.
- *When completing Billing Break assignments, enter "SOF" in this block.*

Medicare/Medicaid: Refer to Medicare guidelines.
Medicare/Medigap: Refer to Medicare guidelines.
MSP: Guidelines for this block are the same as for Medicare.

TRICARE: A signature here authorizes payment of benefits to the physician (if the physician accepts assignment) and release of medical information for claims processing. Have the patient or the authorized representative sign and date this block. If the patient has signed a consent form, "Signature on File" or "SOF" can be typed here. Be sure the form includes both authorizations mentioned above. The form must be current, may be lifetime, and must be in the physician's file. When the patient's representative signs, the relationship to the patient **must** be indicated. If the signature is by mark (X), a witness must sign his or her name and enter the address next to the mark.
- *When completing Billing Break assignments, enter "SOF" in this block.*

CHAMPVA: Refer to TRICARE guidelines.

Workers' Compensation: No signature is required.

Block 13

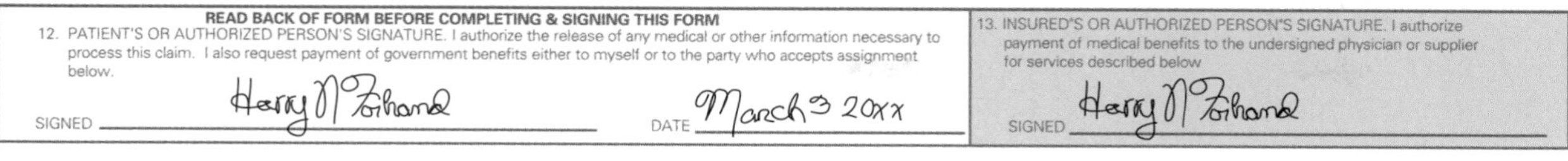

READ BACK OF FORM BEFORE COMPLETING & SIGNING THIS FORM
12. PATIENT'S OR AUTHORIZED PERSON'S SIGNATURE. I authorize the release of any medical or other information necessary to process this claim. I also request payment of government benefits either to myself or to the party who accepts assignment below.
SIGNED Harry M. Forehand DATE March 3 20xx
13. INSURED'S OR AUTHORIZED PERSON'S SIGNATURE. I authorize payment of medical benefits to the undersigned physician or supplier for services described below
SIGNED Harry M. Forehand

or

READ BACK OF FORM BEFORE COMPLETING & SIGNING THIS FORM
12. PATIENT'S OR AUTHORIZED PERSON'S SIGNATURE. I authorize the release of any medical or other information necessary to process this claim. I also request payment of government benefits either to myself or to the party who accepts assignment below.
SIGNED SOF DATE
13. INSURED'S OR AUTHORIZED PERSON'S SIGNATURE. I authorize payment of medical benefits to the undersigned physician or supplier for services described below
SIGNED SOF

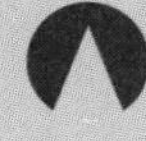

All Private Payers: Patient's signature is required when benefits are assigned. "SOF" may be listed if the patient's signature is on file.
- *When completing Billing Break assignments, enter "SOF" in this block.*

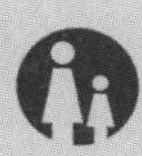

Medicaid: Leave blank.

Medicare: Leave blank.
Medicare/Medicaid: Leave blank.
Medicare/Medigap: For participating provider, a signature here authorizes payment of "mandated" Medigap benefits when required Medigap information is included in Blocks 9 through 9d. List the signature of the patient or authorized representative, or list "SOF" if the signature is on file as a separate Medigap authorization.
- *When completing Billing Break assignments, enter "SOF" in this block.*

MSP: The signature of the patient or authorized representative should appear in this block or list "SOF" if the signature is on file for benefits assigned from the primary carrier.
- *When completing Billing Break assignments, enter "SOF" in this block.*

TRICARE: Leave blank.

CHAMPVA: Leave blank.

Workers' Compensation: Leave blank. All payment goes directly to the physician.

Block 14

14. DATE OF CURRENT: MM DD YY 03 01 20XX — ILLNESS (First symptom) OR INJURY (Accident) OR PREGNANCY	15. IF PATIENT HAS HAD SAME OR SIMILAR ILLNESS GIVE FIRST DATE MM DD YYYY	16. DATES PATIENT UNABLE TO WORK IN CURRENT OCCUPATION MM DD YYYY FROM — TO
17. NAME OF REFERRING PHYSICIAN OR OTHER SOURCE PERRY CARDI MD	17a. I.D. NUMBER OF REFERRING PHYSICIAN 67805027XX	18. HOSPITALIZATION DATES RELATED TO CURRENT SERVICES MM DD YYYY FROM — TO
19. RESERVED FOR LOCAL USE		20. OUTSIDE LAB? YES [X] NO $ CHARGES

All Private Payers: Enter the eight-digit date the patient's first symptoms occurred from the current illness, if stated in the medical record; date of injury or accident; or for pregnancy, first day of last menstrual period. For chiropractic treatment, enter the eight-digit date that treatment began.

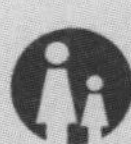

Medicaid: Leave blank.

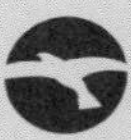

Medicare: Enter the eight-digit date the patient's first symptoms occurred from the current illness, if stated in the medical record; date of injury or accident; or for pregnancy, first day of last menstrual period. For chiropractic treatment, enter the eight-digit date that treatment began.
Medicare/Medicaid: Refer to Medicare guidelines.
Medicare/Medigap: Refer to Medicare guidelines.
MSP: Refer to Medicare guidelines.

TRICARE: Enter the eight-digit date the patient's first symptoms occurred from the current illness, if stated in the medical record; date of injury or accident; or for pregnancy, first day of last menstrual period. For chiropractic treatment, enter the eight-digit date that treatment began.

CHAMPVA: Refer to TRICARE guidelines.

Workers' Compensation: Enter first date of injury, accident, or industrial illness; it should coincide with the date specified in the Doctor's First Report of Injury.

Block 15

14. DATE OF CURRENT: MM DD YY 03 01 20XX — ILLNESS (First symptom) OR INJURY (Accident) OR PREGNANCY	15. IF PATIENT HAS HAD SAME OR SIMILAR ILLNESS GIVE FIRST DATE MM DD YYYY	16. DATES PATIENT UNABLE TO WORK IN CURRENT OCCUPATION MM DD YYYY FROM — TO
17. NAME OF REFERRING PHYSICIAN OR OTHER SOURCE PERRY CARDI MD	17a. I.D. NUMBER OF REFERRING PHYSICIAN 67805027XX	18. HOSPITALIZATION DATES RELATED TO CURRENT SERVICES MM DD YYYY FROM — TO
19. RESERVED FOR LOCAL USE		20. OUTSIDE LAB? YES [X] NO $ CHARGES

All Private Payers: Enter date when patient had same or similar illness, if applicable, and documented in the medical record.

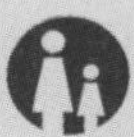

Medicaid: Leave blank.

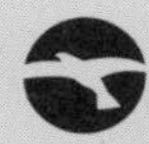

Medicare: Leave blank.
Medicare/Medicaid: Leave blank.
Medicare/Medigap: Leave blank.
MSP: Leave blank.

TRICARE: Enter date when patient had same or similar illness, if applicable and documented in the medical record.

CHAMPVA: Refer to TRICARE guidelines.

Workers' Compensation: Enter date if appropriate and documented in the medical record.

Block 16

14. DATE OF CURRENT: MM DD YY 03 01 20XX ◀ ILLNESS (First symptom) OR INJURY (Accident) OR PREGNANCY	15. IF PATIENT HAS HAD SAME OR SIMILAR ILLNESS GIVE FIRST DATE MM DD YYYY	16. DATES PATIENT UNABLE TO WORK IN CURRENT OCCUPATION FROM MM DD YYYY TO MM DD YYYY
17. NAME OF REFERRING PHYSICIAN OR OTHER SOURCE PERRY CARDI MD	17a. I.D. NUMBER OF REFERRING PHYSICIAN 67805027XX	18. HOSPITALIZATION DATES RELATED TO CURRENT SERVICES FROM MM DD YYYY TO MM DD YYYY
19. RESERVED FOR LOCAL USE		20. OUTSIDE LAB? ☐ YES ☒ NO $ CHARGES

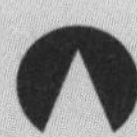

All Private Payers: Enter dates patient is employed but cannot work in current occupation. *From:* Enter first *full* day patient was unable to perform job duties. *To:* Enter last day patient was disabled before returning to work.

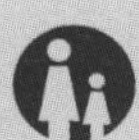

Medicaid: Leave blank.

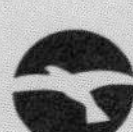

Medicare: Enter eight-digit dates patient is employed but cannot work in current occupation. *From:* Enter first *full* day patient was unable to perform job duties. *To:* Enter last day patient was disabled before returning to work.
Medicare/Medicaid: Refer to Medicare guidelines.
Medicare/Medigap: Refer to Medicare guidelines.
MSP: Refer to Medicare guidelines.

TRICARE: Refer to Medicare guidelines.

CHAMPVA: Refer to Medicare guidelines.

Workers' Compensation: May be completed but is not mandatory and must be verified with documentation in Doctor's First Report of Injury. *From:* Enter first *full* day patient was unable to perform job duties. *To:* Enter last day patient was disabled before returning to work.

- *When completing Billing Break assignments, enter information when documented in the medical record.*

Block 17

14. DATE OF CURRENT: MM DD YY 03 01 20XX	ILLNESS (First symptom) OR INJURY (Accident) OR PREGNANCY	15. IF PATIENT HAS HAD SAME OR SIMILAR ILLNESS GIVE FIRST DATE MM DD YYYY	16. DATES PATIENT UNABLE TO WORK IN CURRENT OCCUPATION FROM MM DD YYYY TO MM DD YYYY
17. NAME OF REFERRING PHYSICIAN OR OTHER SOURCE PERRY CARDI MD		17a. I.D. NUMBER OF REFERRING PHYSICIAN 67805027XX	18. HOSPITALIZATION DATES RELATED TO CURRENT SERVICES FROM MM DD YYYY TO MM DD YYYY
19. RESERVED FOR LOCAL USE			20. OUTSIDE LAB? YES [X] NO $ CHARGES

All Private Payers: Enter complete name and degree of referring physician, when applicable. Do not list other referrals (i.e., family or friends).

Medicare: Enter the name and degree of the referring or ordering physician on all claims for Medicare-covered services and items resulting from a physician's order or referral. Use a separate claim form for each referring and/or ordering physician.

Surgeon: A surgeon must complete this block. When the patient has not been referred, enter the sugeon's name. On an assistant surgeon's claim, enter the primary surgeon's name.

Referring physician: A physician who requests a service for the beneficiary for which payment may be made under the Medicare program. When a physician extender (e.g., nurse practitioner) refers a patient for a consultative service, enter the name of the physician supervising the physician extender.

Ordering physician: A physician who orders nonphysician services for the patient, such as diagnostic radiology/laboratory/pathology tests, pharmaceutical services, durable medical equipment (DME), parenteral and enteral nutrition, or immunosuppressive drugs, and consultations.

When the ordering physician is also the performing physician (e.g., the physician who actually performs the in-office laboratory tests), the performing physician's name and assigned UPIN/NPI number must appear in Blocks 17 and 17a.

When a patient is referred to a physician who also orders and performs a diagnostic service, *a separate claim form* is required for the diagnostic service.

- Enter the original referring physician's name and NPI in Blocks 17 and 17a of the first claim form.
- Enter the ordering (performing) physician's name and NPI in Blocks 17 and 17a of the second claim form.

Medicare/Medicaid: Refer to Medicare guidelines.
Medicare/Medigap: Refer to Medicare guidelines.
MSP: Refer to Medicare guidelines.

TRICARE: Enter name, degree, and address (optional) of referring provider. This is required for all consultation claims. If the patient was referred from a Military Treatment Facility (MTF), enter the name of the MTF and attach DD Form 2161 or SF 513, "Referral for Civilian Medical Care."

CHAMPVA: Refer to TRICARE guidelines.

Workers' Compensation: Indicate name and degree of referring provider.

Block 17a

14. DATE OF CURRENT: MM DD YY 03 01 20XX ◀ ILLNESS (First symptom) OR INJURY (Accident) OR PREGNANCY	15. IF PATIENT HAS HAD SAME OR SIMILAR ILLNESS GIVE FIRST DATE MM DD YYYY	16. DATES PATIENT UNABLE TO WORK IN CURRENT OCCUPATION FROM MM DD YYYY TO MM DD YYYY
17. NAME OF REFERRING PHYSICIAN OR OTHER SOURCE PERRY CARDI MD	17a. I.D. NUMBER OF REFERRING PHYSICIAN 67805027XX	18. HOSPITALIZATION DATES RELATED TO CURRENT SERVICES FROM MM DD YYYY TO MM DD YYYY
19. RESERVED FOR LOCAL USE		20. OUTSIDE LAB? ☐ YES ☒ NO $ CHARGES

All Private Payers: Enter the referring physician's UPIN/NPI number.

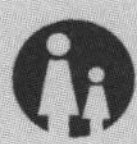

Medicaid: Enter the referring physician's UPIN/NPI number.

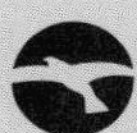

Medicare: Enter the HCFA-assigned UPIN/NPI of the referring or ordering physician (or the supervising physician for a physician extender) as detailed in Medicare Block 17. Temporary "surrogate" NPIs are issued until permanent ones are assigned for physicians in the following categories: residents and interns, retired physicians, nonphysicians (nurse practitioners, clinical nurse specialists, other state licensed nonphysicians), Veterans Affairs/US Armed Services, Public Health/Indian Health Services, and any physician not meeting the just described criteria for a surrogate that has not been issued an NPI.
Medicare/Medicaid: Refer to Medicare guidelines.
Medicare/Medigap: Refer to Medicare guidelines.
MSP: Refer to Medicare guidelines.

TRICARE: Enter the referring physician's state license number. If the patient is referred from a military treatment facility, leave blank.

CHAMPVA: Refer to TRICARE guidelines.

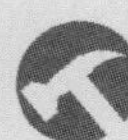

Workers' Compensation: Leave blank.

Block 18

14. DATE OF CURRENT: MM DD YY 03 01 20XX ◀ ILLNESS (First symptom) OR INJURY (Accident) OR PREGNANCY	15. IF PATIENT HAS HAD SAME OR SIMILAR ILLNESS GIVE FIRST DATE MM DD YYYY	16. DATES PATIENT UNABLE TO WORK IN CURRENT OCCUPATION FROM MM DD YYYY TO MM DD YYYY
17. NAME OF REFERRING PHYSICIAN OR OTHER SOURCE PERRY CARDI MD	17a. I.D. NUMBER OF REFERRING PHYSICIAN 67805027XX	18. HOSPITALIZATION DATES RELATED TO CURRENT SERVICES FROM MM DD YYYY TO MM DD YYYY
19. RESERVED FOR LOCAL USE		20. OUTSIDE LAB? ☐ YES ☒ NO $ CHARGES

All Payers: Complete this block when a medical service is furnished as a result of, or subsequent to, a related (inpatient) hospitalization, skilled nursing facility, or nursing home visit. Do not complete for outpatient hospital services, ambulatory surgery, or emergency department services. Enter eight-digit admitting and discharge dates. If the patient is still hospitalized at the time of the billing, enter 8 zeros in the "TO" field.

Block 19

14. DATE OF CURRENT: MM DD YY 03 01 20XX — ILLNESS (First symptom) OR INJURY (Accident) OR PREGNANCY	15. IF PATIENT HAS HAD SAME OR SIMILAR ILLNESS GIVE FIRST DATE MM DD YYYY	16. DATES PATIENT UNABLE TO WORK IN CURRENT OCCUPATION FROM MM DD YYYY TO MM DD YYYY
17. NAME OF REFERRING PHYSICIAN OR OTHER SOURCE PERRY CARDI MD	17a. I.D. NUMBER OF REFERRING PHYSICIAN 67805027XX	18. HOSPITALIZATION DATES RELATED TO CURRENT SERVICES FROM MM DD YYYY TO MM DD YYYY
19. RESERVED FOR LOCAL USE		20. OUTSIDE LAB? ☐ YES ☒ NO — $ CHARGES

All Private Payers: This block may be completed in a number of different ways depending on commercial carrier guidelines. Some common uses are:

- Enter the word "ATTACHMENT" when an operative report, discharge summary, invoice, or other attachment is included.
- Enter an explanation regarding unusual services or unlisted services.
- Enter all applicable modifiers when modifier -99 is used in Block 24D (e.g., 99–80 51). If -99 appears with more than one procedure code, list the line number (24–1, 2, 3, and so on) for each -99 listed (see Example D–2).
- Enter the drug name and dosage when submitting a claim for Not Otherwise Classified (NOC) drugs. Enter the word "ATTACHMENT" and attach the invoice.
- Describe the supply when the code 99070 is used.
- Enter the x-ray date for chiropractic treatment.

Example D–2

2–80 51 3–80 51

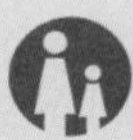

Medicaid: Check with the regional fiscal intermediary who may have special guidelines for entries in this block.

- *When completing Billing Break assignments, refer to private payer guidelines.*

Medicare: Although the block is labeled "Reserved for Local Use," HCFA guidelines state it may be completed in a number of different ways depending on the circumstances of the services provided to the patient. This block can only contain up to three conditions per claim. Some common uses are:

- Enter the attending physician's NPI and the eight-digit date of the patient's latest visit for claims submitted by a physical or occupational therapist, psychotherapist, chiropractor, or podiatrist.
- Enter the drug's name and dosage when submitting a claim for Not Otherwise Classified (NOC) drugs. Enter the word "ATTACHMENT" and include a copy of the invoice.
- Describe the procedure for *unlisted procedures.* If there is not sufficient room in this block, send an attachment.
- Enter all applicable modifiers when modifier −99 is used in Block 24D (e.g., 99–80 51). If −99 appears with more than one procedure code, list the line number (1, 2, 3, and so on) for each −99 listed (see Example D–2).
- Enter "Homebound" when an independent laboratory renders an electrocardiogram or collects a specimen from a patient who is homebound or institutionalized.
- Enter the statement "Patient refuses to assign benefits" when a Medicare beneficiary refuses to assign benefits to a participating provider. No payment to the physician will be made on the claim in this case.
- Enter "Testing for hearing aid" when submitting a claim to obtain an intentional denial from Medicare as the primary payer for hearing aid testing and a secondary payer is involved.
- Enter the specific dental surgery for which a dental examination is being performed.
- Enter the name and dosage when billing for low osmolar contrast material for which there is no Level 2 HCPCS code.
- Enter the eight-digit assumed and relinquished dates of care for each provider when providers share postoperative care for global surgery claims.

- Enter the statement "Attending physician, not hospice employee" when a physician gives service to a hospice patient but the hospice in which the patient resides does not employ the physician.

Medicare/Medicaid: Refer to Medicare guidelines.
Medicare/Medigap: Refer to Medicare guidelines.
MSP: Refer to Medicare guidelines.

TRICARE: Generally this block is reserved for local use (e.g., to indicate referral authorization number or enter x-ray date for chiropractic treatment).

CHAMPVA: Refer to TRICARE guidelines.

Workers' Compensation: Leave blank.

Block 20

14. DATE OF CURRENT: MM DD YY 03 01 20XX ◄ ILLNESS (First symptom) OR INJURY (Accident) OR PREGNANCY	15. IF PATIENT HAS HAD SAME OR SIMILAR ILLNESS GIVE FIRST DATE MM DD YYYY	16. DATES PATIENT UNABLE TO WORK IN CURRENT OCCUPATION FROM MM DD YYYY TO MM DD YYYY
17. NAME OF REFERRING PHYSICIAN OR OTHER SOURCE PERRY CARDI MD	17a. I.D. NUMBER OF REFERRING PHYSICIAN 67805027XX	18. HOSPITALIZATION DATES RELATED TO CURRENT SERVICES FROM MM DD YYYY TO MM DD YYYY
19. RESERVED FOR LOCAL USE		20. OUTSIDE LAB? ☐ YES ☒ NO $ CHARGES

All Private Payers: Enter "yes" or "no" when billing diagnostic laboratory tests. *NO* means the tests were performed by the billing physician/laboratory. *YES* means that the laboratory test was performed *outside* of the physician's office and that the physician is billing for the laboratory service. If "yes," enter purchase price of the test in the Charges portion of this block and complete Block 32.

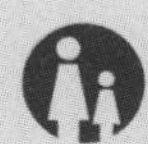

Medicaid: Check "no"; outside laboratories must bill direct.

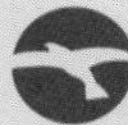

Medicare: Enter "yes" or "no" when billing diagnostic laboratory tests. *NO* means the tests were performed by the billing physician/laboratory. *YES* means that the laboratory test was performed *outside* of the physician's office and that the physician is billing for the laboratory service. If "yes," enter purchase price of the test in the Charges portion of this block and complete Block 32. *Clinical laboratory services must be billed to Medicare on an assigned basis.*
Medicare/Medicaid: Refer to Medicare guidelines.
Medicare/Medigap: Refer to Medicare guidelines.
MSP: Refer to Medicare guidelines.

TRICARE: Refer to Medicare guidelines.

CHAMPVA: Refer to Medicare guidelines.

Workers' Compensation: Refer to Medicare guidelines.

Block 21

21. DIAGNOSIS OR NATURE OF ILLNESS OR INJURY. (RELATE ITEMS 1,2,3 OR 4 TO ITEM 24E BY LINE)

1. 382 . 00
2. ___ . ___
3. ___ . ___
4. ___ . ___

22. MEDICAID RESUBMISSION CODE | ORIGINAL REF. NO.

23. PRIOR AUTHORIZATION NUMBER

24. A DATE(S) OF SERVICE From MM DD YY	To MM DD YY	B Place of Service	C Type of Service	D PROCEDURES, SERVICES, OR SUPPLIES (Explain Unusual Circumstances) CPT/HCPCS | MODIFIER	E DIAGNOSIS CODE	F $ CHARGES	G DAYS OR UNITS	H EPSDT Family Plan	I EMG	J COB	K RESERVED FOR LOCAL USE
1											

INFORMATION

ICD-9-CM
382.00 Acute suppurative otitis media without spontaneous rupture of ear drum

All Payers: Enter up to four diagnostic codes in priority order, with the primary diagnosis in the first position. Codes must be carried out to their highest degree of specificity. Do not use decimal points or add any code narratives unless required in your locale. Code only the conditions or problems that the physician is actively treating and that relate directly to the services billed.

Block 22

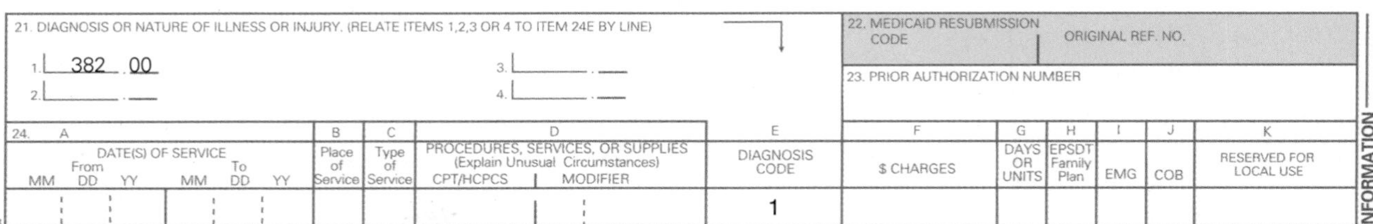

21. DIAGNOSIS OR NATURE OF ILLNESS OR INJURY. (RELATE ITEMS 1,2,3 OR 4 TO ITEM 24E BY LINE)

1. 382 . 00
2. ___ . ___
3. ___ . ___
4. ___ . ___

22. MEDICAID RESUBMISSION CODE | ORIGINAL REF. NO.

23. PRIOR AUTHORIZATION NUMBER

24. A DATE(S) OF SERVICE From MM DD YY	To MM DD YY	B Place of Service	C Type of Service	D PROCEDURES, SERVICES, OR SUPPLIES (Explain Unusual Circumstances) CPT/HCPCS | MODIFIER	E DIAGNOSIS CODE	F $ CHARGES	G DAYS OR UNITS	H EPSDT Family Plan	I EMG	J COB	K RESERVED FOR LOCAL USE
1					1						

INFORMATION

All Private Payers: Leave blank.

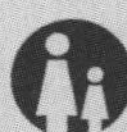

Medicaid: Complete for resubmission.

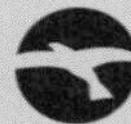

Medicare: Leave blank.
Medicare/Medicaid: Refer to Medicaid guidelines.
Medicare/Medigap: Leave blank.
MSP: Leave blank.

TRICARE: Leave blank

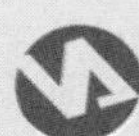

CHAMPVA: Leave blank.

Workers' Compensation: Leave blank.

Block 23

21. DIAGNOSIS OR NATURE OF ILLNESS OR INJURY. (RELATE ITEMS 1,2,3 OR 4 TO ITEM 24E BY LINE)

1. 382 . 00
2. ___ . ___
3. ___ . ___
4. ___ . ___

22. MEDICAID RESUBMISSION CODE | ORIGINAL REF. NO.

23. PRIOR AUTHORIZATION NUMBER

24. A DATE(S) OF SERVICE From MM DD YY To MM DD YY	B Place of Service	C Type of Service	D PROCEDURES, SERVICES, OR SUPPLIES (Explain Unusual Circumstances) CPT/HCPCS | MODIFIER	E DIAGNOSIS CODE	F $ CHARGES	G DAYS OR UNITS	H EPSDT Family Plan	I EMG	J COB	K RESERVED FOR LOCAL USE
1				1						

INFORMATION

All Private Payers: Enter the professional or peer review organization (PRO) 10-digit prior authorization number when applicable.

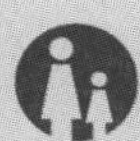

Medicaid: Enter the Professional (Peer) Review Organization (PRO) 10-digit prior authorization or precertification number for procedures requiring PRO prior approval. If billing for an investigational device, enter the Investigational Device Exemption (IDE) number.

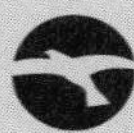

Medicare: Although this block is labeled "Prior Authorization Number," CMS guidelines state it may be completed in a number of different ways depending on the circumstances of the services provided to the patient. Some common uses are:

- Enter the Professional (Peer) Review Organization (PRO) 10-digit prior authorization or precertification number for procedures requiring PRO prior approval.
- Enter the Investigational Device Exemption (IDE) number if billing for an investigational device.
- Enter the 10-digit CLIA (Clinical Laboratory Improvement Amendments) federal certification number when billing for laboratory services billed by a physician office laboratory.
- Enter the 6-digit Medicare provider number of the hospice or home health agency (HHA) when billing for care plan oversight services.

Medicare/Medicaid: Refer to Medicare guidelines.
Medicare/Medigap: Refer to Medicare guidelines.
MSP: Refer to Medicare guidelines.

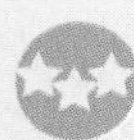

TRICARE: Enter the Professional (Peer) Review Organization (PRO) 10-digit prior authorization or precertification number for procedures requiring PRO prior approval. If billing for an investigational device, enter the Investigational Device Exemption (IDE) number. Attach a copy of the authorization.

CHAMPVA: Refer to TRICARE guidelines.

Workers' Compensation: Leave blank.

Blocks 24A through 24K may not contain more than six detail lines. If the case requires more than six detail lines, put the additional information on a separate claim form and treat it as an independent claim totaling all charges on each claim. Claims cannot be "continued" from one to another. Do not list a procedure on the claim form for which there is no charge.

Block 24A

24.	A DATE(S) OF SERVICE From MM DD YY	To MM DD YY	B Place of Service	C Type of Service	D PROCEDURES, SERVICES, OR SUPPLIES (Explain Unusual Circumstances) CPT/HCPCS	MODIFIER	E DIAGNOSIS CODE	F $ CHARGES	G DAYS OR UNITS	H EPSDT Family Plan	I EMG	J COB	K RESERVED FOR LOCAL USE
1	030320XX		11		99203		1	70 92	1			12	458977XX
2													
3													
4													
5													
6													

25. FEDERAL TAX I.D. NUMBER	SSN	EIN	26. PATIENT'S ACCOUNT NO.	27. ACCEPT ASSIGNMENT? (For govt. claims, see back)	28. TOTAL CHARGE	29. AMOUNT PAID	30. BALANCE DUE
74 10640XX	☐	☒	010	☒ YES ☐ NO	$ 70 92	$	$ 70 92

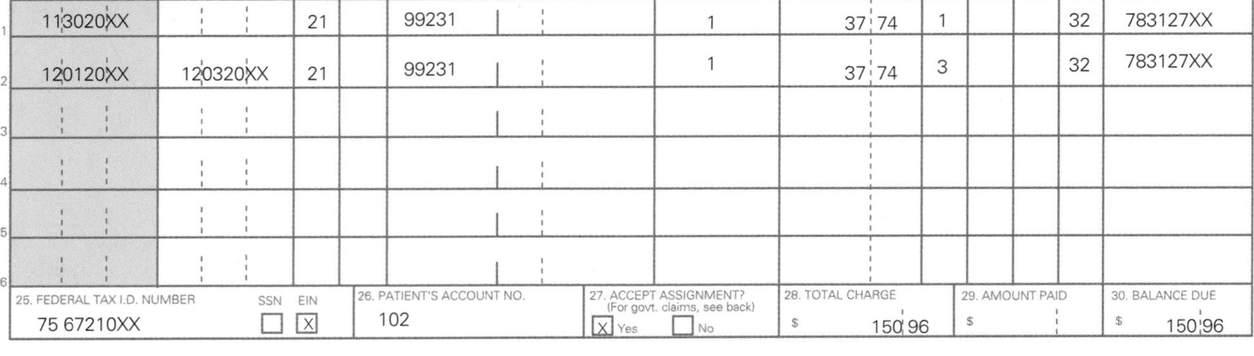

24.	A DATE(S) OF SERVICE From MM DD YY	To MM DD YY	B Place of Service	C Type of Service	D PROCEDURES, SERVICES, OR SUPPLIES (Explain Unusual Circumstances) CPT/HCPCS	MODIFIER	E DIAGNOSIS CODE	F $ CHARGES	G DAYS OR UNITS	H EPSDT Family Plan	I EMG	J COB	K RESERVED FOR LOCAL USE
1	113020XX		21		99231		1	37 74	1			32	783127XX
2	120120XX	120320XX	21		99231		1	37 74	3			32	783127XX
3													
4													
5													
6													

25. FEDERAL TAX I.D. NUMBER	SSN	EIN	26. PATIENT'S ACCOUNT NO.	27. ACCEPT ASSIGNMENT? (For govt. claims, see back)	28. TOTAL CHARGE	29. AMOUNT PAID	30. BALANCE DUE
75 67210XX	☐	☒	102	☒ Yes ☐ No	$ 150 96	$	$ 150 96

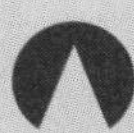

All Private Payers: Enter the month, day, and year (eight digits with no spaces) for each procedure, service, or supply reported in Block 24D. Make sure the dates shown are no earlier than the date of the current illness if listed in Block 14. If the "from" and "to" dates are the same, enter only the "from" date. Enter the "to" date when reporting a consecutive range of dates for the same procedure code. Use a separate line for each month. Some third party payers may use different date formats (e.g., December 4, 20XX = 20001204).

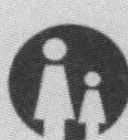

Medicaid: Enter an eight-digit "from" date (month, day, and year with no spaces) for each service or supply. Leave "to" date blank. No date ranging is allowed for consecutive dates.

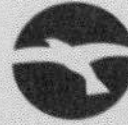

Medicare: Enter the month, day, and year (eight digits with no spaces) for each procedure, service, or supply reported in Block 24D. Make sure the dates shown are no earlier than the date of the current illness if listed in Block 14. If the "from" and "to" dates are the same, enter only the "from" date. Enter the "to" date when reporting a consecutive range of dates for the same procedure code. Use a separate line for each month except when reporting weekly radiation therapy, durable medical equipment, or oxygen rental.
Medicare/Medicaid: Refer to Medicare guidelines.
Medicare/Medigap: Refer to Medicare guidelines.
MSP: Refer to Medicare guidelines.

TRICARE: Enter the month, day, and year (eight digits with no spaces) for each procedure, service, or supply reported in Block 24D. Make sure the dates shown are no earlier than the date of the current illness if listed in Block 14. If the "from" and "to" dates are the same, enter only the "from" date. Enter the "to" date when reporting a consecutive range of dates for the same procedure code. Use a separate line for each month.

CHAMPVA: Refer to TRICARE guidelines.

Workers' Compensation: Enter the month, day, and year (eight digits with no spaces) for each procedure, service, or supply reported in Block 24D. Date ranging is not the preferred format for consecutive dates.

Block 24B

	24. A DATE(S) OF SERVICE From MM DD YY	To MM DD YY	B Place of Service	C Type of Service	D PROCEDURES, SERVICES, OR SUPPLIES (Explain Unusual Circumstances) CPT/HCPCS	MODIFIER	E DIAGNOSIS CODE	F $ CHARGES	G DAYS OR UNITS	H EPSDT Family Plan	I EMG	J COB	K RESERVED FOR LOCAL USE
1	030320XX		11		99203		1	70 92	1			12	458977XX
2													
3													
4													
5													
6													

25. FEDERAL TAX I.D. NUMBER	SSN	EIN	26. PATIENT'S ACCOUNT NO.	27. ACCEPT ASSIGNMENT? (For govt. claims, see back)	28. TOTAL CHARGE	29. AMOUNT PAID	30. BALANCE DUE
74 10640XX	☐	☒	010	☒ Yes ☐ No	$ 70 92	$	$ 70 92

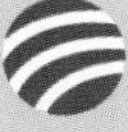

All Payers: Enter the appropriate "Place of Service" code shown in Figure D–1. Identify by location where the service was performed or an item was used. Use the inpatient hospital code only when a service is provided to a patient admitted to the hospital for an overnight stay. Enter the name, address, and provider number of the hospital in Block 32.

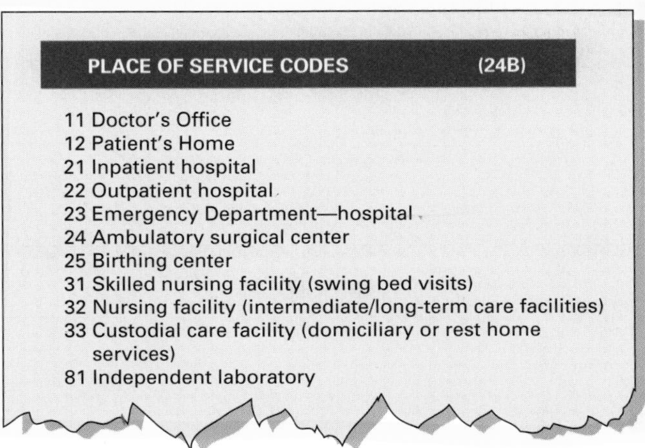

PLACE OF SERVICE CODES (24B)

11 Doctor's Office
12 Patient's Home
21 Inpatient hospital
22 Outpatient hospital
23 Emergency Department—hospital
24 Ambulatory surgical center
25 Birthing center
31 Skilled nursing facility (swing bed visits)
32 Nursing facility (intermediate/long-term care facilities)
33 Custodial care facility (domiciliary or rest home services)
81 Independent laboratory

Figure D–1

Block 24C

	24. A DATE(S) OF SERVICE From MM DD YY	To MM DD YY	B Place of Service	C Type of Service	D PROCEDURES, SERVICES, OR SUPPLIES (Explain Unusual Circumstances) CPT/HCPCS	MODIFIER	E DIAGNOSIS CODE	F $ CHARGES	G DAYS OR UNITS	H EPSDT Family Plan	I EMG	J COB	K RESERVED FOR LOCAL USE
1	030320XX		11		99203		1	70 92	1			12	458977XX
2													
3													
4													
5													
6													

25. FEDERAL TAX I.D. NUMBER	SSN	EIN	26. PATIENT'S ACCOUNT NO.	27. ACCEPT ASSIGNMENT? (For govt. claims, see back)	28. TOTAL CHARGE	29. AMOUNT PAID	30. BALANCE DUE
74 10640XX	☐	☒	010	☒ Yes ☐ No	$ 70 92	$	$ 70 92

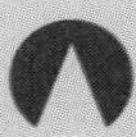

All Private Payers: Leave blank.

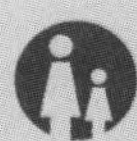

Medicaid: Enter the appropriate "Type of Service" code from Figure D–2.

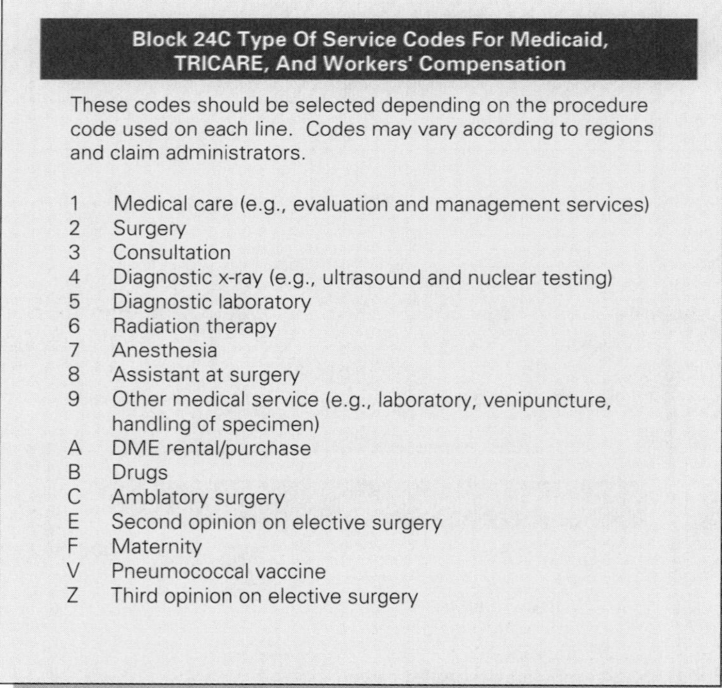

Block 24C Type Of Service Codes For Medicaid, TRICARE, And Workers' Compensation

These codes should be selected depending on the procedure code used on each line. Codes may vary according to regions and claim administrators.

1	Medical care (e.g., evaluation and management services)
2	Surgery
3	Consultation
4	Diagnostic x-ray (e.g., ultrasound and nuclear testing)
5	Diagnostic laboratory
6	Radiation therapy
7	Anesthesia
8	Assistant at surgery
9	Other medical service (e.g., laboratory, venipuncture, handling of specimen)
A	DME rental/purchase
B	Drugs
C	Amblatory surgery
E	Second opinion on elective surgery
F	Maternity
V	Pneumococcal vaccine
Z	Third opinion on elective surgery

Figure D–2

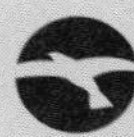

Medicare: Leave blank. "Type of Service" codes are used on Medicare Remittance Advice (RA) documents and electronic claims.
Medicare/Medicaid: Refer to Medicare guidelines.
Medicare/Medigap: Refer to Medicare guidelines.
MSP: Refer to Medicare guidelines.

TRICARE: Enter the appropriate "Type of Service" code from Figure D–2. Codes may vary according to regions and claim administrators.

- *When completing Billing Break assignments, use the codes shown in Figure D–2.*

CHAMPVA: Refer to guidelines for TRICARE.

Workers' Compensation: Enter the appropriate "Type of Service" code shown in Figure D–2. These codes may not be used or may vary according to regions and claim administrators.

- *When completing Billing Break assignments, use the codes shown in Figure D–2.*

Block 24D

24. A DATE(S) OF SERVICE From MM DD YY	To MM DD YY	B Place of Service	C Type of Service	D PROCEDURES, SERVICES, OR SUPPLIES (Explain Unusual Circumstances) CPT/HCPCS	MODIFIER	E DIAGNOSIS CODE	F $ CHARGES	G DAYS OR UNITS	H EPSDT Family Plan	I EMG	J COB	K RESERVED FOR LOCAL USE
1 030320XX		11		99203		1	70 92	1			12	458977XX
2												
3												
4												
5												
6												

25. FEDERAL TAX I.D. NUMBER	SSN	EIN	26. PATIENT'S ACCOUNT NO.	27. ACCEPT ASSIGNMENT? (For govt. claims, see back)	28. TOTAL CHARGE	29. AMOUNT PAID	30. BALANCE DUE
74 10640XX	☐	☒	010	☒ Yes ☐ No	$ 70 92	$	$ 70 92

CPT 99203 Office visit, new patient

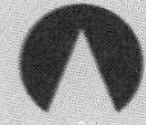

All Private Payers: Enter the appropriate CPT/HCPCS code for each procedure, service, or supply and applicable modifier without a hyphen. If it is necessary to use more than two modifiers with a procedure code, enter modifier -99 in Block 24D and list applicable modifiers in Block 19.

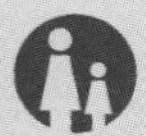

Medicaid: Enter the appropriate CPT/HCPCS code for each procedure, service, or supply and applicable modifier without a hyphen.

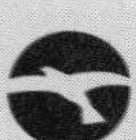

Medicare: Enter CPT/HCPCS code and applicable modifiers without a hyphen for procedures, services, and supplies without a narrative description. When procedure codes do not require modifiers, leave modifier area blank—do not enter 00 or any other combination. For multiple surgical procedures, list the procedure with the highest fee first. For unlisted procedure codes, include a narrative description in Block 19 (e.g., 99499, "Unlisted Evaluation and Management Service"). If information

does not fit in Block 19, include an attachment. When entering an unlisted surgery code, submit the operative notes with the claim as an attachment.
Medicare/Medicaid: Refer to Medicare guidelines.
Medicare/Medigap: Refer to Medicare guidelines.
MSP: Refer to Medicare guidelines.

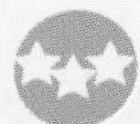

TRICARE: Enter the appropriate CPT/HCPCS code for each procedure, service, or supply and applicable modifier without a hyphen. If it is necessary to use more than two modifiers with a procedure code, enter modifier -99 in Block 24D and list applicable modifiers in Block 19. When Not Otherwise Classified (NOC) codes are submitted (e.g., supplies and injections), provide a narrative of the service in Block 19 or on an attachment.

CHAMPVA: Refer to TRICARE guidelines.

Workers' Compensation: Enter appropriate RVS codes and applicable modifiers (without a hyphen) used in your state or region.

- *When completing Billing Break assignments, use appropriate CPT codes.*

Block 24E

21. DIAGNOSIS OR NATURE OF ILLNESS OR INJURY. (RELATE ITEMS 1,2,3 OR 4 TO ITEM 24E BY LINE)
1. 382 . 00
2. ___ . __
3. ___ . __
4. ___ . __

22. MEDICAID RESUBMISSION CODE | ORIGINAL REF. NO.

23. PRIOR AUTHORIZATION NUMBER

24.	A DATE(S) OF SERVICE From MM DD YY	To MM DD YY	B Place of Service	C Type of Service	D PROCEDURES, SERVICES, OR SUPPLIES (Explain Unusual Circumstances) CPT/HCPCS	MODIFIER	E DIAGNOSIS CODE	F $ CHARGES	G DAYS OR UNITS	H EPSDT Family Plan	I EMG	J COB	K RESERVED FOR LOCAL USE
1	03 03 20XX		11		99203		1	70 92	1			12	458977XX
2													
3													
4													
5													
6													

25. FEDERAL TAX I.D. NUMBER	SSN	EIN	26. PATIENT'S ACCOUNT NO.	27. ACCEPT ASSIGNMENT? (For govt. claims, see back)	28. TOTAL CHARGE	29. AMOUNT PAID	30. BALANCE DUE
74 10640XX	☐	☒	010	☒ Yes ☐ No	$ 70 92	$	$ 70 92

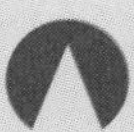

All Private Payers: Enter only one diagnosis code reference "pointer" number per line item (unless you have verified that independent carriers allow more than one) linking the diagnostic code listed in Block 21. When multiple services are performed, enter the corresponding diagnostic reference number for each service (e.g., 1, 2, 3, or 4). DO NOT USE ACTUAL ICD-9-CM CODES IN THIS BLOCK.

- *When completing Billing Break, more than one diagnosis reference "pointer" number per line item is allowed (leave one space between numbers).*

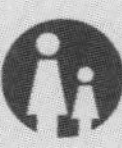

Medicaid: Refer to Medicare guidelines. In some states, completion may not be required.

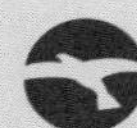

Medicare: Enter only one diagnosis code reference "pointer" number per line item linking the diagnostic codes listed in Block 21. When multiple services are performed, enter the corresponding diagnostic reference number for each service (e.g., 1, 2, 3, or 4). DO NOT USE ACTUAL ICD-9-CM CODES IN THIS BLOCK.
Medicare/Medicaid: Refer to Medicare guidelines.
Medicare/Medigap: Refer to Medicare guidelines.
MSP: Refer to Medicare guidelines.

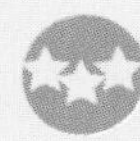

TRICARE: Enter the diagnosis reference number (i.e., indicating up to four ICD-9-CM codes) as shown in Block 21 to relate the date of service and the procedures performed to the appropriate diagnosis. If multiple procedures are performed, enter the diagnosis code reference number for each service.

CHAMPVA: Refer to TRICARE guidelines.

Workers' Compensation: Enter all appropriate diagnosis code reference "pointer" numbers from Block 21 to relate appropriate diagnosis to date of service and procedures performed. A maximum of four diagnosis pointers may be referenced. Place commas between multiple diagnosis reference pointers on the same line.

Block 24F

	24. A DATE(S) OF SERVICE From MM DD YY	To MM DD YY	B Place of Service	C Type of Service	D PROCEDURES, SERVICES, OR SUPPLIES (Explain Unusual Circumstances) CPT/HCPCS	MODIFIER	E DIAGNOSIS CODE	F $ CHARGES	G DAYS OR UNITS	H EPSDT Family Plan	I EMG	J COB	K RESERVED FOR LOCAL USE
1	030320XX		11		99203		1	70 92	1			12	458977XX
2													
3													
4													
5													
6													

25. FEDERAL TAX I.D. NUMBER	SSN EIN	26. PATIENT'S ACCOUNT NO.	27. ACCEPT ASSIGNMENT? (For govt. claims, see back)	28. TOTAL CHARGE	29. AMOUNT PAID	30. BALANCE DUE
74 10640XX	☐ SSN ☒ EIN	010	☒ Yes ☐ No	$ 70 92	$	$ 70 92

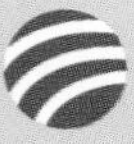

All Payers: Enter the fee for each listed service from the appropriate fee schedule. DO NOT ENTER DOLLAR SIGNS OR DECIMAL POINTS. ALWAYS INCLUDE CENTS. If the same service is performed on consecutive days, list the fee for one service in this block and the number of units (times it was performed) in Block 24G (see bottom graphic for Block 24A). The total for consecutive services should be computed and added into the claim total shown in Block 28.

- *When completing Billing Break assignments for private, Medicaid, TRICARE, and workers' compensation cases, use the* ***Mock Fee.*** *For Medicare participating provider cases, use the* ***Participating Provider Fee.*** *For nonparticipating provider cases, use the* ***Limiting Charge.***

Block 24G

	24. A DATE(S) OF SERVICE From MM DD YY	To MM DD YY	B Place of Service	C Type of Service	D PROCEDURES, SERVICES, OR SUPPLIES (Explain Unusual Circumstances) CPT/HCPCS	MODIFIER	E DIAGNOSIS CODE	F $ CHARGES	G DAYS OR UNITS	H EPSDT Family Plan	I EMG	J COB	K RESERVED FOR LOCAL USE
1	030320XX		11		99203		1	70 92	1			12	458977XX
2													
3													
4													
5													
6													

25. FEDERAL TAX I.D. NUMBER	SSN	EIN	26. PATIENT'S ACCOUNT NO.	27. ACCEPT ASSIGNMENT? (For govt. claims, see back)	28. TOTAL CHARGE	29. AMOUNT PAID	30. BALANCE DUE
74 10640XX	☐	☒	010	☒ Yes ☐ No	$ 70 92	$	$ 70 92

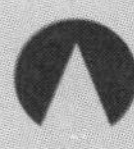

All Private Payers: Enter the number of days or units that apply to each line of service. This block is important for calculating multiple visits, anesthesia minutes, or oxygen volume (see bottom graphic for Block 24A).

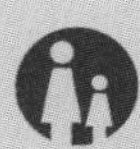

Medicaid: Each service must be listed on separate lines (no date ranging). Indicate that each service was performed one time by listing "1" in this block. List number of visits in 1 day.

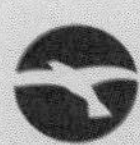

Medicare: Enter the number of days or units that apply to each line of service. This block is important for calculating multiple visits, number of miles, units of supplies including drugs, anesthesia minutes, or oxygen volume. For example, when a physician reports consecutive hospital care services using CPT code number 99231, on December 1, 2, and 3, it would be totalled and shown as on page 532. See the Medicare Manual for reporting anesthesia time/units and for rounding out figures when billing gas and liquid oxygen units.
Medicare/Medicaid: Refer to Medicare guidelines.
Medicare/Medigap: Refer to Medicare guidelines.
MSP: Refer to Medicare guidelines.

TRICARE: Refer to guidelines for Medicare.

CHAMPVA: Refer to Medicare guidelines.

Workers' Compensation: Refer to Medicare guidelines.

Block 24H

24. A DATE(S) OF SERVICE From MM DD YY	To MM DD YY	B Place of Service	C Type of Service	D PROCEDURES, SERVICES, OR SUPPLIES (Explain Unusual Circumstances) CPT/HCPCS	MODIFIER	E DIAGNOSIS CODE	F $ CHARGES	G DAYS OR UNITS	H EPSDT Family Plan	I EMG	J COB	K RESERVED FOR LOCAL USE
1 030320XX		11		99203		1	70 92	1			12	458977XX
2												
3												
4												
5												
6												

25. FEDERAL TAX I.D. NUMBER	SSN	EIN	26. PATIENT'S ACCOUNT NO.	27. ACCEPT ASSIGNMENT? (For govt. claims, see back)	28. TOTAL CHARGE	29. AMOUNT PAID	30. BALANCE DUE
74 10640XX	☐	☒	010	☒ Yes ☐ No	$ 70 92	$	$ 70 92

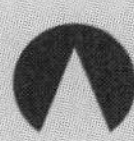

All Private Payers: Leave blank.

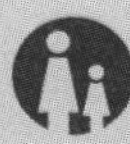

Medicaid: EPSDT means early, periodic, screening, diagnosis, and treatment and this refers to a Medicaid service program for children 12 years of age or younger. Enter "E" for EPSDT services or "F" for family planning services, if applicable.

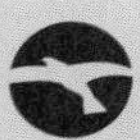

Medicare: Leave blank.
Medicare/Medicaid: Leave blank.
Medicare/Medigap: Leave blank.
MSP: Leave blank.

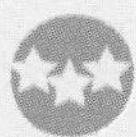

TRICARE: Leave blank.

CHAMPVA: Leave blank.

Workers' Compensation: Leave blank.

Block 24I

	24. A DATE(S) OF SERVICE From MM DD YY	To MM DD YY	B Place of Service	C Type of Service	D PROCEDURES, SERVICES, OR SUPPLIES (Explain Unusual Circumstances) CPT/HCPCS	MODIFIER	E DIAGNOSIS CODE	F $ CHARGES	G DAYS OR UNITS	H EPSDT Family Plan	I EMG	J COB	K RESERVED FOR LOCAL USE
1	030320XX		11		99203		1	70 92	1			12	458977XX
2													
3													
4													
5													
6													

25. FEDERAL TAX I.D. NUMBER	SSN EIN	26. PATIENT'S ACCOUNT NO.	27. ACCEPT ASSIGNMENT? (For govt. claims, see back)	28. TOTAL CHARGE	29. AMOUNT PAID	30. BALANCE DUE
74 10640XX	☐ SSN ☒ EIN	010	☒ Yes ☐ No	$ 70 92	$	$ 70 92

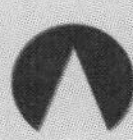

All Private Payers: Leave blank.

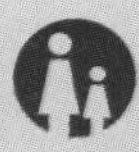

Medicaid: EMG stands for the word “emergency” and means that the service was rendered in a hospital emergency department. Enter “X” if emergency care is provided in an emergency department.

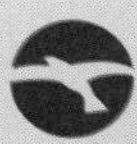

Medicare: Leave blank.
Medicare/Medicaid: Leave blank.
Medicare/Medigap: Leave blank.
MSP: Leave blank.

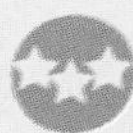

TRICARE: Enter “X” in this block to indicate that the service was provided in a hospital emergency department.

CHAMPVA: Enter “X” in this block to indicate that the service was provided in a hospital emergency department.

Workers’ Compensation: Leave blank.

Block 24J

	24. A DATE(S) OF SERVICE From MM DD YY	To MM DD YY	B Place of Service	C Type of Service	D PROCEDURES, SERVICES, OR SUPPLIES (Explain Unusual Circumstances) CPT/HCPCS	MODIFIER	E DIAGNOSIS CODE	F $ CHARGES	G DAYS OR UNITS	H EPSDT Family Plan	I EMG	J COB	K RESERVED FOR LOCAL USE
1	030320XX		11		99203		1	70 92	1			12	458977XX
2													
3													
4													
5													
6													

25. FEDERAL TAX I.D. NUMBER	SSN	EIN	26. PATIENT'S ACCOUNT NO.	27. ACCEPT ASSIGNMENT? (For govt. claims, see back)	28. TOTAL CHARGE	29. AMOUNT PAID	30. BALANCE DUE
74 10640XX	☐	☒	010	☒ Yes ☐ No	$ 70 92	$	$ 70 92

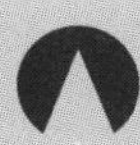

All Private Payers: Refer to the note under Block 24K.

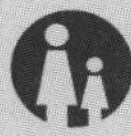

Medicaid: COB means coordination of benefits. Enter "X" if applicable, when the patient has other insurance.

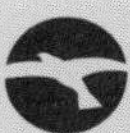

Medicare: Refer to the note for Block 24K.
Medicare/Medicaid: Refer to the note for Block 24K
Medicare/Medigap: Refer to the note for Block 24K.
MSP: Refer to the note for Block 24K.

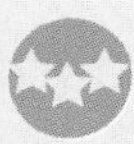

TRICARE: Enter "X," if applicable, when the patient has other insurance.

CHAMPVA: Leave blank.

Workers' Compensation: Leave blank.

Block 24K

24. A DATE(S) OF SERVICE From MM DD YY	To MM DD YY	B Place of Service	C Type of Service	D PROCEDURES, SERVICES, OR SUPPLIES (Explain Unusual Circumstances) CPT/HCPCS	MODIFIER	E DIAGNOSIS CODE	F $ CHARGES	G DAYS OR UNITS	H EPSDT Family Plan	I EMG	J COB	K RESERVED FOR LOCAL USE
1 030320XX		11		99203		1	70 92	1			12	458977XX
2												
3												
4												
5												
6												

25. FEDERAL TAX I.D. NUMBER	SSN	EIN	26. PATIENT'S ACCOUNT NO.	27. ACCEPT ASSIGNMENT? (For govt. claims, see back)	28. TOTAL CHARGE	29. AMOUNT PAID	30. BALANCE DUE
74 10640XX	☐	☒	010	☒ Yes ☐ No	$ 70 92	$	$ 70 92

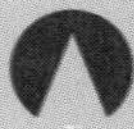

All Private Payers: Enter the CMS-assigned Provider Identification Number (PIN) or National Provider Identifier (NPI) for each line of service when the performing physician/supplier is in a *group practice* and billing under a group I.D. number. An individual physician's PIN/NPI is not required if he or she is in solo practice or when billing under his or her individual I.D. number. **Note:** *Enter the first two digits of the PIN/NPI in Block 24J. Enter the remaining eight digits of the PIN/NPI in Block 24K, including the two-digit location identifier.*

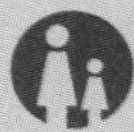

Medicaid: Leave blank.

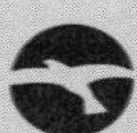

Medicare: Enter the CMS-assigned Performing Provider Identification Number (PPIN) or National Provider Identifier (NPI) for each line of service when the performing physician/supplier is in a *group practice* and billing under a group I.D. number. An individual physician's PPIN/NPI is not required if he or she is in solo practice or when billing under his or her individual I.D. number. **Note:** *Enter the first two digits of the PPIN/NPI in Block 24J. Enter the remaining eight digits of the PPIN/NPI in Block 24K, including the two-digit location identifier.*
Medicare/Medicaid: Refer to Medicare guidelines.
Medicare/Medigap: Refer to Medicare guidelines.
MSP: Refer to Medicare guidelines.

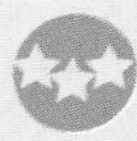

TRICARE: Enter the attending physician's state license number. The state license number is an alpha character followed by six numeric digits. If there are not six digits, enter appropriate number of zero(s) after the alpha character (i.e., A1234 would be A001234).

CHAMPVA: Refer to TRICARE guidelines.

Workers' Compensation: Leave blank.

Block 25

25. FEDERAL TAX I.D. NUMBER SSN EIN	26. PATIENT'S ACCOUNT NO.	27. ACCEPT ASSIGNMENT? (For govt. claims, see back)	28. TOTAL CHARGE	29. AMOUNT PAID	30. BALANCE DUE
74 10640XX ☐ ☒	010	☒ YES ☐ NO	$ 70 92	$	$ 70 92

31. SIGNATURE OF PHYSICIAN OR SUPPLIER INCLUDING DEGREES OR CREDENTIALS (I certify that the statements on the reverse apply to this bill and are made a part thereof)	32. NAME AND ADDRESS OF FACILITY WHERE SERVICECS WERE RENDERED (If other than home or office)	33. PHYSICIAN'S, SUPPLIER'S BILLING NAME, ADDRESS, ZIP CODE & PHONE #
CONCHA ANTRUM MD 030320XX SIGNED DATE	SAME	COLLEGE CLINIC 4567 BROAD AVENUE WOODLAND HILLS XY 12345 0001 555 486 9002 PIN# GRP# 3664021CC

reference initials

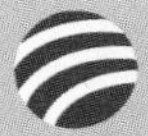

All Payers: Enter the physician/supplier's federal tax I.D. This number may be the Employer Identification Number (EIN) or Social Security Number (SSN). Check the corresponding box.

- A Medicaid case may or may not require a physician's tax I.D. number, depending on individual state guidelines.
- In a Medicare/Medigap case, the physician's federal tax I.D. number is required for Medigap transfer.
- *When completing Billing Break assignments, enter the physician's EIN number and check the appropriate box.*

Block 26

25. FEDERAL TAX I.D. NUMBER SSN EIN	26. PATIENT'S ACCOUNT NO.	27. ACCEPT ASSIGNMENT? (For govt. claims, see back)	28. TOTAL CHARGE	29. AMOUNT PAID	30. BALANCE DUE
74 10640XX ☐ ☒	010	☒ ☐	$ 70 92	$	$ 70 92

31. SIGNATURE OF PHYSICIAN OR SUPPLIER INCLUDING DEGREES OR CREDENTIALS (I certify that the statements on the reverse apply to this bill and are made a part thereof)	32. NAME AND ADDRESS OF FACILITY WHERE SERVICECS WERE RENDERED (If other than home or office)	33. PHYSICIAN'S, SUPPLIER'S BILLING NAME, ADDRESS, ZIP CODE & PHONE #
CONCHA ANTRUM MD 030320XX SIGNED DATE	SAME	COLLEGE CLINIC 4567 BROAD AVENUE WOODLAND HILLS XY 12345 0001 555 486 9002 PIN# GRP# 3664021CC

reference initials

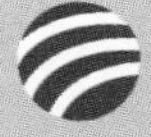

All Payers: Enter the patient's account number assigned by the physician's accounting system. Do not use dashes or slashes. When Medicare is billed electronically, this block must be completed.

- *When completing Billing Break assignments, list the patient account number when provided.*

Block 27

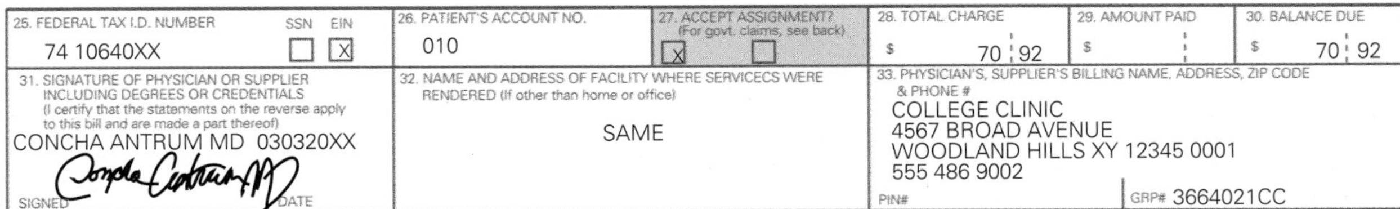

25. FEDERAL TAX I.D. NUMBER SSN EIN	26. PATIENT'S ACCOUNT NO.	27. ACCEPT ASSIGNMENT? (For govt. claims, see back)	28. TOTAL CHARGE	29. AMOUNT PAID	30. BALANCE DUE
74 10640XX ☐ ☒	010	☒ ☐	$ 70 92	$	$ 70 92

31. SIGNATURE OF PHYSICIAN OR SUPPLIER INCLUDING DEGREES OR CREDENTIALS (I certify that the statements on the reverse apply to this bill and are made a part thereof)	32. NAME AND ADDRESS OF FACILITY WHERE SERVICECS WERE RENDERED (If other than home or office)	33. PHYSICIAN'S, SUPPLIER'S BILLING NAME, ADDRESS, ZIP CODE & PHONE #
CONCHA ANTRUM MD 030320XX SIGNED DATE	SAME	COLLEGE CLINIC 4567 BROAD AVENUE WOODLAND HILLS XY 12345 0001 555 486 9002 PIN# GRP# 3664021CC

reference initials

All Private Payers: Check "yes" or "no" to indicate whether the physician accepts assignment of benefits. If yes, then the physician agrees to accept the allowed amount paid by the third party plus any copayment and/or deductible as payment in full.

- *When completing Billing Break assignments, check "yes."*

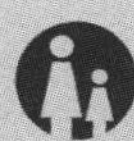

Medicaid: Check "yes."

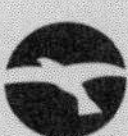

Medicare: Check "yes" or "no" to indicate whether the physician accepts assignment of benefits. If yes, then the physician agrees to accept the allowed amount paid by the third party plus any copayment or deductible as payment in full. If this field is left blank, "no" is assumed, and a participating physician's claim will be denied. The following provider/supplier must file claims on an assignment basis:

- Clinical diagnostic laboratory services performed in physician's office.
- Physicians wishing to accept assignment on clinical laboratory services but not other services should submit two separate claims, one "assigned" for laboratory and one "nonassigned" for other services. Submit all charges on a nonassigned claim, as indicated in Block 27, and write "I accept assignment for the clinical laboratory tests" at the bottom of Block 24.
- Participating physician/supplier services.
- Physician's services to Medicare/Medicaid patients.
- Services of: physician assistants, nurse practitioners, clinical nurse specialists, nurse midwives, certified registered nurse anesthetists, clinical psychologists, clinical social workers.
- Ambulatory surgical center services.
- Home dialysis supplies and equipment paid under Method II (monthly capitation payment).

When completing Billing Break assignments, check "yes."

Medicare/Medicaid: Check "yes."

Medicare/Medigap: Check "yes."

MSP: Check "yes" or "no" to indicate whether the physician accepts assignment of benefits for primary insurance and Medicare.

- *When completing Billing Break assignments, check "yes."*

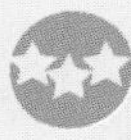

TRICARE: Refer to Medicare guidelines. However, participation in TRICARE may be made on a case-by-case basis.

CHAMPVA: Refer to Medicare guidelines.

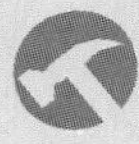

Workers' Compensation: Leave blank.

Block 28

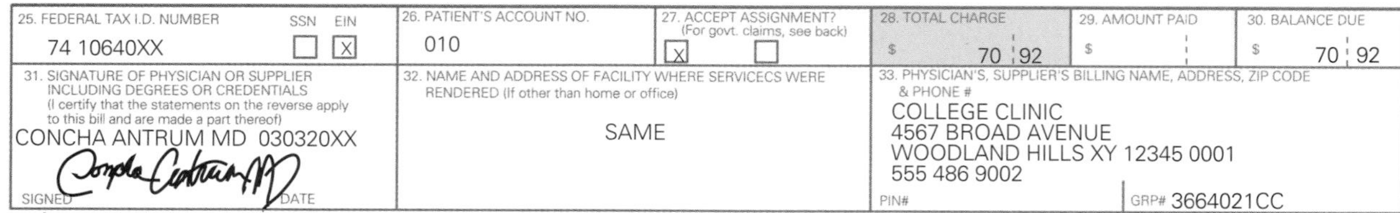

25. FEDERAL TAX I.D. NUMBER SSN EIN
74 10640XX ☐ ☒

26. PATIENT'S ACCOUNT NO.
010

27. ACCEPT ASSIGNMENT? (For govt. claims, see back)
☒ ☐

28. TOTAL CHARGE
$ 70 92

29. AMOUNT PAID
$

30. BALANCE DUE
$ 70 92

31. SIGNATURE OF PHYSICIAN OR SUPPLIER INCLUDING DEGREES OR CREDENTIALS (I certify that the statements on the reverse apply to this bill and are made a part thereof)
CONCHA ANTRUM MD 030320XX
SIGNED DATE

32. NAME AND ADDRESS OF FACILITY WHERE SERVICECS WERE RENDERED (If other than home or office)
SAME

33. PHYSICIAN'S, SUPPLIER'S BILLING NAME, ADDRESS, ZIP CODE & PHONE #
COLLEGE CLINIC
4567 BROAD AVENUE
WOODLAND HILLS XY 12345 0001
555 486 9002
PIN# GRP# 3664021CC

reference initials

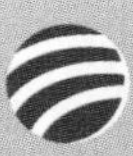

All Payers: Enter total charges for services listed in Block(s) 24F. If more than one unit is listed in Block 24G, multiply the number of units by the charge and add the amount into the total charge (see page 532, bottom). Do not enter dollar signs or decimal points. Always include cents.

Block 29

25. FEDERAL TAX I.D. NUMBER / SSN EIN	26. PATIENT'S ACCOUNT NO.	27. ACCEPT ASSIGNMENT? (For govt. claims, see back)	28. TOTAL CHARGE	29. AMOUNT PAID	30. BALANCE DUE
74 10640XX ☐ ☒	010	☒ ☐	$ 70 92	$	$ 70 92
31. SIGNATURE OF PHYSICIAN OR SUPPLIER INCLUDING DEGREES OR CREDENTIALS (I certify that the statements on the reverse apply to this bill and are made a part thereof) CONCHA ANTRUM MD 030320XX SIGNED DATE	32. NAME AND ADDRESS OF FACILITY WHERE SERVICECS WERE RENDERED (If other than home or office) SAME		33. PHYSICIAN'S, SUPPLIER'S BILLING NAME, ADDRESS, ZIP CODE & PHONE # COLLEGE CLINIC 4567 BROAD AVENUE WOODLAND HILLS XY 12345 0001 555 486 9002 PIN# GRP# 3664021CC		

reference initials

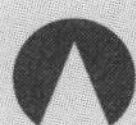

All Private Payers: Enter only the amount paid for the charges listed on the claim.

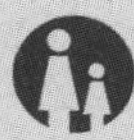

Medicaid: Enter only the payment on claim by a third party payer, excluding Medicare.

Medicare: Enter only the amount paid for the charges listed on the claim.
Medicare/Medicaid: Refer to Medicare guidelines.
Medicare/Medigap: Enter only the amount paid for charges listed on the claim.
MSP: Enter only the amount paid for charges listed on the claim. It is mandatory to enter amount paid by primary carrier and attach an explanation of benefits document when billing Medicare.

TRICARE: Enter only amount paid by other carrier for the charges listed on the claim. If the amount includes payment by any other health insurances, the other health insurance explanation of benefits, work sheet, or denial showing the amounts paid must be attached to the claim. Payment from the beneficiary should not be included.

CHAMPVA: Refer to TRICARE guidelines.

Workers' Compensation: Leave blank.

Block 30

25. FEDERAL TAX I.D. NUMBER / SSN EIN	26. PATIENT'S ACCOUNT NO.	27. ACCEPT ASSIGNMENT? (For govt. claims, see back)	28. TOTAL CHARGE	29. AMOUNT PAID	30. BALANCE DUE
74 10640XX ☐ ☒	010	☒ ☐	$ 70 92	$	$ 70 92
31. SIGNATURE OF PHYSICIAN OR SUPPLIER INCLUDING DEGREES OR CREDENTIALS (I certify that the statements on the reverse apply to this bill and are made a part thereof) CONCHA ANTRUM MD 030320XX SIGNED DATE	32. NAME AND ADDRESS OF FACILITY WHERE SERVICECS WERE RENDERED (If other than home or office) SAME		33. PHYSICIAN'S, SUPPLIER'S BILLING NAME, ADDRESS, ZIP CODE & PHONE # COLLEGE CLINIC 4567 BROAD AVENUE WOODLAND HILLS XY 12345 0001 555 486 9002 PIN# GRP# 3664021CC		

reference initials

All Private Payers: Enter balance due on claim (Block 28 less Block 29).

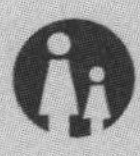

Medicaid: Leave blank or enter balance due on claim depending on individual state guidelines.

- *When completing Billing Break assignments, enter the balance due.*

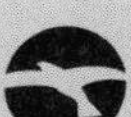

Medicare: Leave blank.
Medicare/Medicaid: Leave blank.
Medicare/Medigap: Leave blank.
MSP: Leave blank.

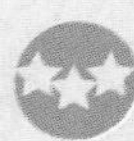

TRICARE: Enter balance due on claim (Block 28 less Block 29).

CHAMPVA: Enter balance due on claim (Block 28 less Block 29).

Workers' Compensation: Enter balance due on claim (Block 28 less Block 29).

Block 31

25. FEDERAL TAX I.D. NUMBER SSN EIN	26. PATIENT'S ACCOUNT NO.	27. ACCEPT ASSIGNMENT? (For govt. claims, see back)	28. TOTAL CHARGE	29. AMOUNT PAID	30. BALANCE DUE
74 10640XX ☐ ☒	010	☒ ☐	$ 70 92	$	$ 70 92
31. SIGNATURE OF PHYSICIAN OR SUPPLIER INCLUDING DEGREES OR CREDENTIALS (I certify that the statements on the reverse apply to this bill and are made a part thereof) CONCHA ANTRUM MD 030320XX SIGNED DATE	32. NAME AND ADDRESS OF FACILITY WHERE SERVICECS WERE RENDERED (If other than home or office) SAME		33. PHYSICIAN'S, SUPPLIER'S BILLING NAME, ADDRESS, ZIP CODE & PHONE # COLLEGE CLINIC 4567 BROAD AVENUE WOODLAND HILLS XY 12345 0001 555 486 9002 PIN# GRP# 3664021CC		

reference initials

All Payers: Type the provider's name and show the signature of the physician or the physician's representative above or below the name. Enter the eight-digit date the form was prepared. Most insurance carriers will accept a stamped signature, but the stamp must be completely inside the block. Do not type the name of the association or corporation.

- *When completing Billing Break assignments, sign the physician's name (as if you were the physician) above or below the typed name.*

Block 32

25. FEDERAL TAX I.D. NUMBER SSN EIN	26. PATIENT'S ACCOUNT NO.	27. ACCEPT ASSIGNMENT? (For govt. claims, see back)	28. TOTAL CHARGE	29. AMOUNT PAID	30. BALANCE DUE
74 10640XX ☐ ☒	010	☒ ☐	$ 70 92	$	$ 70 92
31. SIGNATURE OF PHYSICIAN OR SUPPLIER INCLUDING DEGREES OR CREDENTIALS (I certify that the statements on the reverse apply to this bill and are made a part thereof) CONCHA ANTRUM MD 030320XX SIGNED DATE	32. NAME AND ADDRESS OF FACILITY WHERE SERVICECS WERE RENDERED (If other than home or office) SAME		33. PHYSICIAN'S, SUPPLIER'S BILLING NAME, ADDRESS, ZIP CODE & PHONE # COLLEGE CLINIC 4567 BROAD AVENUE WOODLAND HILLS XY 12345 0001 555 486 9002 PIN# GRP# 3664021CC		

reference initials

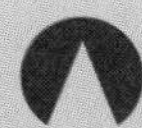

All Private Payers: Enter the word "SAME" in the center of the block if the facility furnishing services is the same as that of the biller listed in Block 33. *If other* than home, office, nursing facility, or community mental health center, enter the name, address, and provider number of the facility (e.g., hospital name for physician's hospital services). For durable medical equipment, enter the *location* where the *order is taken*. If a test is performed by a mammography screening center, enter the six-digit certification number approved by the Food and Drug Administration (FDA). When billing for purchased diagnostic tests performed outside the physician's office but billed by the physician, enter the facility's name, address, and CMS-assigned NPI where the test was performed.

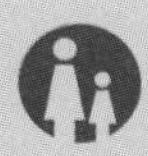

Medicaid: Refer to Medicare guidelines when completing this block; however, use Medicaid facility provider number.

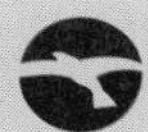

Medicare: Enter "SAME" in the center of the block if the facility furnishing services is the same as that of the biller listed in Block 33. *If other* than home, office, nursing facility, or community mental health center, enter the name, address, and provider number of the facility (e.g., hospital name for physician's hospital services). For hospital services performed by a physician, the Medicare provider number must be preceded by "HSP." For durable medical equipment, enter the *location* where the *order is taken*. If the test is performed by a mammography screening center, enter the six-digit FDA-approved certification number. When billing for purchased diagnostic tests performed outside the physician's office but billed by the physician, enter the facility's name, address, and CMS-assigned NPI where the test was performed.
Medicare/Medicaid: Refer to Medicare guidelines.
Medicare/Medigap: Refer to Medicare guidelines.
MSP: Refer to Medicare guidelines.

TRICARE: Refer to private payer guidelines. For partnership providers, indicate the name of the Military Treatment Facility.

CHAMPVA: Refer to private payer guidelines.

Workers' Compensation: Refer to private payer guidelines.

Block 33

25. FEDERAL TAX I.D. NUMBER SSN EIN	26. PATIENT'S ACCOUNT NO.	27. ACCEPT ASSIGNMENT? (For govt. claims, see back)	28. TOTAL CHARGE	29. AMOUNT PAID	30. BALANCE DUE
74 10640XX ☐ ☒	010	☒ ☐	$ 70 92	$	$ 70 92

31. SIGNATURE OF PHYSICIAN OR SUPPLIER INCLUDING DEGREES OR CREDENTIALS (I certify that the statements on the reverse apply to this bill and are made a part thereof)	32. NAME AND ADDRESS OF FACILITY WHERE SERVICECS WERE RENDERED (If other than home or office)	33. PHYSICIAN'S, SUPPLIER'S BILLING NAME, ADDRESS, ZIP CODE & PHONE #
CONCHA ANTRUM MD 030320XX SIGNED Concha Antrum MD DATE	SAME	COLLEGE CLINIC 4567 BROAD AVENUE WOODLAND HILLS XY 12345 0001 555 486 9002 PIN# GRP# 3664021CC

reference initials

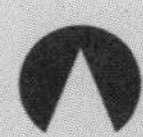

All Private Payers: Refer to Medicare guidelines.

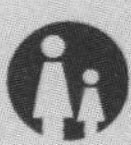

Medicaid: Refer to Medicare guidelines except use Medicaid's facility provider number.

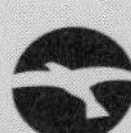

Medicare: Enter the name, address, and telephone number for the physician, clinic, or supplier billing for services. Either enter the PIN/NPI for a performing physician or supplier who is *not* a member of a group practice in the lower left section of the block or enter the *group number* for a performing physician or supplier who belongs to a group practice and is billing under the group I.D. number in the right lower section of the block.
Medicare/Medicaid: Refer to Medicare guidelines.
Medicare/Medigap: Refer to Medicare guidelines.
MSP: Refer to Medicare guidelines.

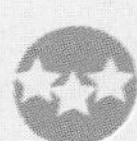

TRICARE: Enter the name, address, and telephone number for the physician, clinic, or supplier billing for services. Radiologists, pathologists, and anesthesiologists may use their billing address if they have no *physical address.* Enter the physician's Tax Identification Number in the lower left section of the block; *the group number is not required.*

- *When completing Billing Break assignments, enter the performing physician's Tax I.D. number in the lower left section of the block.*

CHAMPVA: Refer to TRICARE guidelines.

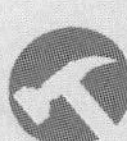

Workers' Compensation: Enter the name, address, and telephone number of the physician. Individual or group provider numbers or state license number are generally required depending on the insurance carrier's requirements.

- *When completing Billing Break assignments, follow Medicare guidelines.*

Bottom of Form

Enter insurance billing specialist's reference initials in lower left corner of the insurance claim form.

PRIVATE PAYER
No secondary coverage

PRIVATE INSURANCE COMPANY NAME
MAILING ADDRESS
CITY STATE ZIP CODE

1. MEDICARE (Medicare #) MEDICAID (Medicaid #) CHAMPUS (Sponsor's SSN) CHAMPVA (VA File #) GROUP Health Plan (SSN or ID) [X] FECA BLK LUNG (SSN) OTHER (ID)

1a. INSURED I.D. NUMBER (FOR PROGRAM IN ITEM 1): 111704521 A482

2. PATIENT'S NAME (Last Name, First Name, Middle Initial): FOREHAND HARRY N

3. PATIENT'S BIRTH DATE MM DD YYYY: 01 06 1946 SEX M [X] F [ ]

4. INSURED'S NAME (LAST NAME, FIRST NAME, MIDDLE INITIAL): SAME

5. PATIENT'S ADDRESS (No., Street): 1456 MAIN STREET

6. PATIENT RELATIONSHIP TO INSURED: Self [X] Spouse [ ] Child [ ] Other [ ]

7. INSURED'S ADDRESS (No, Street)

CITY: WOODLAND HILLS STATE: XY

8. PATIENT STATUS: Single [ ] Married [X] Other [ ]

CITY STATE

ZIP CODE: 12345 0000 TELEPHONE (Include Area Code): 555 490 9876

Employed [X] Full-Time Student [ ] Part-Time Student [ ]

ZIP CODE TELEPHONE (INCLUDE AREA CODE) ( )

9. OTHER INSURED'S NAME (Last Name, First Name, Middle Initial)

10. IS PATIENT'S CONITION RELATED TO:

11. INSURED'S POLICY GROUP OR FECA NUMBER

a. OTHER INSURED'S POLICY OR GROUP NUMBER

a. EMPLOYMENT? (CURRENT OR PREVIOUS) [ ] YES [X] NO

a. INSURED'S DATE OF BIRTH MM DD YYYY SEX M [ ] F [ ]

b. OTHER INSURED'S DATE OF BIRTH MM DD YY SEX M [ ] F [ ]

b. AUTO ACCIDENT? [ ] YES [X] NO PLACE (State)

b. EMPLOYER'S NAME OR SCHOOL NAME

c. EMPLOYER'S NAME OR SCHOOL NAME

c. OTHER ACCIDENT? [ ] YES [X] NO

c. INSURANCE PLAN NAME OR PROGRAM NAME

d. INSURANCE PLAN NAME OR PROGRAM NAME

10d. RESERVED FOR LOCAL USE

d. IS THERE ANOTHER HEALTH BENEFIT PLAN? [ ] YES [X] NO *If yes,* return to and complete item 9 a-d

READ BACK OF FORM BEFORE COMPLETING & SIGNING THIS FORM

12. PATIENT'S OR AUTHORIZED PERSON'S SIGNATURE. I authorize the release of any medical or other information necessary to process this claim. I also request payment of government benefits either to myself or to the party who accepts assignment below.

SIGNED *Harry N Forehand* DATE *March 3 20xx*

13. INSURED'S OR AUTHORIZED PERSON'S SIGNATURE. I authorize payment of medical benefits to the undersigned physician or supplier for services described below

SIGNED *Harry N Forehand*

14. DATE OF CURRENT: MM DD YY 03 01 20XX ILLNESS (First symptom) OR INJURY (Accident) OR PREGNANCY

15. IF PATIENT HAS HAD SAME OR SIMILAR ILLNESS GIVE FIRST DATE MM DD YYYY

16. DATES PATIENT UNABLE TO WORK IN CURRENT OCCUPATION FROM MM DD YYYY TO MM DD YYYY

17. NAME OF REFERRING PHYSICIAN OR OTHER SOURCE: PERRY CARDI MD

17a. I.D. NUMBER OF REFERRING PHYSICIAN: 67805027XX

18. HOSPITALIZATION DATES RELATED TO CURRENT SERVICES FROM MM DD YYYY TO MM DD YYYY

19. RESERVED FOR LOCAL USE

20. OUTSIDE LAB? [ ] YES [X] NO $ CHARGES

21. DIAGNOSIS OR NATURE OF ILLNESS OR INJURY. (RELATE ITEMS 1,2,3 OR 4 TO ITEM 24E BY LINE)

1. 382 00
2.
3.
4.

22. MEDICAID RESUBMISSION CODE ORIGINAL REF. NO.

23. PRIOR AUTHORIZATION NUMBER

24. A DATE(S) OF SERVICE From MM DD YY	To MM DD YY	B Place of Service	C Type of Service	D PROCEDURES, SERVICES, OR SUPPLIES (Explain Unusual Circumstances) CPT/HCPCS	MODIFIER	E DIAGNOSIS CODE	F $ CHARGES	G DAYS OR UNITS	H EPSDT Family Plan	I EMG	J COB	K RESERVED FOR LOCAL USE
030320XX		11		99203		1	70 92	1			12	458977XX

25. FEDERAL TAX I.D. NUMBER: 74 10640XX SSN [ ] EIN [X]

26. PATIENT'S ACCOUNT NO.: 010

27. ACCEPT ASSIGNMENT? (For govt. claims, see back) [X] YES [ ] NO

28. TOTAL CHARGE: $ 70 92

29. AMOUNT PAID: $

30. BALANCE DUE: $ 70 92

31. SIGNATURE OF PHYSICIAN OR SUPPLIER INCLUDING DEGREES OR CREDENTIALS (I certify that the statements on the reverse apply to this bill and are made a part thereof)
CONCHA ANTRUM MD 030320XX
SIGNED *Concha Antrum MD* DATE

32. NAME AND ADDRESS OF FACILITY WHERE SERVICECS WERE RENDERED (If other than home or office)
SAME

33. PHYSICIAN'S, SUPPLIER'S BILLING NAME, ADDRESS, ZIP CODE & PHONE #
COLLEGE CLINIC
4567 BROAD AVENUE
WOODLAND HILLS XY 12345 0001
555 486 9002
PIN# GRP# 3664021CC

reference initials

Figure D–3 Front side of the Health Insurance Claim Form (HCFA-1500) illustrated in red ink to comply with Optical Character Recognition (OCR) guidelines. This form is approved by the American Medical Association's Council on Medical Service. The illustration shown is for completion for a private insurance carrier with no secondary coverage. An initial examination was performed by Dr. Antrum at College Clinic for acute suppurative otitis media. The patient was referred by Dr. Cardi. Third party payer, state, and local guidelines vary and may not always follow the visual guide presented here.

BECAUSE THIS FORM IS USED BY VARIOUS GOVERNMENT AND PRIVATE HEALTH PROGRAMS, SEE SEPARATE INSTRUCTIONS ISSUED BY APPLICABLE PROGRAMS.

NOTICE: Any person who knowingly files a statement of claim containing any misrepresentation or any false, incomplete or misleading information may be guilty of a criminal act punishable under law and may be subject to civil penalties.

REFERS TO GOVERNMENT PROGRAMS ONLY

MEDICARE AND CHAMPUS PAYMENT: A patient's signature requests that payment be made and authorizes release of any information necessary to process the claim and certifies that the information provided in Blocks 1 through 12 is true, accurate and complete. In the case of a Medicare claim, the patient's signature authorizes any entity to release to Medicare medical and nonmedical information, including employment status, and whether the person has employer group health insurance, liability, no-fault, worker's compensation or other insurance which is responsible to pay for the services for which the Medicare claim is made. See 42 CFR 411.24(a). If item 9 is completed, the patient's signature authorizes release of the information to the health plan or agency shown. In Medicare assigned or CHAMPUS participation cases, the physician agrees to accept the charge determination of the Medicare carrier or CHAMPUS fiscal intermediary as the full charge determination of the Medicare carrier or CHAMPUS fiscal intermediary if this is less than the charge submitted. CHAMPUS is not a health insurance program but makes payment for health benefits provided through certain affiliations with the Uniformed Services. Information on the patient's sponsor should be provided in those items captioned in "Insured', i.e., items 1a, 4, 6, 7, 9, and 11.

BLACK LUNG AND FECA CLAIMS

The provider agrees to accept the amount paid by the Government as payment in full. See Black Lung and FECA instructions regarding required procedure and diagnosis coding systems.

SIGNATURE OF PHYSICIAN OR SUPPLIER (MEDICARE, CHAMPUS, FECA AND BLACK LUNG)

I certify that the services shown on this form were medically indicated and necessary for the health of the patient and were personally furnished by me or were furnished incident to my professional service by my employee under my immediate supervision, except as otherwise expressly permitted by Medicare or CHAMPUS regulations.

For services to be considered as "incident" to a physician's professional service, 1) they must be rendered under the physician's immediate personal supervision by his/her employee, 2) they must be an integral, although incidental part of a covered physician's service, 3) they must be of kinds commonly furnished in physician's offices, and 4) the services of nonphysicians must be included on the physician's bills.

For CHAMPUS claims, I further certify that I (or any employee) who rendered services am not an active duty member of the Uniformed Services or a civilian employee of the United States Government or a contract employee of the United States Government, either civilian or military (refer to 5 USC 5536). For Black-Lung claims, I further certify that the services performed were for a Black Lung-related disorder.

No Part B Medicare benefits may be paid unless this form is received as required by existing law and regulations (42 CFR 424.32).

NOTICE: Any one who misrepresents or falsifies essential information to receive payment from Federal funds requested by this form may upon conviction be subject to fine and imprisonment under applicable Federal laws.

NOTICE TO PATIENT ABOUT THE COLLECTION AND USE OF MEDICARE, CHAMPUS, FECA, AND BLACK LUNG INFORMATION

(PRIVACY ACT STATEMENT)

We are authorized by HCFA, CHAMPUS and OWCP to ask you for information needed in the administration of the Medicare, CHAMPUS, FECA, and Black Lung programs. Authority to collect information is in section 205(a), 1862, 1872 and 1874 of the Social Security Act as amended, 42 CFR411.24(a) and 424.5(a) (6), and 44 USC 3101; CFR 101 et seq and 10 USC 1079 and 1086; 5 USC 8101 et seq; and 30 USC 901 et seq; 38 USC 613; E.O. 9397.

The information we obtain to complete claims under these programs is used to identify you and to determine your eligibility. It is also used to decide if the services and supplies you received are covered by these programs and to insure that proper payment is made.

The information may also be given to other providers of services, carriers, intermediaries, medical review boards, health plans, and other organizations or Federal agencies, for the effective administration of Federal provisions that require other third parties payers to pay primary to Federal program, and as otherwise necessary to administer these programs. For example, it may be necessary to disclose information about the benefits you have used to a hospital or doctor. Additional disclosures are made through routine uses for information contained in systems of records.

FOR MEDICARE CLAIMS: See the notice modifying system No. 09-70-0501, titled 'Carrier Medicare Claims Record,' published in the Federal Register, Vol. 55 No. 177, page 37549, Wed., Sept. 12, 1990, or as updated and republished.

FOR OWCP CLAIMS: Department of Labor, Privacy Act of 1974, "Republication of Notice of Systems of Records," Federal Register, Vol. 55 No. 40, Wed., Feb. 28, 1990, See ESA-5, ESA-6, ESA-12, ESA-13, ESA-30, or as updated and republished.

FOR CHAMPUS CLAIMS: PRINCIPLE PURPOSE(S): To evaluate eligibility for medical care provided by civilian sources and to issue payment upon establishment of eligibility and determination that the services/supplies received are authorized by law.

ROUTINE USE(S): Information from claims and related documents may be given to the Dept. of Veterans Affairs, the Dept. of Health and Human Services and/or the Dept. of Transportation consistent with their statutory administrative responsibilities under CHAMPUS/CHAMPVA; to the Dept. of Justice for representation of the Secretary of Defense in civil actions; to the Internal Revenue Service, private collection agencies, and consumer reporting agencies in connection with recoupment claims; and to Congressional Offices in response to inquiries made at the request of the person to whom a record pertains. Appropriate disclosures may be made to other federal, state, local, foreign government agencies, private business entities, and individual providers of care, on matters relating to entitlement, claims adjudication, fraud, program abuse, utilization review, quality assurance, peer review, program integrity, third-party liability, coordination of benefits, and civil and criminal litigation related to the operation of CHAMPUS.

DISCLOSURES: Voluntary; however, failure to provide information will result in delay in payment or may result in denial of claim. With the one exception discussed below, there are no penalties under these programs for refusing to supply information. However, failure to furnish information regarding the medical services rendered or the amount charged would prevent payment of claims under these programs. Failure to furnish any other information, such as name or claim number, would delay payment of the claim. Failure to provide medical information under FECA could be deemed an obstruction.

It is mandatory that you tell us if you know that another party is responsible for paying for your treatment. Section 1128B of the Social Security Act and 31 USC 3801-3812 provide penalties for withholding this information.

You should be aware that P.L. 100-503, the "Computer Matching and Privacy Protection Act of 1988," permits the government to verify information by way of computer matches.

MEDICAID PAYMENTS (PROVIDER CERTIFICATION)

I hereby agree to keep such records as are necessary to disclose fully the extent of services provided to individuals under the State's Title XIX plan and to furnish information regarding any payments claimed for providing such services as the State Agency or Dept. of Health and Humans Services may request.

I further agree to accept, as payment in full, the amount paid by the Medicaid program for those claims submitted for payment under that program, with the exception of authorized deductible, coinsurance, co-payment or similar cost-sharing charge.

SIGNATURE OF PHYSICIAN (OR SUPPLIER): I certify that the services listed above were medically indicated and necessary to the health of this patient and were personally furnished by me or my employee under my personal direction.

NOTICE: This is to certify that the foregoing information is true, accurate and complete. I understand that payment and satisfaction of this claim will be from Federal and State funds, and that any false claims, statements, or documents, or concealment of a material fact, may be prosecuted under applicable Federal or State laws.

Public reporting burden for this collection of information is estimated to average 15 minutes per response, including time for reviewing instructions, searching existing date sources, gathering and maintaining data needed, and completing and reviewing the collection of information. Send comments regarding this burden estimate or any other aspect of this collection of information, including suggestions for reducing the burden, to HCFA, Office of Financial Management, P.O. Box 26684, Baltimore, MD 21207; and to the Office of Management and Budget, Paperwork Reduction Project (OMB-0938-0008), Washington, D.C. 20503.

Figure D–4 Back side of the Health Insurance Claim Form (HCFA-1500) showing various instructions for government programs, physician requirements, collection of information, record keeping, and so forth.

MEDICAID
No secondary coverage

MEDICAID FISCAL INTERMEDIARY NAME
MAILING ADDRESS
CITY STATE ZIP CODE

1. MEDICARE / MEDICAID / CHAMPUS / CHAMPVA / GROUP Health Plan / FECA BLK LUNG / OTHER — [ ] (Medicare #) [X] (Medicaid #) [ ] (Sponsor's SSN) [ ] (VA File #) [ ] (SSN or ID) [ ] (SSN) [ ] (ID)

1a. INSURED I.D. NUMBER (FOR PROGRAM IN ITEM 1): 276835090

2. PATIENT'S NAME (Last Name, First Name, Middle Initial): ABRAMSON ADAM

3. PATIENT'S BIRTH DATE MM DD YYYY: 02 12 1995 SEX M [X] F [ ]

4. INSURED'S NAME (LAST NAME, FIRST NAME, MIDDLE INITIAL)

5. PATIENT'S ADDRESS (No., Street): 760 FINCH STREET

6. PATIENT RELATIONSHIP TO INSURED: Self [ ] Spouse [ ] Child [ ] Other [ ]

7. INSURED'S ADDRESS (No, Street)

CITY: WOODLAND HILLS STATE: XY

8. PATIENT STATUS: Single [ ] Married [ ] Other [ ]; Employed [ ] Full-Time Student [ ] Part-Time Student [ ]

CITY STATE

ZIP CODE: 12345 TELEPHONE (Include Area Code): 555 482 6789

ZIP CODE TELEPHONE (INCLUDE AREA CODE) ( )

9. OTHER INSURED'S NAME (Last Name, First Name, Middle Initial)

10. IS PATIENT'S CONITION RELATED TO:

11. INSURED'S POLICY GROUP OR FECA NUMBER

a. OTHER INSURED'S POLICY OR GROUP NUMBER

a. EMPLOYMENT? (CURRENT OR PREVIOUS) [ ] YES [X] NO

a. INSURED'S DATE OF BIRTH MM DD YYYY SEX M [ ] F [ ]

b. OTHER INSURED'S DATE OF BIRTH MM DD YY SEX M [ ] F [ ]

b. AUTO ACCIDENT? [ ] YES [X] NO PLACE (State)

b. EMPLOYER'S NAME OR SCHOOL NAME

c. EMPLOYER'S NAME OR SCHOOL NAME

c. OTHER ACCIDENT? [X] YES [ ] NO

c. INSURANCE PLAN NAME OR PROGRAM NAME

d. INSURANCE PLAN NAME OR PROGRAM NAME

10d. RESERVED FOR LOCAL USE

d. IS THERE ANOTHER HEALTH BENEFIT PLAN? [ ] YES [ ] NO *If yes,* return to and complete item 9 a-d

READ BACK OF FORM BEFORE COMPLETING & SIGNING THIS FORM

12. PATIENT'S OR AUTHORIZED PERSON'S SIGNATURE. I authorize the release of any medical or other information necessary to process this claim. I also request payment of government benefits either to myself or to the party who accepts assignment below.

SIGNED ______ DATE ______

13. INSURED'S OR AUTHORIZED PERSON'S SIGNATURE. I authorize payment of medical benefits to the undersigned physician or supplier for services described below.

SIGNED ______

14. DATE OF CURRENT: MM DD YY — ILLNESS (First symptom) OR INJURY (Accident) OR PREGNANCY

15. IF PATIENT HAS HAD SAME OR SIMILAR ILLNESS GIVE FIRST DATE MM DD YYYY

16. DATES PATIENT UNABLE TO WORK IN CURRENT OCCUPATION FROM MM DD YYYY TO MM DD YYYY

17. NAME OF REFERRING PHYSICIAN OR OTHER SOURCE

17a. I.D. NUMBER OF REFERRING PHYSICIAN

18. HOSPITALIZATION DATES RELATED TO CURRENT SERVICES FROM MM DD YYYY TO MM DD YYYY

19. RESERVED FOR LOCAL USE

20. OUTSIDE LAB? [ ] YES [X] NO $ CHARGES

21. DIAGNOSIS OR NATURE OF ILLNESS OR INJURY. (RELATE ITEMS 1,2,3 OR 4 TO ITEM 24E BY LINE)

1. 931
2.
3.
4.

22. MEDICAID RESUBMISSION CODE — ORIGINAL REF. NO.

23. PRIOR AUTHORIZATION NUMBER

24. A DATE(S) OF SERVICE From MM DD YY	To MM DD YY	B Place of Service	C Type of Service	D PROCEDURES, SERVICES, OR SUPPLIES (Explain Unusual Circumstances) CPT/HCPCS	MODIFIER	E DIAGNOSIS CODE	F $ CHARGES	G DAYS OR UNITS	H EPSDT Family Plan	I EMG	J COB	K RESERVED FOR LOCAL USE
071420XX		23	1	99282		1	37 02	1			X	
071420XX		23	2	69200		1	49 93	1			X	

25. FEDERAL TAX I.D. NUMBER: 71 32061XX SSN [ ] EIN [X]

26. PATIENT'S ACCOUNT NO.: 030

27. ACCEPT ASSIGNMENT? (For govt. claims, see back) [X] YES [ ] NO

28. TOTAL CHARGE: $ 86 95

29. AMOUNT PAID: $

30. BALANCE DUE: $ 86 95

31. SIGNATURE OF PHYSICIAN OR SUPPLIER INCLUDING DEGREES OR CREDENTIALS (I certify that the statements on the reverse apply to this bill and are made a part thereof)
PEDRO ATRICS MD 071420XX
SIGNED DATE

32. NAME AND ADDRESS OF FACILITY WHERE SERVICECS WERE RENDERED (If other than home or office)
COLLEGE HOSPITAL
4500 BROAD AVENUE
WOODLAND HILLS XY 12345 0001
HSC 43700F

33. PHYSICIAN'S, SUPPLIER'S BILLING NAME, ADDRESS, ZIP CODE & PHONE #
COLLEGE CLINIC
4567 BROAD AVENUE
WOODLAND HILLS XY 12345 0001
555 486 9002
PIN# GRP# HSC12345F

reference initials

Figure D–5 Medicaid case with no secondary coverage emphasizing basic elements needed for filing a claim. The patient received services from Dr. Atrics in the emergency room of College Hospital for a foreign body in the ear.

MEDICARE
No secondary coverage

MEDICARE FISCAL INTERMEDIARY NAME
MAILING ADDRESS
CITY STATE ZIP CODE

1. MEDICARE [X] (Medicare #) MEDICAID [ ] (Medicaid #) CHAMPUS [ ] (Sponsor's SSN) CHAMPVA [ ] (VA File #) GROUP Health Plan [ ] (SSN or ID) FECA BLK LUNG [ ] (SSN) OTHER [ ] (ID)

1a. INSURED I.D. NUMBER (FOR PROGRAM IN ITEM 1): 123 45 6789A

2. PATIENT'S NAME (Last Name, First Name, Middle Initial): HUTCH BILL

3. PATIENT'S BIRTH DATE MM DD YYYY: 05 07 1910 SEX M [X] F [ ]

4. INSURED'S NAME (LAST NAME, FIRST NAME, MIDDLE INITIAL)

5. PATIENT'S ADDRESS (No., Street): 8888 MAIN STREET

6. PATIENT RELATIONSHIP TO INSURED: Self [ ] Spouse [ ] Child [ ] Other [ ]

7. INSURED'S ADDRESS (No, Street)

CITY: WOODLAND HILLS STATE: XY

8. PATIENT STATUS: Single [X] Married [ ] Other [ ]

CITY STATE

ZIP CODE: 12345 TELEPHONE (Include Area Code): 555) 732 1544

Employed [ ] Full-Time Student [ ] Part-Time Student [ ]

ZIP CODE TELEPHONE (INCLUDE AREA CODE) ( )

9. OTHER INSURED'S NAME (Last Name, First Name, Middle Initial)

10. IS PATIENT'S CONITION RELATED TO:

11. INSURED'S POLICY GROUP OR FECA NUMBER: NONE

a. OTHER INSURED'S POLICY OR GROUP NUMBER

a. EMPLOYMENT? (CURRENT OR PREVIOUS) [ ] YES [X] NO

a. INSURED'S DATE OF BIRTH MM DD YYYY SEX M [ ] F [ ]

b. OTHER INSURED'S DATE OF BIRTH MM DD YY SEX M [ ] F [ ]

b. AUTO ACCIDENT? [ ] YES [X] NO PLACE (State)

b. EMPLOYER'S NAME OR SCHOOL NAME

c. EMPLOYER'S NAME OR SCHOOL NAME

c. OTHER ACCIDENT? [ ] YES [X] NO

c. INSURANCE PLAN NAME OR PROGRAM NAME

d. INSURANCE PLAN NAME OR PROGRAM NAME

10d. RESERVED FOR LOCAL USE

d. IS THERE ANOTHER HEALTH BENEFIT PLAN? [ ] YES [ ] NO *If yes*, return to and complete item 9 a-d

READ BACK OF FORM BEFORE COMPLETING & SIGNING THIS FORM

12. PATIENT'S OR AUTHORIZED PERSON'S SIGNATURE. I authorize the release of any medical or other information necessary to process this claim. I also request payment of government benefits either to myself or to the party who accepts assignment below.

SIGNED SOF DATE

13. INSURED'S OR AUTHORIZED PERSON'S SIGNATURE. I authorize payment of medical benefits to the undersigned physician or supplier for services described below

SIGNED

14. DATE OF CURRENT: MM DD YY — ILLNESS (First symptom) OR INJURY (Accident) OR PREGNANCY

15. IF PATIENT HAS HAD SAME OR SIMILAR ILLNESS GIVE FIRST DATE MM DD YYYY

16. DATES PATIENT UNABLE TO WORK IN CURRENT OCCUPATION FROM MM DD YYYY TO MM DD YYYY

17. NAME OF REFERRING PHYSICIAN OR OTHER SOURCE: GERALD PRACTON MD

17a. I.D. NUMBER OF REFERRING PHYSICIAN: 46278897XX

18. HOSPITALIZATION DATES RELATED TO CURRENT SERVICES FROM MM DD YYYY TO MM DD YYYY

19. RESERVED FOR LOCAL USE

20. OUTSIDE LAB? [ ] YES [X] NO $ CHARGES

21. DIAGNOSIS OR NATURE OF ILLNESS OR INJURY. (RELATE ITEMS 1,2,3 OR 4 TO ITEM 24E BY LINE)

1. 487 . 0
2.
3.
4.

22. MEDICAID RESUBMISSION CODE ORIGINAL REF. NO.

23. PRIOR AUTHORIZATION NUMBER

24. A DATE(S) OF SERVICE From MM DD YY	To MM DD YY	B Place of Service	C Type of Service	D PROCEDURES, SERVICES, OR SUPPLIES (Explain Unusual Circumstances) CPT/HCPCS	MODIFIER	E DIAGNOSIS CODE	F $ CHARGES	G DAYS OR UNITS	H EPSDT Family Plan	I EMG	J COB	K RESERVED FOR LOCAL USE
031020XX		11		99205		1	132 28	1			64	211067XX

25. FEDERAL TAX I.D. NUMBER: 75 67321XX SSN [ ] EIN [X]

26. PATIENT'S ACCOUNT NO.: 040

27. ACCEPT ASSIGNMENT? (For govt. claims, see back) [X] YES [ ] NO

28. TOTAL CHARGE $ 132 28

29. AMOUNT PAID $

30. BALANCE DUE $

31. SIGNATURE OF PHYSICIAN OR SUPPLIER INCLUDING DEGREES OR CREDENTIALS (I certify that the statements on the reverse apply to this bill and are made a part thereof)
BRADY COCCIDIOIDES 031020XX
SIGNED DATE

32. NAME AND ADDRESS OF FACILITY WHERE SERVICECS WERE RENDERED (If other than home or office): SAME

33. PHYSICIAN'S, SUPPLIER'S BILLING NAME, ADDRESS, ZIP CODE & PHONE #
COLLEGE CLINIC
4567 BROAD AVENUE
WOODLAND HILLS XY 12345 0001
555 486 9002
PIN# GRP# 3664021CC

reference initials

Figure D–6 Medicare case with no secondary coverage. The patient is referred by Dr. Practon and seen as a new patient by Dr. Coccidioides at College Clinic for influenza with pneumonia. The physician has accepted assignment and the patient's signature is on file.

MEDICARE/MEDICAID
(primary) (secondary)
Crossover claim

MEDICAID FISCAL INTERMEDIARY NAME
MAILING ADDRESS
CITY STATE ZIP CODE

1. MEDICARE [X] (Medicare #) MEDICAID [X] (Medicaid #) CHAMPUS [ ] (Sponsor's SSN) CHAMPVA [ ] (VA File #) GROUP Health Plan [ ] (SSN or ID) FECA BLK LUNG [ ] (SSN) OTHER [ ] (ID)

1a. INSURED I.D. NUMBER (FOR PROGRAM IN ITEM 1)
660 46 2715A

2. PATIENT'S NAME (Last Name, First Name, Middle Initial)
JOHNSON KATHRYN

3. PATIENT'S BIRTH DATE MM DD YYYY 09 07 1937 SEX M [ ] F [X]

4. INSURED'S NAME (LAST NAME, FIRST NAME, MIDDLE INITIAL)

5. PATIENT'S ADDRESS (No., Street)
218 VEGA DRIVE

6. PATIENT RELATIONSHIP TO INSURED Self [ ] Spouse [ ] Child [ ] Other [ ]

7. INSURED'S ADDRESS (No, Street)

CITY WOODLAND HILLS STATE XY

8. PATIENT STATUS Single [ ] Married [X] Other [ ]
Employed [ ] Full-Time Student [ ] Part-Time Student [ ]

CITY STATE

ZIP CODE 12345 TELEPHONE (Include Area Code) 555) 482 9112

ZIP CODE TELEPHONE (INCLUDE AREA CODE) ( )

9. OTHER INSURED'S NAME (Last Name, First Name, Middle Initial)

10. IS PATIENT'S CONITION RELATED TO:

11. INSURED'S POLICY GROUP OR FECA NUMBER
NONE

a. OTHER INSURED'S POLICY OR GROUP NUMBER

a. EMPLOYMENT? (CURRENT OR PREVIOUS) [ ] YES [X] NO

a. INSURED'S DATE OF BIRTH MM DD YYYY SEX M [ ] F [ ]

b. OTHER INSURED'S DATE OF BIRTH MM DD YY SEX M [ ] F [ ]

b. AUTO ACCIDENT? [ ] YES [X] NO PLACE (State)

b. EMPLOYER'S NAME OR SCHOOL NAME

c. EMPLOYER'S NAME OR SCHOOL NAME

c. OTHER ACCIDENT? [ ] YES [X] NO

c. INSURANCE PLAN NAME OR PROGRAM NAME

d. INSURANCE PLAN NAME OR PROGRAM NAME

10d. RESERVED FOR LOCAL USE
MCD016745289

d. IS THERE ANOTHER HEALTH BENEFIT PLAN? [ ] YES [ ] NO *If yes,* return to and complete item 9 a-d

READ BACK OF FORM BEFORE COMPLETING & SIGNING THIS FORM

12. PATIENT'S OR AUTHORIZED PERSON'S SIGNATURE. I authorize the release of any medical or other information necessary to process this claim. I also request payment of government benefits either to myself or to the party who accepts assignment below.

SIGNED Kathryn Johnson DATE 10/1/xx

13. INSURED'S OR AUTHORIZED PERSON'S SIGNATURE. I authorize payment of medical benefits to the undersigned physician or supplier for services described below

SIGNED

14. DATE OF CURRENT: MM DD YY ILLNESS (First symptom) OR INJURY (Accident) OR PREGNANCY

15. IF PATIENT HAS HAD SAME OR SIMILAR ILLNESS GIVE FIRST DATE MM DD YYYY

16. DATES PATIENT UNABLE TO WORK IN CURRENT OCCUPATION FROM MM DD YYYY TO MM DD YYYY

17. NAME OF REFERRING PHYSICIAN OR OTHER SOURCE
BRADY COCCIDIOIDES MD

17a. I.D. NUMBER OF REFERRING PHYSICIAN
64211067XX

18. HOSPITALIZATION DATES RELATED TO CURRENT SERVICES FROM MM DD YYYY TO MM DD YYYY

19. RESERVED FOR LOCAL USE

20. OUTSIDE LAB? [ ] YES [X] NO $ CHARGES

21. DIAGNOSIS OR NATURE OF ILLNESS OR INJURY. (RELATE ITEMS 1,2,3 OR 4 TO ITEM 24E BY LINE)

1. 172 . 7
2.
3.
4.

22. MEDICAID RESUBMISSION CODE ORIGINAL REF. NO.

23. PRIOR AUTHORIZATION NUMBER
7680560012

24. A DATE(S) OF SERVICE From MM DD YY	To MM DD YY	B Place of Service	C Type of Service	D PROCEDURES, SERVICES, OR SUPPLIES (Explain Unusual Circumstances) CPT/HCPCS	MODIFIER	E DIAGNOSIS CODE	F $ CHARGES	G DAYS OR UNITS	H EPSDT Family Plan	I EMG	J COB	K RESERVED FOR LOCAL USE
101220XX		24		11600		1	195 06	1			50	307117XX

25. FEDERAL TAX I.D. NUMBER SSN EIN
74 60789XX [ ] [X]

26. PATIENT'S ACCOUNT NO.
050

27. ACCEPT ASSIGNMENT? (For govt. claims, see back) [X] YES [ ] NO

28. TOTAL CHARGE $ 195 06

29. AMOUNT PAID $

30. BALANCE DUE $

31. SIGNATURE OF PHYSICIAN OR SUPPLIER INCLUDING DEGREES OR CREDENTIALS (I certify that the statements on the reverse apply to this bill and are made a part thereof)
COSMO GRAFF MD 100320XX
SIGNED Cosmo Graff MD DATE

32. NAME AND ADDRESS OF FACILITY WHERE SERVICECS WERE RENDERED (If other than home or office)
WOODLAND HILLS AMBULATORY CENTER
1229 CENTER STREET
WOODLAND HILLS XY 12345 0001
HSP 54321F

33. PHYSICIAN'S, SUPPLIER'S BILLING NAME, ADDRESS, ZIP CODE & PHONE #
COLLEGE CLINIC
4567 BROAD AVENUE
WOODLAND HILLS XY 12345 0001
555 486 9002
PIN# GRP# 3664021CC

reference initials

Figure D–7 Medicare claim completed for crossover to Medicaid (Medicare primary, Medicaid secondary payer). The patient is referred by Dr. Coccidioides to Dr. Graff, who performs an excision of a malignant lesion on the lower limb. The procedure takes place at Woodland Hills Ambulatory Center.

MEDICARE/MEDICAID
(primary) (secondary)
Crossover claim

MEDICARE FISCAL INTERMEDIARY NAME
MAILING ADDRESS
CITY STATE ZIP CODE

1. MEDICARE [X] (Medicare #) MEDICAID [ ] (Medicaid #) CHAMPUS [ ] (Sponsor's SSN) CHAMPVA [ ] (VA File #) GROUP Health Plan [X] (SSN or ID) FECA BLK LUNG [ ] (SSN) OTHER [ ] (ID)

1a. INSURED I.D. NUMBER (FOR PROGRAM IN ITEM 1)
419 16 7272A

2. PATIENT'S NAME (Last Name, First Name, Middle Initial)
BARNES AGUSTA E

3. PATIENT'S BIRTH DATE MM DD YYYY 09 07 1917 SEX M [X] F [ ]

4. INSURED'S NAME (LAST NAME, FIRST NAME, MIDDLE INITIAL)

5. PATIENT'S ADDRESS (No., Street)
356 ENCINA AVENUE

6. PATIENT RELATIONSHIP TO INSURED Self [ ] Spouse [ ] Child [ ] Other [ ]

7. INSURED'S ADDRESS (No, Street)

CITY WOODLAND HILLS STATE XY

8. PATIENT STATUS Single [X] Married [ ] Other [ ]
Employed [ ] Full-Time Student [ ] Part-Time Student [ ]

CITY STATE

ZIP CODE 12345 0000 TELEPHONE (Include Area Code) 555) 467 2646

ZIP CODE TELEPHONE (INCLUDE AREA CODE) ( )

9. OTHER INSURED'S NAME (Last Name, First Name, Middle Initial)
SAME

10. IS PATIENT'S CONITION RELATED TO:

11. INSURED'S POLICY GROUP OR FECA NUMBER
NONE

a. OTHER INSURED'S POLICY OR GROUP NUMBER
MEDIGAP 419167272

a. EMPLOYMENT? (CURRENT OR PREVIOUS) [ ] YES [X] NO

a. INSURED'S DATE OF BIRTH MM DD YYYY SEX M [ ] F [ ]

b. OTHER INSURED'S DATE OF BIRTH MM DD YY SEX M [ ] F [ ]

b. AUTO ACCIDENT? [ ] YES [X] NO PLACE (State)

b. EMPLOYER'S NAME OR SCHOOL NAME

c. EMPLOYER'S NAME OR SCHOOL NAME

c. OTHER ACCIDENT? [ ] YES [X] NO

c. INSURANCE PLAN NAME OR PROGRAM NAME

d. INSURANCE PLAN NAME OR PROGRAM NAME
CALFCA002

10d. RESERVED FOR LOCAL USE

d. IS THERE ANOTHER HEALTH BENEFIT PLAN? [ ] YES [ ] NO *If yes*, return to and complete item 9 a-d

READ BACK OF FORM BEFORE COMPLETING & SIGNING THIS FORM

12. PATIENT'S OR AUTHORIZED PERSON'S SIGNATURE. I authorize the release of any medical or other information necessary to process this claim. I also request payment of government benefits either to myself or to the party who accepts assignment below.

SIGNED Agusta Barnes DATE 11/21/xx

13. INSURED'S OR AUTHORIZED PERSON'S SIGNATURE. I authorize payment of medical benefits to the undersigned physician or supplier for services described below

SIGNED Agusta Barnes

14. DATE OF CURRENT: MM DD YY ILLNESS (First symptom) OR INJURY (Accident) OR PREGNANCY

15. IF PATIENT HAS HAD SAME OR SIMILAR ILLNESS GIVE FIRST DATE MM DD YYYY

16. DATES PATIENT UNABLE TO WORK IN CURRENT OCCUPATION FROM MM DD YYYY TO MM DD YYYY

17. NAME OF REFERRING PHYSICIAN OR OTHER SOURCE
GASTON INPUT MD

17a. I.D. NUMBER OF REFERRING PHYSICIAN
32783127XX

18. HOSPITALIZATION DATES RELATED TO CURRENT SERVICES FROM MM DD YYYY TO MM DD YYYY

19. RESERVED FOR LOCAL USE

20. OUTSIDE LAB? [ ] YES [X] NO $ CHARGES

21. DIAGNOSIS OR NATURE OF ILLNESS OR INJURY. (RELATE ITEMS 1,2,3 OR 4 TO ITEM 24E BY LINE)
1. 786 59
2.
3.
4.

22. MEDICAID RESUBMISSION CODE ORIGINAL REF. NO.

23. PRIOR AUTHORIZATION NUMBER

24. A DATE(S) OF SERVICE From MM DD YY	To MM DD YY	B Place of Service	C Type of Service	D PROCEDURES, SERVICES, OR SUPPLIES (Explain Unusual Circumstances) CPT/HCPCS	MODIFIER	E DIAGNOSIS CODE	F $ CHARGES	G DAYS OR UNITS	H EPSDT Family Plan	I EMG	J COB	K RESERVED FOR LOCAL USE
112120XX		11		93350		1	183 31	1			67	805027XX
112120XX		11		93017		1	68 90	1			67	805027XX

25. FEDERAL TAX I.D. NUMBER 70 64217XX SSN [ ] EIN [X]

26. PATIENT'S ACCOUNT NO. 060

27. ACCEPT ASSIGNMENT? (For govt. claims, see back) [X] YES [ ] NO

28. TOTAL CHARGE $ 252 21

29. AMOUNT PAID $

30. BALANCE DUE $

31. SIGNATURE OF PHYSICIAN OR SUPPLIER INCLUDING DEGREES OR CREDENTIALS (I certify that the statements on the reverse apply to this bill and are made a part thereof)
PERRY CARDI MD 112220XX
SIGNED Perry Cardi M.D. DATE

32. NAME AND ADDRESS OF FACILITY WHERE SERVICECS WERE RENDERED (If other than home or office)
SAME

33. PHYSICIAN'S, SUPPLIER'S BILLING NAME, ADDRESS, ZIP CODE & PHONE #
COLLEGE CLINIC
4567 BROAD AVENUE
WOODLAND HILLS XY 12345 0001
555 486 9002
PIN# GRP# 3664021CC

reference initials

Figure D–8 Medicare claim completed for crossover to a Medigap insurance carrier (Medicare primary, Medigap secondary payer). Dr. Input refers the patient to Dr. Cardi, who performs a 2D echocardiogram and cardiovascular stress test (tracing only) for tightness and pressure in the patient's chest.

OTHER INSURANCE/MEDICARE-MSP
(primary) (secondary)

OTHER INSURANCE COMPANY NAME
MAILING ADDRESS
CITY STATE ZIP CODE

1. MEDICARE [X] (Medicare #) MEDICAID [ ] (Medicaid #) CHAMPUS [ ] (Sponsor's SSN) CHAMPVA [ ] (VA File #) GROUP Health Plan [X] (SSN or ID) FECA BLK LUNG [ ] (SSN) OTHER [ ] (ID)

1a. INSURED I.D. NUMBER (FOR PROGRAM IN ITEM 1): 609 24 5523A

2. PATIENT'S NAME (Last Name, First Name, Middle Initial): BLAIR GWENDOLYN

3. PATIENT'S BIRTH DATE MM DD YYYY: 09 01 1931 SEX M [ ] F [X]

4. INSURED'S NAME (LAST NAME, FIRST NAME, MIDDLE INITIAL): BLAIR GWENDOLYN

5. PATIENT'S ADDRESS (No., Street): 416 RICHMOND STREET

6. PATIENT RELATIONSHIP TO INSURED: Self [X] Spouse [ ] Child [ ] Other [ ]

7. INSURED'S ADDRESS (No, Street): SAME

CITY: WOODLAND HILLS STATE: XY

8. PATIENT STATUS: Single [ ] Married [X] Other [ ]; Employed [X] Full-Time Student [ ] Part-Time Student [ ]

CITY STATE

ZIP CODE: 12345 0000 TELEPHONE (Include Area Code): 555) 459 1519

ZIP CODE TELEPHONE (INCLUDE AREA CODE) ( )

9. OTHER INSURED'S NAME (Last Name, First Name, Middle Initial)

a. OTHER INSURED'S POLICY OR GROUP NUMBER

b. OTHER INSURED'S DATE OF BIRTH MM DD YY SEX M [ ] F [ ]

c. EMPLOYER'S NAME OR SCHOOL NAME

d. INSURANCE PLAN NAME OR PROGRAM NAME

10. IS PATIENT'S CONITION RELATED TO:

a. EMPLOYMENT? (CURRENT OR PREVIOUS) [ ] YES [X] NO

b. AUTO ACCIDENT? [ ] YES [X] NO PLACE (State)

c. OTHER ACCIDENT? [ ] YES [X] NO

10d. RESERVED FOR LOCAL USE

11. INSURED'S POLICY GROUP OR FECA NUMBER: 7845931Q

a. INSURED'S DATE OF BIRTH MM DD YYYY SEX M [ ] F [ ]

b. EMPLOYER'S NAME OR SCHOOL NAME: CITY LIBRARY

c. INSURANCE PLAN NAME OR PROGRAM NAME: ABC INSURANCE COMPANY

d. IS THERE ANOTHER HEALTH BENEFIT PLAN? [ ] YES [ ] NO *If yes,* return to and complete item 9 a-d

READ BACK OF FORM BEFORE COMPLETING & SIGNING THIS FORM

12. PATIENT'S OR AUTHORIZED PERSON'S SIGNATURE. I authorize the release of any medical or other information necessary to process this claim. I also request payment of government benefits either to myself or to the party who accepts assignment below.

SIGNED SOF DATE

13. INSURED'S OR AUTHORIZED PERSON'S SIGNATURE. I authorize payment of medical benefits to the undersigned physician or supplier for services described below

SIGNED SOF

14. DATE OF CURRENT: MM DD YY ILLNESS (First symptom) OR INJURY (Accident) OR PREGNANCY

15. IF PATIENT HAS HAD SAME OR SIMILAR ILLNESS GIVE FIRST DATE MM DD YYYY

16. DATES PATIENT UNABLE TO WORK IN CURRENT OCCUPATION FROM MM DD YYYY TO MM DD YYYY

17. NAME OF REFERRING PHYSICIAN OR OTHER SOURCE: GERALD PRACTON MD

17a. I.D. NUMBER OF REFERRING PHYSICIAN: 46278897XX

18. HOSPITALIZATION DATES RELATED TO CURRENT SERVICES FROM MM DD YYYY TO MM DD YYYY

19. RESERVED FOR LOCAL USE

20. OUTSIDE LAB? [ ] YES [X] NO $ CHARGES

21. DIAGNOSIS OR NATURE OF ILLNESS OR INJURY. (RELATE ITEMS 1,2,3 OR 4 TO ITEM 24E BY LINE)

1. 110 1
2.
3.
4.

22. MEDICAID RESUBMISSION CODE ORIGINAL REF. NO.

23. PRIOR AUTHORIZATION NUMBER

24. A DATE(S) OF SERVICE From MM DD YY	To MM DD YY	B Place of Service	C Type of Service	D PROCEDURES, SERVICES, OR SUPPLIES (Explain Unusual Circumstances) CPT/HCPCS	MODIFIER	E DIAGNOSIS CODE	F $ CHARGES	G DAYS OR UNITS	H EPSDT Family Plan	I EMG	J COB	K RESERVED FOR LOCAL USE
031520XX		11		99243	25	1	103 51	1			54	022287XX
031520XX		11		11750		1	193 45	1			54	022287XX

25. FEDERAL TAX I.D. NUMBER: 62 74109XX SSN [ ] EIN [X]

26. PATIENT'S ACCOUNT NO.: 070

27. ACCEPT ASSIGNMENT? (For govt. claims, see back) [X] YES [ ] NO

28. TOTAL CHARGE: $ 296 96

29. AMOUNT PAID: $ 100 00

30. BALANCE DUE: $

31. SIGNATURE OF PHYSICIAN OR SUPPLIER INCLUDING DEGREES OR CREDENTIALS (I certify that the statements on the reverse apply to this bill and are made a part thereof)

NICK PEDRO DPM 031620XX

SIGNED Nick Pedro DPM DATE

32. NAME AND ADDRESS OF FACILITY WHERE SERVICECS WERE RENDERED (If other than home or office): SAME

33. PHYSICIAN'S, SUPPLIER'S BILLING NAME, ADDRESS, ZIP CODE & PHONE #
COLLEGE CLINIC
4567 BROAD AVENUE
WOODLAND HILLS XY 12345 0001
555 486 9002
PIN# GRP# 3664021CC

reference initials

Figure D–9 Template for a case in which a private insurance carrier (ABC Insurance Company) is primary and Medicare is the secondary payer (MSP). Dr. Practon has referred the patient to Dr. Pedro for an office consultation at College Clinic. Dr. Pedro performs a partial excision of nail matrix for onychomycosis at the same session.

TRICARE
No seconday coverage

TRICARE FISCAL INTERMEDIARY
MAILING ADDRESS
CITY STATE ZIP CODE

1. MEDICARE (Medicare #) ☐ MEDICAID (Medicaid #) ☐ CHAMPUS (Sponsor's SSN) ☒ CHAMPVA (VA File #) ☐ GROUP Health Plan (SSN or ID) ☐ FECA BLK LUNG (SSN) ☐ OTHER (ID) ☐

1a. INSURED I.D. NUMBER (FOR PROGRAM IN ITEM 1): 581147211

2. PATIENT'S NAME (Last Name, First Name, Middle Initial): SMITH SUSAN J

3. PATIENT'S BIRTH DATE (MM DD YYYY): 03 16 1976 SEX M ☐ F ☒

4. INSURED'S NAME (LAST NAME, FIRST NAME, MIDDLE INITIAL): SMITH WILLIAM D

5. PATIENT'S ADDRESS (No., Street): 420 MAPLE STREET

6. PATIENT RELATIONSHIP TO INSURED: Self ☐ Spouse ☒ Child ☐ Other ☐

7. INSURED'S ADDRESS (No, Street): SAME

CITY: WOODLAND HILLS STATE: XY

8. PATIENT STATUS: Single ☐ Married ☒ Other ☐; Employed ☐ Full-Time Student ☐ Part-Time Student ☐

CITY: STATE:

ZIP CODE: 12345 0000 TELEPHONE (Include Area Code): 555) 789 9698

ZIP CODE: TELEPHONE (INCLUDE AREA CODE): ( )

9. OTHER INSURED'S NAME (Last Name, First Name, Middle Initial)

a. OTHER INSURED'S POLICY OR GROUP NUMBER

b. OTHER INSURED'S DATE OF BIRTH MM DD YY SEX M ☐ F ☐

c. EMPLOYER'S NAME OR SCHOOL NAME

d. INSURANCE PLAN NAME OR PROGRAM NAME

10. IS PATIENT'S CONITION RELATED TO:

a. EMPLOYMENT? (CURRENT OR PREVIOUS) ☐ YES ☒ NO

b. AUTO ACCIDENT? ☐ YES ☒ NO PLACE (State)

c. OTHER ACCIDENT? ☐ YES ☒ NO

10d. RESERVED FOR LOCAL USE

11. INSURED'S POLICY GROUP OR FECA NUMBER

a. INSURED'S DATE OF BIRTH (MM DD YYYY): 06 12 1974 SEX M ☒ F ☐

b. EMPLOYER'S NAME OR SCHOOL NAME: USN

c. INSURANCE PLAN NAME OR PROGRAM NAME: TRICARE/CHAMPUS

d. IS THERE ANOTHER HEALTH BENEFIT PLAN? ☐ YES ☒ NO *If yes*, return to and complete item 9 a-d

READ BACK OF FORM BEFORE COMPLETING & SIGNING THIS FORM

12. PATIENT'S OR AUTHORIZED PERSON'S SIGNATURE. I authorize the release of any medical or other information necessary to process this claim. I also request payment of government benefits either to myself or to the party who accepts assignment below.

SIGNED SOF DATE

13. INSURED'S OR AUTHORIZED PERSON'S SIGNATURE. I authorize payment of medical benefits to the undersigned physician or supplier for services described below

SIGNED

14. DATE OF CURRENT: ILLNESS (First symptom) OR INJURY (Accident) OR PREGNANCY (MM DD YY): 06 28 20XX

15. IF PATIENT HAS HAD SAME OR SIMILAR ILLNESS GIVE FIRST DATE MM DD YYYY

16. DATES PATIENT UNABLE TO WORK IN CURRENT OCCUPATION FROM 07 21 20XX TO 09 17 20XX

17. NAME OF REFERRING PHYSICIAN OR OTHER SOURCE: ADAM LANGERHANS MD

17a. I.D. NUMBER OF REFERRING PHYSICIAN: G05783X

18. HOSPITALIZATION DATES RELATED TO CURRENT SERVICES FROM 07 21 20XX TO 09 17 20XX

19. RESERVED FOR LOCAL USE

20. OUTSIDE LAB? ☐ YES ☒ NO $ CHARGES

21. DIAGNOSIS OR NATURE OF ILLNESS OR INJURY. (RELATE ITEMS 1,2,3 OR 4 TO ITEM 24E BY LINE)

1. 650
2.
3.
4.

22. MEDICAID RESUBMISSION CODE ORIGINAL REF. NO.

23. PRIOR AUTHORIZATION NUMBER

24. A DATE(S) OF SERVICE From MM DD YY	To MM DD YY	B Place of Service	C Type of Service	D PROCEDURES, SERVICES, OR SUPPLIES (Explain Unusual Circumstances) CPT/HCPCS	MODIFIER	E DIAGNOSIS CODE	F $ CHARGES	G DAYS OR UNITS	H EPSDT Family Plan	I EMG	J COB	K RESERVED FOR LOCAL USE
062820XX		21	1	59400		1	1864 30	1				AO1817X

25. FEDERAL TAX I.D. NUMBER: 72 57130XX SSN ☐ EIN ☒

26. PATIENT'S ACCOUNT NO.: 080

27. ACCEPT ASSIGNMENT? (For govt. claims, see back) ☒ YES ☐ NO

28. TOTAL CHARGE: $ 1864 30

29. AMOUNT PAID: $

30. BALANCE DUE: $ 1864 30

31. SIGNATURE OF PHYSICIAN OR SUPPLIER INCLUDING DEGREES OR CREDENTIALS (I certify that the statements on the reverse apply to this bill and are made a part thereof)
BERTHA CAESAR MD 081020XX
SIGNED Bertha Caesar MD DATE

32. NAME AND ADDRESS OF FACILITY WHERE SERVICECS WERE RENDERED (If other than home or office)
COLLEGE HOSPITAL
4500 BROAD AVENUE
WOODLAND HILLS XY 12345 0001
95 0731067

33. PHYSICIAN'S, SUPPLIER'S BILLING NAME, ADDRESS, ZIP CODE & PHONE #
COLLEGE CLINIC
4567 BROAD AVENUE
WOODLAND HILLS XY 12345 0001
555 486 9002
PIN# 72 57130XX GRP#

reference initials

Figure D-10 TRICARE Standard claim with no secondary coverage. The patient is referred by Dr. Langerhans to Dr. Caesar, who follows the patient during pregnancy and performs a normal vaginal delivery at College Hospital. The patient is disabled and unable to work from July 21, 20XX to September 17, 20XX.

CHAMPVA
No secondary coverage

CHAMPVA INSURANCE COMPANY NAME
MAILING ADDRESS
CITY STATE ZIP CODE

1. MEDICARE (Medicare #) [ ] MEDICAID (Medicaid #) [ ] CHAMPUS (Sponsor's SSN) [ ] CHAMPVA (VA File #) [X] GROUP Health Plan (SSN or ID) [ ] FECA BLK LUNG (SSN) [ ] OTHER (ID) [ ]

1a. INSURED I.D. NUMBER (FOR PROGRAM IN ITEM 1): 560 12 4444

2. PATIENT'S NAME (Last Name, First Name, Middle Initial): DEXTER BRUCE R

3. PATIENT'S BIRTH DATE (MM DD YYYY): 03 13 1934 SEX: M [X] F [ ]

4. INSURED'S NAME (LAST NAME, FIRST NAME, MIDDLE INITIAL): DEXTER BRUCE R

5. PATIENT'S ADDRESS (No., Street): 226 IRWIN ROAD

6. PATIENT RELATIONSHIP TO INSURED: Self [X] Spouse [ ] Child [ ] Other [ ]

7. INSURED'S ADDRESS (No, Street): SAME

CITY: WOODLAND HILLS STATE: XY

8. PATIENT STATUS: Single [X] Married [ ] Other [ ]; Employed [ ] Full-Time Student [ ] Part-Time Student [ ]

CITY: STATE: XY

ZIP CODE: 12345 0000 TELEPHONE (Include Area Code): 555) 497 1338

ZIP CODE: TELEPHONE (INCLUDE AREA CODE): ( )

9. OTHER INSURED'S NAME (Last Name, First Name, Middle Initial)

a. OTHER INSURED'S POLICY OR GROUP NUMBER

b. OTHER INSURED'S DATE OF BIRTH (MM DD YY) SEX M [ ] F [ ]

c. EMPLOYER'S NAME OR SCHOOL NAME

d. INSURANCE PLAN NAME OR PROGRAM NAME

10. IS PATIENT'S CONITION RELATED TO:

a. EMPLOYMENT? (CURRENT OR PREVIOUS) [X] YES [ ] NO

b. AUTO ACCIDENT? [ ] YES [X] NO PLACE (State)

c. OTHER ACCIDENT? [ ] YES [X] NO

10d. RESERVED FOR LOCAL USE

11. INSURED'S POLICY GROUP OR FECA NUMBER: 023

a. INSURED'S DATE OF BIRTH (MM DD YYYY) SEX M [ ] F [ ]

b. EMPLOYER'S NAME OR SCHOOL NAME: USAF

c. INSURANCE PLAN NAME OR PROGRAM NAME

d. IS THERE ANOTHER HEALTH BENEFIT PLAN? [ ] YES [X] NO *If yes,* return to and complete item 9 a-d

READ BACK OF FORM BEFORE COMPLETING & SIGNING THIS FORM

12. PATIENT'S OR AUTHORIZED PERSON'S SIGNATURE. I authorize the release of any medical or other information necessary to process this claim. I also request payment of government benefits either to myself or to the party who accepts assignment below.

SIGNED SOF DATE

13. INSURED'S OR AUTHORIZED PERSON'S SIGNATURE. I authorize payment of medical benefits to the undersigned physician or supplier for services described below

SIGNED

14. DATE OF CURRENT: (MM DD YY) ILLNESS (First symptom) OR INJURY (Accident) OR PREGNANCY

15. IF PATIENT HAS HAD SAME OR SIMILAR ILLNESS GIVE FIRST DATE (MM DD YYYY)

16. DATES PATIENT UNABLE TO WORK IN CURRENT OCCUPATION: FROM 07 29 20XX TO 07 31 20XX

17. NAME OF REFERRING PHYSICIAN OR OTHER SOURCE: GERALD PRACTON MD

17a. I.D. NUMBER OF REFERRING PHYSICIAN: C01402X

18. HOSPITALIZATION DATES RELATED TO CURRENT SERVICES: FROM TO

19. RESERVED FOR LOCAL USE

20. OUTSIDE LAB? [ ] YES [X] NO $ CHARGES

21. DIAGNOSIS OR NATURE OF ILLNESS OR INJURY. (RELATE ITEMS 1,2,3 OR 4 TO ITEM 24E BY LINE)

1. 600 0
2.
3.
4.

22. MEDICAID RESUBMISSION CODE ORIGINAL REF. NO.

23. PRIOR AUTHORIZATION NUMBER

24. A DATE(S) OF SERVICE From MM DD YY	To MM DD YY	B Place of Service	C Type of Service	D PROCEDURES, SERVICES, OR SUPPLIES (Explain Unusual Circumstances) CPT/HCPCS	MODIFIER	E DIAGNOSIS CODE	F $ CHARGES	G DAYS OR UNITS	H EPSDT Family Plan	I EMG	J COB	K RESERVED FOR LOCAL USE
072920XX		21	2	52601		1	1193 53	1				C06430X

25. FEDERAL TAX I.D. NUMBER: 77 86531XX SSN [ ] EIN [X]

26. PATIENT'S ACCOUNT NO.: 090

27. ACCEPT ASSIGNMENT? (For govt. claims, see back) [ ] YES [ ] NO

28. TOTAL CHARGE: $ 1193 53

29. AMOUNT PAID: $

30. BALANCE DUE: $ 1193 53

31. SIGNATURE OF PHYSICIAN OR SUPPLIER INCLUDING DEGREES OR CREDENTIALS (I certify that the statements on the reverse apply to this bill and are made a part thereof)
GENE ULIBARRI MD 073020XX
SIGNED *Gene Ulibarri MD* DATE

32. NAME AND ADDRESS OF FACILITY WHERE SERVICECS WERE RENDERED (If other than home or office)
COLLEGE HOSPITAL
4500 BROAD AVENUE
WOODLAND HILLS XY 12345 0001
95 0731067

33. PHYSICIAN'S, SUPPLIER'S BILLING NAME, ADDRESS, ZIP CODE & PHONE #
COLLEGE CLINIC
4567 BROAD AVENUE
WOODLAND HILLS XY 12345 0001
555 486 9002
PIN# 77 86531XX GRP#

reference initials

Figure D–11 CHAMPVA claim with no secondary coverage. Dr. Practon has referred the patient to Dr. Ulibarri, who performs a transurethral resection of the prostate gland at College Hospital for benign prostatic hypertrophy. The patient is hospitalized from July 29, 20XX through July 31, 20XX.

WORKERS' COMPENSATION

WORKERS' COMPENSATION INSURANCE COMPANY NAME
MAILING ADDRESS
CITY STATE ZIP CODE

1. MEDICARE (Medicare #) MEDICAID (Medicaid #) CHAMPUS (Sponsor's SSN) CHAMPVA (VA File #) GROUP Health Plan (SSN or ID) FECA BLK LUNG (SSN) OTHER [X] (ID)

1a. INSURED I.D. NUMBER (FOR PROGRAM IN ITEM 1): 667289

2. PATIENT'S NAME (Last Name, First Name, Middle Initial): BARTON PETER A

3. PATIENT'S BIRTH DATE MM DD YYYY: 01 14 1976 SEX M [X] F [ ]

4. INSURED'S NAME (LAST NAME, FIRST NAME, MIDDLE INITIAL): D F CONSTRUCTION

5. PATIENT'S ADDRESS (No., Street): 14890 DAISY AVENUE

6. PATIENT RELATIONSHIP TO INSURED: Self [ ] Spouse [ ] Child [ ] Other [X]

7. INSURED'S ADDRESS (No, Street): 1212 HARDROCK PLACE

CITY: WOODLAND HILLS STATE: XY

8. PATIENT STATUS: Single [ ] Married [ ] Other [ ]

CITY: WOODLAND HILLS STATE: XY

ZIP CODE: 12345 0000 TELEPHONE (Include Area Code): 555) 427 7698

Employed [X] Full-Time Student [ ] Part-Time Student [ ]

ZIP CODE: 12345 0000 TELEPHONE (INCLUDE AREA CODE): 555) 427 8200

9. OTHER INSURED'S NAME (Last Name, First Name, Middle Initial)

10. IS PATIENT'S CONITION RELATED TO:

11. INSURED'S POLICY GROUP OR FECA NUMBER

a. OTHER INSURED'S POLICY OR GROUP NUMBER

a. EMPLOYMENT? (CURRENT OR PREVIOUS) [X] YES [ ] NO

a. INSURED'S DATE OF BIRTH MM DD YYYY SEX M [ ] F [ ]

b. OTHER INSURED'S DATE OF BIRTH MM DD YY SEX M [ ] F [ ]

b. AUTO ACCIDENT? [ ] YES [X] NO PLACE (State)

b. EMPLOYER'S NAME OR SCHOOL NAME

c. EMPLOYER'S NAME OR SCHOOL NAME

c. OTHER ACCIDENT? [ ] YES [X] NO

c. INSURANCE PLAN NAME OR PROGRAM NAME

d. INSURANCE PLAN NAME OR PROGRAM NAME

10d. RESERVED FOR LOCAL USE

d. IS THERE ANOTHER HEALTH BENEFIT PLAN? [ ] YES [ ] NO *If yes,* return to and complete item 9 a-d

READ BACK OF FORM BEFORE COMPLETING & SIGNING THIS FORM

12. PATIENT'S OR AUTHORIZED PERSON'S SIGNATURE. I authorize the release of any medical or other information necessary to process this claim. I also request payment of government benefits either to myself or to the party who accepts assignment below.

SIGNED ______ DATE ______

13. INSURED'S OR AUTHORIZED PERSON'S SIGNATURE. I authorize payment of medical benefits to the undersigned physician or supplier for services described below

SIGNED ______

14. DATE OF CURRENT: MM DD YY 01 04 20XX ILLNESS (First symptom) OR INJURY (Accident) OR PREGNANCY

15. IF PATIENT HAS HAD SAME OR SIMILAR ILLNESS GIVE FIRST DATE MM DD YYYY

16. DATES PATIENT UNABLE TO WORK IN CURRENT OCCUPATION MM DD YYYY FROM 01 04 20XX TO 03 27 20XX

17. NAME OF REFERRING PHYSICIAN OR OTHER SOURCE

17a. I.D. NUMBER OF REFERRING PHYSICIAN

18. HOSPITALIZATION DATES RELATED TO CURRENT SERVICES MM DD YYYY FROM TO

19. RESERVED FOR LOCAL USE

20. OUTSIDE LAB? [ ] YES [ ] NO $ CHARGES

21. DIAGNOSIS OR NATURE OF ILLNESS OR INJURY. (RELATE ITEMS 1,2,3 OR 4 TO ITEM 24E BY LINE)

1. 718 31
2. ___
3. ___
4. ___

22. MEDICAID RESUBMISSION CODE ORIGINAL REF. NO.

23. PRIOR AUTHORIZATION NUMBER

24. A DATE(S) OF SERVICE From MM DD YY	To MM DD YY	B Place of Service	C Type of Service	D PROCEDURES, SERVICES, OR SUPPLIES (Explain Unusual Circumstances) CPT/HCPCS	MODIFIER	E DIAGNOSIS CODE	F $ CHARGES	G DAYS OR UNITS	H EPSDT Family Plan	I EMG	J COB	K RESERVED FOR LOCAL USE
022720XX		11	1	29055		1	150 51	1				

25. FEDERAL TAX I.D. NUMBER: 74 65412XX SSN [ ] EIN [X]

26. PATIENT'S ACCOUNT NO.: 100

27. ACCEPT ASSIGNMENT? (For govt. claims, see back) YES NO

28. TOTAL CHARGE: $ 150 51

29. AMOUNT PAID: $

30. BALANCE DUE: $ 150 51

31. SIGNATURE OF PHYSICIAN OR SUPPLIER INCLUDING DEGREES OR CREDENTIALS (I certify that the statements on the reverse apply to this bill and are made a part thereof)
RAYMOND SKELETON MD 022820XX
SIGNED Raymond Skeleton MD DATE

32. NAME AND ADDRESS OF FACILITY WHERE SERVICECS WERE RENDERED (If other than home or office)
SAME

33. PHYSICIAN'S, SUPPLIER'S BILLING NAME, ADDRESS, ZIP CODE & PHONE #
COLLEGE CLINIC
4567 BROAD AVENUE
WOODLAND HILLS XY 12345 0001
555 486 9002
PIN# GRP# 3664021CC

reference initials

Figure D–12 Workers' compensation claim for a patient receiving a shoulder spica cast for a dislocated shoulder. Dr. Skeleton states that the patient is unable to perform regular work duties from January 4, 20XX to March 27, 20XX.

Appendix E

Glossary

Chapter number(s) is shown in parentheses after each term.

Abuse (1): Incidents or practices, not usually considered fraudulent, that are inconsistent with accepted sound medical business or fiscal practices.

Accepting assignment (11): An agreement in which a Medicare participating physician agrees to accept 80% of the approved charge from the fiscal intermediary and 20% of the approved charge from the patient, after the $100 deductible has been met.

Accident (13): An unexpected happening causing injury traceable to a definite time and place.

Accounts receivable (3): Total amount of money owed for professional services rendered.

Active duty service member (ADSM) (12): Active member of the United States government military services (e.g., Army, Navy, Air Force, Marines, Coast Guard).

Actual charge (9): The fee the physician charges for his or her service at the time the insurance claim is submitted to the insurance company or government payer.

Acute (4): Refers to a medical condition that runs a short but relatively severe course.

Add-on code (6): A code noted in CPT by a cross symbol (+) that represents an additional procedure done with a primary procedure. It must be listed along with the primary procedure code number, referred to as the "parent code."

Adjudication (13): Final determination of the issues involving settlement of an insurance claim, also known as a claim settlement.

Adverse effect (4): Unfavorable, detrimental, or pathologic reaction to a drug that occurs when appropriate doses are given to humans for prophylaxis (prevention of disease), diagnosis, or therapy.

Age analysis (14): Procedure of systematically arranging the accounts receivable, by age, from the date of service.

Allowed amount (9): Maximum dollar value the insurance company assigns to each procedure or service on which payment is based. Typically a percent (e.g., 80%) of the allowed amount is paid by the insurance carrier.

American Association of Medical Assistants (AAMA) (1): National organization composed of medical assistants, medical assisting students, and medical assisting educators with state and local chapters. It promotes education for clinical and administrative medical assistants, has established educational requirements for national certification and continuing education requirements for recertification, and is recognized by the American Medical Association.

Anesthesia (6): The partial or complete absence of normal sensation in the body. Anesthesia induced for medical purposes may be topical, local, regional, or general.

Appeal (15): Request for a review of an insurance claim that has been underpaid or denied by an insurance company to receive additional payment.

Assignment (3, 11, 12): Transfer, after an event insured against, of an individual's legal right to collect an amount payable under an insurance contract. For Medicare, an agreement in which a patient assigns to the physician the right to receive payment from the fiscal intermediary. Under this agreement, the physician must agree to accept 80% of the allowed amount as payment in full, once the deductible has been met. For TRICARE, providers who accept assignment agree to accept 75% or 80% of the TRICARE allowable charge as the full fee, collecting the deductible and 20% or 25% of the allowable charge from the patient.

Attending physician (7): Medical staff member who is legally responsible for the care and treatment given to a patient.

Audit (7): Formal, methodical examination or review done to inspect, analyze, and scrutinize the way something is being done (e.g., bookkeeping practices, medical record documentation, insurance claim filing).

Audit trail (8): Paper trail or path left by a transaction when it is processed.

Authorized provider (12): Physician or other individual authorized provider of care or a hospital or supplier approved by TRICARE to provide medical care and supplies.

Back up (7): Duplicate data file: tape, CD-ROM, disk, or ZIP disk used to record data; it may be used to complete or redo an operation if the primary equipment fails.

Balance (3, 9): Amount owed on a credit transaction; also known as the outstanding or unpaid balance.

Bankruptcy (14): Condition under which a person or corporation is declared unable to pay debts.

Beneficiary (12): Individual entitled to receive insurance policy or government program health care benefits; also known as *participant*, *subscriber*, *dependent*, *enrollee*, or *member*.

Benefit period (11, 13): Period of time for which payments for Medicare inpatient hospital benefits are available. A benefit period begins the first day an enrollee is given inpatient hospital care (nursing care or rehabilitation services) by a qualified provider and ends when the enrollee has not been an inpatient for 60 consecutive days; in workers' compensation cases the maximum amount of time that benefits will be paid to the injured or ill person for the disability.

Benign tumor (4): Neoplasm (growth) that does not have the properties of invasion and metastasis.

Bilateral procedure (6): A surgical procedure performed on both sides of the body or organ.

Birthday law (2): Legal state statute to determine coordination of benefits for primary and secondary carriers of dependent children covered under both parents' insurance plans. The health plan of the parent whose birthday (month and day, not year) falls earlier in the calendar year pays first, and the plan of the other person covering the dependent is the secondary payer.

Blanket bond (1): Insurance that provides coverage for all employees, regardless of job title, in the event of a financial loss to the employer by the act of an employee.

Blue Cross (9): Insurance programs that provide protection against the costs of hospital, surgical, and professional care. Most are nonprofit organizations and other managed care plans for their subscribers. Blue Cross plans contract with the federal government as an administrative agency for federal health programs.

Blue Shield (9): Insurance programs that provide protection against the costs of hospital care, surgery, and other items of medical care. Most are nonprofit organizations offering prepaid health care services for their subscribers.

Bonding (1): An insurance contract by which, in return for a state fee, a bonding agency guarantees payment of a certain sum to an employer in the event of a financial loss to the employer by the act of a specified employee or by some contingency over which the employer has no control.

Bundled code (6): Grouping of more than one component (service procedure) into one CPT code.

By report (BR) (13): Documentation in the form of a report submitted with the claim when the notation BR follows the procedure code description. This term is sometimes seen in workers' compensation fee schedules.

Capitation (9): System of payment used by managed care plans in which physicians and hospitals are paid a fixed, per capita amount for each patient enrolled over a stated period of time, regardless of the type and number of services provided; reimbursement to the hospital on a per-member/per-month basis to cover costs for the members of the plan.

Carcinoma in situ (4): Malignant growth that is localized or confined to the site of origin without invasion of neighboring tissues.

Carrier-direct system (8): Electronic transmission of insurance claims from the physician to the insurance company.

Carve outs (9): Medical services not included within the capitation rate as benefits of a managed care contract; may be contracted for separately.

Case manager (13): Registered or licensed vocational nurse assigned to a workers' compensation case to supervise the administration of medical or ancillary services provided to the patient.

Cash flow (1): In a medical practice, the amount of *actual* cash generated and available for use by the medical practice within a given period of time.

Catastrophic cap (12): Maximum dollar amount that a member has to pay under TRICARE or CHAMPVA in any fiscal year or enrollment period for covered medical bills.

Catchment area (12): In the TRICARE program, an area, defined by ZIP codes, that is approximately 40 miles in radius surrounding each United States military treatment facility.

Categorically needy (10): Aged, blind, or disabled individuals or families and children who meet financial eligibility requirements for Aid to Families with Dependent Children, Supplemental Security Income, or an optional state supplement.

Centers for Medicare and Medicaid Services (CMS) (11): Formerly known as the Health Care Financing Administration (HFCA), CMS divides responsibilities among three divisions: the Center for Medicare Management, the Center for Beneficiary Choices, and the Center for Medicaid and State Operations.

Certification (1): Statement issued by a board or association verifying that a person meets professional standards.

CHAMPVA (12): The Civilian Health and Medical Program of the Department of Veterans Affairs is a program for veterans with total, permanent, service-connected disabilities or surviving spouses and dependents of veterans who died of service-connected disabilities.

Chief complaint (4): Patient's statement describing symptoms, problems, or conditions as the reason for seeking health care services from a physician.

Chronic (4): Refers to a medical condition that persists over a long period of time.

Churning (1): Physicians seeing a high volume of patients—more than medically necessary—to increase revenue. May be seen in fee-for-service or managed care environments.

Claim (2): Bill sent to an insurance carrier requesting payment for services rendered.

Claims examiner (13): In industrial cases, a representative of the insurer who investigates, evaluates, and negotiates the patient's insurance claim and acts for the company in the settlement of claims.

Clean claim (8): A completed insurance claim form submitted within the program time limit that contains all the necessary information without deficiencies so it can be processed and paid promptly.

Clearinghouse (8): Third-party administrator (TPA) that receives insurance claims from the physician's office, performs software edits, and redistributes the claims electronically to various insurance carriers.

Closed fracture (6): Fracture of the bone with no skin wound.

Closed treatment (6): Alignment of a fracture without the site opened for surgical intervention.

Coal miners (13): Persons whose work is digging coal, a solid mineral, in an underground mine.

Coding specialist (1): Expert in coding diagnoses and procedures using diagnostic and procedural code books.

Coinsurance (2): A cost-sharing requirement under a health insurance policy providing that the insured will assume a percentage of the costs for covered services. For Medicare, after application of the yearly deductible, the portion of the approved amount (20%) for which the beneficiary is responsible.

Collection ratio (14): Relationship between the amount of money owed and the amount of money collected in reference to the doctor's accounts receivable.

Combination code (4): A code from one section of the procedural code book combined with a code from another section that is used to completely describe a procedure performed.

Comorbidity (7): Underlying condition or other condition that exists along with the condition for which the patient is receiving treatment.

Competitive Medical Plan (CMP) (9): State-licensed health plan similar to a health maintenance organization (HMO) that delivers comprehensive, coordinated services to voluntarily enrolled members on a prepaid capitated basis. CMP status may be granted by the federal government for the enrollment of Medicare beneficiaries into managed care plans, without having to qualify as an HMO.

Compliance program (7): A management plan composed of policies and procedures to accomplish uniformity, consistency, and conformity in medical record keeping that fulfills official requirements.

Component code (6): The portion of a service described before the semicolon (;) of a CPT comprehensive code, together with the portion of a service described by the indented (component) code.

Comprehensive code (6): Single procedural code that describes or covers two or more CPT component codes that are bundled together as one unit.

Compromise and release (C and R) (13): An agreement arrived at, whether in or out of court, for settling a workers' compensation case after the patient has been declared permanent and stationary.

Computer billing (14): Producing statements via a computer system.

Concurrent care (7): Provision of similar services (e.g., hospital visits) to the same patient by more than one physician on the same day. Usually, there is the presence of a separate physical disorder.

Concurrent condition (4): Disorder that coexists with the primary condition, complicating the treatment and management of the primary disorder; also referred to as *comorbidity*.

Confidential communication (1): Privileged communication that may be disclosed only with the patient's permission.

Consultation (5): Services rendered by a physician whose opinion or advice is requested by another physician or agency in the evaluation or treatment of a patient's illness or a suspected problem.

Consulting physician (7): Provider whose opinion or advice regarding evaluation and/or management of a specific problem is requested by another physician.

Continuity of care (1, 7): Continued treatment of a patient who is referred by one physician to another for the same condition.

Contract (2): Legally enforceable agreement (insurance policy).

Contractural adjustment (9): Difference between the allowed amount and the billed amount that is credited to an account as agreed upon in the insurance contract with the provider of service.

Conversion factor (9): The dollars and cents amount that is established for one unit as applied to a service or procedure. This unit is then used to convert various services/procedures into fee-schedule payment amounts by multiplying the relative value unit by the conversion factor.

Cooperative care (12): Term used when a patient is seen by a civilian physician or hospital for services cost-shared by TRICARE.

Coordination of benefits (COB) (2): Two insurance carriers working together and coordinating the payment of their benefits, so that there is no duplication of benefits paid between the primary insurance carrier and the secondary insurance carrier.

Copayment (copay) (2): Specific dollar amount to be collected when services are received (e.g., $10).

Correct coding initiative (CCI) (11): Federal legislation that attempts to eliminate unbundling or other inappropriate reporting of procedural codes for professional medical services rendered to patients.

Cost-share (12): The portion of the allowable charge (20% or 25%) after the deductible has been met that the TRICARE patient is responsible for.

Counseling (5): Discussion between the physician and a patient, family, or both concerning a diagnosis, recommended studies or tests, treatment options, risks and benefits of treatment, patient and family education, and so on.

Courtesy adjustment (11): Credit entry posted to a patient's account for a debt that has been determined to be uncollectible. In the Medicare program, this is the difference between the amount charged and the approved amount.

Covered services (10): Specific services and supplies for which the insurance plan (Medicaid) will provide reimbursement. These consist of a combination of mandatory and optional services stated in the plan.

CPT (5, 6): See *Current Procedural Terminology*.

Credit (3): 1. From the Latin *credere*, meaning "to believe" or "to trust"; trust in regard to financial obligation. 2. Accounting entry reflecting payment by a debtor (patient) of a sum received on his or her account.

Credit card (14): Card issued by an organization and devised for the purpose of obtaining money, property, labor, or services on credit.

Creditor (3): Person to whom money is owed.

Critical care (5): Intensive care provided in a variety of acute life-threatening conditions requiring constant bedside attention by a physician.

Crossover claim (8, 11): Bill for services rendered to a patient receiving benefits simultaneously from Medicare and Medicaid or from Medicare and a Medigap plan. Medicare pays first and then determines the amounts of unmet Medicare deductible and coinsurance to be paid by the secondary insurance carrier. The claim is automatically transferred (electronically) to the secondary insurance carrier for additional payment; also known as *claims transfer*.

***Current Procedural Terminology* (CPT) (5, 6):** Reference book using a five-digit numerical system to identify and code procedures and services established by the American Medical Association.

Cycle billing (14): System of billing accounts at spaced intervals during the month based on breakdown of accounts by alphabet, account number, insurance type, or date of first service.

Day sheet (3): Register for recording daily business transactions (charges, payments, adjustments); also known as daily log.

Debit card (14): Card permitting bank customers to withdraw from any affiliated automated teller machine (ATM) and to make cashless purchases from funds on deposit without incurring revolving finance charges for credit.

Debt (14): Legal obligation to pay money.

Debtor (3): Person owing money.

Deductible (2): Specific dollar amount that must be paid each calendar or fiscal year by the insured before a medical insurance plan or government program begins covering health care costs.

Defense Enrollment Eligibility Reporting System (DEERS) (12): An electronic database used to verify beneficiary eligibility for those individuals in TRICARE programs.

Delinquent claim (15): Insurance claim submitted to an insurance company for which payment is overdue.

Denied claim (15): Insurance claim submitted to an insurance company for which payment has been rejected owing to a technical error or medical coverage policy issue.

Dependents (2): Spouse and children of the insured. Under some insurance policies, parents, other family members, and domestic partners may be covered as dependents.

Deposition (13): Process of taking a witness's sworn testimony out of court; usually done by an attorney.

Diagnosis (4): Identification of a disease, syndrome, or condition by scientific evaluation of history, physical signs, symptoms, tests, and procedures.

Digital signature (8): In an electronic document, a signature that consists of lines of text or a text box stating the signer's name, date/time, and a statement indicating a signature has been attached from within a software application.

Dingy claim (8): Insurance claim that cannot be processed because of the type of software program used to transmit the claim; it may be incompatible with the receiving system.

Direct referral (9): Simplified authorization request form completed and signed by a physician and handed to the patient at the time of referral.

Dirty claim (8): Claim submitted with errors or one that requires manual processing to resolve problems or is rejected for payment.

Disability income insurance (13): Form of health insurance that provides periodic payments to replace income when the insured is unable to work as a result of illness, injury, or disease—not as a result of a work-related accident or condition.

Discount (9): Reduction of a normal charge based on a specific amount of money or a percentage of the charge.

Disenrollment (9): Member's voluntary cancellation of membership in a managed care plan.

Documentation (7): Detailed chronologic recording of pertinent facts and observations about a patient's health as seen in chart notes and medical reports; entries in the medical record such as prescription refills, telephone calls, and other pertinent data.

Downcoding (6): Coding system used by the physician's office does not match the coding system used by the insurance company receiving the claim. The insurance company computer system converts the code submitted to the closest code in use, which is usually down one level from the submitted code, generating decreased payment.

Dun messages (14): Messages or phrases to inform or remind a patient about a delinquent account.

Durable medical equipment (DME) number (8): Group or individual provider number used when submitting bills for specific medical supplies, devices, and equipment to the Medicare fiscal intermediary for reimbursement.

E codes (4): Classification of ICD-9-CM coding used to describe environmental events, circumstances, and conditions as the external cause of injury, poisoning, and other adverse effects.

Early and Periodic Screening, Diagnosis, and Treatment (EPSDT) (10): Program of prevention, early detection, and treatment of welfare children who are younger than age 21 years. In New York, this is called the Child Health Assurance Program (CHAP).

Elective surgery (6): Surgical procedure that may be scheduled in advance, is not an emergency, and is discretionary on the part of the physician and patient.

Electronic claim (8): Insurance claim submitted to the insurance carrier via a central processing unit (CPU), tape diskette, direct data entry, direct wire, dial-in telephone, digital fax, or personal computer download or upload.

Electronic claims processor (ECP) (8): Individual who converts insurance claims to standardized electronic format and transmits electronic insurance claims data to the insurance carrier or clearinghouse to help the physician receive payment; sometimes referred to as *electronic claims professional.*

Electronic claim submission (ECS) (8): Insurance claims prepared on a computer and submitted via modem (telephone lines) to the insurance carrier's computer system; also called *electronic media claims (EMC).*

Electronic data interchange (EDI) (8): Process by which understandable data items are sent back and forth via computer linkages between two or more entities that function alternatively as sender and receiver.

Electronic signature (8): Any mark or symbol accepted by both parties to show intent, approval of, or responsibility for computer document content.

Eligibility (2): Qualifying factors that must be met before a patient receives benefits (medical services) under a specified insurance plan, government program, or managed care plan.

Emancipated minor (2): Person younger than 18 years of age who lives independently, is totally self-supporting, and possesses decision-making rights.

Embezzlement (1): Willful act by an employee of taking possession of an employer's money.

Emergency (5): A sudden, unexpected medical condition, or the worsening of a condition, that poses a threat to life, limb, or sight and requires immediate treatment (e.g., shortness of breath, chest pain, drug overdose).

Emergency care (5): Health care services provided to prevent serious impairment of bodily functions or serious dysfunction to any body organ or part. Advanced life support may be required. Not all care provided in an emergency department of a hospital can be termed "emergency care."

Employer identification number (EIN) (8): An individual's federal tax identification number issued by the Internal Revenue Service for income tax purposes.

Encounter form (3): All-encompassing billing form personalized to the practice of the physician. It may be used when a patient submits an insurance claim; also called *charge slip, communicator, fee ticket, multipurpose billing form, patient service slip, routing form, superbill,* and *transaction slip.*

Endoscopy (6): Insertion of a flexible fiberoptic tube, referred to as a scope, through a small incision into a body cavity or into a natural body orifice (opening), such as the ears, nose, mouth, vagina, urethra, or anus. An endoscopic procedure may be diagnostic, may be performed for the purpose of visualization and determination of the disease process, or may be surgical, including incisions, repairs, and excisions.

End-stage renal disease (ESRD) (11): Chronic kidney disease requiring dialysis or kidney transplant. To qualify for Medicare coverage, an individual must be fully or currently insured under Social Security or the railroad retirement system or be the dependent of an insured person. Eligibility for Medicare coverage begins with the third month after the beginning of a course of renal dialysis. Coverage may begin sooner if the patient participates in a self-care dialysis training program or receives a kidney transplant without dialysis.

Eponym (4): Name of a disease, anatomical structure, operation, or procedure, usually derived from the name of a place where it first occurred or a person who discovered or first described it.

Ergonomic (13): Science and technology that seeks to fit the anatomic and physical needs of the worker to the workplace.

Established patient (5): Individual who has received professional services within the past 3 years from the physician or another physician of the same specialty who belongs to the same group practice.

Ethics (1): Standards of conduct generally accepted as a moral guide for behavior by which an insurance billing or coding specialist may determine the appropriateness of his or her conduct in a relationship with patients, the physician, coworkers, the government, and insurance companies.

Etiology (4): Cause of a disease; the study of the cause of a disease.

Etiquette (1): Customs, courtesy, and manners of the medical profession.

Evaluation and Management services (5): Services provided by the physician in a variety of settings (e.g., physician's office, hospital, patient's home) to evaluate the patient and manage the patient's condition; previously referred to as *office, hospital,* or *home visits.*

Exclusions (2, 13): Provisions written into the insurance contract denying coverage or limiting the scope of coverage.

Exclusive provider organization (EPO) (9): Type of managed health care plan that combines features of HMOs and PPOs. It is referred to as exclusive because it is offered to large employers who agree not to contract with any other plan. EPOs are regulated under state health insurance laws.

Explanation of benefits (EOB) (3, 15): A document detailing services billed and describing payment determinations; also known in Medicare, Medicaid, and some other programs as a *remittance advice*. In the TRICARE program, it is called a *summary payment voucher*.

Expressed contract (2): Verbal or written agreement.

External audit (7): A review done after claims have been submitted (retrospective review) of medical and financial records by an insurance company or Medicare representative to investigate suspected fraudulent and abusive billing practices.

Extraterritorial (13): State laws effective outside the state by either specific provision or court decision. For workers' compensation, benefits under a state law that apply to a compensable injury of an employee hired in one state but injured outside that state.

Facility provider number (8): Number assigned to a facility (e.g., hospital, laboratory, radiology office, nursing facility) to be used by the facility to bill for services, or by the performing physician to report services done at that location.

Fascimile (FAX) (7): Electronic process for transmitting written and graphic matter over telephone lines.

Family history (FH) (7): Review of medical events in the patient's family, including diseases that may be hereditary or that place the patient at risk.

Fee for service (9): Method of payment in which the patient pays according to an established schedule of fees for each professional service performed.

Fee schedule (9, 13): List of charges or established allowances for specific medical services and procedures. See also *Relative value studies (RVS)*.

Fiscal intermediary (FI) (11): Organization under contract to the government that handles claims under Medicare Part A and/or Part B from hospitals, skilled nursing facilities, home health agencies, and/or providers of medical services and supplies. For TRICARE and CHAMPVA, the insurance company that handles the claims for care received within a particular state or country; also known as *fiscal agent*, *fiscal carrier*, or a *claims processor*.

Fixation (6): Use of internal and/or external hardware (e.g., pins, rods, plates, wires) to keep a bone in place; also referred to as instrumentation.

Formal referral (9): Authorization request (telephone, fax, or completed form) required by the managed care organization contract to determine medical necessity and grant permission before services are rendered or procedures performed.

Foundation for medical care (FMC) (9): Organization of physicians sponsored by a state or local medical association concerned with the development and delivery of medical services and the cost of health care.

Fracture manipulation (6): Manual stretching or applying pressure or traction to realign a broken bone; also referred to as a *reduction*.

Fraud (1): An intentional misrepresentation of the facts to deceive or mislead another.

Gatekeeper (9): In the managed care system, a physician who controls patient access to specialists and diagnostic testing services.

Global surgery policy (6): Medicare policy relating to surgical procedures in which preoperative and postoperative visits (24 hours before [major] and day of [minor]), usual intraoperative services, and complications not requiring an additional trip to the operating room are included in one fee.

Group provider number (8): Number assigned to a group of physicians submitting claims under the group name and reporting income under one name; used instead of the individual physician's number (PIN) for the performing provider.

Guarantor (2): Individual responsible for payment of the medical bill.

Health benefits advisor (HBA) (12): Government employee responsible for helping all military health system beneficiaries in the TRICARE program obtain medical care.

Health Care Financing Administration Common Procedure Coding System (HCPCS) (5): Now referred to as Healthcare Common Procedure Coding System. Three-tier coding system developed by the Centers for Medicare and Medicaid Services (CMS), formerly HCFA, used for reporting physician/supplier services and procedures. Level I codes are national CPT codes, Level II codes are HCPCS national codes used to report items not covered under CPT, and Level III codes are HCPCS regional/local codes used to identify new procedures or items for which there is no national code. Pronounced "hick-picks."

Health Care Finder (HCF) (12): Health care professionals, generally registered nurses, who are located at TRICARE Service Centers to act as a liaison between military and civilian providers, verify eligibility, determine availability of services, coordinate care, facilitate the transfer of records, and perform first-level medical review.

Health insurance (2): Contract between the policyholder and/or member and insurance carrier or government program to reimburse the policyholder and/or member for all or a portion of the cost of medical care rendered by health care professionals; generic term also applies to lost income arising from illness or injury; also known as *accident and health insurance* or *disability income insurance*.

Health Insurance Claim Form (HCFA-1500) (8): Now known as CMS-1500. Universal insurance claim form developed and approved by the American Medical Association Council on Medical Service and the Centers for Medicare and Medicaid Services, formerly the Health Care Financing Administration. It is used by physicians and other professionals to bill outpatient services and supplies to TRICARE, Medicare, and some Medicaid programs as well as most private insurance carriers and managed care plans.

Health maintenance organization (HMO) (9): The oldest of all prepaid health plans. A comprehensive health care financing and delivery organization that provides a wide range of health care services with an emphasis on preventive medicine to enrollees within a geographic area through a panel of providers. Primary care physician "gatekeepers" are usually reimbursed via capitation.

History of present illness (HPI) (7): Chronologic description of the development of the patient's present illness from the first sign and/or symptom or from the previous encounter to the present.

Hospice (11): Public agency or private organization primarily engaged in providing pain relief, symptom management, and supportive services to terminally ill patients and their families in their own homes or in a home-like center.

Implied contract (2): Contract between physician and patient not manifested by direct words but implied or deduced from the circumstance, general language, or conduct of the patient.

Incomplete claim (8): Any Medicare claim missing required information; such claims are identified to the provider so they may be resubmitted.

Indemnity (2): Benefits paid to insured; also known as *reimbursement.*

Indented code (6): Codes listed after stand-alone codes whose descriptions have a dependent status. To read the description, you must first read the description of the stand-alone code that comes before the semicolon (;) and then continue with the indented description listed by the subsequent code (indented code).

Independent (or Individual) Practice Association (IPA) (9): Type of MCO in which a program administrator contracts with a number of physicians who agree to provide treatment to subscribers in their own offices. Physicians are not employees of the MCO and are not paid salaries. They receive reimbursement on a capitation or fee-for-service basis; also referred to as a *medical capitation plan.*

Injury (13): In a workers' compensation policy, this term signifies any trauma or damage to a body part or disease, arising out of and occurring in the course of employment.

Inpatient (5): Term used when a patient is admitted to the hospital for overnight stay.

Inquiry (15): See *Tracer.*

Insurance adjuster (13): Individual at the workers' compensation insurance carrier overseeing an industrial case, authorizing diagnostic testing and medical treatment, and communicating with the provider of medical care.

Insurance balance bill (14): Billing statement that is sent to the patient after his or her insurance company has paid its portion of the claim.

Insurance claim number (11): Social Security number of the wage earner, which appears on the Medicare identification card.

Insurance policy (2): Legally enforceable agreement; also known as *insurance contract.*

Insured (2): Individual or organization protected in case of loss under the terms of an insurance policy.

Intermediate care facilities (ICFs) (11): Institutions furnishing health-related care and services to individuals who do not require the degree of care provided by acute care hospitals.

Internal review (7): Process of going over financial documents in the medical office before and after billing insurance carriers to determine documentation deficiencies or errors.

***International Classification of Diseases, Ninth Revision, Clinical Modification* (ICD-9-CM) (4):** Diagnostic code book that uses a system for classifying diseases and operations to facilitate collection of uniform and comparable health information. A code system to replace this is ICD-10, which is being modified for use in the United States.

Internet (8): Large interconnected message-forwarding system linking academic, commercial, government, and military computer networks all over the world.

Invalid claim (8): Any Medicare claim that contains complete, necessary information but is illogical or incorrect (e.g., listing an incorrect provider number for a referring physician). Invalid claims are identified to the provider and may be resubmitted.

Itemized statement (14): Detailed summary of all transactions of a patient's account: dates of service, detailed charges, payments (copayments and deductibles), date the insurance claim was submitted, adjustments, and account balance.

Key components (5): Three elements necessary for many evaluation and management services (history, physical examination, and medical decision making).

Late effect (4): Residual effect after the acute phase of an illness or injury has ended.

Ledger card (3): Individual account indicating charges, payments, adjustments, and balances owed for services rendered.

Lien (13): Claim on the property of another as security for a debt. In litigation cases, it is a legal promise to satisfy a debt owed by the patient to the physician out of any proceeds received on the case.

Local area network (LAN) (8): Interlink of multiple computers contained within a room or building that allows sharing of files and devices such as printers.

Lost claim (15): Insurance claim that cannot be located after sending it to an insurer.

Main term (4): In a diagnostic statement, the condition.

Major medical (2): Health insurance policy designed to offset heavy medical expenses resulting from catastrophic or prolonged illness or injury.

Malignant tumor (4): Neoplasm (abnormal growth) that has the properties of invasion and metastasis (i.e., transfer of diseases from one organ to another). The word "carcinoma" (CA) refers to a cancerous or malignant tumor.

Managed care organization (MCO) (9): Generic term applied to managed care plans, such as EPOs, HMOs, and PPOs. MCOs are usually prepaid group plans, and physicians are typically paid by the capitation method.

Manifestation (4): Characteristic sign or symptom associated with an illness.

Manual billing (14): Processing statements by hand; may involve typing statements or photocopying the patient's ledger and placing it in a window envelope, which then becomes the statement.

Maternal and Child Health Programs (MCHP) (10): State service organization to assist children younger than 21 years of age who have conditions leading to health problems.

Medicaid (MCD) (10): Federally aided and state-operated and administered program that provides medical benefits for certain low-income persons in need of health and medical care; known as *Medi-Cal* in California.

Medi-Cal (10): California's version of the nationwide program known as Medicaid. See *Medicaid.*

Medical insurance billing specialist (1): Employee who works for a physician or in a health care facility and handles source documents, codes procedures and diagnoses, processes insurance claims, and follows up on delayed reimbursement and delinquent accounts.

Medical-legal (ML) evaluation (13): In workers' compensation, the independent assessment of an employee that results in the preparation of a narrative medical report prepared and attested to in accordance with the state labor code.

Medical necessity (7): Performance of services and procedures that are consistent with the diagnosis in accordance with standards of good medical practice, performed at the proper level, and provided in the most appropriate setting. Medical necessity *must* be established (via diagnostic and/or other information presented on the individual claim under consideration) before the carrier may make payment.

Medical record (7): Written or graphic information documenting facts and events during the rendering of patient care.

Medical service order (13): Authorization given to the physician, either written or verbal, to treat an injured or ill employee.

Medically indigent (10): See *Medically needy.*

Medically needy (MN) (10): Persons in need of financial assistance and/or whose income and resources will not allow them to pay for the costs of medical care; also called *medically indigent* in some states.

Medicare Part A (11): Hospital benefits of a nationwide health insurance program for persons age 65 years and older and certain disabled or blind individuals regardless of income, administered by CMS, formerly HCFA. Local Social Security offices take applications and supply information about the program.

Medicare Part B (11): Medical insurance of a nationwide health insurance program for persons age 65 years and older and certain disabled or blind individuals regardless of income, administered by CMS, formerly HCFA. Local Social Security offices take applications and supply information about the program.

Medicare Part C (11): Medicare + Choice plans offer a number of health care options in addition to those available under Medicare Part A and Part B. Plans may include health maintenance organizations, fee-for-service plans, provider-sponsored organizations, religious fraternal benefit societies, and Medicare medical savings accounts.

Medicare/Medicaid (Medi-Medi) (11): Refers to an individual who receives medical benefits from both Medicare and Medicaid programs; sometimes referred to as a *Medi-Medi case.*

Medicare Secondary Payer (MSP) (11): Primary insurance plan of a Medicare beneficiary that must pay for medical services first before Medicare is sent a claim.

Medigap (MG) (11): Specialized Medicare supplemental insurance policy regulated by the federal government and devised for the Medicare beneficiary. It typically covers the deductible and copayment amounts not covered under the Medicare policy; also known as *Medifill.*

Mentor (1): Guide or teacher who offers advice, criticism, wisdom, guidance, and perspective to an inexperienced but promising protégé to help reach a life goal.

Military retiree (service retiree) (12): Individual who is retired from a career in the armed forces; also known as *service retiree.*

Military treatment facilities (MTFs) (12): All uniformed service hospitals; also known as *military hospitals* or *uniformed service hospitals.*

Modifier (5, 6): In CPT coding, a two-digit add-on or five-digit number placed after the usual procedure code number to indicate circumstances in which a procedure as performed differs in some way from that described by its usual five-digit code. In HCPCS Level II coding, a one- or two-digit alpha or alphanumeric character placed after the usual Level I or II code.

Morbidity (7): Diseased condition or state.

Mortality (7): Cause of death. Mortality rate is the number of deaths in a given time or place.

Multipurpose billing form (3): See *Encounter form.*

Multiskilled health practitioner (MSHP) (1): Individual cross-trained to provide more than one function, often in more than one discipline. These combined functions can be found in a broad spectrum of health-related jobs, ranging in complexity and including both clinical and administrative functions. The terms *multiskilled, multicompetent,* and *cross-trained* can be used interchangeably.

National drug code (NDC) (5): Eleven-digit drug product identifier code identifying manufacturer, repackager or distributor, drug product (strength, dosage, and formulation), and package size. Used to bill for drugs when transmitting insurance claims electronically.

National provider identifier (NPI) (8): A Medicare lifetime 10-digit number that when adopted will replace the provider identification number (PIN) and the unique physician identification number (UPIN).

Neoplasm (4): Spontaneous new growth of tissue forming an abnormal mass; also known as a tumor; may be benign or malignant.

Network HMO (9): Managed care organization that contracts with two or more group of practices to provide health services.

Networking (1): Exchange of information or services among individuals, groups, or institutions; making use of professional contacts.

New patient (NP) (5): Individual who has not received any professional services from the physician or another physician of the same specialty who belongs to the same group practice within the past 3 years.

No charge (NC) (9): Waiving of the entire fee owed for professional care.

Nonavailability statement (NAS) (12): Statement issued upon request and signed by the commanding officer before treatment when the military treatment facility cannot provide inpatient care and the patient lives in a certain ZIP code near a military hospital. INAS is an acronym for inpatient nonavailability statement.

Nondisability (ND) claim (13): Claim for on-the-job injury that requires medical care but does not result in loss of working time or income.

Nonprivileged information (1): Information consisting of ordinary facts unrelated to the treatment of the patient. The patient's authorization is not required to disclose the data unless the record is in a specialty hospital or in a special service unit of a general hospital, such as the psychiatric unit.

Nursing facility (NF) (11): Specially qualified facility that has the staff and equipment to provide skilled nursing care and related services that are medically necessary to a patient's recovery; formerly known as *skilled nursing facility.*

Objective findings (7): That which can be determined by either seeing (visual), feeling (palpation), smelling, listening to (auscultation), or measuring (i.e., size or test results).

Observation status (5): Patient not formally admitted to the hospital, instead admitted to "observation status" while his or her condition is being observed and a decision is made regarding admittance or discharge. The patient need not be in a separate observation area in the hospital to meet the observation criteria.

Occupational illness (or disease) (13): Abnormal condition or disorder caused by environmental factors associated with employment. It may be caused by inhalation, absorption, ingestion, or direct contact.

Occupational Safety and Health Administration (OSHA) (13): Federal agency that regulates and investigates safety and health standards in work locations.

Open accounts (14): Accounts from which charges are made from time to time and payment is expected within a specified period without a formal written contract.

Open fracture (6): Broken bone with an open skin wound; also referred to as a *compound fracture.*

Open treatment (6): Treatment of a fracture in which the site is surgically opened.

Optical character recognition (OCR) (8): Device that can read typed characters at very high speed and convert them to digitized files that can be saved on disk; also known as *intelligent character recognition* (ICR).

Ordering physician (7): Physician ordering nonphysician services for a patient (e.g., diagnostic laboratory tests, pharmaceutical services, or durable medical equipment). Ordering physician may also be the treating/performing physician.

Other claim (8): Medicare claim that requires investigation or development on a prepayment basis to determine if Medicare is the primary or secondary carrier.

Other health insurance (OHI) (12): Health care coverage for TRICARE beneficiaries through an employer, an association, or a private insurer. A student in the family may have a health care plan through school.

Outpatient (5): Patient who receives services in a health care facility, such as a physician's office, clinic, urgent care center, emergency department, or ambulatory surgical center.

Overpayment (15): Money paid over and above the amount due by the insurance carrier or the patient.

Paper claim (8): Any insurance claim submitted on paper, including those optically scanned and converted to an electronic form by the insurance carrier.

Partial disability (13): Disability from an illness or injury that prevents an insured person from performing one or more of the functions of his or her regular job.

Participating provider (par) (9): Physician who has a contractual agreement with an insurance plan to render care to eligible beneficiaries and bills the insurance carrier directly.

Partnership program (12): Program that lets TRICARE-eligible individuals receive inpatient or outpatient treatment from civilian providers of care in a military hospital, or from uniformed services providers of care in civilian facilities.

Password (1): Combination of letters and/or numbers selected by individuals, reported to management, and assigned to access computer data.

Past history (PH) (7): Patient's past experiences with illnesses, operations, injuries, and treatments.

Patient registration form (3): Questionnaire designed to collect demographic data and essential facts about medical insurance coverage for each patient seen for professional services; also called *patient information form.*

Peer review (9, 15): One or more physicians using federal guidelines to evaluate another physician in regard to the quality and efficiency of medical care. This is done to discover over- or misutilization of a plan's benefits.

Peer review organization (PRO) (11): State-based group of practicing physicians paid by the federal government to review cases to determine appropriateness and quality of care of Medicare patients.

Pending claim (8): Insurance claim held in suspense owing to review or other reason. These claims may be cleared for payment or denied.

Percutaneous treatment (6): Treatment of a fracture in which the site is neither open nor closed. The fracture is not visualized so fixation is placed across the fracture site using x-ray.

Performing physician (7): Provider who renders a service to a patient; also known as *treating physician.*

Permanent and stationary (P & S) (13): Phrase used when a workers' compensation patient's condition has become stabilized and no improvement is expected. It is only after this declaration that a case can be rated for a compromise and release.

Permanent disability (PD) (13): Illness or injury (impairment of the normal use of a body part) expected to continue for the lifetime of the injured worker that prevents the person from performing the functions of his or her occupation, therefore, impairing his or her earning capacity.

Personal bond (1): Insurance that provides coverage for individuals who handle large sums of money during business transactions.

Petition (13): Formal written request commonly used to indicate an appeal.

Phantom billing (1): Billing for services not performed.

Physical examination (PE or PX) (7): Objective inspection and/or testing of organ systems or body areas of a patient by a physician.

Physician extenders (3): Health care personnel trained to provide medical care under the direct or indirect supervision of a physician (e.g., nurse practitioners, nurse midwives, physician assistants, and nurse anesthetists).

Physician provider group (PPG) (9): Physician-owned business that has the flexibility to deal with all forms of contract medicine and still offer its own packages to business groups, unions, and the general public.

Physician's fee profile (9): Compilation of each physician's charges for specific professional services and the payments made to the physician over a given period of time.

Ping-ponging (1): Excessive referrals to other providers for unnecessary services.

Point-of-service (POS) option (12): Option under TRICARE Prime that allows self-referral for any TRICARE-covered nonemergency services outside the prime network of providers.

Point-of-service (POS) plan (9): Managed care plan in which members are given a choice as to how to receive services, whether through an HMO, PPO, or fee-for-service plan. The decision is made at the time the service is needed (i.e., "at the point of service"); sometimes referred to as *open-ended HMOs, swing-out HMOs, self-referral options,* or *multiple option plans.*

Poisoning (4): Condition resulting from a drug or chemical substance overdose or from the wrong drug or agent given or taken in error.

Position-schedule bond (1): Insurance that provides coverage for a designated job title rather than a named individual.

Post (3): Record or transfer financial entries, debit or credit, to an account (e.g., day sheet, ledger, bank deposit slip, chest register, or journal).

Preauthorization (2): Requirement in some health insurance plans to obtain permission for a service or procedure before it is done and to determine whether the insurance program agrees it is medically necessary.

Precertification (2): To determine benefits (surgery, tests, hospitalization) under a patient's health insurance policy.

Predetermination (2): To determine before treatment the maximum dollar amount the insurance company will pay for surgery, consultations, postoperative care, and so forth.

Preferred Provider Organization (PPO) (9): Type of health benefit program in which enrollees receive the highest level of benefits when they obtain services from a physician, hospital, or other health care provider designated by their program as a "preferred provider." Enrollees may receive substantial, although reduced, benefits when they obtain care from a provider of their own choosing who is not designated as a "preferred provider" by their program.

Premium (2): Cost of insurance coverage paid annually, semiannually, or monthly to keep the policy in force.

Prepaid group practice model (9): Plan under which health services are delivered at one or more locations by participating physicians who either contract with an HMO or who are employed by an HMO.

Prepaid health plan (2): Health care program in which a specified set of health benefits is provided in exchange for a yearly fee or fixed periodic payments.

Prevailing charge (9): Fee that is most frequently charged in an area by a group of specialty physicians. The top of this range establishes an overall limitation on the charges that a carrier, which considers prevailing charges in reimbursement, will accept as reasonable for a given service without special justification.

Preventive medicine (5): Services provided to prevent the occurrence of illness, injury, and disease.

Primary care manager (PCM) (12): Physician who is responsible for coordinating and managing all the TRICARE beneficiary's health care unless there is an emergency.

Primary care physician (PCP) (9): Physician (e.g., family practitioner, general practitioner, pediatrician, obstetrician/gynecologist, or general internist) who oversees the care of patients in a managed health care plan (HMO or PPO) and refers patients to see specialists (e.g., cardiologist, oncologists, surgeons) for services as needed; also known as a *gatekeeper.*

Primary diagnosis (4): Initial identification of the condition or chief complaint for which the patient is treated in an outpatient medical setting.

Principal diagnosis (4): Condition established after study that is chiefly responsible for the admission of the patient to the hospital.

Prior approval (10): Evaluation of a provider request for a specific service to determine medical necessity and appropriateness of the care; also called *prior authorization* in some states.

Privileged information (1): All data related to the treatment and progress of the patient that can be released only when written authorization of the patient or guardian is obtained.

Procedure coding (5): Standardized method used to transform written descriptions of procedures and professional services into numeric designations (code numbers).

Professional component (PC) (6): Portion of a test or procedure (containing both a professional and technical component) that the physician performs, such as interpreting an electrocardiogram (ECG), reading an x-ray, or making an observation and determination using a microscope.

Professional courtesy (9): Exemption from charges for professional services; rarely used in current medicine.

Professional review organization (PRO) (9): Organization formed to determine the assurance of the quality and operation of health care using a process called *peer review.*

Prolonged services (5): Services that go beyond the usual time alloted in either inpatient or outpatient settings.

Prompt payment laws (15): State statutes designed to govern actions of insurers and third party payers to pay insurance claims in a timely manner; also outlines actions collectors can take against insurance companies if statutes are not followed.

Prospective payment system (PPS) (11): Method of payment for Medicare hospital insurance based on diagnosis-related groups (a fixed dollar amount for each type of illness based on diagnosis).

Provider (3): Individual or facility that provides health care services.

Provider identification number (PIN) (8): Carrier-assigned number used by physicians when submitting insurance claims for services.

Qualitative analysis (6): Referring to a test that determines the presence of an agent within the body.

Quantitative analysis (6): Referring to a test that determines the amount or percentage of an agent that is present within the body.

Reasonable fee (11): Amount on which payment is based for participating physicians in the Medicare program.

Rebill (15): Subsequent request for payment for an overdue bill sent to either the insurance company or patient.

Recipients (10): In the Medicaid program, persons who receive the state benefits under this program.

Reciprocity (10): Mutual exchange of privileges or services; in the Medicaid program it applies to an individual who obtains medical services while out of the state in which he or she receives benefits.

Referral (5): Transfer of specific or total care of a patient from one physician to another. In managed care, a request for authorization for a specific service.

Referring physician (7): Physician who sends the patient for testing or treatment noted on the insurance claim when it is submitted by the physician performing the service.

Registration (1): Entry in an official registry or record that lists names of persons in an occupation who have satisfied specific requirements, attaining a certain level of education, and paying a fee.

Reimbursement (3): Repayment; term used when insurance payment is pending.

Rejected claim (8): Insurance claim submitted to an insurance carrier that is discarded by the system because of a technical error (omission or erroneous information) or because it does not follow Medicare instructions. It is returned to the provider for correction or change so that it may be processed properly for payment.

Relative value studies (scale) (RVS) (9): List of coded procedures that are assigned unit values that indicate the value of one procedure over another.

Relative value unit (RVU) (9): Monetary value assigned to each service based on the amount of physician work, practice expenses, and the cost of professional liability insurance. These three RVUs are then adjusted according to geographic area and used in a formula to determine Medicare fees.

Remittance advice (RA) (3): Document detailing services billed and describing payment determination issued to providers of the Medicare or Medicaid program; also known in some programs as an *explanation of benefits.*

Resource-based relative value scale (RBRVS) (9): System that ranks physician services by units and provides a formula to determine a Medicare fee schedule.

Respite care (11): Short-term inpatient hospital stay for a terminally ill patient to give temporary relief to the patient's primary caregiver.

***Respondeat superior* (1):** "Let the master answer." Refers to a physician's liability in certain cases for the wrongful acts of his or her assistant(s) or employee(s).

Review of systems (ROS) (7): Inventory of body systems obtained through a series of questions that is used to identify signs and/or symptoms that the patient might be experiencing or has experienced.

Running balance (3): Amount owed on a credit transaction; also known as *outstanding* or *unpaid balance.*

Secondary diagnosis (4): Reason subsequent to the primary diagnosis for an office or hospital encounter that may contribute to the condition or define the need for a higher level of care but is not the underlying cause. There may be more than one secondary diagnosis.

Second-injury fund (13): Special fund that assumes all or part of the liability for benefits provided to a worker because of the combined effect of a work-related impairment and a preexisting condition; also known as *subsequent injury fund (SIF).*

Self-referral (9): Patient in a managed care plan who refers himself or herself to a specialist. The patient may be required to inform the primary care physician.

Separate procedure (6): Procedure that is an integral part of a larger procedure and does not need a separate code, unless performed independently and not immediately related to other services.

Service benefit program (12): Program (e.g., TRICARE) that provides benefits without a contract guaranteeing the indemnification of an insured party against a specific loss; there are no premiums.

Share of cost (10): Amount some patients must pay each month before they can be eligible for Medicaid; also known as *liability* or *spend down.*

Skip (14): Debtor who has moved and neglected to give a forwarding address (i.e., skipped town).

Social history (SH) (7): Age-appropriate review of a patient's past and current activities (e.g., smoking, diet intake, alcohol use).

Social Security Disability Insurance (SSDI) (13): Entitlement program for disabled workers or self-employed individuals.

Social Security Number (SSN) (8): Number assigned to each individual by the federal government for identification purposes; used as a tax identification number.

Sponsor (12): For the TRICARE program, the service person, either active duty, retired, or deceased, whose relationship makes the patient (dependent) eligible for TRICARE.

Staff model (9): Type of HMO in which the health plan hires physicians directly and pays them a salary.

Stand-alone code (6): Procedure code that has a full description.

Star procedure (6): In CPT, surgical procedures with a star symbol (*) indicate minor surgical services with specific guidelines different from guidelines for nonstarred surgical procedures.

State Disability Insurance (SDI) (13): Insurance that covers off-the-job injury or sickness and is paid for by deductions from a person's paycheck. This program is administered by a state agency and is sometimes known as *Unemployment Compensation Disability (UCD).*

State license number (8): Number issued to a physician who has passed the state medical examination indicating his or her right to practice medicine in the state where issued.

Statute of limitations (14): Time limit established for filing lawsuits; may vary from state to state.

Subjective information (7): Data that cannot be measured, typically referred to as "symptoms."

***Subpoena* (7):** "Under penalty." A writ that commands a witness to appear at a trial or other proceeding and give testimony.

Sub rosa films (13): Videotapes made without the knowledge of the subject; used to investigate suspicious claims in workers' compensation cases.

Subscriber (2): Contract holder covered by an insurance plan, who either has coverage through his or her place of employment or has purchased coverage directly from the plan or affiliate. This term is used primarily in Blue Cross and Blue Shield programs.

Supplemental insurance (8): Secondary insurance policy that covers only what the primary insurance does not cover.

Supplemental Security Income (SSI) (11): Program of income support for low-income aged, blind, and disabled persons established by Title XVI of the Social Security Act.

Surgical package (6): One fee applied to unstarred surgical procedure code numbers that include services other than the operation, such as local infiltration, digital block, or topical anesthesia, and normal, uncomplicated postoperative care (referred to as a "package").

Suspended claim (15): Insurance claim held by the insurance carrier as pending because of either an error or the need for additional information.

Symptom (4): Change in normal bodily function; any indication of disease perceived by the patient.

Technical component (TC) (6): Portion of a test or procedure (containing both a technical and a professional component) that refers to the use of the equipment and its operator that performs the test or procedure, such as ECG machine and technician, radiography machine and technician, and microscope and technician.

Temporary disability (TD) (13): Period following a work-related injury during which the employee is unable to perform all or part of his or her work duties for a period of time.

Temporary disability insurance (TDI) (13): See *State Disability Insurance (SDI).*

Tertiary care (9): Services requested by a specialist from another specialist.

Test panel (6): Grouping of a number of laboratory tests (represented by individual codes) that are usually performed together and reported using one CPT code. The most common tests done to investigate a specific disease or organ have been included in test panels.

Third party liability (13): Third party liability exists if an entity (not connected with the employer) is the cause and is liable to pay the medical cost for injury, disease, or disability of a person hurt during the performance of his or her occupation.

Third party subrogation (13): Legal process by which an insurance company seeks from a third party, who has caused a loss, recovery of the amount paid to the policyholder.

Time limit (2): Amount of time from the date of service to the date the insurance claim can be filed with the insurance company.

Total disability (13): Term that varies in meaning from one disability insurance policy to another. An example of a liberal definition might read, "The insured must be unable to perform the major duties of his or her specific occupation."

Total, permanent service-connected disabilities (12): Disabilities that are permanent in nature and incurred by a service member while on active duty.

Tracer (15): An inquiry made to an insurance company to locate the status of an insurance claim (i.e., claim in review, claim never received, and so forth).

Treating physician (7): Provider that renders a service to a patient; also known as *performing physician.*

TRICARE Extra (12): Preferred provider organization type of TRICARE option in which the individual does not have to enroll or pay an annual fee. On a visit-by-visit basis, the individual may seek care from an authorized network provider and received a discount on services and reduced cost-share (copayment).

TRICARE For Life (TFL) (12): Health care program that offers additional TRICARE benefits as a supplementary payer to Medicare for uniformed service retirees, their spouses, and survivors age 65 or older.

TRICARE Prime (12): Voluntary HMO-type option for TRICARE beneficiaries.

TRICARE Service Center (12): Office staffed by TRICARE Health Care Finders and beneficiary service representatives.

TRICARE Standard (12): Health care program offered to spouses and dependents of service personnel with uniform benefits and fees implemented nationwide by the federal government.

Unbundling (6): Practice of using numerous CPT codes to identify procedures normally covered by a single code; also known as *itemizing, fragmented billing, exploding,* or *à la carte medicine.*

Unemployment compensation disability (UCD) (13): See *State Disability Insurance (SDI).*

Unique provider identification number (UPIN) (8): Number issued by the Medicare fiscal intermediary to each physician who renders medical services to Medicare recipients; used for identification purposes on the HCFA-1500 claim form.

Upcoding (6): Deliberate manipulation of CPT codes for increased payment.

Usual, customary, and reasonable (UCR) (9): Method used by insurance companies to establish their fee schedules in which three fees are considered in calculating payment: (1) the usual fee is the fee typically submitted by the physician; (2) the customary fee falls within the range of usual fees charged by providers of similar training in a geographic area; and (3) the reasonable fee meets the aforementioned criteria or is considered justifiable because of special circumstances.

Utilization review (UR) (9): Process, based on established criteria, of reviewing and controlling the medical necessity for services and providers' use of medical care resources. Reviews are carried out by allied health care personnel at predetermined times during the hospital stay. In managed care systems, such as an HMO, reviews are done to establish medical necessity, thus curbing costs; also called *utilization* or *management control.*

V codes (4): Subclassification of ICD-9-CM coding used to identify health care encounters that occur for reasons other than illness or injury and to identify patients whose injury or illness is influenced by special circumstances or problems.

Verbal referral (9): Referral carried out via a telephone call from the primary care physician to the referring physician.

Veteran (12): Any person who has served in the armed forces of the United States, especially in time of war; is no longer in the service; and has received an honorable discharge.

Voluntary disability insurance (13): Self-insured disability insurance plan used in lieu of a state plan, where a majority of employees voluntarily consent to be covered.

Waiting period (WP) (2, 13): For disability insurance, the initial period of time when a disabled individual is not eligible to receive benefits even though unable to work; for workers' compensation, the days that must elapse before workers' compensation weekly income benefits become payable.

Waiver of premium (13): Disability insurance policy provision that states an employee does not have to pay any premiums while disabled; also known as *elimination period.*

Wide area network (WAN) (8): Interconnected computers that cover a large geographic area (e.g., America Online).

Workers' compensation (WC) insurance (13): Contract that insures a person against on-the-job injury or illness. The employer pays the premium for his or her employees.

Work hardening (13): Individualized program of therapy using simulated or real job duties to build up strength and improve the worker's endurance to be able to work up to 8 hours per day. Sometimes work site modifications are instituted to get the employee back to gainful employment.

Yo-yoing (1): Calling patients back for repeated and unnecessary follow-up visits.

Appendix F

College Clinic Form File

Make photocopies of all forms as indicated for use in future exercises. Additional photocopies may be made so that one can be used as a rough draft and one for final completion. Remember to complete forms using legible penmanship or typewriter as these may be placed into your job portfolio.

Form Number	Form Title	Approximate Number of Copies Needed
01	College Clinic Letterhead	2
02	Business Envelope	1
03	U.S. Postal Service Form	1
04	Insurance Predetermination Form	1
05	Patient Registration Form	1
06	Partially Completed Patient Registration Form	1
07	Ledger Card/Statement	13
08	Diagnostic Code Worksheet	3
09	HCFA-1500 Insurance Claim Form	12
10	Assignment Score Sheet	2
11	Performance Evaluation Checklist	12
12	Medical Record Coding Sheet	10
13	Treatment Authorization Request Form	1
14	TRICARE Preauthorization/Referral Request Form	1
15	Doctor's First Report of Occupational Injury and Illness Form	1
16	Insurance Claim Tracer	1
17	Ledger—Kenneth Kozak	1
18	Ledger—Larry Slomkowski	1
19	Ledger—Julie Vale	1

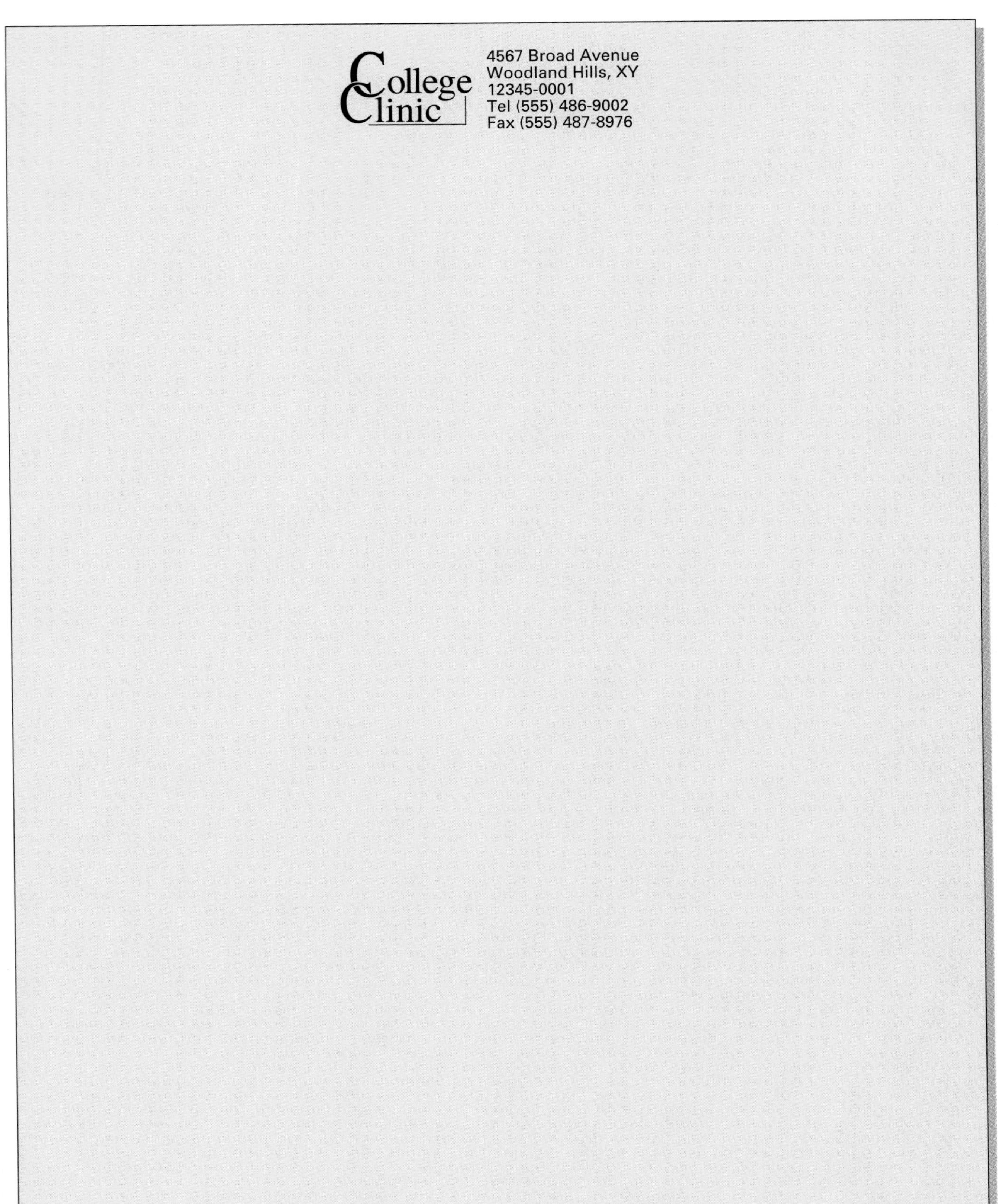
College Clinic
4567 Broad Avenue
Woodland Hills, XY
12345-0001
Tel (555) 486-9002
Fax (555) 487-8976

FORM 01

FORM 02

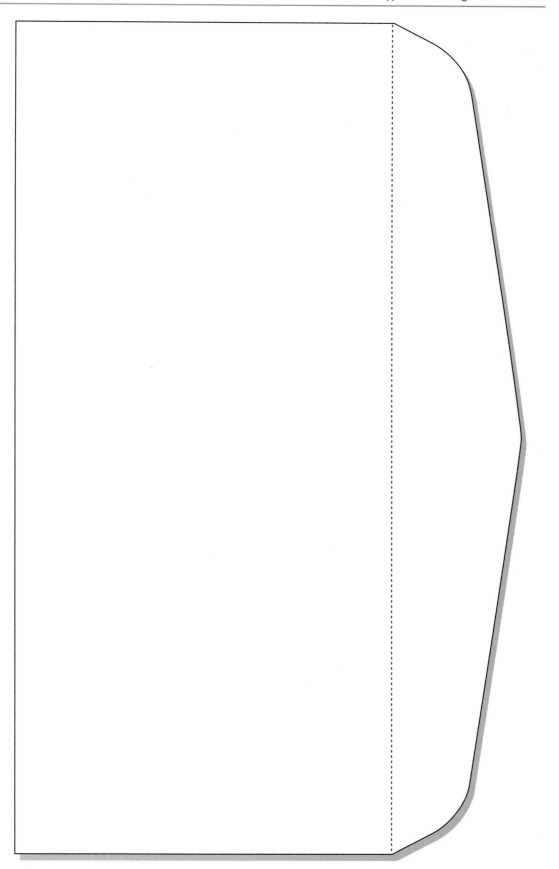

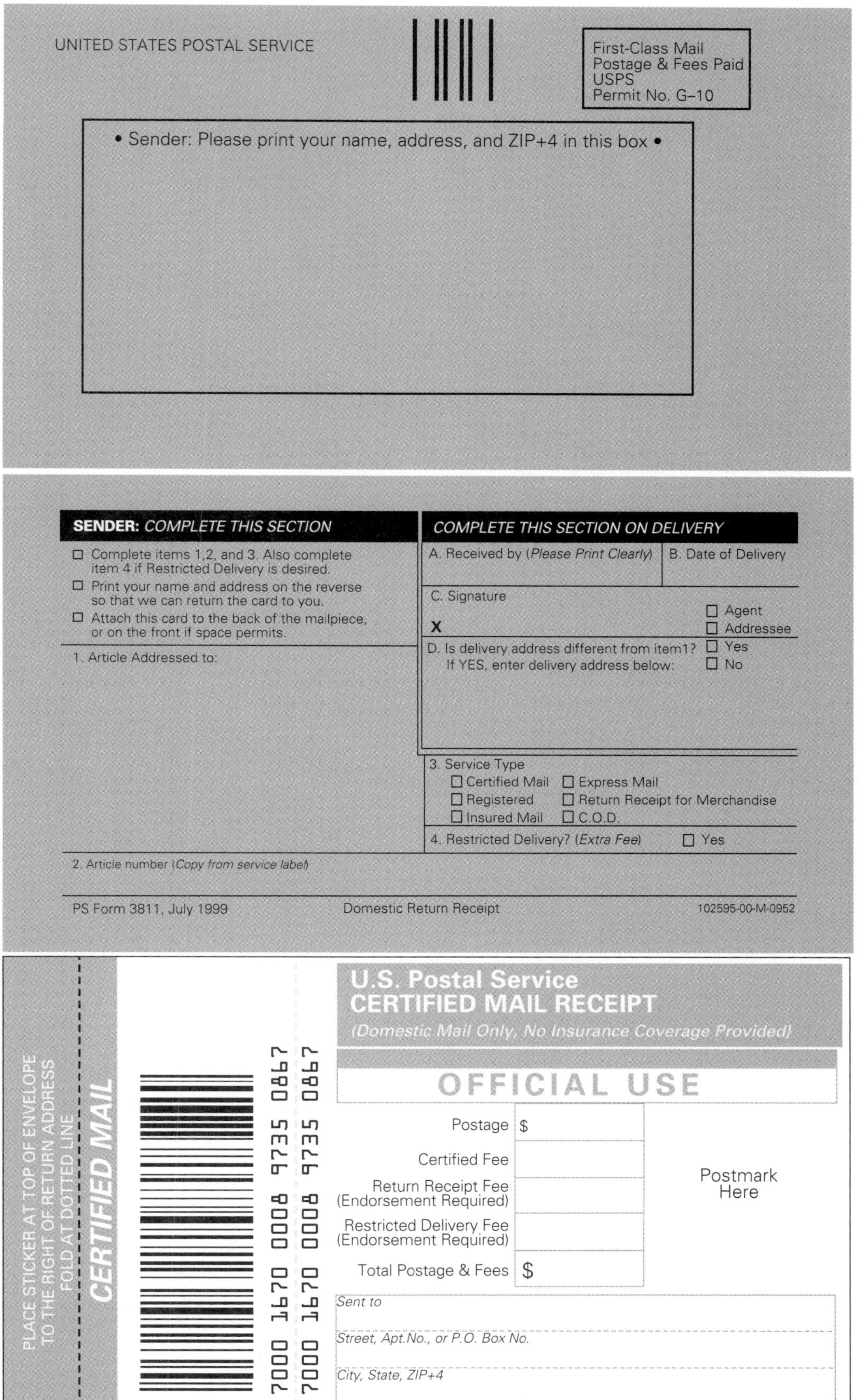
UNITED STATES POSTAL SERVICE

First-Class Mail
Postage & Fees Paid
USPS
Permit No. G–10

• Sender: Please print your name, address, and ZIP+4 in this box •

SENDER: *COMPLETE THIS SECTION*

☐ Complete items 1,2, and 3. Also complete item 4 if Restricted Delivery is desired.
☐ Print your name and address on the reverse so that we can return the card to you.
☐ Attach this card to the back of the mailpiece, or on the front if space permits.

1. Article Addressed to:

COMPLETE THIS SECTION ON DELIVERY

A. Received by (*Please Print Clearly*) B. Date of Delivery

C. Signature
X ☐ Agent ☐ Addressee

D. Is delivery address different from item1? ☐ Yes
If YES, enter delivery address below: ☐ No

3. Service Type
☐ Certified Mail ☐ Express Mail
☐ Registered ☐ Return Receipt for Merchandise
☐ Insured Mail ☐ C.O.D.

4. Restricted Delivery? (*Extra Fee*) ☐ Yes

2. Article number (*Copy from service label*)

PS Form 3811, July 1999 Domestic Return Receipt 102595-00-M-0952

PLACE STICKER AT TOP OF ENVELOPE TO THE RIGHT OF RETURN ADDRESS
FOLD AT DOTTED LINE

CERTIFIED MAIL

7000 1670 0008 9735 0867
7000 1670 0008 9735 0867

U.S. Postal Service
CERTIFIED MAIL RECEIPT
(Domestic Mail Only, No Insurance Coverage Provided)

OFFICIAL USE

Postage	$
Certified Fee	
Return Receipt Fee (Endorsement Required)	
Restricted Delivery Fee (Endorsement Required)	
Total Postage & Fees	$

Postmark Here

Sent to

Street, Apt.No., or P.O. Box No.

City, State, ZIP+4

PS Form 3800, May 2000 See Reverse for Instructions

FORM 03

College Clinic
4567 Broad Avenue
Woodland Hills, XY
12345-0001

Phone: 555/486-9002 Fax: 555/487-8976

INSURANCE PREDETERMINATION FORM

Raymond Skeleton MD
physician

Patient: Mason Roberts
Telephone # (555) 486-2233
Address: 2400 Lighthouse Way
Date of Birth 11-15-60
City Woodland Hills State XY
ZIP 12345
Social Security # 421-XX-1491
Accident Yes____ No ✓
Insurance Company ABC Insurance Co
Member # 215497T
Insurance Co. Address 4500 Center Street
Los Alamos, XY 12345
Group # 1201
Telephone # (555) 986-4700
Policy holder Mason Roberts
Relationship to insured: Self X Spouse____ Child____ Other____
Type of coverage: HMO____ PPO____ 80/20____ 70/30____ Other:____
Procedure/Service Aspiration and injection of bone cyst (CPT 20615)
Diagnosis Solitary bone cyst (ICD-9-CM 733.21)

BENEFITS:

Coverage effective date: From________ To________
Maximum benefit or benefit limitation:________
Pre-existing exclusions: ________
Second opinion requirements: Yes____ No____
Major medical Yes____ No____
Precertification/Preauthorization Yes____ No____
Deductible Yes____ No____ Amount $________
Reference #________
Per family: Yes____ No____ Amount $________
Authorized by:________
Deductible paid to date: Amount $________
Out of pocket expense limit: Amount $________
Per:________

COVERAGE:

Procedures/Services

			COVERAGE DETAILS AND LIMITS
Office visits	YES ____	NO ____	________
Consultations	YES ____	NO ____	________
ER visits	YES ____	NO ____	________
X-ray	YES ____	NO ____	________
Laboratory	YES ____	NO ____	________
Office surgery	YES ____	NO ____	________
Hospital surgery	YES ____	NO ____	________
Anesthesia	YES ____	NO ____	________
DME			________

Physician payment schedule: RVS____ RBRVS____ UCR____ Other____

Payment sent to: Provider____ Patient ____ Time limit after submssion?________
Verification by:________ Date:________

FORM 04

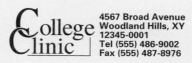

4567 Broad Avenue
Woodland Hills, XY
12345-0001
Tel (555) 486-9002
Fax (555) 487-8976

REGISTRATION
(PLEASE PRINT)

Account #________________ Today's Date: ________________

PATIENT INFORMATION

Name ______________________________ Soc. Sec. # ________________
Last Name First Name Initial

Address ______________________________ Home Phone ________________

City ________________ State ________ Zip ________________

Single___ Married___ Separated___ Divorced___ Sex M___ F___ Birthdate ________________

Patient Employed by ______________________________ Occupation ________________

Business Address ______________________________ Business Phone ________________

Spouse's Name ________________ Employed by ________ Occupation ________________

Business Address ______________________________ Business Phone ________________

Reason for Visit ________________ If accident: Auto____ Employment____ Other________

By whom were you referred? ______________________________

In case of emergency, who should be notified? ______________________________ Phone ________________
Name Relation to Patient

PRIMARY INSURANCE

Insured/Subscriber ______________________________
Last Name First Name Initial

Relation to Patient ________________ Birthdate ________ Soc. Sec.# ________________

Address (if different from patient's) ______________________________

City ________________ State ________ Zip ________________

Insurance Company ______________________________

Insurance Address ______________________________

Insurance Identification Number ________________ Group # ________________

ADDITIONAL INSURANCE

Is patient covered by additional insurance? Yes ______ No ______

Subscriber Name ________________ Relation to Patient ________ Birthdate ________________

Address (if different from patient's) ______________________________ Phone ________________

City ________________ State ________ Zip ________________

Subscriber Employed by ______________________________ Business Phone ________________

Insurance Company ______________________________ Soc. Sec. # ________________

Insurance Address ______________________________

Insurance Identification Number ________________ Group # ________________

ASSIGNMENT AND RELEASE

I, the undersigned, certify that I (or my dependent) have insurance coverage with ______________________________ and assign
Name of Insurance Company(ies)

directly to Dr. ________________ insurance benefits, if any, otherwise payable to me for services rendered. I understand that I am financially responsible for all charges whether or not paid by insurance. I hereby consent for the doctor to release all information necessary to secure the payment of benefits. I authorize the use of this signature on all insurance submissions.

______________________________ ________________ ________________
Responsible Party Signature Relationship Date

ORDER # 58-8426 @BIBBERO SYSTEMS, INC. •PETALUMA, CALIFORNIA• TO REORDER CALL TOLL FREE (800)242-9330

FORM 05

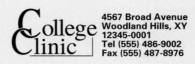

4567 Broad Avenue
Woodland Hills, XY
12345-0001
Tel (555) 486-9002
Fax (555) 487-8976

REGISTRATION
(PLEASE PRINT)

Account # 0296 Today's Date: 08/05/XX

PATIENT INFORMATION

Name Young (Last Name) Eunice (First Name) L. (Initial) Soc. Sec. # 286-XX-1400

Address 1400 Vega Drive Home Phone (555) 486-0927

City Woodland Hills State XY Zip 12345

Single___ Married ✓ Separated___ Divorced___ Sex M___ F ✓ Birthdate 02-19-74

Patient Employed by Malibu Design Center Occupation Interior Decorator

Business Address 209 Beach Blvd. Malibu XY 12345 Business Phone (555) 296-0404

Spouse's Name Gary Young Employed by Point Loma Tech Occupation Engineer

Business Address 7219 First Street Point Loma, XY Business Phone (555) 386-2000

Reason for Visit Wrist pain If accident: Auto___ Employment___ Other ✓

By whom were you referred? Mother - Beatrice Yim

In case of emergency, who should be notified? Gary Young (Name) Husband (Relation to Patient) Phone (555) 296-0404

PRIMARY INSURANCE

Insured/Subscriber ___ Last Name ___ First Name ___ Initial

Relation to Patient ___ Birthdate ___ Soc. Sec.# ___

Address (if different from patient's) ___

City ___ State ___ Zip ___

Insurance Company ___

Insurance Address ___

Insurance Identification Number ___ Group # ___

ADDITIONAL INSURANCE

Is patient covered by additional insurance? Yes___ No ✓

Subscriber Name ___ Relation to Patient ___ Birthdate ___

Address (if different from patient's) ___ Phone ___

City ___ State ___ Zip ___

Subscriber Employed by ___ Business Phone ___

Insurance Company ___ Soc. Sec. # ___

Insurance Address ___

Insurance Identification Number ___ Group # ___

ASSIGNMENT AND RELEASE

I, the undersigned, certify that I (or my dependent) have insurance coverage with Health Net (Name of Insurance Company(ies)) and assign directly to Dr. Gerald Practon insurance benefits, if any, otherwise payable to me for services rendered. I understand that I am financially responsible for all charges whether or not paid by insurance. I hereby consent for the doctor to release all information necessary to secure the payment of benefits. I authorize the use of this signature on all insurance submissions.

Gary C Young (Responsible Party Signature) Husband (Relationship) 8-05-XX (Date)

ORDER # 58-8426 ©BIBBERO SYSTEMS, INC. • PETALUMA, CALIFORNIA • TO REORDER CALL TOLL FREE (800)242-9330

FORM 06

STATEMENT

College Clinic
4567 Broad Avenue
Woodland Hills, XY 12345-0001
Tel: (555) 486-9002
Fax: (555) 487-8976

Phone No. (H) ________________ (W) ________________ Birthdate: ________________
Insurance Co. ________________ Policy No. ________________

DATE	REFERENCE	PROFESSIONAL SERVICE DESCRIPTION	CHARGE	CREDITS		CURRENT BALANCE
				Payments	Adjustments	

Due and payable within 10 days.

Pay last amount in balance column ⇧

Key: PF: Problem-focused
EPF: Expanded problem-focused
D: Detailed
SF: Straightfoward
L: Low complexity
M: Moderate complexity
CON: Consultation
HX: History
PX: Phys Exam
ED: Emergency Dept.
HC: House call
HV: Hospital visit

FORM 07

Diagnostic Code Worksheet

DIAGNOSTIC STATEMENT	MAIN TERM	SUBTERM	SUBSUBTERM	ADDITIONAL SUBTERMS	CODE	Verified in Volume 1

FORM 08

PLEASE DO NOT STAPLE IN THIS AREA

PICA

HEALTH INSURANCE CLAIM FORM

PICA

CARRIER

PATIENT AND INSURED INFORMATION

1. MEDICARE (Medicare #) MEDICAID (Medicaid #) CHAMPUS (Sponsor's SSN) CHAMPVA (VA File #) GROUP Health Plan (SSN or ID) FECA BLK LUNG (SSN) OTHER (ID)

1a. INSURED I.D. NUMBER (FOR PROGRAM IN ITEM 1)

2. PATIENT'S NAME (Last Name, First Name, Middle Initial)

3. PATIENT'S BIRTH DATE MM DD YYYY SEX M F

4. INSURED'S NAME (LAST NAME, FIRST NAME, MIDDLE INITIAL)

5. PATIENT'S ADDRESS (No., Street)

6. PATIENT RELATIONSHIP TO INSURED Self Spouse Child Other

7. INSURED'S ADDRESS (No, Street)

CITY STATE

8. PATIENT STATUS Single Married Other

CITY STATE

ZIP CODE TELEPHONE (Include Area Code) ( )

Employed Full-Time Student Part-Time Student

ZIP CODE TELEPHONE (INCLUDE AREA CODE) ( )

9. OTHER INSURED'S NAME (Last Name, First Name, Middle Initial)

10. IS PATIENT'S CONITION RELATED TO:

11. INSURED'S POLICY GROUP OR FECA NUMBER

a. OTHER INSURED'S POLICY OR GROUP NUMBER

a. EMPLOYMENT? (CURRENT OR PREVIOUS) YES NO

a. INSURED'S DATE OF BIRTH MM DD YYYY SEX M F

b. OTHER INSURED'S DATE OF BIRTH MM DD YY SEX M F

b. AUTO ACCIDENT? YES NO PLACE (State)

b. EMPLOYER'S NAME OR SCHOOL NAME

c. EMPLOYER'S NAME OR SCHOOL NAME

c. OTHER ACCIDENT? YES NO

c. INSURANCE PLAN NAME OR PROGRAM NMAE

d. INSURANCE PLAN NAME OR PROGRAM NAME

10d. RESERVED FOR LOCAL USE

d. IS THERE ANOTHER HEALTH BENEFIT PLAN? YES NO *If yes*, return to and complete item 9 a-d

READ BACK OF FORM BEFORE COMPLETING & SIGNING THIS FORM

12. PATIENT'S OR AUTHORIZED PERSON'S SIGNATURE. I authorize the release of any medical or other information necessary to process this claim. I also request payment of government benefits either to myself or to the party who accepts assignment below.

SIGNED ______ DATE ______

13. INSURED'S OR AUTHORIZED PERSON'S SIGNATURE. I authorize payment of medical benefits to the undersigned physician or supplier for services described below

SIGNED ______

PHYSICIAN OR SUPPLIER INFORMATION

14. DATE OF CURRENT: MM DD YY ILLNESS (First symptom) OR INJURY (Accident) OR PREGNANCY (LMP)

15. IF PATIENT HAS HAD SAME OR SIMILAR ILLNESS GIVE FIRST DATE MM DD YYYY

16. DATES PATIENT UNABLE TO WORK IN CURRENT OCCUPATION FROM MM DD YYYY TO MM DD YYYY

17. NAME OF REFERRING PHYSICIAN OR OTHER SOURCE

17a. I.D. NUMBER OF REFERRING PHYSICIAN

18. HOSPITALIZATION DATES RELATED TO CURRENT SERVICES FROM MM DD YYYY TO MM DD YYYY

19. RESERVED FOR LOCAL USE

20. OUTSIDE LAB? YES NO $ CHARGES

21. DIAGNOSIS OR NATURE OF ILLNESS OR INJURY. (RELATE ITEMS 1,2,3 OR 4 TO ITEM 24E BY LINE)

1. ______ 3. ______

2. ______ 4. ______

22. MEDICAID RESUBMISSION CODE ORIGINAL REF. NO.

23. PRIOR AUTHORIZATION NUMBER

24. A DATE(S) OF SERVICE From MM DD YY To MM DD YY	B Place of Service	C Type of Service	D PROCEDURES, SERVICES, OR SUPPLIES (Explain Unusual Circumstances) CPT/HCPCS MODIFIER	E DIAGNOSIS CODE	F $ CHARGES	G DAYS OR UNITS	H EPSDT Family Plan	I EMG	J COB	K RESERVED FOR LOCAL USE

25. FEDERAL TAX I.D. NUMBER SSN EIN

26. PATIENT'S ACCOUNT NO.

27. ACCEPT ASSIGNMENT? (For govt. claims, see back) YES NO

28. TOTAL CHARGE $

29. AMOUNT PAID $

30. BALANCE DUE $

31. SIGNATURE OF PHYSICIAN OR SUPPLIER INCLUDING DEGREES OR CREDENTIALS (I certify that the statements on the reverse apply to this bill and are made a part thereof)

SIGNED DATE

32. NAME AND ADDRESS OF FACILITY WHERE SERVICECS WERE RENDERED (If other than home or office)

33. PHYSICIAN'S, SUPPLIER'S BILLING NAME, ADDRESS, ZIP CODE & PHONE #

PIN# GRP#

(APPROVED BY AMA COUNCIL ON MEDICAL SERVICE 8/88)

PLEASE PRINT OR TYPE

APPROVED OMB-0938-0008 FORM HCFA-1500 (12-90), FRM RRB-1500, APPROVED OMB-1215-0055 FORM OWCP-1500, APPROVED OMB-0720-0001 (CHAMPUS)

FORM 09

Weigh Your Progress!

ASSIGNMENT SCORE SHEET

KEY
SS = Study Session
EE = Exercise Exchange
BB = Billing Break

DATE ASSIGNED	DATE COMPLETED	ASSIGNMENT SS/EE/BB	STUDENT SCORE	POSSIBLE SCORE	PERCENT	COMMENTS
1/1/01	*1/8/01*	*SS # 1-16*	*15*	*16*	*94%*	

Divide the student score by the amount possible to obtain a percentage (15 ÷ 16 = 94%)

FORM 10

PERFORMANCE EVALUATION CHECKLIST

Billing Break No. ______________

Student Name: ________________________________ Date: ________________

Performance Objective

Task: Given access to all necessary equipment and information, the student will complete a HCFA-1500 health insurance claim form.

Standards: Claim Productivity Management
Time__________ minutes
Note: Time element may be given by instructor

Directions: See Billing Break assignment

NOTE TIME BEGAN__________ **NOTE TIME COMPLETED**__________

PROCEDURE STEPS	ASSIGNED POINTS	STEP PERFORMED SATISFACTORY	COMMENTS
1. Assembled HCFA-1500 claim form, patient record E/M code slip, ledger card, typewriter or computer, pen or pencil, and code books.	________	________	________
2. Posted ledger card correctly.	________	________	________
3. Proofread form for spelling and typographical errors while form remained in typewriter or on computer screen.	________	________	________
4. Points earned for corrrect completion of HCFA-1500 block-by-block data (see next page).	________	________	________
TOTAL	________	________	________

FORM 11a

PERFORMANCE EVALUATION CHECKLIST

BLOCK	INCORRECT	MISSING	NOT NEEDED	REMARKS	BLOCK	INCORRECT	MISSING	NOT NEEDED	REMARKS
1					18				
1A					19				
2					20				
3					21				
4									
5					22				
6					23				
7					24A				
8					24B				
					24C				
9					24D				
9A									
9B									
9C					24E				
9D									
					24F				
10A					24G				
10B					24H, 24I				
10C					24J				
10D					24K				
11					25, 26				
11A					27				
11B					28				
11C					29				
11D									
12					30				
13									
14					31				
15									
16					32				
17									
17A					33				
					Reference Initials				

TOTAL POINTS EARNED: ____________ TOTAL POINTS POSSIBLE: ____________

Evaluator's signature ____________________________ NEED TO REPEAT: ____________

Comments: ____

____

FORM 11b

MEDICAL RECORD CODING WORKSHEET

DOS	Symptom/code	Diagnosis/code	Services and Procedures /code
______	1.__________/________	1.__________/________	1.__________/________
______	2.__________/________	2.__________/________	2.__________/________
______	3.__________/________	3.__________/________	3.__________/________
______	4.__________/________	4.__________/________	4.__________/________
______	5.__________/________	5.__________/________	5.__________/________
______	6.__________/________	6.__________/________	6.__________/________

FORM 12

MANAGED CARE PLAN AUTHORIZATION REQUEST

TO BE COMPLETED BY PRIMARY CARE PHYSICIAN OR OUTSIDE PROVIDER

Health Net ☐ Met Life ☐
Pacificare ☐ Travelers ☐
Secure Horizons ☐ Pru Care ☐

Member No. ______________

Patient Name: ______________ Date: ______________

M____ F____ Birthdate ______________ Home telephone number ______________

Address ______________

Primary Care Physician ______________ Provider ID# ______________

Referring Physician ______________ Provider ID# ______________

Referred to ______________ Address ______________

______________ Office telephone number ______________

Diagnosis Code ______________ Diagnosis ______________

Diagnosis Code ______________ Diagnosis ______________

Treatment Plan: ______________

Authorization requested for procedures/tests/visits:

Procedure Code ______________ Description ______________

Procedure Code ______________ Description ______________

Facility to be used: ______________ Estimated length of stay ______________

Office ☐ Outpatient ☐ Inpatient ☐ Other ☐

List of potential consultants (i.e., anesthetists, assistants, or medical/surgical):

____

Physician's signature ______________

TO BE COMPLETED BY PRIMARY CARE PHYSICIAN

PCP Recommendations: ______________ PCP Initials ______________

Date eligibility checked ______________ Effective date ______________

TO BE COMPLETED BY UTILIZATION MANAGEMENT

Authorized ______________ Not authorized ______________

Deferred ______________ Modified ______________

Authorization Request # ______________

Comments: ______________

FORM 13

TRICARE PREAUTHORIZATION/REFERRAL REQUEST FORM

Do not schedule procedures or appointments prior to receiving authorization.

TRICARE Service Center ______________________ Fax No.______________________

HCF/CRN ______________________ Telephone No. ______________________

Request is: ☐ Emergent ☐ Urgent ☐ Routine
☐ Referral/consult ☐ Preauthorization ☐ Second Opinion

Sponsor's Name ______________________ Sponsor's SSN ______________________

Sponsor's Date of Birth ______________________ Sex: ☐ Male ☐ Female

____

Patient's Last Name First Name Middle Initial Telephone No.

____

Address City State ZIP Code Date of Birth

Plan: ☐ Prime ☐ Extra ☐ Standard ☐ TSP ☐ TPR ☐ SHCP

Other Insurance ☐ Yes ☐ No If yes, specify: ______________________

Requesting MD/DO (if not PCM): ______________________ TIN No. ______________________

Contact person: ______________________ Phone No. ______________________ Fax No. ______________________

Refer to facility (name): ______________________ Phone No. ______________________

Refer to provider (name): ______________________ Specialty: ______________________

Provider phone no. ______________________ TIN# ______________________ Suffix______________________

Place of service: ☐ Inpatient ☐ Outpatient Anticipated date(s) of service______________________

PCM: ______________________ Telephone no. ______________________

Diagnosis (description): ______________________ ICD-9-CM Code ______________________

CPT Code: ______________ Units: ______________ Description: ______________________

CPT Code: ______________ Units: ______________ Description: ______________________

CPT Code: ______________ Units: ______________ Description: ______________________

Request CANNOT be processed without the following: (1) Clinical history, (2) previous treatment, (3) plan of treatment, (4) supporting lab and x-ray reports, etc.

____

____

____

____

____

____

FORM 14

DOCTOR'S FIRST REPORT OF OCCUPATIONAL INJURY OR ILLNESS

Within 5 days of initial examination, for every occupational injury or illness, send 2 copies of this report to the employer's workers' compensation insurance carrier or the self-insured employer. Failure to file a timely doctor's report may result in assessment of a civil penalty. In the case of diagnosed or suspected pesticide poisoning, send a copy of this report to Division of Labor Statistics and Research.

1. INSURER NAME AND ADDRESS

2. EMPLOYER NAME Policy No.

3. Address No. and Street City Zip

4. Nature of business (e.g., food manufacturing, building construction, retailer of women's clothes)

5. PATIENT NAME (first name, middle initial, last name) | 6. Sex ☐ Male ☐ Female | 7. Date of birth Mo. Day Yr.

8. Address No. and Street City Zip | 9. Telephone Number

10. Occupation (Specific job title) | 11. Social Security Number

12. Injured at: No. and Street City County

13. Date and hour of injury or onset of illness Mo. Day Yr. Hour ____ a.m. ____ p.m. | 14. Date last worked Mo. Day Yr.

15. Date and hour of first examination or treatment Mo. Day Yr. Hour ____ a.m. ____ p.m. | 16. Have you (or your office) previously treated patient? ☐ Yes ☐ No

Patient please complete this portion, if able to do so. Otherwise, doctor please complete immediately. Inability or failure of a patient to complete this portion shall not affect his/her rights to workers' compensation under the Labor Code.

17. DESCRIBE HOW THE ACCIDENT OR EXPOSURE HAPPENED (Give specific object, machinery or chemical)

18. SUBJECTIVE COMPLAINTS (Describe fully.)

19. OBJECTIVE FINDINGS

A. Physical examination

B. X-ray and laboratory results (state if none or pending.)

20. DIAGNOSIS (If occupational illness specify etiologic agent and duration of exposure.) Chemical or toxic compounds involved? ☐ Yes ☐ No

ICD-9 Code ________

21. Are your findings and diagnosis consistent with patient's account of injury or onset of illness? ☐ Yes ☐ No If "no" please explain.

22. Is there any other current condition that will impede or delay patient's recovery? ☐ Yes ☐ No If "yes" please explain.

23. TREATMENT REQUIRED

24. If further treatment required, specify treatment plan/estimated duration.

25. If hospitalized as inpatient, give hospital name and location Date admitted Mo. Day Yr. Estimated stay

26. WORK STATUS–Is patient able to perform usual work? ☐ Yes ☐ No

If "no," date when patient can return to: Regular work ___/___/___

Modified work ___/___/___ Specify restrictions ________

Doctor's signature ________ License number ________

Doctor's name and degree ________ IRS number ________

Address ________ Telephone number ________

FORM 15

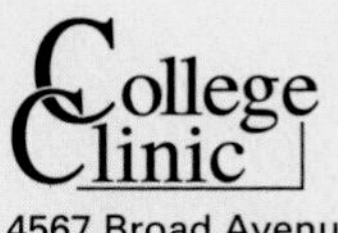

Telephone (555) 486-9002

4567 Broad Avenue
Woodland Hills, XY
12345-0001

Fax (555) 487-8976

INSURANCE CLAIM TRACER

INSURANCE COMPANY NAME ______________________ DATE ______________

ADDRESS ____

Patient: ______________________

Insured: ______________________

Employer: ______________________

Policy/certificate no. ______________________

Group name/no. ______________________

Date of initial claim submission: ______________

Amount of claim: ______________________

> An inordinate amount of time has passed since the submission of our original claim. We have not received a request for additional information and still await payment of this assigned claim. Please review the attached duplicate and process for payment within 7 days.

If there is any difficulty with this claim, please check the reason below and return this letter to our office. Thank you.

- ☐ No record of claim.
- ☐ Claim received and payment is in process.
- ☐ Claim is in suspense (comment please).
- ☐ Claim is in review (comment please).
- ☐ Additional information needed (comment please)
- ☐ Claim paid. Date: __________ Amount:$ ______________ To whom: ______________
- ☐ Claim denied (comment please).

Comments: ____

____

____

Thank you for your assistance in this important matter. Please contact the insurance specialist named below if you have any questions regarding this claim.

______________________ Insurance Specialist (555) 486-9002 Ext. ________

______________________ Treating Physician

FORM 16

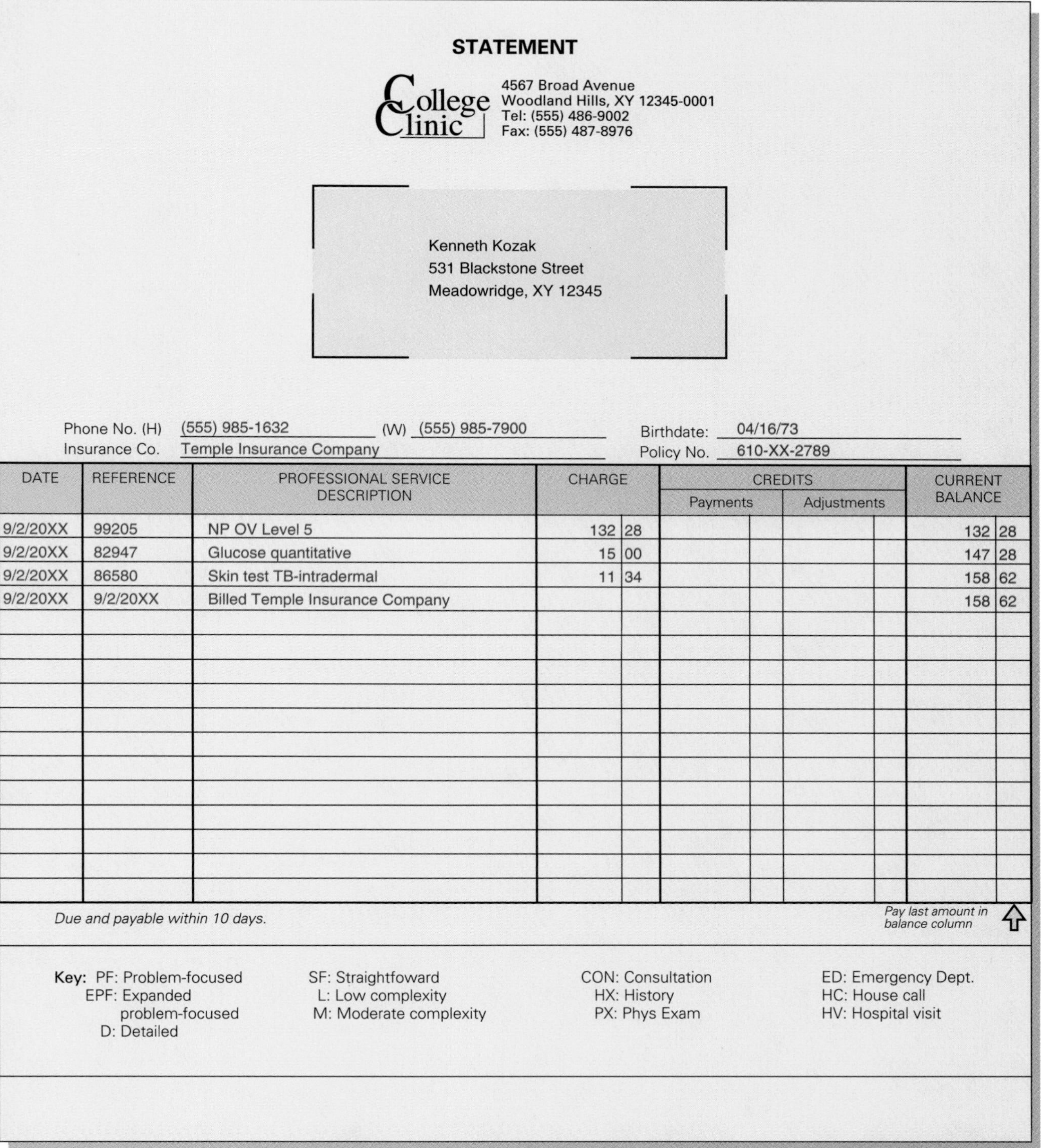

STATEMENT

College Clinic
4567 Broad Avenue
Woodland Hills, XY 12345-0001
Tel: (555) 486-9002
Fax: (555) 487-8976

Kenneth Kozak
531 Blackstone Street
Meadowridge, XY 12345

Phone No. (H) (555) 985-1632 (W) (555) 985-7900 Birthdate: 04/16/73
Insurance Co. Temple Insurance Company Policy No. 610-XX-2789

DATE	REFERENCE	PROFESSIONAL SERVICE DESCRIPTION	CHARGE		CREDITS				CURRENT BALANCE	
					Payments		Adjustments			
9/2/20XX	99205	NP OV Level 5	132	28					132	28
9/2/20XX	82947	Glucose quantitative	15	00					147	28
9/2/20XX	86580	Skin test TB-intradermal	11	34					158	62
9/2/20XX	9/2/20XX	Billed Temple Insurance Company							158	62

Due and payable within 10 days.

Pay last amount in balance column

Key: PF: Problem-focused
EPF: Expanded problem-focused
D: Detailed
SF: Straightfoward
L: Low complexity
M: Moderate complexity
CON: Consultation
HX: History
PX: Phys Exam
ED: Emergency Dept.
HC: House call
HV: Hospital visit

FORM 17

STATEMENT

College Clinic
4567 Broad Avenue
Woodland Hills, XY 12345-0001
Tel: (555) 486-9002
Fax: (555) 487-8976

Larry Slomkowski
12 Ramona Place
Orange Grove, XY 12345

Phone No. (H) (555) 967-6111 (W) (555) 486-1616 Birthdate: 03/10/69
Insurance Co. Temple Insurance Company Policy No. 886-XX-7940

DATE	REFERENCE	PROFESSIONAL SERVICE DESCRIPTION	CHARGE		CREDITS Payments		CREDITS Adjustments		CURRENT BALANCE	
2/12/20XX	99202	NP OV Level 2	51	91					51	91
2/12/20XX	2/12/20XX	Billed Temple Insurance Company							51	91
3/25/20XX	Ck #4890	ROA Temple Ins. Co. (2/12/20XX)			41	23			10	68
3/25/20XX	2/12/20XX	Billed Patient							10	68
4/10/20XX	Ck #302	ROA Patient			10	68			0	0
9/5/20XX	99212	Est Pt OV Level 2	28	55					28	55
9/5/20XX	9/5/20XX	Billed Temple Insurance Company							28	55

Due and payable within 10 days.

Pay last amount in balance column

Key: PF: Problem-focused
EPF: Expanded problem-focused
D: Detailed
SF: Straightfoward
L: Low complexity
M: Moderate complexity
CON: Consultation
HX: History
PX: Phys Exam
ED: Emergency Dept.
HC: House call
HV: Hospital visit

FORM 18

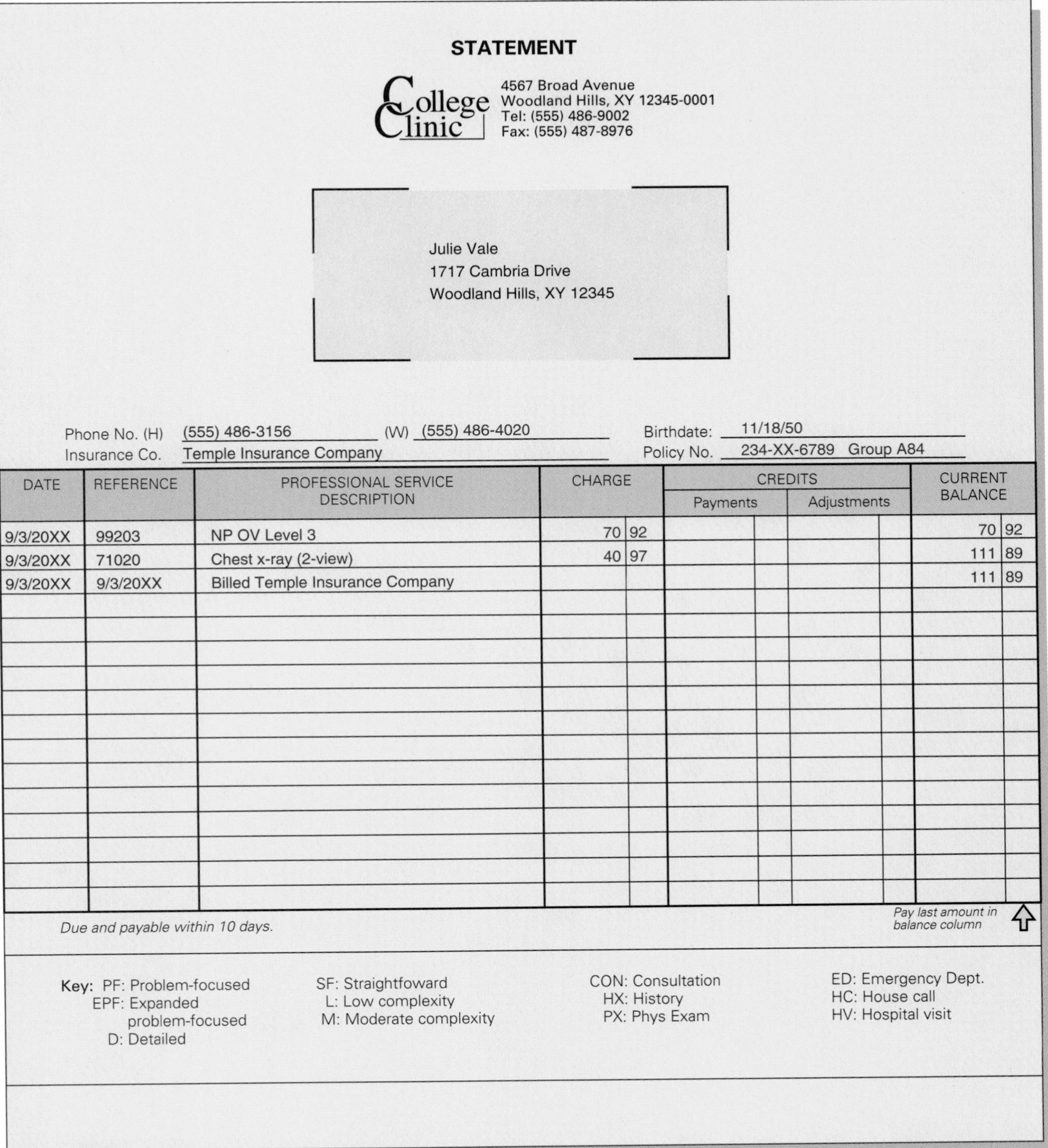

STATEMENT

College Clinic
4567 Broad Avenue
Woodland Hills, XY 12345-0001
Tel: (555) 486-9002
Fax: (555) 487-8976

Julie Vale
1717 Cambria Drive
Woodland Hills, XY 12345

Phone No. (H) (555) 486-3156 (W) (555) 486-4020 Birthdate: 11/18/50
Insurance Co. Temple Insurance Company Policy No. 234-XX-6789 Group A84

DATE	REFERENCE	PROFESSIONAL SERVICE DESCRIPTION	CHARGE		CREDITS Payments		CREDITS Adjustments		CURRENT BALANCE	
9/3/20XX	99203	NP OV Level 3	70	92					70	92
9/3/20XX	71020	Chest x-ray (2-view)	40	97					111	89
9/3/20XX	9/3/20XX	Billed Temple Insurance Company							111	89

Due and payable within 10 days.

Pay last amount in balance column ⇧

Key: PF: Problem-focused
EPF: Expanded problem-focused
D: Detailed
SF: Straightfoward
L: Low complexity
M: Moderate complexity
CON: Consultation
HX: History
PX: Phys Exam
ED: Emergency Dept.
HC: House call
HV: Hospital visit

FORM 19

Appendix

G

Student Software Challenge *Installation and Operating Instructions*

Since many medical practices use computer technology to perform financial operations, user-friendly computer software is included with the *Medical Insurance Billing and Coding* worktext. It is designed to create a realistic approach to completing the HCFA-1500 insurance claim form. All relevant documents appear on screen and may be printed for 10 patient cases that escalate in difficulty. Key terms are integrated into the cases, and definitions may be accessed from a glossary.

The main objective is to complete the HCFA-1500 insurance claim form for each case and insert accurate data, including diagnostic and procedural code numbers. This mimics real office claims processing. The HCFA-1500 form has been created in an open-entry format, making it easy to move between the related patient forms and corresponding blocks on the HCFA form. By working through the cases, the student will challenge coding skills, computer skills, and critical thinking skills.

An ongoing summary of scores achieved on completed cases may be brought up on screen to keep the student and instructor informed of progress made. Detailed scoring reports may be printed so that the instructor has access to the information from time to time. The software also allows the user to complete the HCFA-1500 claim form for all Billing Break assignments and print it out for evaluation. This method of learning will help the student produce perfect completed insurance claims in a fun and challenging way.

MINIMUM SYSTEM REQUIREMENTS

Operating System:	Windows 95 or 98 only
Computer:	IBM and compatible PCs with 80486/66 or Pentium CPU MS-DOS 5.0 or 6.0
Optimal Screen Requirements:	sVGA or higher graphics adapter operating in 640 × 480, 256-color mode
Other Requirements:	CD-ROM drive Mouse
Memory:	16 MB RAM

SITE LICENSE

A single-user license agreement appears on the last page in this worktext. To order a site license for this program, contact your local sales representative or customer service at (800) 222-9570; technical support (800) 692-9010.

INSTALLING THE PROGRAM

The software may be installed on individual computers and is network compatible with most networks, including Novell Netware 4.1 and Windows NT Server 4.0.

Before you can use the software, you must install it on your hard drive. The installer decompresses and copies files from the *Student Software Challenge* CD-ROM onto your hard drive or network and creates a Medical Insurance folder.

Steps to Install the *Student Software Challenge* on a Computer Running Windows 95 or 98

1. Turn off virus protection, disk-security, and other open programs prior to installing *Student Software Challenge*.
2. Insert the *Student Software Challenge* CD-ROM into the CD-ROM drive.
3. Launch the *Student Software Challenge* installer by double-clicking the file called "install.exe" on the CD-ROM. Launch the installer by selecting **Run** from the Start menu, type d:\Setup.exe in the Command Line (where "d" represents your CD-ROM drive), and press **Enter.** If necessary, substitute the appropriate drive letter for your CD-ROM drive.
4. Follow the installation instructions that appear on your screen. There are several options during installation.
   - ***Minimum install.*** *The default installation option is used to install only those files needed to run the program from the CD-ROM. As the student uses the program, any student data files will need to be saved to a floppy disk. The user can instead select to save files to the hard drive by selecting "minimum install, save to hard drive." If the floppy disk option is chosen, the student must have his or her disk to log-on and use the program. Installing the CD-ROM runtime version requires approximately 1 MB of free hard-drive space.*
   - ***Full install.*** *The full installation option installs the entire program on the hard drive. Installing the entire program requires approximately 23 MB of free hard-drive space and will enhance the software's performance. Again, the user can select whether to save files to a floppy disk or to the hard drive.*
5. Select the location where the program will be installed. The default location is C:\MI7. Use the Browse feature to change the drive or directory in which the software will be installed. The installation program automatically detects whether there is adequate free space available on the hard drive. If there is not enough space available, a prompt appears directing you to select another location. *Note:* To install the software to a network hard drive, use the Browse feature to locate the network drive.

6. Once installation is complete, a program folder will appear on the user's desktop. Click "Medical Insurance Software Challenge" to start the program. For future use, the user can drag the "Medical Insurance Software Challenge" icon onto his or her desktop for easy access. The program is also accessible via Start/Programs/Medical Insurance/Medical Insurance Software Challenge.

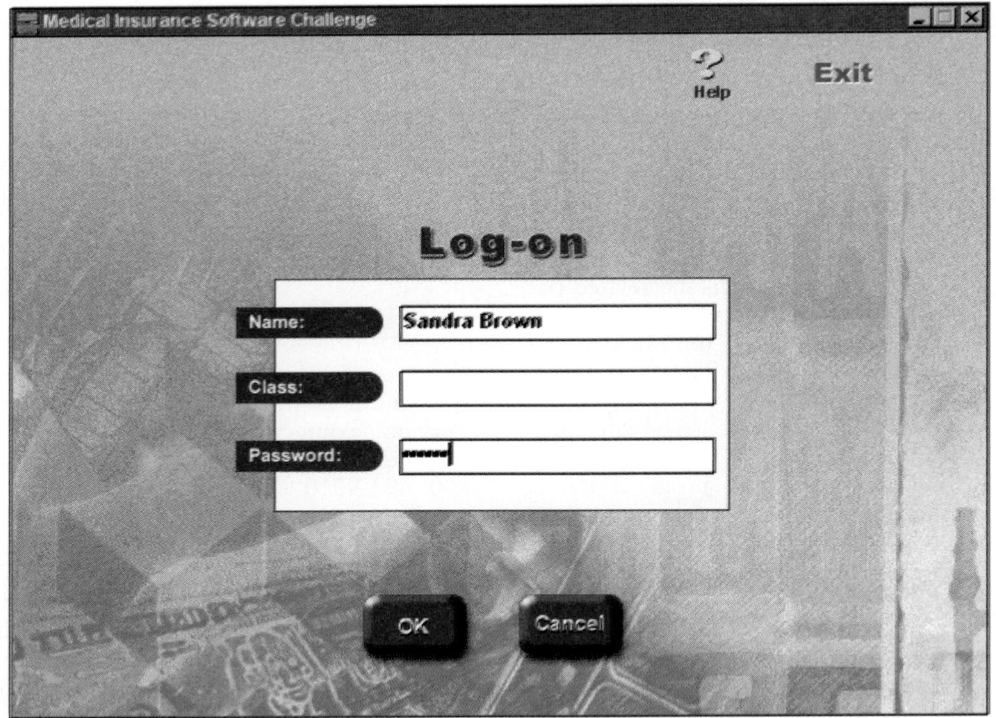

Figure G–1. Log-on screen.

LOGGING ON TO *STUDENT SOFTWARE CHALLENGE*

First-Time Log-on Steps

1. If the installation is configured to store student data on data disk, insert the data diskette in the diskette drive before logging on. If no diskette is detected, the program will prompt for it. *Note:* The program will accept blank, formatted data diskettes as student data diskettes.
2. The program will begin with a list of students. The class list is organized alphabetically, last name first, from A to Z. There are two buttons available: [OK] and [New].
3. If your name does not appear in the student list, click **New** to self-register. The program will branch to the log-on registration screen, at which point you will be prompted to register.

3a. **First Name.** This required field can contain up to 20 characters and is case sensitive.

3b. **Last Name.** This field can contain up to 20 characters and is case sensitive.

3c. **Class.** This optional field may be used to enter the name of the class and is limited to a maximum of 30 characters. It is case sensitive.

3d. **Password.** The password field is required and can include a password up to 10 characters. It is case insensitive. There is a prompt to verify the password when entered for the first time.

4. After completing the self-registration, a data file with your unique information will be created in the drive and directory specified at installation.

Subsequent Log-on Steps

- If the installation is configured to store student data on data disk, the data disk must be inserted in the disk drive before logging on. If no disk is detected, the program will prompt for it.
- When starting the program in subsequent sessions, select (highlight) your name from the list and click **OK.** A log-on screen will appear; enter your password in the field provided and click **OK.**

USING THE *STUDENT SOFTWARE CHALLENGE*

After logging onto the software, the Patient Cases menu will display. If this is the first time you are using the software, a brief introduction and instructions will display in a dialog on top of the Patient Cases menu. Print (if possible) or close the instructions after reading them. If you have used the software before and were in the middle of an exercise when you last worked with the program, a bookmark allows you to bypass the Patient Cases menu. Click **Continue where you left off** to return to the case on which you were last working. Click **Restart from beginning of case** to restart the case. This will erase all information previously entered in the case. Click **Cancel** to go to the Patient Cases menu.

The Patient Cases menu (Fig. G–2) includes 10 patient case folders organized alphabetically by the patient's last name.

The case numbers indicate the order of difficulty and coincide with the patient's account numbers. The menu also includes an eleventh file folder labeled "Other Patients." This feature is described in detail on page 620.

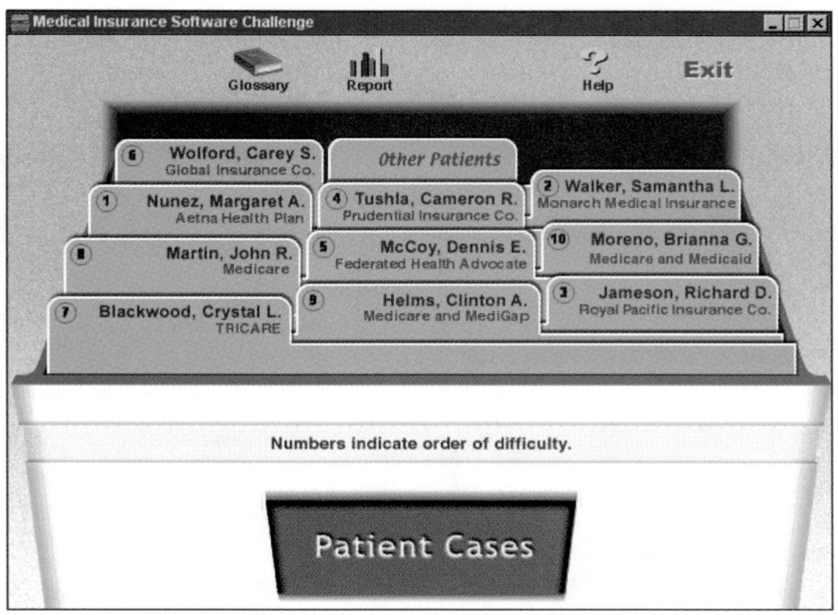

Figure G–2. Patient Cases Menu.

Button Bar

The software includes several buttons on the button bar. Click to access the following information:

- **Patients.** Go to the Patient Cases menu.
- **Glossary.** Go to the Glossary to define an abbreviation or look up a word.
- **Report.** Access a report listing the cases completed and view scores of your work.
- **Print.** Produce hard copy of the information forms or an HCFA-1500 form.
- **Help.** Obtain program-software information on the current displayed screen.
- **Exit.** Quit the program. A prompt to confirm your selection will appear.

Working with Patient Cases

PATIENT CASES SCREEN. Six basic insurance cases may be chosen by name or number in order of difficulty. Cases 1 through 6 are completed using general third party payer guidelines.

Four advanced insurance cases may be chosen by name or insurance type (TRICARE, Medicare, Medicare/Medigap, and Medi-Medi). These cases, 7 through 10, are numbered in order of difficulty and completed using specific program guidelines.

The Other Patients file may be chosen to complete the HCFA-1500 insurance claim form for a case the instructor may choose or for any Billing Break assignments.

1. Select a patient case. A screen with four folders will display.
    - **Patient Information Form.** This data is needed to complete the top portion of the HCFA-1500 insurance claim form (Fig. G–3).
    - **Encounter Form.** This form is used for Cases 1 through 5.
    - **Medical Record.** This form is used for Cases 6 through 10. This document gives you realistic medical history and progress notes about the patient. Information is extracted directly from the chart note to code diagnoses and procedures when completing the HCFA-1500 insurance claim form (Fig. G–4).
    - **Physician Information File.** The clinic/physician file contains important data about the clinic physicians and the demographic information and reference numbers needed to complete the HCFA-1500 insurance claim form (Fig. G–5).
    - **HCFA-1500 Claim Form.** Allows entry of data in a free-form style (Fig. G–6).
2. Click on the folder tabs to display the contents of the folder.
3. View a different part of the information forms by placing your cursor on the form, clicking and holding down the mouse button (a hand will appear), and dragging the form until the part you are looking for is in view.

   OR

   Use the scroll bar at the right and bottom sides of the form to scroll horizontally and vertically to lo-

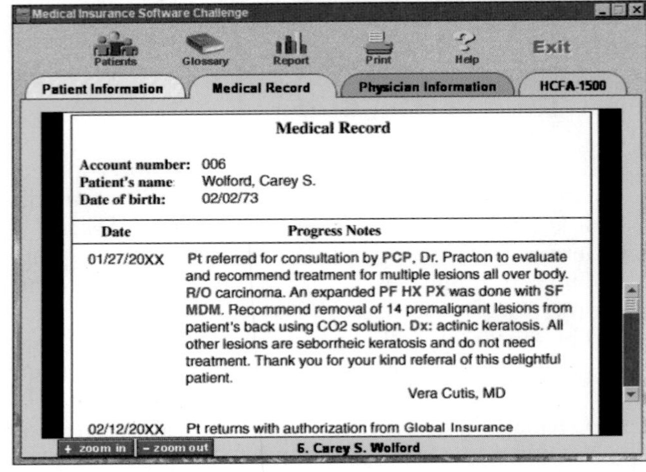

Figure G–4. Medical Record Screen.

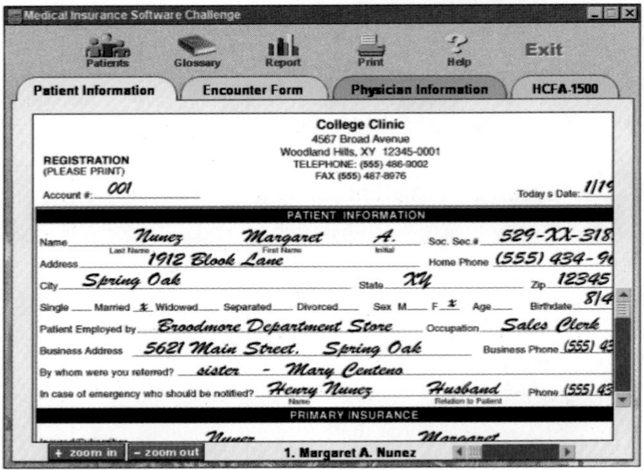

Figure G–3. Patient Information Screen.

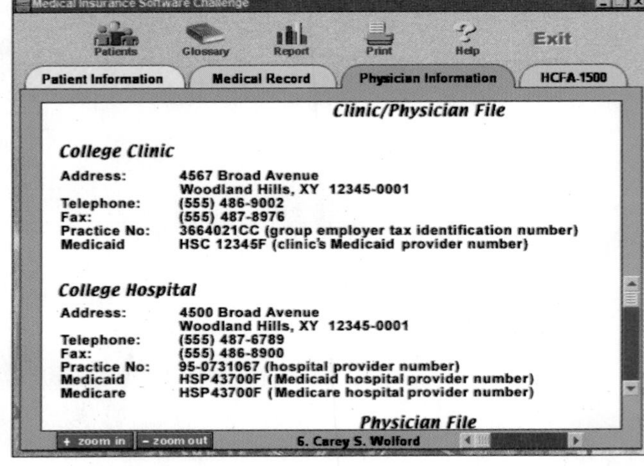

Figure G–5. Physician Information Screen.

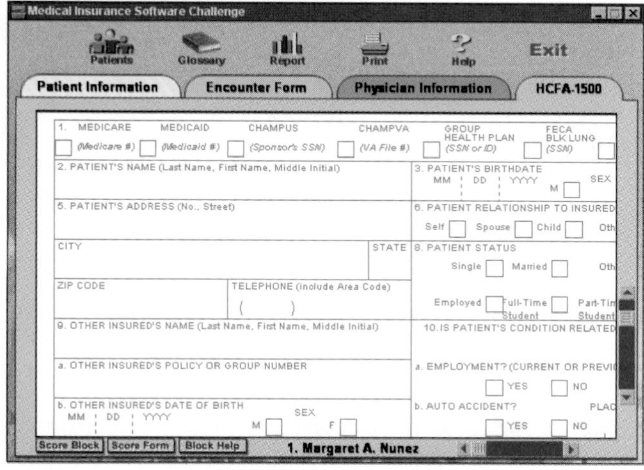

Figure G–6. HCFA-1500 Form.

cate different sections of the form. The information forms may be enlarged or decreased in size by using the "+ 200m in" and "− 200m out" features.

4. On the HCFA-1500 form you may click in a field to enter information and/or tab from one field to the next to enter information. Always hit **Tab** after entering information to save it in the case. Use the information provided in the first three folders to complete the HCFA-1500 insurance claim form. You can return to the information forms at any time while completing the HCFA-1500 form for the selected case. It is preferable to print information forms if a printer is connected to your computer.
5. Check your work on a specific block by placing your cursor in the block and clicking the **Score Block** button. The software will score the selected block and provide feedback on your performance. You have two chances to complete the block correctly.

- **Block Help** found in claim completion provides formatting details and reviews specific insurance guidelines for:
  - *Private insurance claims*
  - *Medicare claims*
  - *TRICARE claims*

  Use Block Help when you are unsure about block requirements or when a block error appears. The dialog will contain three buttons for selecting the type of insurance for which you need Block Help. The default is Private. You can change the default by clicking on one of the other selections.
- Click the **Score Form** button when you have completed the form. The software will score the form and display feedback on your performance.
- After scoring the form, blocks containing errors will appear in blue. You have two chances to look for and correct errors and score the form. Individual blocks that have been previously scored may be changed, but will only *reflect the score after the second change.* Click **Score Form** twice before printing.
- Print the HCFA-1500 form from the patient case screen by clicking on the **Print** button on the button bar. If you print the form from the Patient Cases screen, your entries will appear as you typed them and errors will be displayed in bold blue. Your performance on the HCFA-1500 form will be recorded in the Report (see Scoring and Reporting).

Scoring and Reporting

- Each completed case will be indicated by a check (✓) mark. Each attempt on a patient case will be scored and reflected as a percentage. The data are stored in the Report. Click **Report** and choose (highlight) the

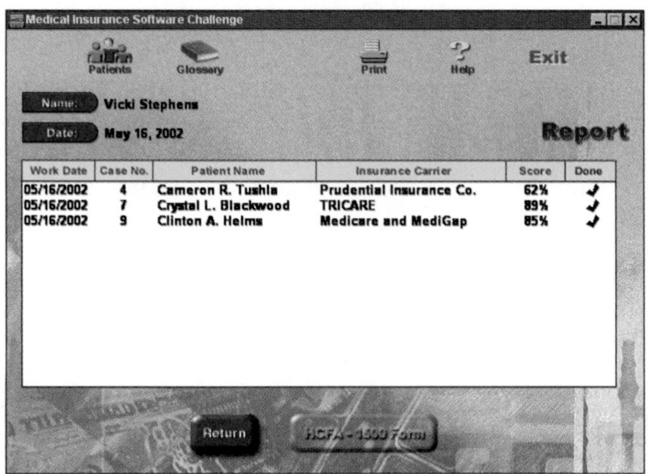

Figure G–7. Report Screen.

case you were working on. Click **HCFA-1500 Form** at the bottom of the screen to go to the Print Preview screen and view or print the corrected form. Blocks completed incorrectly will display the correct answer as follows:
An error on the *first attempt* that was corrected on the second attempt will be displayed in **blue bold text.**
An error on the *second attempt* or first attempt errors that were never corrected will be displayed in ***blue bold italic.***

- When using a black and white printer, compare the printout with this screen and highlight all errors (bold and italic blue print) so they are easily distinguished. Performance data will be stored in the Report as follows:
Full credit (1 point) for completing a field on the *first try*, **half credit** (½ point) for completing a field on the *second try*, **no credit** for incorrect entries *after the second attempt*. **Penalty** of ½ point for filling in fields that are not required on either first or second attempt.
- The Report also stores the HCFA-1500 forms for patients that you created in the Other Patients section of the software. Although these forms are not scored, they are included in the report so that you can access the data even if you have deleted the patient. For these forms, only the Work Date and Patient Name columns are completed. Each entry includes the following information:
    - ***Work date.*** *This is the date the case was worked on. In the case of bookmarked cases that were started on one day and completed on another, the work date is the date on which the case was started. If you continue a case on a subsequent date, the Work Date will appear on the HCFA-1500 form as well as "Today's Date."*
    - ***Case number.*** *The number that appears on the patient folder in the Patient Cases menu.*
    - ***Patient name.*** *The patient name that appears on the patient folder in the Patient Cases menu.*
    - ***Insurance carrier.*** *The name of the insurance carrier that appears on the patient folder in the Patient Cases menu.*
    - ***Score.*** *The score shows the percentage of fields of the total form that you completed correctly on the first try (1 point) and second try (½ point).*
    - ***Completed.*** *This column displays a checkmark for those cases 1 through 10 that have been completed.*

Other Patients

- **Add other patients** by clicking on the *"Other Patients"* folder tab on the Patient Cases menu. A list of the *Other Patients* will display. The *Other Patients* file folder tab on the Patient Cases menu allows you to add up to 50 patients and complete HCFA-1500 forms for them. These patients may be chosen from the Billing Break exercises or may be cases created by the instructor. The first time you use this feature, the list will be empty.
- **Add a new patient** by clicking on the **New Patient** button. The New Patient Registration screen will display. Enter the first name and then the last name of the new patient and click **OK.** The patient's name will be added to the Other Patients list. Select (highlight) a patient, click **OK,** and a blank HCFA-1500 form will display. If you leave the HCFA-1500 form in progress, your work will be saved.
- **Delete patients** by selecting a name in the list and clicking the **Delete Patient** button. A prompt to confirm the deletion will appear. If you delete a patient from the Other Patients list, you can still display the form for that patient from the Report (see Scoring and Reporting). Remember you can add up to 50 patients to the Other Patients list. Once the limit is reached, you will be prompted to delete patients from the list before adding new ones. To return to the Patient Cases menu, click the **Cancel** button. To return to the Patient Cases menu, click the **Patients** button on the button bar.

Using the Glossary

A comprehensive list of 200 key terms and abbreviations can be *accessed from all screens* in the software except the log-on sequence. It includes a Find text entry field that searches on multiple characters and then displays its definition.

- Click on the **Glossary** button bar to access the Glossary.
- Type the first few characters of the word in the Find field to search for a word. The Glossary will automatically scroll to the first term beginning with those characters and display its definition.
- Click on a term or abbreviation that is displayed in green in the Patient's Medical Record to automatically go to the Glossary and read the definition.
- Click the **Return** button on the Glossary screen to return to the previous screen.

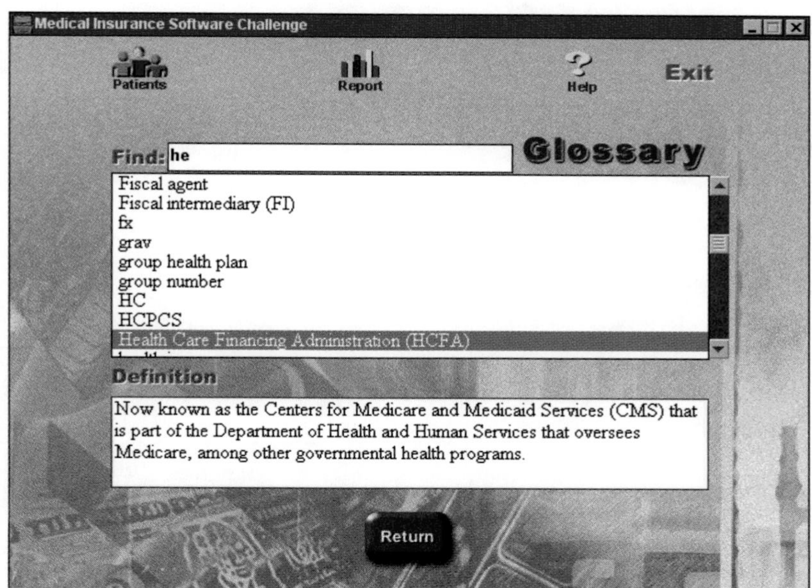

Figure G–8. Glossary Screen.

Index

Note: Page numbers followed by the letter b refer to boxed material. Those followed by the letter f refer to figures, and those followed by t refer to tables.

A

D

E

I

J

K

L

M

N

O

P

Q

R

S

T

U

V

W

Y